Leslie with

from us both,

Lorna
and Brian

12.3.80

# ADAMS & MAEGRAITH:
# CLINICAL TROPICAL DISEASES

# ADAMS & MAEGRAITH:

# CLINICAL
# TROPICAL DISEASES

## BRIAN MAEGRAITH

*From the Liverpool School of
Tropical Medicine*

with contributions by
S.G.BROWNE
H.M.GILLES
H.A.REID
W.P.STAMM

*SEVENTH EDITION*

BLACKWELL SCIENTIFIC PUBLICATIONS
OXFORD LONDON EDINBURGH MELBOURNE

© 1964, 1966, 1971, 1976, 1980 by
Blackwell Scientific Publications
Editorial Offices:
Osney Mead, Oxford, OX2 0EL
8 John Street, London, WC1N 2ES
9 Forrest Road, Edinburgh, EH1 2QH
214 Berkeley Street, Carlton
Victoria 3053, Australia

First published 1953
Second edition 1960
Third edition 1964
Fourth edition 1966
Fifth edition 1971
Sixth edition 1976
Seventh edition 1980

Distributed in U.S.A. by
Blackwell Mosby Book Distributors
11830 Westline Industrial Drive
St Louis, Missouri 63141,
in Canada by
Blackwell Mosby Book Distributors
86 Northline Road, Toronto
Ontario, M48 3E5,
and in Australia by
Blackwell Scientific Book Distributors
214 Berkeley Street, Carlton
Victoria 3053


Printed in Great Britain at
The Alden Press, Oxford
and bound by
Kemp Hall Bindery
Oxford

British Library
Cataloguing in Publication Data

Adams, Alfred Robert Davies
Clinical tropical diseases.—7th ed.
1. Tropical medicine
I. Title II. Maegraith, Brian Gilmore
616.9'88'3      RC961
ISBN 0-632-00536-X

This edition is dedicated to the memory of
PROFESSOR CHARLES STUART LEITHEAD CBE
for many years a distinguished and
much loved member of the
Department of Tropical Medicine, and subsequently
Professor of Medicine and co-founder of the
Medical School at Addis Ababa, Ethiopia

# CONTENTS

vii

# Contents

Yellow fever: virus hepatitis; dengue; sandfly fever; haemorrhagic fevers; Asian haemorrhagic fevers; African and American haemorrhagic fevers (Lassa fever, Marburg and Ebola fevers); meningo-encephalitis

Ascariasis; enterobiasis; strongyloidiasis; larva migrans; gnathostomiasis; eosinophilic encephalo-meningitis; trichuriasis; capillariasis; anisakiasis; flukes: hepatic, intestinal, lung; tape worms: cyclophyllidean and pseudophyllidean

# ACKNOWLEDGEMENTS FOR
# SEVENTH EDITION

In editing this edition I have again been greatly helped by friends and colleagues. Valuable sections have been written by Professor H.M.Gilles and Dr H.A.Reid, from the Liverpool School, by Dr S.G.Browne, The Leprosy Study Centre, London, and by Air Vice-Marshal W.P.Stamm.

I acknowledge with thanks permission to publish text figures and photographs from the following sources:

*Annals of Tropical Medicine and Parasitology*, School of Tropical Medicine, Liverpool.
*British Encyclopaedia of Medical Practice*, Butterworth, London.
*The Lancet*, London.
*Pathological Processes in Malaria and Blackwater Fever*, by B.G.Maegraith, 1948; *Bone Lesions in Yaws*, by C.J.Hackett, 1951, both Blackwell Scientific Publications, Oxford.
Roche Products Limited, Welwyn Garden City, Herts., England.
*Symptoms and Signs in Clinical Medicine*, E.Noble Chamberlain; *Textbook of Medicine*, ed. E.Noble Chamberlain, both John Wright & Sons Ltd., Bristol, 1951.
*Transactions Royal Society of Tropical Medicine and Hygiene*, London.
*Clinical Methods in Tropical Medicine*, by B.G.Maegraith and C.S. Leithead, Cassell & Co. Ltd., London.

Photographs and line drawings, for which we are most grateful, were supplied by the following: the late Professor D.B.Blacklock, the late Col. B.Blewitt, Mr J.Brady, Sir Clement Chesterman, the late Mr D.Dagnall, Dr Z.Farid, Mr J.E.Friend, Dr H.Foy, Dr M.Gelfand, Professor H.M.Gilles, Dr C.J.Hackett, Dr D.B.Jelliffe, Professor W.E.Kershaw, Dr C. da Silva Lacaz, the late Dr W.H.P.Lightbody, Dr D.S.McLaren, Dr Ch.Mofidi, Dr R.H.Mole, Dr S.Na-Nakorn, Dr H.Peaston, Professor W.Peters, the late Professor B.Platt, Dr D.R.Seaton, Dr J.Weir, Dr T.H.White.

I am also indebted to Dr A.B.Christie and E.&S.Livingstone, Ltd. for permission to reproduce a passage from the book *Infectious Diseases, Epidemiology and Clinical Practice*, First Edition.

I am obliged for the help afforded us by the staffs of various libraries, including that of the Royal Society of Medicine and the Harold Cohen Library, Liverpool, and especially by Miss U.M.Nottage, Librarian of the Liverpool School of Tropical Medicine.

Finally, I wish to pay thankful tribute to the skilful and patient secretarial assistance of Miss Olive Williams, and to my wife for her support.

*Liverpool 1978*                                    BRIAN MAEGRAITH

# PREFACE TO SEVENTH EDITION

The text of this book is designed essentially for the physician who has to deal with the sick patient.

Information regarding methods used in clinical pathological diagnosis is included in places to enable the physician to understand what is going on and how and why the specimens he collects from his patients are manipulated.

I have adhered to the alphabetical arrangement of subjects as far as possible. My experience has been that this has been found useful for the clinicians and has now been generally accepted.

As usual, there are no references. Those interested in details of specific points can always find them; if not, they do not really need them. In any case, in what is intended as a short practical book, references would clutter up and considerably expand the text.

Some reviewers of previous editions have suggested that, because of the increasing complexity of the subject, it might be advisable to convert the book into a multi-author compendium. While accepting some very special collaboration where I considered it was needed, I believe that multiplicity of authorship in this particular book would lead, as it often does, to massive increase in size, irregular standards of contribution, and loss of rhythm.

*Disease on the move.* This book was originally written for the doctor in, or going to, the tropics and other areas of the disadvantaged world. In the modern jet age, as importation of disease by travellers and immigrants rapidly increases, much of the text is also of practical value for the doctor in the temperate and developed world.

The geographical distribution of the major diseases has thus been given in some detail, largely to define the endemicity, but also to assist the reader to identify possible sources of infection which may be carried from the areas mentioned (exported) to other parts of the world (imported), where the particular disease may not exist or is uncommon.

The export/import of disease in this manner today affects every doctor who examines a patient, wherever he may be. Movement of people, singly or in groups, has become a vital factor in the practice of medicine, since, at any time, a doctor may be faced with a disease brought from some other country, or from another area of his own country, about which he is totally ignorant. The recognition of diseases imported in this way is very important to the patient concerned and sometimes to the community as well.

The point to be made, therefore, is that in the routine examination and interrogation of every patient, the doctor, or nurse, or whoever sees him first, must automatically obtain his geographical history.

The major element in spreading disease across the world has been the aeroplane. When this book was first written travel on the present scale was just beginning. The majority still travelled by sea and, in the course of long voyages, people coming from endemic areas developed clinical signs of infections they may have acquired and were usually expertly diagnosed by watchful doctors on the ship or at the port of entry by the health authorities. A man coming from West Africa arriving in Liverpool with a fever was regarded as suffering from malaria until it was proved otherwise. The sea voyages were long enough to cover the incubation period of most infectious diseases.

Today it has all changed and the public health barriers which were so effective for sea travel are largely useless in air travel. A man may be infected with malignant malaria in the Far East and be home in England the same day, looking and feeling well and a fortnight away from the disease which will appear at the end of the incubation period.

The size of the problem can be seen from the statistics of international movement. In 1977 over 400 million people moved from one country to another by air. Most of these were businessmen, often making frequent trips abroad, or holiday makers, lured into the sun by glossy brochures, which carefully ignored any reference to possible health risks. Relatively few travelled by sea, except on cruises, which carried their own risks at the ports visited and on the subsidiary trips ashore.

In both sea and air travel, there are the crews to be considered, regularly exposed to infections in out-of-the-way endemic areas, and the others, missionaries, teachers, servicemen, who work for long periods abroad.

All these could import disease in themselves and so could visitors from infected areas, or those who pass through infected areas on the way, possibly merely for refuelling. Some visitors from endemic areas are on short visits only, others have come for work and stay for long periods as immigrants.

The matter has become a world problem. It is just as important for Singapore as it is for Britain.

Medical hazards are not limited to the diseases discussed in this book. *Any* disease can be exported from an endemic area and imported into another country. The European takes his cold *to* Africa and returns with malaria *from* Africa. Malaria is especially important in this respect, but so is pulmonary tuberculosis. There is much to be said for the view that tuberculosis is the most serious of all imported diseases in areas such as Britain, in which the disease has been controlled. Immigrants, living in 'colonies' in the towns of England have spread the disease to the point where it is estimated that over half the cases have actually been infected in the host country.

The difficulties and dangers of the export/import of disease will not be solved until the diseases themselves are stamped out from the endemic regions, or until adequate and permanent protection can be offered to the individual and the community.

As things are today, the best that can be done is to make surveillance a success, so that in every country the diagnosis and management of imported disease are quick and sure, and that information reaches the health authorities immediately.

The doctor must therefore be fully aware of the possibility of import of disease in every patient he sees, every visitor, every immigrant he examines.

It would help if members of the travelling public were also warned of the risks they run when they go abroad, and of the need to consult a doctor, should they become ill on return, and tell him *exactly* where they have been and when. Every help in this respect should be given by those concerned with travel, from Agents to Airlines.

The vital questions the doctor must ask his patient are:

For the indigenous traveller returned home: *Where have you been and when?*

For the immigrant: *Where have you come from and when?*

For the visitor from abroad: *Both questions.*

Doctors of any country cannot be turned into experts in geographical medicine overnight. Nevertheless, they must be aware of the possibility of meeting imported disease in their next patient and of the possible risks to the patient and the community.

A doctor can get the geographical history of his patient by intelligent questioning and should be prepared to consider major diseases such as malaria. The medical implications of the patient's travels may not be clear to him and he should seek specialist help.

We hope this book will provide some of the diagnostic and therapeutic information that the doctors concerned may require.

In order to help both the profession and the traveller, methods of protection against some infections and the natural hazards of the disadvantaged world are also included.

*Liverpool 1978*                                     BRIAN MAEGRAITH

# PREFACE TO FIRST EDITION

For some time we have felt the need for a handbook giving that information essential for the clinical diagnosis and the treatment of those diseases which occur primarily in the tropics. It is to fill this need that we have ventured to produce this volume. Our aim has been to supply essential facts as dogmatically and concisely as we can; where possible we have avoided speculation. We have made no attempt to provide information of an encyclopaedic nature. None other than the most brief descriptions are given of the organisms causing disease, their identification, and the vectors that convey them; such information is readily available in the text books on bacteriology and parasitology.

A.R.D.ADAMS
B.G.MAEGRAITH

# 1

## AMOEBIASIS AND OTHER PROTOZOAL INTESTINAL INFECTIONS

### (Contributed by W.P.Stamm)

#### DEFINITION

Amoebiasis is the state of harbouring an amoeba. By far the commonest potentially lethal parasite of man is *Entamoeba histolytica*. The parasite may behave as a commensal or invade the tissues of the intestinal wall, or spread elsewhere. Patients may also be infected with free-living amoebae (Naegleria and Acanthamoeba); but these primarily infect the central nervous system.

## AMOEBIASIS DUE TO *E. HISTOLYTICA*

### GEOGRAPHICAL DISTRIBUTION

*E. histolytica* infection of man is of world-wide distribution. It is most prevalent in ill-sanitated areas, particularly in warm climates. The World Health Organization estimates that 10 per cent of the world population are infected with *E. histolytica*.

### AETIOLOGY

*The parasite*

*E. histolytica* is a natural parasite of man. It can be transmitted to other animals including monkeys but it is doubtful if it occurs in them naturally. Laboratory animals including baby rats and guinea pigs can be infected by intracaecal inoculation of trophozoites; such models are used for the study of the infection and the assay of anti-amoebic compounds. The parasite can be cultured *in vitro*, using various media in which there are associated bacteria or *Trypanosoma cruzi*; by special techniques subcultures of *E. histolytica* can be induced to grow axenically (without bacterial or other associates) and these cultures are particularly useful for the production of antigens.

The trophozoites living in the lumen of the large intestine multiply by binary fission. Some eventually encyst and are passed in the faeces. These are the infective stages of the parasite and develop further on being swallowed by a new host. In the terminal ileum or in the first part of the colon, the cyst hatches and liberates a four-nucleated amoeba; this divides into four single-nucleated entamoebae which establish themselves in the first instance anywhere in the lumen of the colon.

I

A

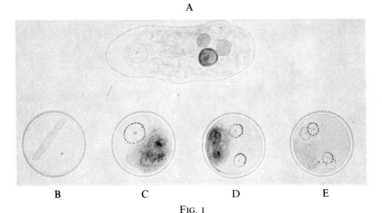

B           C           D           E

Fɪɢ. ɪ

*E. histolytica.* A, Vegetative amoeba; B, Unstained cyst showing chromidial bar; C, D, E, Iodine-stained cysts, C and D showing glycogen mass. (Diameter of cysts, 14 μm.)

[From E.Noble Chamberlain, *A Textbook of Medicine,* John Wright & Sons Ltd., Bristol, 1951]

The *E. histolytica* trophozoite is a large actively motile organism. The cytoplasm consists of an outer clear translucent zone of ectoplasm and an inner, densely granular endoplasm containing a spherical nucleus within which is a single large granule (karyosome). The endoplasm contains food vacuoles within which may be bacteria and ingested erythrocytes (when invasion has taken place as in amoebic dysentery). The trophozoite moves freely by extension of the ectoplasm into large finger-like bulbous pseudo-podia into which flow the endoplasm and contents.

The mean diameter is about 20 μm, with very considerable variation from organism to organism. The former separation into 'small' and 'large' races is no longer regarded as valid. *E. hartmanni,* which has a small cyst (10 μm or less) with four nuclei and smaller trophozoites, is now recognized as a separate and non-pathogenic species. Small trophozoites of *E. histolytica* may sometimes be found in the non-dysenteric stool and be confused with *E. hartmanni.*

The recently formed cyst of *E. histolytica* has a mean diameter of 10–12 μm. It has only one nucleus and the cytoplasm contains an indefinite glycogen mass and one or more characteristic refractile or chromidial bars up to 5 μm in length. As the cyst matures to become infective the nucleus divides and the glycogen and chromidial bars disappear. The mature cyst has four nuclei.

In diarrhoeic and dysenteric forms of amoebiasis, trophozoites are carried rapidly through the intestinal lumen and are discharged in the faeces. In infections where there is no diarrhoea the amoebae form cysts which are passed in the faeces after a slow passage through the bowel. Thus trophozoites are normally found in acute intestinal infections with diarrhoeic or dysenteric stools and cysts are found in the normal stools in intermissions or in non-invasive infections. Purgation in the latter case may lead to a temporary discharge of trophozoites.

The infective form of *E. histolytica* is the cyst. The trophozoites derived therefrom may or may not invade the wall of the intestine. Trophozoites may eventually invade extra-intestinal tissues.

The infection is transmitted as a result of the host swallowing mature cysts in contaminated food and drink. Man is the only effective reservoir. Food handling by infected persons, flies, direct faecal contact, are all factors in determining the incidence of the infection in a given area. Occasional outbreaks have resulted from special circumstances, such as leakage of sewage containing cysts into drinking water.

The cysts remain viable and infective for up to 10 days in faeces. They are killed by desiccation, so that dust is not infective. They are also killed by heat greater than 55° C so that boiled water is safe. The amount of chlorine needed to purify ordinary water is insufficient to kill cysts. Chlorination at high level is effective but water must be subsequently dechlorinated before use.

*E. histolytica* is more prevalent in the tropics than in temperate regions. This is probably a reflection on the poor sanitation and health education in the crowded tropical and emergent countries. The infection is sometimes equally prevalent in temperate areas under insanitary conditions.

Vegetables and fruits eaten raw are a common source of infection, especially in areas where human faeces are used as fertilizer, as in parts of the Far East. It has not been determined whether such infection results from application of faeces immediately before harvesting or from washing the vegetables in infected water.

Direct contact with faeces containing cysts, usually on a basis of person to person, is an important means of infection, especially in groups of people in institutions where personal hygiene and sanitation are poor. Food handlers are suspected of being involved in transmission but their importance is uncertain, although cysts will live in faecal dirt under fingernails for about an hour. In liquid foods they may survive for days.

The prevalence of infection in many areas of the world has not been established. Prevalence rates vary widely from place to place. Rates for the sophisticated countries including Western Europe are generally low; in some areas, such as parts of North Wales, the prevalence may be as much as 10 per cent. In Central and South America, the Middle East, North Africa and many parts of tropical Africa, and the Far East according to the locality (and the validity of the statistics) the rates vary from 30 to 80 per cent. A high prevalence of infection can be regarded as an indication of frequent transmission which is in turn evidence of poor conditions of sanitation and health education.

The incidence of clinical amoebiasis also varies widely from one area to another, but is usually roughly in line with the local prevalence of infection.

Variations in pathogenicity seem to depend on the relevant strain of parasite and on geographical and host factors (see below).

On the whole, the chances of developing clinical amoebiasis seem to be greater after infection with a strain in the tropics than with one in Europe. This may be dependent on the physiological and pathogenic activity of the relevant parasite or on factors such as frequency of reinfection, the prevailing colonic bacteria or the type of food.

In regions of high endemicity children may show a higher rate of clinical amoebiasis than adults. It is not known whether this is due to the size of the infecting dose, the frequency of reinfection, or the absence of immunity. Humoral immune bodies may be detected in individuals invaded by *E. histolytica* but there is no evidence whether these are protective.

Host differences, including race, are sometimes suggested as affecting the issue of an infection. Thus, the Bantu in some areas of South Africa develop a particularly severe form of amoebic dysentery. This was formerly believed to be associated with a low protein high carbohydrate diet, but it has been found that well-fed members of the same group in urban areas also get very severe amoebic dysentery. The clinical picture may be due to genetic factors. On the other hand, it may be due merely to the high degree of pathogenicity in the infecting strain of parasite.

Clinical amoebiasis in areas of high endemicity is much commoner in adult males than in females. This sex difference in prevalence is not obvious in children, suggesting that the difference in adults is largely dictated by opportunity of infection.

PATHOLOGY

*Pathogenicity*
Infection acquired in temperate regions is commonly commensal but may be invasive.

The pathogenicity or otherwise of a strain of *E. histolytica* is not understood. Some strains are probably more invasive than others. Thus, parasites producing large cysts are found most commonly in infections with clinical effects and parasites producing smallcysts (less than 10 $\mu$m in diameter) are correspondingly rare. However, there is no real evidence that the pathogenicity of true *E. histolytica* is reflected in the size of the trophozoite or the cyst. Many of the recorded cases in which small cysts were passed and no signs developed are now believed to have been infected with the non-pathogenic parasite *E. hartmanni*.

The view that *E. histolytica* always invades the gut wall irrespective of whether symptoms are produced is not acceptable on the evidence. *E. histolytica* may remain as a commensal in the intestine for years without invading the tissues. Serological evidence indicates that it may invade the gut tissues without producing clinical signs or symptoms; this may account for the development of an amoebic liver abscess without a history of intestinal disturbance or infection. Infection without tissue invasion and infection without symptoms may both lead to the passage of cysts in the stool; it is believed that the two conditions may be distinguishable in that detectable antibodies are formed subsequent to the tissue invasion but not when infection is confined to the contents of the intestinal lumen.

There are undoubtedly host factors concerned in the invasion after infection. The growth and multiplication of the amoebae in the gut lumen probably depend on suitable accompanying bacterial flora being present; this is indicated by the disappearance of an infection which may follow the use of antibiotics which alter the flora but have no direct action on the amoebae. In extra-intestinal tissues the amoebae do not need bacterial associates and flourish in bacteriologically sterile conditions. There is experimental evidence that multiplication of *E. histolytica,* and sometimes its invasive powers, can be influenced by the host diet; thus a milk diet decreases the efficiency of an invasive parasite directly injected as trophozoites into the guinea pig caecum and deficiency of vitamin C increases it. No clear evidence of this exists in man.

There appear to exist avirulent and virulent strains of *E. histolytica,* the former being non-invasive, the latter invasive. This has been confirmed experimentally in regard to invasiveness of strains in animals but the precise differences between the avirulent and virulent strains have not been clearly determined. A virulent strain maintained for months *in vitro* may lose its virulence but this can be restored by animal passage. The life cycle is the same in the avirulent and virulent parasites and, apart from the presence of the enzyme carboxypeptidase in the former and its absence in the latter, few consistent differences have been detected in the parasites.

*Pathology in man*
The amoeba penetrates the lining of the intestinal wall through and between the epithelial cells which show some degree of autolysis arising from the activity of their own lysosomes.

The organisms multiply in the subepithelial tissues and penetrate laterally by lysis of the cells. At this stage there may be some bacterial invasion of the affected tissue with inflammatory response. Otherwise there is some light lymphocytic accumulation at the advancing edges of the lesion. The epithelial surface ulcerates and the ulcer remains shallow for some time as the spread of the process into the submucosa is limited by the muscularis mucosae, on which collections of lymphocytes, plasma cells, and sometimes polymorphs accumulate. This barrier finally breaks down and the amoebae, with or without bacteria, invade the submucosa. The lesion is at first lined by scattered lymphocytes beyond the advancing lateral front of active amoebae; in this area the local blood vessels dilate and may themselves be invaded by the amoebae. The lesion extends circumferentially and by metastatic spread along the local lymphatic vessels to the submucosal lymph nodes; in this way secondary lesions may be induced some distance from the initial point of invasion.

Ulcers are formed in the intestinal wall as a result of this process, or from the extension to the surface of metastatic lesions. The ulcers may appear small macroscopically with overhanging undermined irregular borders, but the lesion is commonly 'flask-shaped' with much larger extension in the submucosal tissues. The affected area is filled with necrotic cellular debris and amoebae are found normally only in the periphery at the advancing edge. The lesion may extend from the surface through the whole thickness of the intestinal wall. In between the lesions the mucosa is undamaged. Invasion of local blood vessels may lead to transport of amoebae to distant tissues to set up extra-intestinal infection which may die out or develop local tissue lesions. In fulminating infections the destruction of all layers of the intestinal wall is extensive and may be confluent, involving large areas of the gut. Complications are common.

Complications of amoebic intestinal abscesses include perforation into the peritoneal cavity leading to amoebic peritonitis, sometimes bacteriologically contaminated. Erosion of large vessels in the ulcerated area may lead to severe bleeding and occlusion may cause local gangrene. Repeated invasion associated with secondary infection may set up progressive inflammatory reactions in the intestinal wall, characterized by oedema and cellular granulation tissue composed of lymphocytes, eosinophils, fibroblasts, and plasma cells, with variable numbers of polymorphs depending on the degree of bacterial infection. The tumour so produced is called an 'amoeboma'. It may contain scattered small abscesses, sometimes with amoebae in the peripheral tissues and with irregular areas of fibrosis.

Lesions are common in the caecum, transverse and sigmoid colon; they also occur in the recto-colonic junction and in the rectal mucosa. They are sometimes found also in the terminal ileum.

Extra-intestinal distribution of amoebae except in direct extensions to the peritoneum or the skin is largely metastatic. Such metastases probably occur repeatedly in the course of development of the intestinal lesions but the parasites seldom survive in the tissues in which they settle.

The commonest extra-intestinal lesions occur in the liver. The liver lesions are of two main types. During acute intestinal infections the liver may undergo a generalized enlargement with tenderness; this has been called 'amoebic hepatitis' but the presence of amoebae in the liver has not been demonstrated; most authorities consider this to be a non-specific effect caused by intestinal toxins and not due to the presence of amoebae in the liver. A similar hepatic tender enlargement can accompany bacillary dysentery and ulcerative colitis.

The second type of lesion is the amoebic 'liver abscess' which may occur with or soon after an intestinal infection but more commonly the clinical manifestations do not appear until years after the probable time of original infection. In about 50 per cent of patients with an amoebic liver abscess there is no history of an intestinal infection.

The lesions of an amoebic liver abscess arise from metastatic amoebae caught up in the small radicals of the portal vein. Local lymphocytic and neutrophilic infiltrations occur and the amoebae may begin to divide. Some lysis of local cells may occur and the process may cease at this point and resolve without further damage. On the other hand, small areas of lytic necrosis may form about metastatic amoebae and may coalesce to form larger lesions, sometimes exaggerated by localized infarct, and ultimately extensive areas of colliquative necrosis with relatively little cellular response. The 'abscess' so formed does not contain pyogenic pus. It is filled with reddish sterile liquid material consisting of the debris of necrotic polygonal and other cells lying amongst the trabeculae of the degenerate matrix. The 'shaggy' periphery is irregular and consists of stroma and layers of compressed liver parenchyma, in which centrilobular congestion is usually evident. There is no fibrotic capsule. Amoebae are often found in large numbers in the tissue at the periphery of the lesion. They occur also in the contents and may be found in most samples of 'pus' removed by needling. Abscesses may be small and multiple but are more commonly large and single and situated in the right lobe.

Experimentally, amoebic liver abscesses can be produced by injection of trophozoites into the portal vein in guinea-pigs which have, or have recently had, chronic amoebic intestinal lesions; they do not occur after inoculation into otherwise normal and uninfected animals although they will develop easily in other animals, especially the hamster, after direct injection into the parenchyma or merely into the peritoneal cavity. The results in guinea-pigs have suggested the view that the tissues of the liver in the gut-infected animals may have been conditioned to accept the amoebae, possibly as a result of local immunosensitivity reactions initiated by the organism (acting as an antigen) when caught up in the portal vein. Such sensitivity reactions are known to cause dynamic impedance to the local circulation which may provide the physical environment needed for amoebic multiplication. It is possible that similar sensitivity reactions are initiating factors in the production of an amoebic abscess in man and may explain the common development of the lesion in periods of remission of long-term amoebic dysentery or colitis.

The process may extend or the abscess rupture into contiguous tissues. Sometimes the infection may be carried by metastatic amoebae to other tissues *via* the blood-stream.

Other forms of extra-intestinal lesions are initiated in a similar fashion by metastatic transport of the amoebae followed by cellular (mostly lymphocytic) reaction. The development depends on the anatomical region. When abscesses form they are bacteriologically sterile and contain the debris of lysed cells and the trophozoites. There is no peripheral fibrosis.

Clinical manifestations of amoebiasis include amoebic dysentery and non-dysenteric amoebic colitis, with or without complications, and ulcerative post-dysenteric colitis and amoeboma, which is a localized form involving the gut wall and sometimes confused clinically with neoplasm. Extra-intestinal amoebic infection leads most commonly to liver abscess or acute non-suppurative hepatic amoebiasis. Other organs may become involved as a sequel to hepatic amoebiasis or without it. Amoebiasis can mimic almost any abdominal or hepatic condition and there are no clinical signs which are pathognomonic of amoebic infection. It is world-wide in distribution and, although not common in temperate climates, it is easy to treat; for these reasons it should always be kept in mind and excluded before unnecessary surgery or dangerous medication is contemplated.

Contrary to common teaching, amoebiasis can exactly produce the clinical pictures of both ulcerative colitis and Crohn's disease; before a definitive diagnosis of either of these conditions is made, amoebiasis should be excluded by serological testing; failure to do this may result in the patient's death from surgery or from fulminating amoebiasis precipitated by steroid medication.

Some infected persons remain asymptomatic. The stools of such carriers may appear normal but microscopic examination reveals cysts of *E. histolytica*. It is thought that in these patients the amoebae remain in the lumen of the gut and do not invade the tissues.

AMOEBIC DYSENTERY

The symptoms of this may appear within a week or two of infection or be delayed for months or years. The onset is usually gradual, with some looseness for a few days followed by evacuation of up to six or eight, but rarely more than a dozen, mucoid blood-stained motions a day. Tenesmus is unusual unless there is a lesion immediately inside the anus. On physical examination there may be no signs of significance. Occasionally, and especially during more acute attacks, there is palpable thickening, with tenderness on pressure, of the caecum or of the descending colon and sigmoid flexure. There is no fever of significance and little prostration. The duration of an attack of amoebic dysentery of ordinary severity may be a few days or it may last for some weeks; it then usually subsides spontaneously. There follows a period of remission which may last days, weeks, months, or even years; during this the patient, not uncommonly, is constipated. In the quiescent period any digestive disturbances and bowel discomforts are commonly ascribed to the infection; often it is doubtful whether they can truly be regarded as due to it. Another attack of dysentery then follows. This sequence of attacks of dysentery followed by intermissions associated with constipation, which may continue for years and even for the duration of the patient's life, constitutes the classical picture of amoebic dysentery. At any time complications, especially an amoebic liver abscess, may develop; they do so in about one-fifth of neglected cases.

In some cases, for instance in patients who are undernourished or are suffering from other debilitating diseases, attacks may be prolonged and may be very severe, sometimes fatal.

Amoebic dysentery is sometimes very acute and fulminating, with sudden onset, swinging fever, chills, sweating and very severe dysentery, dehydration, and prostration. In such cases the stools are liquid, with flecks of faecal matter and variable amounts of blood and mucus. There may be severe intestinal haemorrhages or perforation, followed by amoebic peritonitis. The mortality in untreated cases is high. Attacks of this kind have frequently been reported in South Africa, usually in Bantu.

### AMOEBIC COLITIS (NON-DYSENTERIC)

The patient complains of irregular episodes of diarrhoea, with the passage of a few loose stools in the day, sometimes containing blood, sometimes mucus, but seldom both. There is thus usually no clear history of dysentery as such. In some cases short periods of diarrhoea and long remissions, often with constipation, may alternate over months and years with little ill health (but usually with a good deal of introversion) and occasionally some slight loss of weight. During the active stages the passage of the stool is usually painless, but many

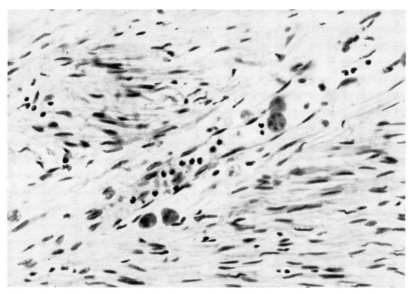

FIG. 2. Amoebic colitis. Amoebae in tissues and within blood vessels. Note relative absence of cellular reaction.

[Courtesy J.Brady]

patients complain of intermittent intestinal pain and discomfort. The picture somewhat resembles that of colonic carcinoma. Patients may give a history resembling that of ulcerative colitis, with chronic looseness of the bowels and irregular passage of stools streaked with mucus, sometimes blood and occasionally pus.

There are few physical signs beyond the stool changes. The colon is often palpable and thickened, especially over the caecum, the descending colon and sigmoid, all of which may be tender, but not focally.

AMOEBOMA

This condition is caused by extension of the infection into the bowel wall at places where there is faecal stasis: the colonic flexures, caecum and rectum. The infection causes inflammatory swelling which increases the stasis which in turn increases the swelling through oedema of the bowel wall. As a result a localized tumour is formed which clinically resembles a neoplasm; even at operation the surgeon may still think he is dealing with a neoplasm and in fact an amoeboma is sometimes superimposed on a neoplasm.

ULCERATIVE POST-DYSENTERIC COLITIS

The clinical picture closely resembles that of ulcerative colitis. There are bouts of irregular abdominal pains and sometimes colic, diarrhoea with blood or mucus, or both, and sometimes with a small amount of pus, followed by relatively normal bowel behaviour. In some cases the loose stools may be continuous. Many patients show a mixed anaemia, with a folic acid deficiency element. The patient is usually introverted and loses weight. Radiology reveals an irritable colon, with irregular spasm and occasional filling defects which may be suggestive of carcinoma.

The condition develops most commonly after years of neglect of amoebic colitis or mild dysentery. It may follow months or years after apparently successful anti-amoebic treatment.

On sigmoidoscopy, the colon is irritable and may go into spasm. The sigmoid mucosa is rough and reddened and may bleed easily. Flecks of mucus and blood are common and there may be small accumulations of pus. Occasional superficial ulcers may be present near the recto-sigmoid junction.

COMPLICATIONS

The direct complications of an intestinal infection are haemorrhage, often considerable, from erosion of a large vessel in the bowel wall; extension of the infection through the bowel wall, with the formation of amoebic granulomata (amoebomata); and frank, sudden perforation. In addition to sudden perforation of an amoebic ulcer, with development of an acute surgical abdomen, a form of slow leakage through an extensively diseased bowel may result in peritonitis. The latter occurs only in the severe fulminating type of amoebic dysentery. All complications are rare in the classical case of average severity. Amoebomata are usually the result of extension of the amoebic infection together with an accompanying bacterial infection. Hard inflammatory tumours therefore form at the site of the lesion and these develop and extend in the abdomen with an accompanying pyrexia. This complication is a serious one and, once established, does not always rapidly respond to specific anti-amoebic treatment; not uncommonly it is mistaken for malignant disease.

EXTRA-INTESTINAL AMOEBIASIS

The commonest remote complication of intestinal amoebiasis is embolic spread of the infection to the liver, via the portal vein. This may result eventually in the formation of an 'abscess'. The stages of liver involvement intermediate to this are not clearly defined. Some authors describe an inflammatory state they call 'diffuse amoebic hepatitis' arising from seeding of the liver with amoebae and associated with liver enlargement and tenderness, but no formation of pus. This not uncommonly develops during a dysenteric attack and responds to anti-amoebic treatment. Other workers are not prepared to accept this as a separate entity, regarding the hepatomegaly as a non-specific inflammatory phenomenon without invasion of the liver by the amoebae.

This issue may be settled experimentally in time, but for the present it is best to limit the description of the clinical effects of amoebic infection of the liver (probably best called hepatic amoebiasis) to the characteristic picture of amoebic liver abscess, which develops years after the probable date of original infection.

There is some resistance to labelling as an abscess the lesion developed in the liver, because the contents are essentially not pus in the sense of polymorphonuclear accumulations, but are composed primarily of lysed tissue cells and other debris. This point is not taken here, where the lesion is labelled and regarded as an 'abscess' and the contents as 'pus'.

HEPATIC AMOEBIASIS: AMOEBIC LIVER ABSCESS

The clinical picture develops most frequently years after acquisition of the original infection. The patient may give a history of dysentery or intermittent loose diarrhoea but there may be no such previous evidence of infection. Only rarely does the picture develop during an attack of dysentery or active colitis, although liver enlargement and tenderness may occur during the attack.

There is usually only one large abscess, but occasionally there are two or more and sometimes many small lesions. The volume of the contents of the lesion may be as much as 500–1500 ml.

In the early stages the patient complains of discomfort and fullness in the liver region. The liver enlarges and becomes tender, the tenderness becoming intensified over the area of the abscess. Moderate fever develops which may at first be intermittent but becomes remittent. Sweating is severe, especially at night. The patient is very anorexic and begins to lose weight. For a time he feels better than his clinical state warrants, but he becomes progressively more toxic and eventually prostrated.

By the time the abscess has formed, there is often a high swinging or intermittent fever, with drenching night sweats. The patient complains of intense discomfort and tenderness over the liver, particularly over the region occupied by the abscess. The liver is often enlarged and tender, sometimes bulging in the abscess area, where the tenderness is intense and very localized. The maximum tenderness is commonly on the right in an intercostal space in the lateral or medial–lateral lines over the lower rib cage. The chest wall and abdomen are sometimes obviously bulging in this area.

Movement of the affected side of the chest is greatly restricted. The patient finds deep breathing painful and the respiration rate is consequently increased. On whichever side of the liver the abscess has developed, the hepatic dullness is increased upwards and, when the lesion is in the right lobe, the shadow is increased upward and on X-ray of the affected side there is immobility of the diaphragm which is usually raised and may be deformed. The liver edge is usually palpable well away from the abscess area and may project two or three fingers' breadth below the costal margin; it is firm and tender.

Jaundice is uncommon. When it occurs it is obstructive in type and is the result of the pressure of the abscess on the biliary ducts. Liver function may otherwise be little disturbed. The results of liver function tests are equivocal. The serum alkaline phosphatase is usually increased and bilirubin is raised if there is biliary obstruction.

Most cases have a moderate degree of leucocytosis, ranging from 12,000 to 15,000 cells per mm$^3$, most of which are polymorphs. The ESR is raised.

There may be signs of pulmonary involvement, usually above the raised immobile diaphragm at the base of the right lung in which there may be some atelectasis; pleural effusion is not uncommon in the same region. When the hepatic lesion has broken through the diaphragm into the lung, the abscess contents may reach the bronchi and the patient develops a cough and may discharge the classical 'anchovy sauce' sputum which usually contains amoebae and lysed liver material.

If the progress of the abscess is not arrested by specific treatment it will erode into adjacent structures; that is, through the diaphragm into the thoracic cavity or into the pericardial sac (especially when the abscess is in the left lobe of the liver); through the peritoneum into the peritoneal cavity; through the chest or abdominal wall to the exterior or into contiguous organs or tissues within the abdomen.

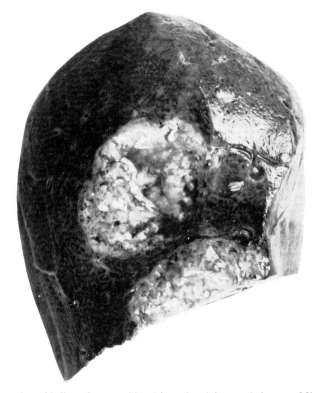

FIG. 3. Amoebic liver abscesses. Note 'shaggy' periphery and absence of fibrosis.
[Courtesy J.Brady]

Embolic spread may result in abscess formation in other organs, some-times in the brain, with localizing signs depending on the area in which the lesion develops. It is probable that most lesions of this sort are derived from an initial amoebic abscess in the liver but primary brain and lung lesions have been reported; in the latter case the pus coughed up in the sputum is creamy white and not anchovy. Cerebral abscess is particularly likely to occur second-ary to amoebic infection of the lung.

### DIAGNOSIS

The certain diagnosis of intestinal amoebiasis is dependent on the demon-stration of the trophozoites in the acute stages and cysts in the remissions. The initial diagnosis of liver abscess and other extra-intestinal manifestations of the infection has often to be made clinically, supported by serological tests.

*Laboratory diagnosis*
The laboratory is concerned with examination of the faeces, pus from

abscesses, sputum and other material and the demonstration of specific antibodies in the tissues and serum of the patient.

*Faeces*
It is best to examine specimens immediately after passage, wet preparations from the stool, or scrapings taken on sigmoidoscopy or proctoscopy are examined in suspension in saline on a warmed microscope slide. It is essential that the microscopist should have expert training and experience in faecal microscopy. When immediate examination of specimens cannot be achieved, aliquots of the specimen should be preserved in polyvinyl alcohol (PVA) for trophozoites, and in 10 per cent formalin for cysts. Trophozoites in PVA can be specifically stained by the indirect immunofluroescent technique. Specimens preserved in this way can be sent by post to a laboratory where the necessary expertise is available.

The stools should always be examined in cases of suspected extra-intestinal spread of *E. histolytica,* in order to establish the presence or otherwise of an intestinal infection; in 50 per cent of patients with an amoebic liver abscess no amoebae can be found in the stools.

'Pus' from a suspected amoebic liver abscess should be examined as a wet preparation immediately after aspiration. Trophozoites usually with ingested erythrocytes will be found in the pus in about 80 per cent of cases in which a clinical diagnosis can be made. They are most easily found in the last of the aspirate. In cases where characteristic 'anchovy sauce' material has been aspirated from the liver, but trophozoites have not been discovered, specific treatment should be commenced, even if cysts are not found in the stools. When typical pus has been obtained, the presence of cysts in the stools, or occasionally trophozoites, inferentially supports the diagnosis.

Trophozoites are usually present in expectorated abscess material, in sputum in pulmonary infections and in pus or exudates from suspected amoebic peritonitis or skin infections.

All materials of this sort, including liver aspirates, should be examined immediately. The parasites quickly die and round up and are extremely difficult to identify in material which has been allowed to stand for more than an hour at room temperature.

In liver aspirates in which parasites cannot easily be detected, the enzyme streptodornase–streptokinase may be added to portions of the whole specimen in a dilution of 10 units to each 1.0 ml of pus. After shaking and incubating for half an hour, the amoebae may be freed from the coagulase and can be identified.

Amoebae can be cultured in appropriate media from faeces containing active trophozoites.

Permanent staining of faecal smears is sometimes useful in searching for amoebae and in identifying them in doubtful cases. The specimens should be prepared from fresh faecal samples and stained by the Heidenhain iron haematoxylin technique. Amoebae can be identified in tissue sections stained with haematoxylin and eosin but are often missed in sections examined by routine methods. Whenever the presence of amoebae is thought to be likely, formalin-fixed sections should be stained by the indirect immunofluorescent technique.

*Immunodiagnostic methods*

Highly specific methods exist for identification of antibodies produced in invasive amoebiasis. The antibodies persist for varying periods after termination of the infection and their identification is thus not necessarily an indication of active infection. Failure to detect antibodies may indicate that invasion has not taken place; this may be the best means of separating the commensal from the invasive infection in individuals passing cysts.

Of the techniques available, the complement fixation test is complicated and less reliable than the more modern methods; the indirect haemagglutination test (IHA) is highly sensitive and specific but it is technically difficult, uneconomic to perform on single sera and a positive result may persist for many years after cure of the patients. The indirect immunofluorescent test is fairly sensitive and specific, it is cheap and easy to perform; it is not as persistent as the IHA but may remain positive for about 3 years. The gel diffusion precipitin test is not as sensitive as the others but it is highly specific and becomes negative within a few months of successful treatment; it is very useful clinically because if a patient has a positive gel diffusion test he almost certainly has active invasive amoebiasis. The cellulose acetate precipitin test gives results similar to the gel diffusion test and the answers are available within 4 hours.

All these tests are nearly 100 per cent positive on sera from patients with an amoebic liver abscess but only about 70 per cent positive in intestinal amoebiasis.

The immunodiagnostic techniques are, however, limited in their general usage because they are dependent on the availability of a reliable antigen which can best be obtained from axenic or at least monoxenic cultures of trophozoites and are expensive to buy commercially.

TREATMENT

*Chemotherapy of amoebiasis*

The aim of chemotherapy is to eradicate the infection with *E. histolytica* wherever the parasite may be in the bowel lumen, the intestinal wall or in extra-intestinal tissues.

Amoebicides in common use vary in efficacy in the sites where the parasites exist. Some are most active in the gut lumen and the gut wall, some are active systemically, others not. It thus may be necessary to use combinations of drugs for destruction of the amoebae. Certain drugs have been developed recently which are active in all sites, thereby simplifying treatment.

Drugs acting directly on *E. histolytica* in the bowel lumen are many. They include quinoline derivatives such as di-iodohydroxyquinoline (diodoquine) and chiniofon, arsenicals such as carbarsone, acetarsol (stovarsol) and Milibis (which is primarily a bismuth compound containing arsenic) and others including diloxanide furoate and paromomycin.

The ideal drug against amoebiasis would be one which is safe, without side effects and acts on the parasite in the lumen and in the gut wall and all other tissues.

*Metronidazole* (Flagyl) is considered to approximate to this. It has powerful activity against the parasite in the tissues and in the lumen. It is well tolerated and non-toxic. It also has the advantage of being given orally, in doses of 800 mg thrice daily for 5 days for amoebic dysentery or colitis (see below).

The following are particularly effective in the tissues.

*Emetine hydrochloride.* This drug is given intramuscularly in a dosage of 1 mg per kg body weight, up to a maximum of 65 mg a day, for up to 10 days. It has a toxic effect on the myocardium and should be used with caution and only in patients confined to bed.

*Dehydroemetine.* This drug has the same action as emetine on *E. histolytica* but is believed to be less toxic; contra-indications are the same. It is given intramuscularly in a dosage of 1.5 mg per kg body weight up to a maximum dose of 90 mg daily for 10 days.

These drugs are excellent for dealing with *E. histolytica* in the tissues, but are less effective against the parasites living in the gut lumen. If used alone in amoebic dysentery, therefore, the relapse rate is high.

The following are most effective in certain tissues.

*Emetine bismuth iodide* (EBI). This may be given for intestinal infection with invasion of the gut tissues, in an oral dosage of 195 mg daily singly or in three divided doses, for 10 days. Side effects include severe nausea, sometimes vomiting, and diarrhoea. Concurrent administration of phenobarbitones is advisable.

EBI will deal with the amoebae in the tissues of the intestinal wall and also with the parasites living in the lumen. Relapse rate following its use is therefore low.

*Chloroquine.* The 4-amino-quinolines are concentrated in the liver and are effective in eradicating amoebae invading it. Chloroquine diphosphate is given in a dosage of 600 mg (base) stat. followed by 300 mg (base) after 6 hours; thereafter: 150 mg (base) twice or thrice daily for 28 days. Headache, blurring of vision with central scotomata, nausea, and vomiting are common side effects, appearing in the later stages of treatment.

Chloroquine is usually given in suspected hepatic amoebiasis as a supportive rather than primary treatment.

*Niridazole.* This drug is discussed in the sections on schistosomiasis and dracunculitis (see pp. 377 and 107). It is a very active tissue amoebicide in doses of 25 mg per kg body weight, up to a maximum dose of 1500 mg daily for 7–10 days. It may have toxic effects including psychoses and epileptiform fits, especially in patients with severe liver damage. It is generally agreed that at present this compound should not be used in the treatment of amoebic liver abscess.

*Antibiotics.* Certain antibiotics act indirectly on amoebae in the gut lumen and tissues, probably by their effect on the intestinal bacterial flora. Of these, the most successful are penicillin, tetracycline, chlortetracycline, and oxytetracycline in the usual dosage of 250 mg 6-hourly for 10 days.

### MANAGEMENT AND TREATMENT OF AMOEBIASIS

#### ASYMPTOMATIC INTESTINAL AMOEBIASIS

There is controversy on whether patients who are asymptomatic and passing cysts of *E. histolytica* should be treated. We do not know whether tissue invasion may subsequently occur if the patient's defences are lowered; we know that 50 per cent of patients with an amoebic liver abscess have no history of symptomatic intestinal amoebiasis; it therefore seems rational to treat all patients who are infected whether symptomatic or asymptomatic.

The most difficult problem is presented by the so-called 'food handlers', the cooks, stewards, or kitchen hands who are asymptomatic but are passing *E. histolytica* cysts. Most of these could be successfully treated, leading to local reduction of transmission. Nevertheless, in the circumstances which usually apply in areas where the prevalence is high and reinfection very likely, routine examination and treatment of food handlers is regarded as an impracticable method of control, since a relatively small proportion of those infected will be identified at any one examination. Intermittent treatment of all food handlers would probably be more successful, but is recommended only when the risk of infection is regarded as very high. Kitchen hygiene, prevention of contamination of foods at source and of the consumption of uncooked foods, especially vegetables and fruits, and adequate supplies of clean water are the most reliable methods of control of infection in groups such as service or constructional personnel working in highly endemic areas. The same principles apply to the exposed individual.

There are several alternatives for treatment which are cheap, safe and well tolerated. The following are effective:

Diloxanide furoate, 500 mg orally thrice daily for 10 days.
Di-iodohydroxyquinoline (diodoquin) 600 mg thrice daily for 21 days.

Tetracycline 250 mg orally every 6 hours for 7 days may be combined with these drugs, but is not usually needed.

Since the passage of cysts is irregular, careful follow-up is needed after attempts to eradicate a symptomless infection, for example in food handlers. Stools should be examined several times, at least a month after treatment. Where re-infection is likely, as in an area of high endemicity, it is doubtful whether such procedures are of any value.

### ACUTE AMOEBIC DYSENTERY

General management includes bed rest in severe cases and the control of dehydration parenterally if necessary. After recovery, adjustment of diet and malnutrition, if present, and health education, are important.

The condition responds rapidly to chemotherapy.

Mild or moderately severe attacks can be treated as outpatients or in-patients by metronidazole, 800 mg orally thrice daily for 5 days.

An alternative is tetracycline, oxytetracycline, or chlortetracycline, 250 mg orally every 6 hours and diloxanide furoate, 500 mg orally thrice daily, both for 10 days. Di-iodohydroxyquinoline (diodoquine), 600 mg orally thrice daily for 21 days, may be given instead of diloxanide. Chloroquine may be added to protect the liver from invasion.

Severe dysentery should be treated with metronidazole, 800 mg orally thrice daily for 5 days. This form of treatment is simple, cheap and usually very effective. As an alternative emetine hydrochloride may be used in a dosage of 1 mg per kg body weight (not exceeding 65 mg in any one day) intramuscularly or subcutaneously as a single dose or in two divided doses, each day for 4–10 days.

Dehydroemetine may be given as an alternative to emetine, in doses of 1.5 mg per kg body weight (not exceeding 90 mg in any one day).

Neither of these drugs should be given to patients with cardiac disease; they are best avoided in pregnancy and in aged patients. They should be given only when the patient is in bed and under supervision.

The emetine injections are stopped once the acute signs have ceased and treatment of the intestinal infection is continued with tetracycline and diloxanide furoate or diodoquine as above, or an arsenical such as carbarsone or milibis.

### AMOEBIC NON-DYSENTERIC COLITIS

Forms of amoebic colitis other than dysentery respond to similar treatment. In most cases good response follows the regime suggested above for mild or moderate dysentery.

AMOEBIC LIVER ABSCESS

Small abscesses will respond to chemotherapy only. Large abscesses require drainage by closed aspiration. Surgical procedures are not advisable and in any case must not be carried out except during full chemotherapy. They may be needed in cases where pus cannot be obtained by aspiration and severe signs persist or when repeated aspiration does not bring relief, as may happen in children or in the presence of multiple abscesses.

*Chemotherapy*

Metronidazole, 800 mg thrice daily for 5 days, is usually adequate. This regimen will also clear any contiguous complication or intestinal infection that may be present. It may be combined with chloroquine (see below).

Alternatively, a combined course may be given, consisting of emetine hydrochloride 65 mg or dehydroemetine, 90 mg intramuscularly as a single dose or in two divided doses daily for 4–12 days depending on the clinical response. Chloroquine 600 mg (base) immediately, followed by 300 mg (base) in 6 hours then 150 mg (base) twice daily for up to 28 days. The possible gut infection is controlled by diloxanide furoate, 500 mg thrice daily for 10 days.

Pain is usually relieved by aspiration, otherwise standard analgesics should be given, for example distalgesic, two tablets three or four times daily.

Abscesses are nearly always bacteriologically sterile. Aspiration, especially when repeated, introduces some risk of secondary infection. Antibiotics, for example penicillin or tetracycline are indicated, depending on the relevant organism. Anti-amoebic chemotherapy must be continued.

*Aspiration*

Aspiration is needed if chemotherapy does not bring relief or if there is a mass with very localized tenderness, or if the abscess appears to be pointing in a particular spot. Big abscesses need aspiration and are indicated by a grossly elevated and immobilized hemidiaphragm (usually right-sided).

The patient is sedated with morphine or pethidine. The site of aspiration is infiltrated with local anaesthetic and the aspiration needle is introduced with full aseptic precautions. A syringe is attached and gentle aspiration applied. The needle should be inserted and withdrawn if no pus is found and should be introduced in several different directions. If no pus is recovered, needling should be repeated in 24 hours. If the volume of pus withdrawn exceeds 200 ml further aspiration is carried out after 48 hours and again after a similar interval if necessary.

After aspiration patients must be carefully watched. A persistent high rise of pulse rate suggests haemorrhage which requires transfusion. In severe haemorrhage surgical operation may be necessary.

*Extension of abscess to contiguous tissues*

Pulmonary and pleural involvement usually responds to anti-amoebic

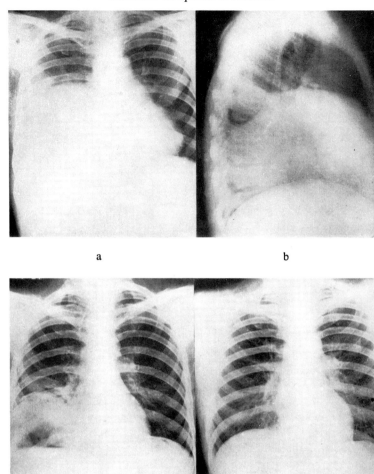

a                                      b

c                                      d

FIG. 4. An enormous liver abscess.

a. and b. Before treatment.
c. Twenty-four hours after aspiration of 6 litres of amoebic liver abscess pus.
d. One month after a course of 12 daily injections of emetine hydrochloride 65 mg.

therapy. Secondary infection requires antibiotics. Amoebic empyema must be aspirated; if aspiration is unsuccessful, surgical continuous drainage with or without rib resection may be needed.

Amoebic pericarditis may follow liver abscess in the left lobe. Repeated aspiration may be needed in suppurative pericarditis.

OTHER FORMS OF EXTRA-INTESTINAL AMOEBIASIS

Metronidazole, 800 mg thrice daily, should be given for 5–10 days in very severe cases, for example, in infections of the skin or peritoneum following rupture of a liver abscess or after surgical interference. Emetine or dehydroemetine may be offered as an alternative for a few days followed by a course of metronidazole for 5–10 days.

## MANAGEMENT

*Prophylaxis.* The patient with an acute attack of amoebic dysentery is passing amoebae and these rapidly die on being voided. They would not cause infection of man even if swallowed. The patient with amoebic dysentery, therefore, can safely be nursed in the general ward without other than the usual attention. When he recovers from his acute attack the stools become formed and may contain cysts—the infective form of the parasite. It is now that he may infect others in the absence of elementary personal hygiene and suitable sanitation. He should be treated as for symptomless amoebiasis.

## TEST OF CURE

No patient is cured, however effectively his clinical condition may have been relieved, until the parasitic infection is eradicated from the large intestine as well as elsewhere. Skilful daily stool examinations, preferably for 10 or 12 days, done within 2 weeks after completion of all amoebicidal drug treatment, will indicate whether sterilization of the infection has in fact been achieved or not. A series of daily stool examinations should be carried out 1 month later to confirm negative results. If amoebae are still present a further course of treatment, preferably with some combination of drugs including one of the tetracycline antibiotics, is indicated. Amoebiasis is not difficult to eradicate completely and within a comparatively short time. An important sign of cure is the early disappearance of rectal abscesses during or subsequent to treatment.

ULCERATIVE POST-DYSENTERIC COLITIS

Amoebicides are useless if *E. histolytica* cannot be demonstrated by thorough stool examination and by sigmoidoscopy.

Management consists of maintaining water:electrolyte balance, adjustment of anaemia, with blood transfusion if necessary, and a maintenance dose of folic acid 5 mg daily. The diet should be high in protein calories and low in roughage. Abdominal colic may be relieved by antispasmodics such as colofac. Steroids may be necessary in refractory cases. It is important to ensure that amoebic infection has been eradicated before giving steroids because steroids given to a patient with amoebic infection can lead to a fulminant form of amoebic dysentery.


## CONTROL

Control measures including food hygiene which are effective against enteric bacterial infections will usually prove effective for amoebiais.

Measures for chemotherapeutic control of infection in individuals are discussed under treatment. Routine examination of food handlers, followed by exclusion or treatment of those infected, is regarded as impracticable in highly endemic areas.

The infective agents are the cysts, which are easily killed by desiccation and heat. The amount of chlorine needed to kill the cysts is considerably greater than that needed for water bacterial purification. If chlorination is used, the water must subsequently be treated to remove the taste.

The prevalence of amoebiasis in a limited area can sometimes be greatly reduced by administration of drugs such as diodoquine. The amount of drug required is usually less than that needed for full therapy. Mass chemotherapy cannot, however, be contemplated in the large areas of high endemicity in the present absence of information about prevalence. The real answer to transmission of amoebiasis is improvement of living standards and levels of health education.


## OTHER AMOEBIC INFECTIONS IN MAN

A meningo-encephalitis, fatal within 10 days of infection, and affecting adolescents who have been swimming in heated pools, has been reported from Australia, the U.S.A., and Europe; it is caused by a 'free-living amoeba' (amoebae which can live apart from a host) of the genus *Naegleria*. Another genus of free-living amoeba, *Acanthamoeba,* has caused more localized and chronic granulomatous cerebral lesions affecting patients of any age. Similar amoebae have been isolated from some patients with corneal ulcers, although in these cases the causative relationship between the amoebae and the lesions has not been clearly established.

The species of *Naegleria* which causes primary amoebic meningo-encephalitis (PAME) is *N. fowleri*. The symptoms are malaise, sore throat and nasal discharge, followed by headache, with rigidity, vomiting, coma and death. Infection is thought to occur via the nasal mucosa, through the cribriform plate to the olfactory nerves. Post-mortem examination of the brain shows a generalized meningo-encephalitis with particular affection of the olfactory bulbs.

Infections with *Acanthamoeba* show a much more localized granulomatous infection in patients of any age, often with a history of cranial trauma, and death may be delayed for months.

Diagnosis can be made by finding the amoebae on microscopical examination of the cerebrospinal fluid; they were missed until 1965 because they were thought to be amoeboid monocytes.

So far, only Amphotericin B given as described on p. 125 has had any successful chemotherapeutic effect.

## OTHER INTESTINAL PROTOZOAL INFECTIONS

## BALANTIDIOSIS

### DEFINITION

Balantidiosis is a comparatively rare condition of parasitization of the large intestine with the large ciliate protozoan parasite *Balantidium coli.* The disease which results is characterized by a severe and chronic form of dysentery.

### GEOGRAPHICAL DISTRIBUTION

The trophozoite of *B. coli* is an oval and flattened ciliate protozoon measuring from 50 to 100 $\mu$m in length and from 50 to 70 $\mu$m in breadth. It produces rounded cysts, measuring about 50 $\mu$m in diameter, which are passed in the stools. The parasite is a common one of pigs and occurs also in guinea-pigs, monkeys and in man. Infection results from swallowing the cysts passed in formed stools by the reservoir hosts, principally the pig. It has no restriction in geographical location.

### PATHOLOGY

While, as in the case of *Entamoeba histolytica, B. coli* in asymptomatic cases of infection may dwell within the lumen of the large bowel, in those cases presenting symptoms it is a tissue-invading organism. On histological section parasites can be seen lying in the mucosa and submucosa of the wall of the large intestine; the presence of parasites causes the development in the overlying mucosa of irregularly rounded ulcers, which have undermined edges and a base composed of necrotic material. In addition to these limited areas of necrosis, haemorrhagic areas without ulceration are to be seen in the mucosa.

### CLINICAL PICTURE

The infection in some cases is asymptomatic and is detected only incidentally on examination of the stools. In most cases of balantidiosis there is dysentery with the passage of bloody mucoid stools; clinically the picture much resembles severe amoebic dysentery. The diagnosis during such an attack is made by finding the trophozoites of the parasite in the stools; during intermissions the cysts will be found.

### TREATMENT

The tetracycline antibiotics are claimed to exert a specific action on the causative parasite. The dose of these for an adult is 500 mg, 8-hourly, for 10 days. Oxytetracycline has been stated to give the best result.

## FLAGELLATE DIARRHOEA

A number of flagellate protozoa commonly parasitize the human intestine. *Giardia lamblia* is one of these which on occasions causes clinical manifestations of its presence in the form of a watery or of a fatty diarrhoea. Indefinite digestive disturbances with evidence of malabsorption of fat, sometimes with the passage of sprue-like stools, are not uncommon in those patients with large numbers of the parasites in the stools. While the organism cannot be regarded as an invariable pathogen, the fact that it adheres by means of a sucking disc to the mucosa of the duodenum lends credence to the view that it may give rise to duodenitis when present in very large numbers. Biopsy of the duodenal mucosa, by means of the Crosby capsule, indeed has shown changes in the villi in those heavily infected. It has also been stated that it may invade the biliary passages by ascent of the common bile duct.

Diagnosis of the infection is made by finding cysts of the parasite in formed stools and vegetative forms in fluid stools.

### TREATMENT

Metronidazole is usually extremely effective, given orally in doses of 800 mg thrice daily for 5 days. Children: aged 9–14, 200 mg thrice daily for 7 days; aged 5–8, 100 mg thrice daily for 7 days; aged 2–4, 100 mg twice daily for 7 days; aged under 2, 100 mg once daily for 7 days.

Patients should be given a bland, mainly fluid, diet. Codeine phosphate, 30 mg thrice daily or kaolin and morphine mixture BPC, 15 ml thrice daily, may be used to relieve diarrhoea and pain in adults.

Malabsorption syndromes are treated by offering a low fat:high protein diet, folic acid, iron and Vitamin B complex plus Vitamin A if required.

Alternatives are chloroquine 300 mg (base), daily for 5 days and mepacrine 100 mg (hydrochloride), thrice daily for 5 days.

## COCCIDIOSIS

The intracellular protozoa *Isospora hominis* and *I. belli,* which some authorities consider identical, sometimes occur in man.

Infective oocysts passed in the faeces or observed in duodenal aspirates are the only stages of the parasite so far identified in human infections. It is believed that the full cycle resembles that of *I. felis* which infects cats. The mature oocyst contains four sporozoites which are liberated in the lumen of the small intestine and penetrate epithelial cells. Schizogony and eventually sporogony take place therein and merozoites penetrate other contiguous cells. In this way shallow lesions are formed which heal easily but may initiate the diarrhoea, which is the major clinical feature.

The infection is found in parts of India, the Middle East, South-east Asia, and the South Pacific. It may also occur in Europe. It follows ingestion of food or drink contaminated with ripe oocysts containing sporozoites. Clinical signs appear in about a month. The patient develops diarrhoea which is usually mild although the stool may sometimes contain blood, pus cells and mucus. There may be colic. Eosinophilia is usual. The episode usually lasts about a week. The clinical picture is self-limited. There is no specific treatment. Oocysts which are elongated and tapering, 20–30 $\mu$m in length, contain within a clear thin wall the segmenting sporoblast or the four fully developed sporozoites. They appear in the faeces a day or two after the onset of diarrhoea and may persist. They are sometimes accompanied by Charcot–Leyden crystals. They may be found in the faeces of apparently healthy individuals. Cysts of *Eimeria* sp. have also been found in human faeces.

(See also Toxoplasmosis.)

# 2

# ANAEMIAS IN THE TROPICS

Anaemia results from excessive loss of blood, increased blood destruction, impaired erythrocyte formation, or any combination of these mechanisms. Efficient correction of an anaemia depends on the discovery of the pathological processes causing it. In the tropics, unfortunately, there are often many aetiological factors in a single individual case. Of these, certain parasitic and helminthic infections and hereditary haemoglobin abnormalities may be readily detectable. Many of the other factors are obscure, as is indicated by the present multiplicity of classifications of so-called 'tropical' anaemias.

Most forms of anaemia which occur in the temperate regions of the world may also appear in the tropics.

A particularly interesting example of local primary haematological conditions is the anaemia associated with idiopathic thrombocytopenia which has been described by many observers in Africa, particularly in East Africa, and has been called onyalai. The characteristic clinical picture is one of sudden onset, bleeding from bullae which appear on mucosal surfaces nearly always in the mouth and the appearance of purpuric spots in the conjunctivae and skin. Bleeding time is increased and the platelet count ranges from 5000 to 50,000. The bone marrow is little changed. It is now considered that onyalai is probably not a specific disease entity but should be regarded as a clinical syndrome with a variety of causes.

Anaemias in the tropics may be broadly classified into those which are associated with normoblastic haemopoiesis and those associated with megaloblastic haemopoiesis. In some anaemias, both forms of haemopoiesis may occur.

*A. Haemopoiesis normal: normoblastic bone marrow*
The following simple and practical classification should be helpful.

I. *Iron deficiency anaemia*
Low intake of Fe.
Impaired absorption of Fe.
Haemorrhage.
Pregnancy.

II. *Anaemia associated with protein malnutrition*

III. *Haemolytic anaemias*
    Haemoglobinopathies.
    G-6-Pd deficiency.
    Vegetable, mineral and animal toxins.
    Malaria. Bartonellosis.
    Hypersplenism.

IV.   *Anaemias associated with infection*
    Hookworm infection.
    Tuberculosis.
    Chronic sepsis, etc.

V. *Anaemias associated with cosmopolitan diseases*
    Reticuloses.
    Malignancy.
    Renal disease, etc.

B. *Haemopoiesis abnormal: megaloblastic bone marrow*

I. *Folic acid deficiency*
    Low intake of folic acid.
    Malabsorption syndromes including sprue and giardiasis.
    Haemolytic states.
    Protein malnutrition.
    Pregnancy.
    Drugs.
    Scurvy.

II. *Vitamin $B_{12}$ (Cyanocobalamin) deficiency*
    Addisonian pernicious anaemia.
    Alteration of intestinal flora.
    Malabsorption syndromes.
    *Diphyllobothrium* infection.

III. *Mixed deficiences*

*Normoblastic anaemias*

*Iron deficiency*. See Hookworm infection (p. 163). Dietary iron deficiency is rare in most parts of the tropics where the intake is usually high, except in infancy and sometimes in pregnancy. Iron loss in sweat or skin desquamation or resulting from interference with intestinal iron absorption is probably of minor importance.

In some areas iron overloading and iron deficiency with or without anaemia may occur concurrently in the same population. Thus, male South

African Bantu commonly develop siderosis, the incidence of which increases with age, whereas infants and females during reproductive life rarely develop siderosis and iron deficiency is common.

The blood picture is characteristically hypochromic and microcytic; it may be normocytic.

The most significant factor in the production of this type of anaemia is the state of the body iron reserves. If these are depleted, normoblastic iron deficiency anaemia may develop in any condition in which there is abnormal physiological demand for iron, for example in pregnancy, or in which there is chronic blood loss. In the latter respect the commonest and most important anaemias occur in hookworm infection. Any other causes of bleeding, such as duodenal ulcer, menorrhagia, or trauma, including viperine snake bite, may have similar results.

In the development of some forms of normoblastic anaemia inadequate and improperly adjusted protein intake may play some part. It is presumed that in these cases the relevant element of the anaemia arises from inadequate synthesis of the globin fraction of the haemoglobin, due to deficiency in the supply of certain essential amino acids.

*Haemolytic anaemias.* These may be associated in all age groups with haemoglobinopathies, thalassaemia or glucose-6-phosphate dehydrogenase deficiency. In holoendemic or hyperendemic areas malaria is the most important single factor in the development of haemolytic anaemia in very young non-immune children and in women in the third trimester of pregnancy (in whom there is some failure of the immune processes). Older children and adults who have achieved some degree of immunity to malaria do not normally acquire severe anaemia from the infection.

Where haemolysis is severe and acute, as in falciparum malaria, black-water fever or bartonellosis, grave anaemia will develop irrespective of the state of the iron reserve and balance. Where the haemolysis is more limited although continuous, as in heavy hookworm infection, the degree of anaemia achieved will depend on the iron reserve and intake and the haemopoietic response on the one hand and the iron and possibly protein loss or availability on the other. The response of the marrow to blood loss may also be restricted or delayed in some infections, for example in acute malaria, in which the escape of young cells from the marrow to the blood is held up so long as erythrocytic forms of the parasite remain in the circulation. Hypersplenism is also involved in the production of anaemia in kala azar or in the portal hypertensive syndrome which develops in schistosomiasis.

*It should be noted that, in some of the forms of apparently normoblastic anaemias discussed above, there may be a masked element of megaloblastic anaemia arising from folic acid deficiency.* This may be detectable only by bone marrow examination. It should always be suspected in cases in which the response to iron therapy is incomplete in terms of the rise of haemoglobin concentration to normal levels.

## Megaloblastic anaemias

*Folic acid deficiency.* Most of the megaloblastic anaemias seen in the tropics are due to folic acid deficiency; serum levels of vitamin $B_{12}$ are usually normal. Megaloblastic anaemia is most commonly found in women. It may result from dietary deficiency of folic acid or from factors which either increase the demand for or diminish the absorption of this substance. It may accompany intestinal disease, for example when a stricture or blind intestinal loop gives rise to stagnation of intestinal contents; it may occur in sprue and other malabsorption syndromes. It is not dependent on the state of the iron reserves.

It is also encountered occasionally in scurvy, protein malnutrition, hookworm infection, sometimes giardiasis, haemolytic states and as a result of ingestion of drugs which are folic acid antagonists, for example anticonvulsants and pyrimethamine in high and prolonged dosage. The prophylactic doses of pyrimethamine normally advised in malaria do not result in folic acid deficiency.

*Vitamin $B_{12}$ (Cyanocobalamin) deficiency.* Addisonian anaemia is very rare in the tropics, but vitamin $B_{12}$ deficiency has been described as a result of alteration of the intestinal flora. Infection with the tapeworm *Diphyllobothrium latum* may initiate severe $B_{12}$ deficiency.

## Anaemias of pregnancy

Anaemia is one of the most serious hazards of pregnancy in the tropics.

*Iron deficiency normoblastic anaemia* results from physiological changes in the mother and the increased demands of the foetus which more than offset the iron savings resulting from the cessation of menstruation.

Women living in highly endemic *Plasmodium falciparum* areas often develop an exacerbation of malaria infection during the third trimester of pregnancy. An increasingly severe normoblastic iron-deficient anaemia results, with which is almost always associated some degree of megaloblastic anaemia arising from folic acid deficiency.

When both elements are present, the anaemia is commonly called *dimorphic*; it requires concurrent treatment of both elements.

*Folic acid deficiency megaloblastic anaemia* is a vital element in the very severe and not infrequently fatal anaemias of females of child-bearing age in the tropics. It is commonly seen in the later stages of pregnancy or in the puerperium (in many cases remission occurs after the birth of the child) and arises from folic acid deficiency or a block in the folic acid–folinic acid mechanism resulting from a variety of causes, not all of which are understood. It is usually associated with some degree of iron-deficiency anaemia. Deficiency of vitamin $B_{12}$ appears to be rare in pregnancy in the tropics except in India and other parts of South Asia; it is much commoner in Europe.

The blood picture which presents in a given patient may be apparently normoblastic or obviously megaloblastic or a combination of both. The examination of the bone marrow is necessary in doubtful cases and is recommended whenever possible.

In any case it is wise to regard anaemia in pregnancy as being dimorphic in some degree and to treat accordingly, always considering the possibility of *P. falciparum* infection.

TREATMENT

The treatment of tropical anaemias will depend upon their aetiology. The routine suggested is:

1. Treatment of the underlying cause of any haematological disturbance, for example, malaria or hookworm.

2. Blood transfusion when necessary. Most anaemias in adults can be treated without transfusion, which is usually reserved for severe haemolytic anaemias occurring, for example, in falciparum malaria. If iron deficiency is present, ferrous sulphate, 600 mg daily in three divided doses may be given for 1–3 months. This should be a routine for women in the third trimester of pregnancy.

3. If folic acid deficiency is present, folic acid, 50 mg should be given daily intramuscularly for 2 successive days, followed by 25 mg orally daily until the blood picture is normal. In the third trimester of pregnancy a maintenance dose of 5 mg thrice daily is advisable.

4. If vitamin $B_{12}$ deficiency is present, 1000 $\mu$g of vitamin $B_{12}$ (Cyanocobalamin) intramuscularly or subcutaneously should be given and repeated in 3 days, thereafter 250 $\mu$g should be given weekly until the blood picture is normal.

5. In pregnancy it is wise to regard anaemia as dimorphic and treat for both iron and folic acid deficiency (2 and 3 above). Treatment with vitamin $B_{12}$ is seldom necessary.

6. See chapter on sickle cell anaemia and haemoglobinopathies (p. 126).

# 3

# BACILLARY DYSENTERY

DEFINITION

Bacillary dysentery is due to infection of the large intestine with one of the pathogenic species of bacteria belonging to the genus *Shigella*. The infection is a local one within the bowel, and it does not spread systemically. The disease caused by it is characterized by colitis, with severe bloody diarrhoea and fever; its course is acute; certain complications remote from the bowel are the result of absorption of toxins. The mortality is high with certain infections.

GEOGRAPHICAL DISTRIBUTION

World-wide and particularly prevalent when sanitation is defective or lacking. The most severe forms of bacillary dysentery are especially associated with the tropics.

AETIOLOGY

Infection with organisms of the genus *Shigella* in nature is peculiar to man. The infection results from swallowing the bacilli, usually in food or water contaminated with infected human faeces. Insanitary and uncleanly habits and the activities of flies facilitate their dissemination by mechanical transference. The bacilli are voided in great numbers in the stools of those actively suffering from an attack of bacillary dysentery; in some cases they continue to be passed in the stools for some time after the attack; symptomless carriers are an occasional source of infection. Under suitable conditions bacillary dysentery tends to occur in epidemics; the severity of these and the associated mortality depend on the species and strain of the causative shigella infection.

Species and varieties of the genus *Shigella* are numerous; those of greatest clinical importance are *S. shigae,* various types of *S. flexneri* and of *S. boydii, S. schmitzii,* and *S. sonnei.* The organism causing the most consistently severe disease is *S. shigae,* which occurs chiefly as a tropical infection; *S. sonnei* is responsible for a mild form of dysentery particularly found in temperate climates. The other species and varieties cause manifestations of all degrees of severity between these two extremes. The identification and the typing of the organisms, which are recovered by bacteriological culture of the stools or proctoscopically obtained swabs, are matters for a properly equipped and staffed laboratory.

## PATHOLOGY

On swallowing dysentery bacilli these may be destroyed by the physiological barrier of the normal gastric juice. This barrier is readily broken down, for example by dilution; the organisms then pass into the small intestine and reach the large bowel. In the large bowel they multiply with great speed; in a severe infection they largely supplant the normal flora of the bowel. Toxins liberated by the bacteria cause inflammatory lesions in the mucosa, which in virulent infections is damaged and is invaded by the organisms. In clinically mild cases of dysentery, however, there is nothing more than a mild inflammation and engorgement of the mucosa of the large intestine; this is of short duration and resolves when the infection is overcome, often within a few days. In more severe cases the inflammation is extensive and pronounced; there is marked engorgement and oedema of the mucosa; and the crests of the folds of the mucosa, lying transversely across the bowel, are denuded, giving rise to narrow and shallow serpiginous ulcers ('snail track' ulcers). These ulcers heal with minimal scarring as the infection is overcome and the inflammation subsides; the bowel ultimately is restored substantially to normal. In the most severe attacks of dysentery, commonly due to *S. shigae* infections, the whole process is exaggerated and the mucosal destruction is deeper and more extensive. Considerable areas of mucosa and submucosa slough. If the patient recovers from such an attack these gross areas of ulceration are repaired by the formation of scar tissue which contracts, causing kinking and deformity of the bowel. Moreover, being covered only by simple epithelium, and being comparatively avascular, the scars are readily injured and secondarily infected by a variety of bacterial organisms. The end result may be a chronic post-dysenteric colitis, from which the primary and causative shigella infection has disappeared.

Rarely, chronic bacillary dysentery may follow an acute attack of bacillary dysentery. This condition is associated with persistence of the causative shigella infection in the bowel. The organisms are passed continuously or intermittently in the stools, from which they can be recovered for culture on suitable media. The lesions in the bowel are of a chronic inflammatory nature, with engorgement, oedema, and recurring ulceration following abscess formation in the mucosa; blockage of crypts containing mucus-secreting glands during the inflammatory process results in their distension and the formation of 'retention cysts'. The abscesses and cysts contain dysentery bacilli, and the liberation of their contents accounts for the periodic appearance of the organisms in the stools.

Absorption of toxins from the intestine is held to be responsible for a variety of inflammatory lesions remote from the intestine. These lesions, which invariably are bacteriologically sterile and never suppurate, affect in particular the eyes, the joints, and peripheral nerves. Conjunctivitis and iridocyclitis, polyarthritis, and peripheral neuritis, are common complications or early sequelae of an attack of bacillary dysentery.

CLINICAL PICTURE

*Traveller's diarrhoea* Most Europeans on first going to the tropics, especially by air, suffer from attacks of diarrhoea. This is commonly referred to as 'the squitters', 'the trots', 'Guppy tummy', 'Delhi belly', and so forth. It may be precipitated by changes in environment, climate and diet (especially the ingestion of 'hot' spiced food, such as is offered in India and Thailand, or of unusual cooking oils), by alterations in the intestinal flora, or by the inhalation and ingestion of trauma-producing matter such as dust and sand. Some episodes may be viral or physiological in origin, but some are probably very mild attacks of bacillary dysentery, which pass undiagnosed.

The incubation period of bacillary dysentery is short. It does not exceed a week, usually is less than 3 days and may even be less than 24 hours. The onset of an attack of average severity is sudden; it is associated with abdominal discomfort, sometimes nausea and vomiting, and a rise in temperature. Within a few hours there are colicky pains and sharp diarrhoea. The first motion passed contains faecal material, but thereafter there is little of this and the motions largely consist of tenacious, blood-stained mucus which is voided in small amounts at very frequent intervals. The naked-eye appearance of the motions has been likened to that of 'red-currant jelly'. Their passage is accompanied by urgency, griping pains and tenesmus, which are distressing. The number of motions voided in 24 hours is considerable and usually exceeds 20; in severe cases there is a continuous desire to defaecate. The fever, which usually is remittent or intermittent, continues throughout most of the attack; this lasts from 1 week to as much as 3 weeks, according to its severity. As the infection is overcome the temperature declines, the intensity of the symptoms diminishes, the amount of blood in the motions lessens, and the number of stools decreases. Visible blood vanishes from the motions, which, though still consisting largely of mucus, become bile-stained before becoming more normal in appearance and consistency with the end of the attack and the entry upon convalescence.

Mild and ambulatory cases of bacillary dysentery are very common and often escape specific diagnosis. Fulminating cases of the disease are particularly associated with shiga infections. In these all the clinical manifestations are exaggerated. The toxaemia and prostration are profound; large amounts of blood may be lost in virtually continuous fluid motions; these contain shreds and pieces of necrotic mucosa; their appearance has been likened to that of 'raw meat choppings'. In such cases the temperature may rise in a day or so to a very high level, or it may not rise at all but become subnormal and the patient dies within a short time.

In a febrile, toxaemic and exhausting disease such as this, which is associated with the continuous loss of fluid, such complications as dehydration, peripheral circulatory failure and renal failure may be expected. These are particularly evident in children and in the elderly, in both of whom bacillary dysentery is a serious and not uncommonly fatal disease. In young children the onset of the disease is not unusually associated with convulsions.

It is towards the end of the acute attack or in early convalescence that the common systemic complications, inflammation of the eyes, joints, or peripheral nerves, make their appearance. These, though not of themselves serious, can cause much discomfort; they resolve after some days or within a week or two, and leave no permanent evidence of their presence.

Serious intra-abdominal complications which may be encountered include severe intestinal haemorrhage, perforation with acute peritonitis and chronic peritonitis; all these are rare. More rare still are pneumoperitoneum, and portal pyaemia with multiple abscess formation in the liver.

Haemorrhoids, which may thrombose, or rectal prolapse are liable to occur during an attack of bacillary dysentery, as in attacks of diarrhoea of any causation.

### DIAGNOSIS

The clinical picture clearly suggests the diagnosis, especially during an epidemic of bacillary dysentery. Simple microscopical examination of the stools should invariably be made; this will reveal the presence of an inflammatory exudate. In this exudate will be found macrophage cells; these must clearly be differentiated from amoebae. Culture for the causative organism should also be done. Material for this is best obtained by rectal swabbing; alternatively, suitable portions of the motions may be selected for the purpose without delay after passage. When the inoculation of media cannot be performed at once, the selected portion of stool may be put in 30 per cent glycerol in isotonic saline. The dysentery bacilli will survive for some days in such a medium, while they die or are overgrown rapidly by other bacteria if left in the stool itself; thus the material can be conveyed to a distant laboratory.

On isolation of a morphologically and culturally distinctive organism it may further be checked by testing for agglutinins in the serum of the patient. The routine serological testing of the patient's serum against standard cultures of *Shigella* is of no help in the diagnosis of bacillary dysentery.

### TREATMENT

Bacillary dysentery is usually a mild and self-limited disease. Most patients recover after a few days of rest, good nursing and oral rehydration. Food should be soft and bland and given frequently in small amounts.

Severe cases need parenteral rehydration, as in cholera, with careful adjustment of electrolytes, including potassium. Where there has been pronounced bleeding, transfusion may be needed.

Routine usage of drugs is unnecessary for mild and moderate cases. There is no convincing evidence that drugs shorten the period of excretion of the organisms. They are thus of no epidemiological value. Nevertheless, in some hospitals in the developed world all bacillary dysentery patients are given tetracyline, ampicillin, or chloramphenicol.

In very severe cases, where chemotherapy is judged necessary to save life, drugs must be given, as far as possible only after drug sensitivity tests have been made.

### Sulphonamides
In the past triple soluble sulphonamides were commonly used, so long as the fluid and electrolyte balance could be maintained. Alternatively, relatively insoluble sulphonamides were given, especially when treatment was in unskilled hands. Of these, sulphaguanidine and phthalyl sulphathiazole (Thiazole) were most used. The adult dose was 3 g immediately, followed after 4 hours by 2 g 4-hourly for 5–7 days. One-third of this dose was given to children under 3 years of age, half the dose up to the age of 10, and two-thirds up to the age of 15.

Sulphonamides should not be used in cases where there is notable dehydration.

### Antibiotics
Of these, the best is tetracycline. Ampicillin, streptomycin, and several others have shown considerable activity and have been used as substitutes for tetracycline when resistance to the latter is present in the organism.

These compounds are used only in the absence of selective drug resistance, which is unfortunately becoming common in areas where drugs have been too freely used.

Tetracycline is given orally in doses of 500 mg 6-hourly for 5–7 days. Children are given doses in proportion to their body weight. Resistance is common. Ampicillin is the best alternative in doses of 500 mg 6-hourly for adults at 100 mg per kg body weight (in 4 divided doses); in children treatment is continued for 5 days.

### Combinations of sulphonamides and antibiotics
Streptotriad (sulphtriad and streptomycin) and guanimycin (sulphaguanidine and streptomycin) have been used successfully.

### Resistance to sulphonamides and antibiotics
The susceptibility of *Shigella* spp. to many of these drugs has become greatly reduced over the last few years. In some areas, 90 per cent of the organisms have become resistant to tetracycline. This is partly due to indiscriminate use of the drug and to transfer of DNA-containing genes coding resistance (the R-factor) from other Gram-negative bacilli, some of which may not be pathogens. Transfer of resistance, which may be multiple, involving several drugs, may occur between *Escherichia coli, Shigella, Salmonella* (including

*S. typhi*), and other organisms of the same class. This transfer of resistance, which depends on the temporary formation of a 'bridge' between one bacterium and another, may occur during a single outbreak or even during the treatment of a single patient. Hence the great importance of limiting the usage of the drugs.

*Dehydration*

Mild cases can be rehydrated orally by giving a dilute solution of salt. Physiological saline diluted 1:4 with water is palatable and accepted by children.

Oral fluid should be given to all patients who can accept it.

In more severe cases, intravenous replacement is essential.

Dehydration, which may be accompanied by acidosis, is a major and rapid cause of death in infants and children in particular. A gravely dehydrated child may have lost up to 20 per cent of its body weight in fluid.

Rehydration should be carried out as for cholera (see p. 59).

Fluid should be given to infants and children parenterally as one-half strength physiological saline or half-strength Darrow's solution (60 mEq sodium, 50 mEq chloride, 18 mEq potassium per litre) or, when acidosis is present, in similar dilutions of compound sodium lactate injection (B.P. 1958). In the young child the deficit in severe dehydration is 120–160 ml per kg body weight. The dehydration is carried out rapidly to begin with, to adjust the intravascular volume. This requires 20 ml per kg body weight in the infant. The deficit is then made up over a period of 6 hours. After this, fluid replacement is adjusted to supplying normal needs and to replacing any continued excessive loss.

Dilution is necessary as the child's kidney is less efficient in salt excretion than is that of an adult. Salt overloading must be avoided and fluid overloading also can be disastrous. If intravenous infusion is impossible subcutaneous infusion, with hyaluronidase, can be substituted. These solutions should also be given orally and will be consumed by children. Judgment is necessary to restore and maintain a correct fluid and electrolyte balance in children but 600 ml of one of the recommended solutions can safely be given subcutaneously as an emergency measure to a clinically dehydrated child suffering from gastroenteritis or dysentery and it may well prove life-saving. Specific drug treatment is also started at once to control the infection.

*Other complications*

Shock and renal failure are treated by standard methods (see pp. 280, 281).

PREVENTION

Bacillary dysentery is essentially a scourge of dirty, overcrowded regions in which human faeces are allowed to contaminate water and food and are accessible to flies. It is thus particularly common in the disadvantaged world, where sanitation is bad and living standards are poor.

Outbreaks also occur in the developed world, mostly due to *S. sonnei* and in localized communities, such as schools and hostels. In these outbreaks the sick patient is more important than the symptomless carrier in spreading the infection. He must be isolated. This is impossible in most of the third world, where the control of bacillary dysentery to the level obtaining in Western Europe must await tremendous improvements in communal and personal hygiene.

The carrier of the organism usually cures himself in days or weeks. If discharge of *Shigella* persists, the carrier should be treated in isolation with a drug to which the relevant organism is known to be sensitive.

Vaccination may one day be possible. Live vaccines of attenuated streptomycin-sensitive *Shigella* have been tried in the field and amongst school children, producing some success, but only strain-specific immunity.

# 4

# BARTONELLOSIS

## DEFINITION

Bartonellosis, Oroya fever and verruga peruana, or Carrion's disease, are due to infection with *Bartonella bacilliformis.* The infection is transmitted by female sandflies (*Phlebotomus* spp.). The disease is characterized by two distinct and consecutive clinical syndromes. The first is Oroya fever, a severe febrile anaemia; the second, the verruga peruana, is characterized by an eruption of small haemangioma-like tumours.

## GEOGRAPHICAL DISTRIBUTION

The disease is remarkably restricted in its distribution, being confined to the continent of South America. There it has been found on the eastern and the western slopes of the Andes in certain narrow valleys in Peru, Ecuador, and Colombia, usually between 610 and 3050 m above sea level.

Bartonellosis normally is endemic in well-defined localities; under certain conditions, such as the congregation of non-immunes in an endemic area, it can become epidemic.

## AETIOLOGY AND PATHOLOGY

Persons of all ages and both sexes are affected. Among the natives of the endemic areas the disease is one of childhood, and as infection confers immunity to reinfection its occurrence in adults is correspondingly low.

The mortality in the untreated is about 40 per cent during the first stage and in some epidemics it has been much higher. The mortality is rarely due to uncomplicated Oroya fever; commonly it is the result of a complicating septicaemic salmonella infection, to which these patients' resistance is peculiarly lowered.

The causative agent, *B. bacilliformis,* has been recovered only from man and the insect vectors. It is a very small extremely pleomorphic bacterium-like organism, which can be found in large numbers in red cells and in cells of the reticulo-endothelium throughout the body during the Oroya fever stage of the disease. It takes the form of minute Gram-negative rods or rounded bodies measuring up to 2 $\mu$m in their greatest diameter; the rods often are slightly curved and some are bipolar; they occur singly, in short chains, or in clusters;

they stain reddish-violet with the Romanovsky stain. They can be cultured in tissue cultures, on blood agar and other enriched media. In fresh preparations of naturally infected blood, and in young cultures *in vitro,* they show motility.

*Phlebotomus verrucarum* is the most widely distributed, numerous and epidemiologically important vector. The vector becomes infective in about 3 days. Transmission takes place in the act of feeding, possibly through infection *via* the proboscis.

In the first non-eruptive, or Oroya fever stage, the essential pathological changes are due to massive invasion of red cells and cells of the reticulo-endothelium by *B. bacilliformis.* There is a severe anaemia and marked reticulo-endothelial proliferation. The skin of patients dying during Oroya fever is wax-like; there may be diffuse or punctate haemorrhages in the mucosae and subcutaneous tissues. There are petechiae in the serous membranes and internal organs. The lymph glands, the spleen and the liver are enlarged. *B. bacilliformis* is present in great numbers in the erythrocytes and in the cytoplasm of endothelial cells throughout the reticulo-endothelial tissues. The infected endothelial cells are swollen and proliferated; some appear actively phagocytic and contain erythrocytes. The endothelial cells of the spleen and the Kupffer cells of the liver are loaded with haemosiderin, which is also deposited in the interstitial spaces. The bone marrow is hyperplastic and megaloblastic. In the liver there are extensive areas of central necrosis; Kupffer cells are hyperplastic and actively phagocytic in the spleen. In the lymph glands there is a proliferation of large, swollen endothelial cells.

In the second eruptive, or verruga peruana stage, the lesions of the skin consist at first of newly formed blood vessels lying in oedematous connective tissue. In the lesions there are haemorrhagic foci and pronounced proliferation of the vascular endothelial cells. The endothelial cells outside the vessels proliferate also and form angioblastic tumours which compress and may obliterate the vessels. In older lesions a fibroblastic reaction occurs, with infiltration with lymphocytes, plasma cells and leucocytes. In some lesions the overlying epidermis disappears and the surface is covered by organized blood clot. Secondary bacterial infection is common.

Subcutaneous nodules, histologically similar to the cutaneous lesions, also form and often undergo central necrosis. *B. bacilliformis* is present in the cytoplasm of the endothelial cells but in smaller numbers than in the initial non-eruptive stage.

### CLINICAL PICTURE

Oroya fever and verruga peruana are stages of the same disease. The eruptive, or second, stage, though commonly a sequel of the first, may appear in its apparent absence; possibly in such cases the non-eruptive Oroya fever stage is so unusually mild as to escape diagnosis.

*Oroya Fever.* The incubation period of Oroya fever is variable; it ranges from 6 days to 4 months; usually it is 3 or 4 weeks.

The onset may be sudden, with high fever and rigors; usually it is insidious, with increasing malaise, headache, severe pains in the joints and bones and intermittent or remittent fever. Nausea, vomiting and diarrhoea are present in association with anorexia and thirst. The blood pressure falls, there is a marked increase in the respiration rate, and the patient suffers from vertigo on attempting to rise. The skin becomes wax-like and the mucous membranes blanched. The patient is prostrated and may be delirious. Pains are troublesome and continuous; in particular they involve the joints and the epiphyses of the long bones.

The fever is intermittent or remittent. It persists with accompanying signs and symptoms in favourable cases for 2–6 weeks.

A severe, rapidly progressive anaemia becomes clinically evident in a few days. The red cell count and whole blood haemoglobin concentration markedly fall. The red cell diameters, volume and thickness all are increased; there is a rise in the reticulocyte count; and normoblasts and megaloblasts appear in the circulating blood as a result of marrow hyperactivity. The blood volume is diminished; the sedimentation rate is much increased. The white cell count is not significantly affected. *B. bacilliformis* is present usually in great numbers in the erythrocytes throughout the Oroya fever stage. The principal cause of mortality is infection with *Salmonella* spp., commonly *S. typhimurium*. This may occur during the stage of massive red cell destruction; usually it occurs in convalescence during regeneration of the red cells with a high reticulosis. In uncomplicated Oroya fever the prognosis is good; it is rather less so in those suffering the salmonella complication when this is suitably controlled by drugs; if the latter is neglected the mortality may be over 90 per cent.

*Verruga peruana.* Sometimes the verrugous stage begins before the attack of Oroya fever has ended. Commonly, from some 2 weeks to 2 months after an attack of Oroya fever multiple verrugous lesions appear on the skin and mucous membranes. In the skin they develop anywhere on the body, but they are particularly prevalent on the face and on the limbs; the mucous membranes of the mouth, nose and eyes may all be affected. Most frequently they take the form of miliary lesions 1–8 mm in diameter; these are raised, hemispherical, bright red, or dusky red swellings covered with a thin layer of shiny skin. Comparable nodules can be felt in the deeper layers of the skin; these grow in size, attain a diameter of some centimetres, and protrude. They may or may not break through the skin surface; in the former event they take the form of red tumours of irregular contour, which may become pedunculated. These latter lesions bleed particularly easily and usually they become secondarily infected ('mulaire' verrugas).

The various types of lesions, the miliary, the nodular and the mulaire, all appear concurrently in successive crops. There may be few or thousands with the miliary type preponderating. Normally they persist for 1–6 months, but sometimes for as long as 2 years. The lesions then heal without scar formation, unless they have been the seat of gross secondary infection.

The clinical pictures of Oroya fever and of verruga peruana, in relation to the area from which the patient comes, usually are characteristic. In the non-eruptive Oroya fever stage the diagnosis can be confirmed by examination of blood films for *Bartonella*. In the verrugous or eruptive stage biopsy of the lesions will reveal the organism in smaller numbers in the endothelial cells.

There is no specific treatment. The anaemia of the Oroya fever stage, while it progresses, may be controlled by suitable blood transfusions.

Chloramphenicol is the most effective drug for control of the usual salmonella infection; it should be given promptly in the usual doses in every case. If given early, it reduces the mortality in a dramatic manner.

# 5

# BRUCELLOSIS

DEFINITION

Diseases caused by infection with species of *Brucella* organisms. Types of the disease are also called Malta fever, Mediterranean fever, and abortus fever. In the subacute form the infection is often known as undulant fever.

AETIOLOGY

*Brucella* spp. are very short Gram-negative rods, the smaller forms of which are coccal in shape. The organisms in culture may appear singly or in short chains. They can be grown readily by incubation at 37° C on serum dextrose agar and sheep blood agar. Brucellosis is essentially a disease of animals. Man acquires the infection by ingestion of or contact with the infected animals and their secretions, including milk. The organisms which infect man are *Brucella melitensis* (Malta fever), *Br. abortus* (Brucellosis or abortus fever), and *Br. suis*. Spread from man to man has not been reported.

*Br. abortus* infects cattle in many parts of the world. The infection in the animal does not usually produce serious disease, but the organisms are excreted in the milk and may continue to be excreted for long periods. Infection of the genital tract leads to abortion and the placenta, amniotic fluid and other discharges, as well as the dead foetus, are all highly infective. The organisms are also excreted in great numbers in the urine and faeces. Drinking milk or coming into contact with any of the infected material or exposure to the dust and environment of the cowshed leads to infection in man; this may occur by the nasopharynx or through the abraded skin or the conjunctivae.

*Br. melitensis* infects goats. The disease in the animals is mild and often inapparent; it does not cause abortion, but the uterine and vaginal discharges become heavily infected. The organisms also escape in the faeces and urine and contaminate the environment. The great danger to man lies in the fact that the milk is heavily infected and remains so for months. Where goats and cattle are herded together the latter may become infected with *Br. melitensis*. In such infections abortion is uncommon but the milk and excrement become heavily infected.

*Br. suis* infects pigs. Suckling pigs are highly susceptible and adults less so; abortion is less common than in *Br. abortus* infection in cattle. The excrement is heavily infected and the environment of infected animals is highly contaminated.

42

Other animals, including horses, are occasionally infected. Outbreaks in pigs have been caused by contact with infection in wild hares. Dogs and cats are resistant and are not concerned in the transmission of the infection to man.

Man becomes infected by drinking infected milk, by direct contact with the products of abortion or parturition, or in the process of tending or slaughtering, and by inhalation of infected dust.

Brucellae are easily destroyed by heat or by exposure to the common disinfectants. Organisms will remain alive in infected, damp, shaded material for weeks and months. They persist in milk until it turns sour. Pasteurization of milk kills them, but fresh milk and milk products such as goat's cheese (unless made from pasteurized milk) are very infective. The organisms persist for long periods in animal faeces and urine and in dirty water, dung-covered floors and walls, and in the dust of infected environments. They are present in the tissues and blood of slaughtered infected animals.

In milk-transmitted infections in some geographical areas, for some reason not known, the disease is much commoner in adults than in children; it is commoner in men than in women. There are special occupational hazards in farmers, shepherds and goatherds, abattoir workers, and veterinarians. Laboratory outbreaks have occurred, in which all three species have been involved; infections with *Br. abortus* in these circumstances are less severe than with *Br. suis* or *Br. melitensis*.

In general, infections with *Br. abortus* in man are the least virulent. Necrosis and suppuration in the tissues occurs most frequently in *Br. suis* infections.

### PATHOLOGY

The *Brucella* organisms are essentially intracellular, multiplying in the cells of the host. This makes them somewhat resistant to chemotherapeutic agents which destroy them when they are extracellular but do not always reach them in their intracellular haunts. After entering the host through the damaged skin or the conjunctivae or following ingestion or inhalation, the organisms are sometimes engulfed by polymorphs or settle in local lymph glands where they enter the reticulo-endothelial cells and later reach the blood stream. From the blood they become localized in the reticulo-endothelial cells of the body, especially in the liver, spleen, bone marrow, lymph nodes and the kidney. In these tissues granulomas form about the foci of infection. These are made up of the hypertrophied reticulo-endothelial cells, lymphocytes, plasma cells, and epithelioid cells; there may be giant cell formation. The granulomas closely resemble those of sarcoidosis and are the basic lesions of brucellosis. They occasionally suppurate, causing local abscesses; this occurs most often in *Br. suis* infections. From time to time degeneration and necrosis of the infected cells is followed by escape of *Brucella* organisms into the blood-stream.

The resulting bacteraemia gives rise to clinical signs, including fever. These may be accompanied by reactions probably initiated by the escape of the products of necrosis or of the organisms in the cells and the release of toxic substances, possibly endotoxins. Periodic release of these products probably determines the irregular repetition of febrile episodes, as seen in the subacute and chronic infections. The reaction of the host is modified in the more prolonged infections by immuno-sensitivity reactions similar to those in tuberculosis.

CLINICAL PICTURE

The incubation period, when it can be measured after a single exposure, usually varies from 1 to 3 weeks; it may be several months.

The disease may present in several patterns. The most severe forms result from *Br. suis* and *Br. melitensis* infections.

The onset of the acute form is commonly insidious with fever appearing over the course of some days. It may be sudden with chills, severe muscle and joint pains and backache, persistent headache, and sometimes fleeting peripheral neuralgia. The temperature rises sharply to peaks of 39.4–40.6° C, swinging considerably. The fever is remittent rather than intermittent. The acute phase is commonly accompanied by drenching sweats, coming on after the peaks of fever have been passed and the temperature is falling to the lower levels of 37.8–38.3° C. The patient rapidly becomes toxic and anxious. He complains of prostration and is anorexic. There may be an irritating cough, with little sputum, but with no physical pulmonary signs. The spleen is often palpable and tender. The liver edge may be tender but there is usually no hepatic enlargement. The patient frequently becomes notably constipated and complains of abdominal discomfort and distension. The lymph glands of the neck may be palpable and tender. There are no really specific signs to account for the patient's obvious illness. Moderate leucopenia is usual, with the granulocytes reduced and relative increase in mononuclear cells. A moderate hypochromic anaemia commonly develops.

The attack lasts for 2 or 3 weeks, then subsides gradually. Convalescence with complete recovery may follow, but recurrences of the clinical picture are common whether or not the patient has been treated. They may appear after only a few days, sometimes weeks or months.

The patient with recurrences passes into the subacute form of the disease, characterized by irregular bouts of fever and return of the joint pains, sweating and splenic enlargement. The joint pains may be general. They are sometimes confined to only one or two large joints or circumscribed areas of the spine; they do not flit from joint to joint as they do in rheumatic fever. As the disease progresses, arthritic changes may develop in the affected joints (see below). This situation may follow an acute attack as described above, but often develops insidiously. The patient is tired and depressed. The episodes of fever and illness last a few days to a week or so and are followed by intervals of weeks or months in which the patient never feels really well, but remains tired and inefficient and may run a low fever in the evenings. In some people the latter picture may continue without the recurrent acute attacks. When the latter occur the disease is often called 'undulant fever'. Again there are seldom very obvious localizing signs and the patient looks and feels ill. Depression and fatigue are part of the syndrome and are often mistaken for neurosis. The spleen is usually enlarged and tender, but often only slightly more than just palpable; the liver edge may be tender but at this stage hepatic enlargement is not characteristic. There may be some irregular lymph gland enlargement.

Splenomegaly is sometimes pronounced. For instance, a picture closely resembling that of visceral leishmaniasis occurs in Kenya, in which there may be gross enlargement of the spleen and relatively less enlargement of the liver. In neglected cases in children splenomegaly may be a prominent feature. In such cases infarcts and perisplenitis may cause episodes of considerable local pain.

The absence of enlargement of the spleen does not rule out the possibility of the infection.

In most patients the disease subsides within 6–12 months and health is gradually restored. In 10–15 per cent of cases the disease becomes chronic.

The classical complications of brucellosis develop during this form of the disease. Of these, spondylitis is one of the commonest. The intervertebral discs become replaced by granulomatous tissue and the cartilages of the contiguous vertebrae are involved. Collapse of the vertebra may follow and occasionally abscesses and even compression myelopathy develop about the affected area. This series of events occurs usually in the lumbar spine leading to severe back pain and sciatica resembling the effects of a 'slipped disc'. Arthritic changes with osteophytes and bony erosion are liable to occur in any of the large joints, especially the shoulder, sacro-iliac, knee, and hip joints. The arthritis usually appears in the large joints and is most commonly uniarticular. Effusion is common and often severe; purulent effusions may develop, especially in *Br. suis* infections. Arthritis may occur in any stage of the disease, acute, chronic or in convalescence. Occasionally it may be the presenting sign; in such cases it may be a polymorphonuclear leucocytosis, rather than leucopenia.

Bone destruction in the spine or big joints, if inadequately managed, may lead to permanent damage and deformity.

Osteomyelitis with abscess formation may occasionally occur in the long bones and the ribs.

In some geographical areas inflammation of the body of the testis and sometimes the epididymis commonly occurs and causes severe clinical epididymo-orchitis which lasts a few days, then subsides, leaving swelling which may persist for weeks. Sterility is not a sequel.

Abortion is not a special risk in any of the infections nor is sterility in the female. This is a point which should be stressed, since the mental effects of the disease may be considerably worsened by the fear of sterility or abortion.

Granulomatous reactions in the kidney, ureters or bladder may produce localized complications with frequency, dysuria and haematuria, but these are uncommon.

Endocarditis, with the clinical picture of bacterial endocarditis, is occasionally caused by brucella infection. Deep venous thrombosis may also occur, especially in patients kept immobile in bed for too long. Pleural effusion occurs occasionally and brucellar empyema has been reported.

*Brucella* may infect any part of the eye, producing granulomatous reactions as elsewhere and causing keratitis and even choroiditis. Severe lesions occur more commonly in *Br. melitensis* infection but are rare in any case. In most infections the patient commonly complains of some blurring of vision, without accompanying clinical signs.

In some patients the infection survives for years. Such persons may provide a history of an acute attack or of an irregular series of attacks, or they may drift slowly into a chronic state of ill health, with occasional evening fevers, persistent backache, pain in other bones and joints, with the picture of osteophytic arthritis appearing radiologically. Depression and fatigue are always present and may be the only indication of illness. In this stage the spleen is usually palpable but seldom becomes very enlarged. The diagnosis at this stage, unless helped by the previous history or by social or occupational evidence may be extremely difficult (see below).

Cirrhosis of the liver has occasionally been attributed to chronic brucellosis, but there is little evidence for this. Where the condition is present in the long-continued infection, it may be more likely that the hepatic damage has resulted from alcohol used to combat the persistent depression.

DIAGNOSIS

*Brucella* spp. can usually be recovered by blood culture during a febrile attack and sometimes when the patient is afebrile. A positive culture is obtained more frequently in *Br. melitensis* than in *Br. abortus* infections. A sample of 5.0 ml venous blood is taken and should be seeded into two flasks of serum broth or liver infusion broth. One of these is treated anaerobically, the other aerobically or under slightly raised $CO_2$ pressure. Subcultures are made every 3–5 days on blood agar. It may be 4–6 weeks before a good growth is obtained.

Agglutinins usually appear in the primary attack by the fifth to eighth day, but may be delayed for several weeks. Zones of inhibition in the lower dilutions of serum are common; they are less pronounced if the serum is kept for a few days before use. The two main antigens A and M occur in all *Brucella,* but in varying amounts. Monospecific sera may be prepared with one or other, to which the species will react. *Br. abortus* and *Br. suis* contain more A than M antigen, and *Br. melitensis* more M than A. It is thus possible to make some differentiation by selective use of antigen absorption in the agglutination test. As normally done, however, the test is group- and not species-specific.

The agglutination reaction is commonly positive by the end of the second week.

A titre of 1 in 80 suggests brucellosis in an acutely ill febrile patient or in one in a suspected subacute stage. Titres of up to 1 in 80 may be found in apparently healthy individuals who have been frequently exposed to infection by drinking raw milk or by their occupation and who have no history of febrile illness. The titre in these circumstances is not highly significant and may remain at this level for years. Much higher titres may be recorded. Titres of 1 in 1000 or over are usually taken as indicative of active infection.

In cases where the titre is around 1 in 80 and where there is some uncertainty about diagnosis, the presence of the microglobulin antibodies (which need the continued existence of the antigen to stimulate their production and are thus indicative of active infection) may be determined by the anti-human globulin (AHG) reaction, in which a suspension of *Brucella* organisms is mixed with the suspected serum and incubated with AHG rabbit serum. Agglutination of the organisms indicates a positive result.

A complement fixation is sometimes used. Occasionally this may be positive when agglutination is negative, but on the whole the results of the reactions run in parallel in the acute infections. The complement fixation titre falls within 6 months of successful treatment or spontaneous cure of the infection.

If the agglutination test (or the complement fixation test) and the AHG are both positive, it is likely that the infection is persisting. If all these are negative, so is the diagnosis.

Sensitivity to the organism may be detected by the intradermal injection of 0.1 ml of 'brucellin', an antigen made from filtrates of broth culture of *Brucella* spp. The reactions to antigens made from the individual species are sometimes specific. A positive reaction is the appearance after 4–36 hours at the injection site of a raised tender erythematous indurated plaque up to 6 mm across. It indicates past or present infection. The test is not therefore of diagnostic value in the clinical assessment of an individual case, but may be useful as an epidemiological tool.

Where there is arthritis with effusion the joint fluid should be withdrawn and examined. Culture of the organisms from this fluid may be easier than from blood and there is evidence that the agglutinin titre is higher than in the corresponding serum. Radiological examination of the spine or affected big joints may reveal the characteristic appearance, including osteophytes. In the early or mild infection there may be no radiological changes visible even when there is severe arthritic involvement with effusion.

### TREATMENT

Chemotherapy is the same for infection with all species of *Brucella*.

The acute febrile case will respond to tetracycline 500 mg 4-hourly or

6-hourly (when tolerance of the drug is poor), given orally each day for 3 weeks. Some physicians give a daily dose of 1.0 g streptomycin intramuscularly over the same periods, but this technique is unpleasant for the patient and there is no good evidence that the combined treatment is more successful than the tetracycline alone. The drug may be given parenterally in very toxic, comatose or delirious patients or where diarrhoea and vomiting are severe. Oxytetracycline is usually preferred to tetracycline (which may discolour or damage the teeth) for treatment in young children in whom, in any case, the disease is usually mild and spontaneous cure frequent.

Trimethoprim-sulphamethoxole (Septrin) has recently been used with success in adult dosage of two tablets twice daily for 3 weeks. The relapse rate is about the same as in other treatments.

Vitamin B complex should be given orally during treatment.

Chemotherapy usually causes a fall of temperature to normal and abatement of signs and symptoms in a few days. Relapse, probably the result of survival of intracellular *Brucella* which escape the chemotherapeutic agents, is common in the first few months. The rate after a year is about 3 per cent.

Acute infections respond better than subacute or chronic.

Corticosteroids may be useful in controlling sensitivity reactions which occasionally appear in the first few days of treatment or in severely toxic states. Cortisone in a dose of 300 mg daily for 3 days is usually adequate.

Relapse requires a further full course of treatment.

In the acute case bed rest and good nursing are essential.

Where there is arthritis involving the spine or a large joint, the general chemotherapeutic treatment described above is needed. Some authors consider that in these circumstances the combination of tetracycline and streptomycin may produce the best results.

Orthopaedic treatment may be needed for spinal or joint lesions. The period of operation and convalescence should be covered by a 3-week course of chemotherapy, as above.

Orchitis usually needs only local supportive measures and relief of pain by analgesics. Surgical treatment is not needed; spontaneous cure occurs in a few weeks and relief is hastened by antibiotic therapy.

Chronic brucellosis is notoriously difficult to eradicate, especially with its overlay of often severe depression and neurosis. A course of tetracycline, as above, should be given and the effect on the agglutination titre and the AHG agglutination test should be watched. Deep-seated intracellular organisms may cause relapse even after apparently successful therapy. A further course of treatment is then needed. Desensitization by gradually increasing doses of *Brucella* antigens has been tried with some success. This must be done with great care, to avoid serious reactions.

### PREVENTION

Pasteurization destroys the organisms and thus milk and products such as cheese made from pasteurized milk are free from infection. Infected meat and meat products are similarly sterilized by heating.

Occupational risks can be reduced by protective clothing and spectacles and by strict personal hygiene. Contact with infected herds should be minimal. Infected animals are detected by serological tests and are usually slaughtered, at any rate in milk herds. In goats and sheep the infection can be controlled by a living attenuated vaccine which is usually given only to animals aged 3–6 months. Killed vaccines are also in use. Attenuated *Br. abortus* vaccine is commonly used in calves. This produces good immunity but has the disadvantage of producing high agglutinin titres which interfere with herd testing. A non-agglutinogenic vaccine made from a rough strain of *Br. abortus* is being tried as an alternative.

Vaccination in man has not been successful. Severe reactions have followed the use of attenuated *Br. abortus* vaccine.

# 6

# CHOLERA

## DEFINITION

Cholera is an acute, self-limited, often fatal, infectious disease of short duration caused by a specific organism, *Vibrio cholerae*, which multiplies in the gut contents but does not invade the blood-stream or tissues. It is characterized by copious watery diarrhoea, vomiting, muscle cramps, severe dehydration, vascular collapse and various complications, especially anuria with acute uraemia.

## GEOGRAPHICAL DISTRIBUTION

The historical endemic regions of classical cholera are in India, Pakistan and China, in areas of poverty and poor sanitation. In recent years the El Tor strain of cholera has appeared in many countries in the Western Pacific and South-east Asian areas, including Japan, Indonesia, Malaysia, Thailand, Kampuchea, the Philippines, Korea, Hong Kong, Burma, India, Bangladesh, Sri Lanka, and Pakistan. It has also occurred in Afghanistan, Iran, the Middle East, parts of Southern and Eastern Europe, and North-eastern, Eastern, Western and Central Subsaharan Africa. Cases have been imported into most Western European countries and Britain.

Traditionally, epidemic and pandemic extensions of cholera have occurred from time to time along established trade routes and other lines of communication. Modern air travel has added a significant factor to the potential distribution of this disease, since it is now possible for carriers and convalescents infected with the El Tor vibrio or persons in the incubation or 'contact-carrier' periods of classical cholera to be transported thousands of miles from the infective source to a susceptible area in a few hours. The infection has been carried to Australia and New Zealand in this way. Fortunately in well-sanititated areas it is easily controlled. Where the sanitary situation is poor it is not.

## AETIOLOGY

The causative organism *V. cholerae* belongs to a group of bacteria which are morphologically similar to but antigenically and biochemically distinct from other vibrios. The cholera vibrio is small, comma-shaped and motile, with a single terminal flagellum. It is Gram-negative and grows easily at $37^\circ$ C in ordinary bacteriological media. There are two biotypes, the classical cholera vibrio and the haemolytic El Tor vibrio. These are antigenically separated into Ogawa and Inaba and the much rarer Hikojima subtypes.

Until recently the classical vibrios were mainly responsible for the disease. Either Ogawa or Inaba subtypes predominated in outbreaks and epidemics and could be broadly differentiated by their H and O agglutinins. The present pandemic, which started in 1958 in Southeast Asia has, however, been largely due to infection with the El Tor vibrio which has invaded the classical cholera endemic areas, where in many instances it has replaced the classical strains, and has spread over most of the world except the Americas. The El Tor organism commonly causes a mild disease in the areas in which it is endemic, such as Sulawesi (where the current pandemic began) but, in the widespread outbreaks it has caused in recent years, the disease has presented in full severity and caused many deaths. For practical purposes, therefore, the El Tor organism is now regarded as identical with the other strains so far as clinical effects are concerned and cholera, as an internationally quarantinable disease, includes Cholera El Tor. In many of the areas in which there have been severe epidemics of El Tor cholera, the organism has become endemic after the subsidence of the outbreak. Cholera has thus become endemic in many countries which were formerly free of the infection, including some in sub-Saharan Africa.

The bacteriological separation of the cholera organisms is sometimes very difficult, thus considerably hampering epidemiological surveys. The antigenic patterns are unstable although *V. cholerae* and *V. cholerae El Tor* possess similar O (somatic) antigens, and the cultural biochemical and physical properties are erratic. The distinction of El Tor from the others on the grounds that it alone can cause *in vitro* haemolysis has been shown to be unreliable, since some strains of El Tor are not haemolytic. At present the organism is most surely separated from the others by haemagglutination tests and by its resistance to bacteriophage (Phage IV) and Polymixin B which destroy the other vibrios and by its abilty to agglutinate chick erythrocytes.

In nature the vibrios are pathogenic only to man. Other animals are not affected. A condition somewhat resembling cholera can, however, be induced by artificial gut infection of young guinea pigs and rabbits and by extracts of the organism or culture media in which it has been grown. The clinical picture has been reproduced in man by administration of such extracts.

In the human case the vibrio grows and multiplies almost entirely in the lumen of the gut. It does not penetrate beyond the submucosa of the intestinal wall and is never found in the blood-stream or in the urine. In the clinical attack it is present in enormous numbers in the faeces and vomitus.

The classical vibrio may be found in the faeces during the incubation period and in the faeces and vomitus during the attack and for about a week thereafter; the El Tor vibrio may persist for several weeks or even months. There are no true 'carriers' of classical cholera, although convalescents or persons who have been in contact with infective material may excrete organisms for up to a week without clinical effects ('contact carriers'). Unfortunately, true carriers of the El Tor vibrio do exist, in whom excretion persists for months or years.

It appears, therefore, that the maintenance of endemicity of cholera must depend on the direct spread of infection from case to case, the mode of transmission being mainly through faeces. Individuals may become infected without showing any clinical evidence of the disease. It is thus not necessary to have overt cases for transmission to occur.

The organism can survive on moist clothing for up to 3 days. It dies rapidly in pure water but survives for days (maximum of 6 weeks) in slightly dirty water containing salts and organic matter. It is easily killed by moderate heat (55° C for half an hour) and acid. The El Tor organism survives longer in water and liquid foodstuffs than do the classical vibrios.

Cholera is primarily a disease of low socio-economic groups living in insanitary conditions and with poor health services, bad water supplies and inadequate or absent sewage disposal.

In such communities the infection spreads most commonly through infected water (including ice and cold drinks) contaminated with faeces. Other potable fluids including milk, cold cooked foods, vegetables sprinkled with water, and uncooked fruits may also be concerned with the spread of infection.

Spread may occur from case to case through direct contact with faeces or vomitus. It may spread from one area of a country to another across borders or along rivers and coastal areas in fishing vessels (as in West Africa).

Transmission is sometimes suspected to occur through the domestic fly.

In endemic areas most cases occur in the hot moist season, possibly because of the mechanical flushing of local filthy water supplies. Thus, the incidence is highest in Bengal in the early rains (May, June and July) and lowest in the dry weather.

Epidemics and outbreaks arise from the introduction of the vibrio by infected individuals. Once the disease is introduced it spreads by the same means as in the endemic area.

In non-endemic areas prevention of the import of the disease is a matter of sanitary control and quarantine of ships and aircraft from infected areas, and the isolation of suspected cases. Where cholera has appeared local water and food supplies must be examined and protected from pollution. Chlorination will rapidly destroy the vibrio in water. Individual drinking and washing supplies should be boiled or chlorinated before use and the strictest attention must be paid to the preparation, purveyance and consumption of food.

Anti-fly precautions should be enforced.

*Resistance to infection.* In a group of individuals exposed to the same source of infection by no means all may become infected. Of those infected some will show the fully developed syndrome, others may have no clinical ill-effects. It is believed that certain individuals may thus present some natural resistance to infection. The acidity of the gastric juice may act as a barrier to infection of the gut, the vibrios being highly susceptible to an acid environment; reduction in gastric acidity may predispose to infection.

Newcomers to the endemic area are believed to be more likely to become infected, but this is not certain. There is little evidence of herd immunity in the sense that it exists in malaria; the local population of an endemic area may be highly susceptible during outbreaks.

The cholera outbreak in a community is self-limited. It tends to die out after reaching its peak. This may be in some measure due to the large number of subclinical cases which develop or to the acquisition of temporary individual immunity. It has been demonstrated, however, that one attack does not protect against subsequent infection, except partially for a very limited period.

In epidemics a smaller proportion of the local population may be infected than might be anticipated. Napier, for instance, pointed out the striking difference between the infection rate of cholera (about one in three) and of smallpox, in an exposed community in which there is free intercommunication.

Antibodies, including agglutinins, and some measure of protection against infection are produced in animals by the inoculation of killed vibrio cultures intramuscularly or subcutaneously.

*Vaccination*

Individual or mass protection by the use of vaccines of dead vibrios, preferably local strains, should be carried out if possible. Individual injection is given in two doses (first dose 0.5 ml and second dose 1.0 ml) a week apart. When vaccination is used for mass protection, for example during an epidemic, a single dose of 1.0 ml is employed.*

Modern vaccines do not usually produce a febrile reaction. The single injection acts as a booster. Visitors to endemic areas should have the double vaccination. Natives in endemic areas usually need only a single injection. The vaccines will reduce overt disease in an individual in about half the vaccinated persons. It is not known whether these individuals nevertheless become infected. Cholera has been reported in individuals who have been repeatedly vaccinated. The partial protection lasts only about 3 months (the international certificate of vaccination is valid for 6 months). Vaccines made from the classical vibrios are effective for a few months against El Tor infection and *vice versa*. The El Tor vaccine protects against the specific infection for about 6 months.

Race, sex and age appear to play little part in the incidence of the disease. Malnutrition and poor health probably predispose to infection, but otherwise healthy subjects are often readily infected.

* Vaccine is standardized to contain 8000 million organisms per 1.0 ml.

PATHOLOGY

*Pathogenesis*

In cholera the organisms remain in the gut and do not invade the bloodstream. In the gut the vibrios multiply rapidly and cause the loss of enormous quantities of water and salt from the tissues through the intestinal epithelium into the lumen and so outside the body. This is the basic physiological lesion. Certain local effects on the gut wall may be produced. There may be some shredding of the epithelium and in the later stages some bleeding into the lumen. Biopsies indicate, however, that the intestinal wall remains essentially intact during the acute attack. There is no excessive loss of protein with the stool.

The mode of action of the infection is not completely understood. It has been shown, however, that poisonous substances or enterotoxins are formed *in vitro* during the growth and lysis of the vibrio, and it is likely that these are involved. The enterotoxin, also called 'choleragen', and now regarded by most authorities as an 'exotoxin' liberated by the vibrios growing on the intact intestinal mucosa, has been shown in animals to affect the permeability of the gut wall to water and electrolytes. Its effect can be neutralized to some extent by antibodies derived from injection of killed cultures of cholera vibrios. The syndrome of cholera arises from selective interference with the physiological properties of the intestinal wall (most pronounced in the duodenum and jejunum), leading to greatly increased flow of water and electrolytes into the lumen, with relatively little reduction in resorption—as indicated by the success of oral replacement therapy. The electrolyte loss is thought to occur mainly via the mucosal crypt cells.

The loss of fluid and electrolytes is rapid and severe. The concentration of sodium chloride in the cholera stool is about the same as that of plasma. Hence the evacuation of large volumes of stool produces severe loss of extracellular fluid and fall in circulating plasma volume. Cellular potassium is also lost; the concentration of the ion in the stool may be five times that in the plasma. The concentration of bicarbonate in the stool also exceeds, sometimes considerably, that in the plasma, consequentially some degree of acidosis develops and may be exacerbated in cases in which vomiting is severe.

The serious dehydration itself affects the circulating plasma volume, which is often further reduced by the appearance of vascular collapse. Haemoconcentration is pronounced in severe cases; there is an equivalent increase in haemoglobin concentration. The viscosity of the blood increases considerably and the efficiency of the circulation is correspondingly diminished.

The information regarding the morbid anatomy of cholera is surprisingly incomplete. The tissue changes are basically non-specific, and the lesions in the internal organs appear to be those which arise from the prevailing dehydration and/or vascular collapse.

Rigor mortis develops rapidly. The muscles are deep red and dehydrated; violent post-mortem contractions may occur. The tissues are dry. The blood is viscid. There may be scattered petechial haemorrhages in the mucous membrane of the intestine and in the pericardium.

Changes in the organs are commoner in cases which have survived to the late stages before death. The anuric and uraemic case may present kidney lesions similar to those often met in other examples of the renal anoxia syndrome. There may be irregular ischaemia of the cortex involving the glomeruli in a patchy manner, some medullary congestion and epithelial degeneration and desquamation, particularly in the cortical tubules, which, together with the collecting tubules, may contain casts of albuminous material and epithelial debris. On the other hand, there may be little evidence of structural change in the kidneys of the anuric case, especially if death has occurred soon after the renal failure. The liver may be congested and show some degenerative lesions, mainly centrilobular. The gall bladder and bile ducts are filled with dark viscid inspissated bile.

Pulmonary oedema may be present in cases with severe uncorrected acidosis, or shock.

*Clinical pathology*

*Stools.* In the fully developed case the stools are watery, of very low specific gravity and contain vibrios and shreds of mucus. The total sodium chloride loss may be as great as 30 g. The stool is invariably alkaline with high potassium and bicarbonate content. Otherwise, it is roughly isotonic.

*Blood cells.* The dehydration and loss of plasma volume cause rapid haemoconcentration. In severe cases the blood is viscid and the erythrocyte count may become as high as 8 million cells per mm$^3$. The white cell count is correspondingly increased.

*Blood.* The viscosity and specific gravity is increased roughly in proportion to the loss of plasma volume. The specific gravity of normal blood is about 1.054. In severe cases at the height of 'fluid loss' it may be 1.060 or even more.

The chemical constituents of the blood depend primarily upon the state of hydration and the successful function or otherwise of the kidneys.

In the severe case the total chloride concentration may be normal or slightly lowered; the sodium is higher in proportion; the potassium is usually unchanged but rises in cases with acute renal failure and sometimes in hypovolaemic shock. Figures for such concentrations are not, however, a reliable guide to total losses or to the replacement required. For example, there is pronounced loss of total chloride per kg of body weight, even when the chloride content of the blood is little changed.

The blood urea nitrogen concentration is raised above the normal range in most cases. In the anuric case it rises steadily to reach very high figures. In recovery from anuria it falls rapidly.

Plasma protein concentration is raised considerably in the severely dehydrated case.

*Urine*. The output is low in all cases. Anuria may develop in some. The specific gravity may be high and the urine deeply pigmented. Nevertheless, the urea and electrolyte content is low and there may be no chloride or sodium. Albumin and casts are present in the acute attack. After recovery the electrolytes return rapidly but owing to the slow recovery of the renal epithelium it may be some time before the concentration of urine is re-established.

CLINICAL PICTURE

Cholera may be mild or severe. It is of short duration, seldom lasting more than 5 days. Infection may be so severe that death results before the classical watery diarrhoea becomes established. On the other hand, infection may be present without clinical signs. The majority of the clinically overt cases are severe. In epidemics the early and late cases are often less severe than those at the height of the outbreak. Occasionally in children there may develop paralytic ileus, with retention of fluid in the intestinal lumen; the syndrome may then develop without the severe diarrhoea (so-called *cholera sicca*).

Infection with the El Tor vibrio may produce a relatively mild form of the disease, which tends to recur in certain geographical areas. It more frequently initiates the full classical picture of severe cholera.

*Incubation period*
The incubation period varies from a few hours to 5 days. Commonly it is about 3 days. There are no prodromal symptoms.

*The classical attack*
The stage of *evacuation* commences with diarrhoea which may at first be mild, but which soon empties the bowel of faeces and changes to the urgent watery diarrhoea of the classical condition. The patient now passes frequent watery stools which amount to little more than large quantities of clear or slightly opalescent fishy-smelling liquid containing practically no faeces. Against a dark background little flecks of mucus can often be seen floating about. This appearance has led to the descriptive name of 'rice water stools'. The stools swarm with vibrios. In the late stages there may be a little blood. The total loss of fluid as stools may be 15–20 litres in 24 hours.

Bowel motions are frequent, effortless, and uncontrolled. Napier refers to them as the painless passage of pints of pale fluid. The stool comes out in spurts, sometimes with considerable force. The general appearance is that of turning a faucet on and off. There is commonly no pain and no colic and the patient is often scarcely aware that he is evacuating his bowel. Contamination of bed clothing is therefore frequent.

Vomiting begins as a rule after the diarrhoea has become established but may precede it. There is no nausea. The patient has little or no control over the vomitus which gushes out with considerable force and volume. The watery vomit is essentially similar in appearance and content to the stool and like the latter contains enormous numbers of vibrios and is highly infective. It constitutes a real danger to the unwary physician.

Evacuation continues for a variable time, but seldom for more than 3 or 4 days. The frequent bowel evacuation and vomiting lead rapidly to tremendous loss of fluid and electrolytes. Within a matter of hours the severely ill patient becomes dehydrated. The whole body seems to shrink; subcutaneous fluid is lost and the pale clammy skin becomes inelastic and stretched over the underlying tissues. The eyes are sunken, the cheeks hollow, the skin tight over the malar prominences. The mouth and tongue are dry; there is extreme thirst; the voice is husky. The patient becomes anxious, foreboding and restless but remains mentally clear. As the dehydration continues, the circulation becomes inefficient. The blood pressures fall, the pulse quickens and may be impalpable at the wrist. The picture now becomes essentially one of dehydration and vascular collapse and closely resembles similar conditions such as severe heat exhaustion in which medical shock has developed. When acidosis is present the patient shows signs of air hunger with deep and sometimes rapid breathing; there is normally some mental confusion and disorientation.

Muscle cramps are common once dehydration has become established. They are severe and painful, frequent, of short duration, and arise particularly in the legs. The abdominal muscles are affected only in the later stages. Tetanic spasms may occur.

The rectal temperature may be raised a little above normal. Skin and oral temperatures are often subnormal.

From the start of the syndrome the urine volume is reduced; as the dehydration proceeds, the urinary output diminishes. Even in relatively mild cases there is oliguria. In severe cases there may be complete anuria which may be only temporary or may pass on to irreversible acute renal failure and uraemia. The deeply pigmented urine has a low electrolyte concentration. It contains albumin and granular tubular casts and may have high specific gravity.

By the time dehydration is manifest the plasma volume is considerably reduced from this alone. When vascular collapse supervenes there is a further reduction. The result is a progressive concentration of the cellular elements of the blood. The specific gravity of the blood is increased with corresponding rise in viscosity.

Death is common at this point from the combined effects of dehydration and shock.

The fate of the patient is determined by the degree and duration of dehydration, evacuation and collapse. With successful replacement therapy, in most cases rehydration is rapid and the patient quickly recovers. The shrivelled shrunken corpse-like appearance disappears in a matter of hours as the tissue fluid is restored. Evacuation and vomiting, if not already stopped in the collapse stage, now cease. The blood pressures and the circulation return to normal.

There may be a moderate but transient febrile period during the recovery stages.

If the collapsed stage has been prolonged or very severe, there may be no circulatory recovery or a temporary reaction stage may be followed by serious and sometimes irreversible changes in vital organ function and the threat to life again becomes urgent.

This is particularly so in cases in which anuria has developed. If the anuria has been of very short duration, reaction may be immediately followed by recovery of urinary flow and renal function. On the other hand, in some cases, especially those in which the anuria has been prolonged, renal failure may persist into acute uraemia. Such cases usually die within a few days. Even in their late stages, however, recovery may occur, as it does in other examples of the renal anoxia syndrome. Occasionally, the anuria of the collapse may be followed by a short period of oliguria in which small volumes of urine containing albumin and casts may be passed; anuria then reappears and the patient dies in uraemia.

In some cases, after brief improvement, the peripheral circulation may fail again and the patient dies of shock. It must be noted that, in many fatal cases the algid stage persists to death and there is no recovery stage.

The whole progress of the cholera case is only a matter of a few days at the most. Recovery is usually rapid; with correct treatment it is often remarkable. Cholera in children follows the same pattern, but there are often additional signs, including fever, very rapid breathing, stupor, and convulsions; cardiac arrhythmias are sometimes pronounced. The mortality is high unless treatment is given early.

*Course and prognosis*
In milder cases there may be an interval of recovery after the collapse stage, followed in turn by the complications of the reaction stage, especially renal or circulatory failure, or both. The very severe case may perish in a few hours. This is especially so in children.

Prognosis depends considerably on the length of time elapsing from onset of the signs to commencement of treatment. The longer the dehydrated patient is left untreated, the worse the prognosis. If dehydration is very severe and shock develops, the outlook is bad. Prognosis is bad if anuria has already developed and persisted for some hours before treatment.

The recovery rate is high with efficient treatment, except in advanced and shocked patients.

Complications of cholera, other than renal failure and shock, are rare. Pneumonia is sometimes described, especially in outbreaks in cold climates, and gangrene of the extremities has been reported in a few neglected cases. There are no sequelae in the recovered case. Once the tissue water–salt balance and the plasma volume have been adjusted, return to normal is very fast, usually a matter of a few days.

The death rate in untreated cases in local outbreaks or in epidemics is very high, often over 50 per cent. The mortality rate is usually higher in children and the aged. Even under epidemic conditions, however, the death rate of patients treated in hospital or by mobile teams is usually not greater than about 5 per cent.

In any outbreak there are many mild cases which recover spontaneously or respond remarkably quickly to treatment and there are probably many more cases without symptoms.

Cholera is more serious in pregnant than in non-pregnant women; dehydration and diarrhoea are more severe. Abortion is common in the third trimester; the foetus usually dies within the first 24 hours of the overt attack.

## DIAGNOSIS

In an outbreak the clinical diagnosis of the individual case is easy. Doubtful cases must be treated as cholera. Any condition leading to acute dehydration with watery diarrhoea and vomitng may be mistaken for cholera. Choleraic and algid falciparum malaria, acute food or chemical poisoning, and heat exhaustion are examples of related clinical pictures.

The diagnosis of an isolated case may be difficult. The presence of vibrios must be confirmed in wet or stained stool preparations. Further identification of the organism is essential. The vibrio can often be isolated by inoculation of specimens of faeces or material from a rectal swab into alkaline peptone water and incubation at $37^\circ$ C for 6 8 hours. The ordinary faecal organisms are partly inhibited by the alkalinity and the vibrio becomes concentrated at the surface of the medium. Further bacteriological identification is then simplified. There are no reliable serological diagnostic tests but vibriocidal, agglutinating and phage neutralizing antibodies may appear in the blood after infection. In the absence of vaccination, limited numbers of cases can be followed up, but this is better done by rectal swabbing and bacterological techniques, with or without previous purging with magnesium sulphate. Organisms may sometimes be obtained by duodenal intubation.

In epidemiological surveys, evidence of infection may be provided by demonstration of individual vibriocidal antibodies. In some parts of Southeast Asia the titres of these antibodies show considerable yearly fluctuations, which are regarded as stimulation of the immune responses by other infections. Antibodies appearing in previously negative persons are considered to indicate persistence of the infection in the area, but bacteriological proof of this is not always obtained.

## TREATMENT

The treatment is essentially a matter of non-specific measures for rehydraton, restoration of the electrolyte balance and correction of acidosis and the maintenance of the corrected fluid and salt balance. Tetracycline is valuable therapeutically and from the public health aspect. It lessens the volume and duration of evacuation and reduces the period of excretion of the vibrio.

Electrolyte balance is restored and rehydration accomplished by intravenous infusion of saline fluids. Acidosis is corrected by the use of infusion fluids containing sodium bicarbonate or lactate. Other measures include the control of oligaemic shock and uraemic anuria.

### TECHNIQUE OF TREATMENT

*Replacement of water and electrolytes: control of acidosis*
The object is to replace the initial loss of fluid and electrolytes as quickly as possible and then to maintain physiological levels and replace any further loss until the evacuation ceases.

*Initial rehydration*
The fluids and electrolytes are usually replaced by intravenous infusion. In very collapsed patients it may be necessary to give the first litre via the external jugular vein and then transfer the needle to a vein in the arm or leg. Oral replacement is now being more widely attempted, even in severe cases (see below).

The replacement volume of infusion needed in a given patient will depend on the initial dehydration. This may be calculated in several ways.

The effects of rehydration can best be judged by clinical observation of the patient, who will transform from a withered shrunken creature to something resembling a human in a matter of a few hours. The skin will lose its tension and regain its elasticity, the blood pressures will rise and the pulse volume improve; frequent check on the quality of the radial pulse will indicate this. The rapid deep breathing (air hunger) will give place to normal respiration and the patient will become less confused as the acidosis is corrected. The lungs must be regularly examined for evidence of pulmonary oedema which can originate from the acidosis or develop during intravenous therapy if the volume given is excessive.

The volume of every specimen of urine passed should be measured. As rehydration develops, the output will increase and the sodium chloride content, which may initially be low, will return to normal. Persistence of very low output may indicate oncoming renal failure.

Where facilities are available, an assessment of the volume of replacement fluid required can be made by serial measurement of the whole blood or plasma specific gravity.

A common calculation is that for every 0.001 rise of the specific gravity of plasma above 1.025, the patient will need an initial amount in ml equivalent to the weight in kg multiplied by 4.

Subsequent infusion will depend on whether the evacuation continues or comes under control.

A rough approximation of the volume needed in the average severe case is to calculate the volume in litres as the equivalent of one-tenth of the body weight in kg. Thus a person weighing 50 kg on admission will need about 5 litres of infusion fluid for initial rehydration.

The first litre of fluid (20–30 ml per kg body weight in children) should be given in 10 minutes. The common practice is to use physiological saline containing lactate, bicarbonate, or acetate to counteract the acidosis.

In children, the initial dose (usually 30 ml per kg body weight Ringer lactate solution) is injected into a peripheral or a scalp vein with a small needle; a further 30 ml per kg body weight is given over the next 3 hours. Thereafter, maintenance replacement of the same solution is given by slow drip. Glucose (5 per cent in water) is offered orally as early as possible.

In the adult, the infusion fluid commonly consists of two volumes of isotonic sodium chloride (0.9 per cent) plus one volume isotonic lactate (1.75 per cent). Sodium bicarbonate (1.4 per cent) may be substituted for the lactate which is expensive and easily grows mouldy when stored. The bicarbonate has to be added to the saline in the form of sterile powder; *it must not be boiled.*

Some workers now use sodium acetate (2.1 per cent of the trihydrated salt).

Potassium loss must be replaced as soon as possible but not until after the first litre of saline has been given. An ECG should be taken where possible to make sure that hyperkalaemia is not present.

A commonly used general-purpose intravenous fluid is 5 g sodium chloride, 4 g sodium bicarbonate, 1 g potassium chloride, all dissolved in 1 litre of sterile water. The mixture must *not* be sterilized by boiling.

After the first litre of saline (plus lactate or bicarbonate or acetate) has been given, 1.0 g of potassium chloride should be added to the fluid (equivalent to 13 mEq per litre), (if the above solution has not been used).

The infusion is continued until up to a total of 5 litres has been given in an adult. The volume needed for children is 20–30 ml per kg for each litre given to the adult.

Saline without added potassium can be given at the rate of 1 litre in 2 hours. If potassium is included, the rate of administration should be slowed to 250 ml per hour.

*Maintenance hydration*
Where there is good clinical evidence of initial rehydration, the evacuation may stop. If it continues, further infusion may be needed if the diarrhoea is not controlled.

Infusion is then given on the basis of an equivalent of the amount of fluid lost in the stools, the volume of which should be measured every 2 hours. There may be as much as 20 litres lost in 24 hours.

In most cases, the diarrhoea slows or stops after initial rehydration and fluid administration can continue by mouth or nasogastric tube. Physiological saline diluted 1:4 with water is acceptable particularly if glucose up to 2 per cent is added. Various formulae are used for oral fluids, containing sodium chloride, sodium bicarbonate, potassium citrate and glucose. In mild or moderate diarrhoea it is usually possible to correct the dehydration and maintain hydration by giving the saline solution orally from the beginning. This inexpensive method is especially useful in rural areas where hospital facilities may not be readily available. The oral fluid recommended by WHO is: sodium chloride 3.5 g; sodium bicarbonate 2.5 g; potassium chloride 1.5 g and glucose 20.0 g, made up in 1 litre of water. Potassium citrate 1.0 g may be preferred to the chloride as it makes the fluid more acceptable to the patient.

The patient is given frequent sips and encouraged to drink for himself.

Not more than 10 mg potassium chloride should be given in 24 hours.

Oral replacement should be tried early, or from the beginning. It can often be successful in severe cases which would formerly have received parenteral replacement. The oral method has obvious advantages in the field in an epidemic.

## MANAGEMENT

Renal failure requires the routine treatment described on pages 280–281.

Moderate hypotension is usually corrected by the saline infusion. Shocked patients are treated on standard lines and with corticosteroids if considered necessary (see p. 280).

L-noradrenaline infusion has been used successfully in combating shock. Coma, which may occur especially in children, can be countered by adding 5–10 per cent glucose to the infusion.

Vomiting usually ceases with the correction of acidosis. Intractable vomiting is rare after initial rehydration. Anti-emetic drugs should be used only as a last resort.

The intense pain of muscular cramps may be difficult to control. The cramps usually subside as the patient becomes rehydrated and the evacuation and vomiting stop. Severe pain may be relieved by analgesics. Morphine is contra-indicated.

Tetany is relieved by intravenous administration of calcium gluconate.

*Chemotherapy*

Tetracycline, given orally in doses of 250 mg 6-hourly for 48 hours (adults and children) is effective in shortening the duration of the diarrhoea. It also renders the stools free from vibrios, as a rule within 24 hours. It is usually started about 3 hours after replacement treatment has commenced, when vomiting has normally stopped. It is not successful as a prophylactic.

Chloramphenicol has the same effect but tetracycline is the drug of choice.

*Progress*

Infusion of saline will usually bring about immense relief in all symptoms including muscle cramps, which may be very violent.

The diarrhoea is usually controlled within 48 hours. If it continues after this period the antibiotic is continued until the diarrhoea stops.

In the active stage the patient is unable to take more than sips of water or glucose solution by mouth. As he improves he may be given glucose drinks, sugared barley, arrowroot, or rice water and buttermilk. He is gradually brought back to a diet of soft rice, potato, fish, etc.

Careful nursing is essential. In the convalescent stage the patient must be kept quiet to avoid the recurrence of vascular collapse.

### CONTROL

Vaccination for prophylaxis is discussed above (p. 53).

Vaccination does not reduce the number of people in a population in an endemic area who excrete the El Tor vibrio.

In an outbreak, contacts and local populations are usually vaccinated, using the single dose technique.

Mobile teams equipped for immediate rehydration therapy have been organized in most endemic areas and in times of epidemics. In addition to the life-saving early rehydration of patients such teams are useful for dealing with contacts, arranging disinfection, control of faeces and water supplies, and for carrying out vaccinations. They have proved immensely successful in recent El Tor epidemics, and are also valuable in helping the early detection of infection.

# 7

# FILARIASES

## FILARIASIS (BANCROFTIAN AND MALAYAN)

### DEFINITION

Infection with parasitic nematodes *Wucheria bancrofti* and *Brugia malayi*, the adults of which inhabit the lymphatic tissues. The clinical effects range from none to elephantiasis.

### GEOGRAPHICAL DISTRIBUTION

Bancroftian filariasis is widely spread in the tropics and subtropics. It occurs in the Caribbean Islands; South America as far south as the Argentine; southern Spain; the African Mediterranean seaboard, West, Central and East Africa; Malagasy Republic; the Middle East, India, Burma, southern China, South Korea; Japan; and South and West Thailand, Malaysia, Indonesia, Papua New Guinea, many Pacific Islands, including Samoa and Fiji. It existed until recently in the southern United States and northern Australia.

Malayan filariasis is more restricted. In some areas it occurs alone, in others it overlaps with bancroftian. It is found in large areas of Malaysia, Thailand, Indonesia, and Papua New Guinea, and in pockets in India, Vietnam, Sri Lanka, and southern China.

### AETIOLOGY

*The causal organisms in the human host*
The development in the human host is practically identical. The adults are fine filiform worms, the females reaching 10 cm in length. The worms may be found coiled together in the larger lymphatics near the aorta, in the pelvis and genitalia and in the lymphatic glands. Mating occurs in these areas. The females are viviparous and embryos are passed in large numbers into the lymphatics. The embryos or microfilariae are sheathed. They ultimately escape from the lymphatics and appear in the peripheral blood.

It probably takes 3–6 months or longer for the larval forms injected by the vector to reach full maturity. It is not known how long the individual adult may survive in the host but it is obviously a matter of years.

The anatomical features of the microfilariae of *W. bancrofti* and *B. malayi* differ in some respects. The differentiation of the one from the other is referred to later (see p. 79).

*Periodicity*
In most endemic areas the microfilariae of *W. bancrofti* appear in greatest numbers in the peripheral blood during the night somewhere between 22.00 and 02.00 hours and may be very scarce during the day, when they probably concentrate in the pulmonary vessels. This nocturnal periodicity has never been satisfactorily explained. It is commoner in regions where the vector is a night feeder. Non-periodic varieties are found in some endemic regions, especially in the Pacific Islands. A sub-periodic strain has recently been identified in western Thailand extending across the Burmese border.

Microfilariae of *B. malayi* exhibit either nocturnal periodicity similar to that of *W. bancrofti* (periodic) or diurnal periodicity with a peak in the early evenings (sub-periodic). In West Malaysia the type of microfilariae predominating in a given region depends largely on the available vectors.

*Transmission*
Bancroftian filariasis is transmitted by the bite of several genera and species of mosquitoes. The most widely distributed vectors are species of *Culex, Aedes* and *Anopheles.*

Malayan filariasis. The periodic form is transmitted by certain species of *Mansonia* breeding in water containing suitable plants, including the water lettuce *Pistia* and certain grasses, and species of *Anopheles* breeding in pools and ditches. It is found in cleared areas such as rice fields suitable for the breeding of these vectors. It infects animals only with difficulty so that man may be regarded as the only significant reservoir. The sub-periodic parasite is transmitted by species of *Mansonia* which breed in forest swamps. Since it is easily transmitted to wild animals, including monkeys, and to domestic cats and dogs, these animals may constitute important reservoirs of infection.

The problems of control thus differ considerably in the two forms of infection.

*The causal organism in the vector*
The insect becomes infected by ingesting human blood containing infective microfilariae. After ingestion the microfilaria escapes from the sheath, penetrates the gut wall of the insect and passes to the thoracic muscles where it undergoes a series of moults. After 2 weeks or more the infective larvae reach the proboscis, the larvae are deposited on the human skin when the insect bites and enter the puncture wound, reaching the subcutaneous lymphatics.

*Epidemiology*
Transmission of bancroftian filariasis in a given area depends on the presence of suitable vectors in large enough numbers and on an adequate human

reservoir of infective microfilariae. The suitability of the human reservoir depends to some extent on the stage of clinical development. Infective microfilariae are found in the blood in large numbers in most cases during the inflammatory and early obstructive stages. In advanced cases of elephantiasis circulating microfilariae are rarely present and the patients are non-infective.

In many regions the main sources of infection are asymptomatic cases in which large numbers of microfilariae may be present in the blood.

The infection of the vector depends to some extent on its habits. Night feeders are likely to be more effective in transmitting filariasis in which there is pronounced nocturnal periodicity. Day feeders are more likely to be concerned with the transmission of non-periodic strains.

Transmission of periodic malayan filariasis depends also on an adequate supply of vectors and human reservoirs. In the sub-periodic forms of the parasite animal reservoirs may also be important.

Continued reinfection over a long period is apparently necessary for the development of the full clinical condition, which occurs much more frequently in natives of endemic areas than in vistors.

There is, however, no racial immunity. Some acquired resistance is thought to be developed and may be responsible for certain manifestations of the disease.

The sexes acquire the disease equally when the risks of infection are equal. The preponderance of infection in one sex often results from increased opportunity of infection, usually arising from occupation.

Clinical filariasis is uncommon in very young children, probably because of the time required by the worms to reach maturity in the host. Microfilariae are seldom found in the blood in children before the age of 3 or 4 years. Very rarely, clinical signs have been observed in children at the end of the first year of life. The later stages of the disease commonly develop in youth or early adult life.

## PATHOLOGY

Pathological changes in the tissues are induced chiefly by the adult worms, living and dead, directly by their presence, or indirectly by the production of some soluble toxic factor. The role of the microfilariae circulating in the blood stream has not been fully ascertained; they play some part in local sensitivity reactions but it is not clear whether they may be concerned directly in the obstructive phases.

Secondary infection may be important in the production of lesions, especially after the death and necrosis of the worm and in the later stages of elephantiasis.

Certain manifestations of the infection, such as the fleeting tissue oedemas and erythemas, arise as sensitivity reactions resulting from the temporary presence of adults and possibly of microfilariae. These immunosensitivity reactions also play some part in the cellular responses involved in the acute lymphangitis and adenitis and in some of the general reactions, including fever, skin rashes, and eosinophilia.

Early inflammatory changes occur in the lymphatic vessels and glands. Obstruction to local lymph flow may result, causing distension of lymph vessels, tissue oedema, and retention of fluid in serous cavities. The final stage is elephantiasis involving the skin and subcutaneous tissues and resulting from chronic obstruction of lymph drainage.

### Inflammatory and early obstructive stages

Changes occur principally in the lymphatic vessels and glands and in the connective tissue. The most marked reactions occur about adult worms lying in lymphatics, especially when the worm has died and started to degenerate. Local reactions may appear, however, in the absence of worms.

The characteristic lesion is a granulomatous lymphangitis, usually slowly progressive but subject to acute exacerbations. It develops in the tissue immediately associated with a lymphatic vessel or a series of vessels in which there may be adult worms and sometimes microfilariae. The tissue becomes infiltrated with lymphocytes, plasma cells, and eosinophils, which may be present in large numbers during the acute stage. When the adult worms are dead reticulo-endothelial cells become mobilized, with the formation of epithelioid nests and giant cells. The local blood vessels are dilated and usually show some cuffing with round cells. Nodules of cellular granulation tissue are formed in this way which press in upon the lumen of the lymphatic vessel and tend to occlude it. The endothelium of the vessels may become hypertrophic, leading to endovascular occlusion or lymph thrombosis. Sometimes the process goes on to necrosis and pus formation. Abscesses may discharge to the surface and lead to the development of persistent sinuses. Finally, the granulomatous tissue and occluded vessels are replaced by fibrous tissue.

Where the lesions develop around superficial lymphatics there is commonly some hard oedema and erythema of the overlying skin.

The affected vessels show clinical signs of obstruction, becoming dilated, distorted, and tense with lymph. The irregular development of granulomatous tissue gives rise to a lobulated mass.

In some regions the dilated vessels may rupture into the surrounding tissues and nearby hollow viscera.

The lesions which develop in the lymph glands are essentially the same as those about the lymphatics. The sinuses may contain adult worms and in the vicinity of these granulomatous tissue develops, with epithelioid cells and giant cells, surrounded by lymphocytes and plasma cells. Eosinophils may be present in large numbers in the periphery of the inflamed area; they are said to be most numerous when the worm is dead. As in the lymphatics, the lesion may proceed to fibrosis or to abscess and sinus formation. Obstruction to local lymph flow results and may lead eventually to elephantiasis.

The obstruction of the flow of lymph from the drainage area brought about by these changes in lymph vessels and glands leads to the development of oedema which is at first soft but eventually becomes firm. The tissues involved may gradually undergo elephantoid changes.

*Elephantiasis*
There is a gradual increase in thickness of all the tissues. The epithelium thickens irregularly in all layers; in some areas the hypertrophy exceeds that in others and warty excrescences develop. The connective and fatty tissues thicken and change into an oedematous myxomatous mass irregularly infiltrated with lymphocytes and eosinophils. The subcutaneous lymphatics and spaces increase in number. They become distended and lobulated and may rupture on to the surface, as in lymph scrotum. In the limbs the muscles at first hypertrophy but later atrophy.

The thickened tissue comes to hang in folds. Elephantoid areas of the skin of the trunk often hang forward on pedicles of normal skin. In the folds of the elephantoid skin secondary infection may invade the deeper tissues and lead to acute inflammation and necrosis and eventually fibrosis. It is difficult to assess the importance of secondary infection in building up the final condition.

In the early stages of elephantiasis there may be acute lymphatic inflammatory episodes similar to those described above. Biopsy may reveal the presence of adult worms and sometimes microfilariae in the lymphatics or glands; X-ray may disclose the presence of calcified worms.

The local lymph glands are nearly always affected.

### CLINICAL PICTURE

*Incubation period*
In natives of endemic regions who are open to repeated reinfection it is not possible to estimate the incubation period, defined as the period between infection and the first clinical signs with or without microfilariae in the blood. Study of individual European cases and cases in troops stationed for short periods in endemic areas in the Pacific during the Second World War has indicated that the period is probably of the order of 8–12 months because of the slow maturation of the worms. Repeated infection appears to be necessary for the development of the full clinical picture.

The clinical features of the early stages of filariasis may be separated to some extent into those which are inflammatory and those which are obstructive. It should be realized, however, that such division is artificial and that all stages may overlap considerably. Many cases of advanced filariasis may give no history of early involvement of the lymphatic system and, on the other hand, obvious infection with blood invasion by microfilariae may exist without any contemporaneous or subsequent development of clinical signs or symptoms.

*The onset*

The condition first appears most commonly in young adults after frequent exposure to reinfection. The onset is usually slow and insidious. Search into the patient's history will, however, often reveal one or more febrile or inflammatory episodes.

*Filarioid or elephantoid fever*

The initial febrile illness is referred to as elephantoid fever. It may start with rigor and a high temperature of the order of 40° C or more. The fever tends to fall after the first day or two and may subside in a few days to a week. There may be only mild fever. There is usually vigorous sweating. For some days before the onset and during the fever the patient suffers from malaise and anorexia. Nausea and vomiting are common during the attack; a feeling of depression often persists after the fever has subsided.

After a variable but short time the fever subsides and the patient may completely recover, only to develop further brief febrile attacks, followed by remissions until the acute inflammatory local reactions appear.

*Inflammatory reactions*

These local reactions are expressions of inflammatory changes in the lymphatic vessels and glands and are very varied in their distribution and intensity. They consist essentially of lymphangitis, lymphadenitis, and abscess formation. They tend to recur in the areas in which they first appeared and to develop into obstructive lesions. The advanced case usually gives a history of a series of local reactions in the parts of the body affected by elephantiasis, but this is not always so.

*Lymphangitis.* Acute involvement of lymphatic vessels is common, especially in the extremities, most freqeuntly the legs. The inflammation is usually accompanied by high fever, sometimes with rigors, and severe toxaemia.

The affected vessels are acutely tender, easily palpable and the overlying skin is usually turgid and erythematous, so that the inflamed vessels are etched on the skin as bright red streaks.

The condition is sometimes accompanied by very itchy, irregular, fleeting, hard erythematous swellings of the skin scattered over the body; these may appear in the absence of local lymphangitis.

The lymphangitis tends to be centrifugal in its distribution. For instance, it commonly starts in the lymphatics near the femoral glands and proceeds downwards in the leg.

In the legs the femoral and malleolar vessels are most frequently affected. The inflammation may be unilateral or bilateral. In the latter case, one side is frequently involved much more severely than the other. The vessels of the spermatic cord and testis are especially susceptible.

Lymphatic vessels anywhere in the body may become involved and cause local effects which may simulate other conditions. For instance, inflammation of abdominal lymphatics may suggest acute abdominal states, with deep tenderness and muscular rigidity.

Sometimes small abscesses may form in the affected vessels or glands and discharge on the surface, leading eventually to the formation of sinuses. This is particularly common in the malleolar regions and in the axillae. Abscesses may contain the remains of dead adult worms. The site of an abscess is often indicated at an early stage by extreme tenderness over the area involved, the so-called 'focal spot'.

*Lymphadenitis.* In association with the lymphangitis there is almost always some local adenitis. This may precede the lymphangitis. The glands are swollen, firm and tender. They remain discreet after the acute episode and may be involved in abscess formation. There is usually some hard oedema of the overlying skin.

The glands most commonly affected are those in the groin and the epitrochlear regions. The latter are commonly enlarged in malayan and pacific infections before any other manifestations of the disease. Such glandular enlargement tends to persist. The glands sometimes contain adult worms living or calcified.

*Funiculitis and Orchitis.* The manifestations are common in bancroftian and extremely rare in malayan filariasis. The first signs of cord or testis involvement are often accompanied by fever but as the condition progresses fever may be absent. Both funiculitis and orchitis tend to recur and subside spontaneously; the pain and tenderness disappear in quiescent periods but some induration remains. Thickening of the cord is one of the earliest signs of filariasis and must always be carefully searched for.

Orchitis begins suddenly with very severe local pain greatly exaggerated by movement and pressure. The patient is completely incapacitated. The organ is enlarged and exquisitely tender. The epididymis is usually swollen and acutely tender; occasionally there may be epididymitis only. The scrotal skin may be oedematous and erythematous and there is almost always an associated severe funiculitis. Orchitis is often unilateral but may be bilateral. It is sometimes associated with acute hydrocoele.

The acute symptoms and signs last a few days and then almost completely subside. After a variable period they recur and the condition progresses through episodes of attack and remission to recovery or to permanent obstructive changes.

In the acute stage the clinical signs of involvement of the cord and epididymis are obvious. The degree of involvement of the body of the testis itself is variable; some authors believe this organ usually escapes damage. In the intervals of quiescence the epididymis may remain enlarged and the cord is usually thickened and nodular (due to infiltration with lymphocytes) along its whole length.

Hydrocoele commonly develops in recurrent cases of orchitis.

The stage of intermittent acute inflammation may stretch over months or years and cover successive advances of the disease towards the fully developed obstructive stage. Within a few months of the onset, however, the two stages usually begin to overlap.

*Obstructive signs*

The obstructive signs develop usually in parts of the body where inflammatory reactions have occurred. They may sometimes appear without previous local inflammation. Obstructive phenomena arise from interference with local lymphatic drainage or circulation and consequent accumulation of fluid within the vessels and in the interstitial tissues. The affected vessels may eventually rupture. Minor obstruction of venous blood flow may be involved in the late stages.

Obstructive signs include oedema, varices of local lymphatic vessels, lymph scrotum, hydrocoele in bancroftian filariasis, and other local accumulations of fluid.

The signs of obstruction to lymph drainage are usually progressive and often associated with irregular bursts of local inflammation involving both vessels and glands.

*Varices.* Distension and varicosity of lymphatic vessels are especially common in the superficial vessels of the femoral, inguinal, and testicular regions. More deeply placed lymphatics such as those of the abdomen are also involved. The appearance of a varix may be the first indication of the disease, but a careful study of the clinical history will usually disclose previous local inflammatory episodes.

The vessels involved are distorted, tense and distended with fluid; superficial vessels may be partly emptied by massage away from the local glands,

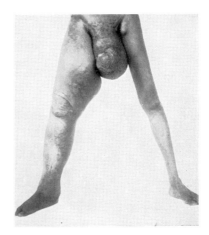

Fig. 5. Bancroftian filariasis.
Elephantiasis of leg and scrotum.
(Note left femoral varix and gland mass.)
[Courtesy Dr. T.H.White]

which are almost always enlarged. Deeper varices such as those in the scrotal vessels may often be felt as collections of tense cords, or may not be discovered until operation, for example at the removal of hydrocoele.

Varices tend to be slowly progressive and are usually painless. There may be occasional periods of acute exacerbation. In periods of quiescence the skin is freely movable over the affected vessels; in exacerbations it may become oedematous and erythematous. Occasionally the whole limb may become oedematous.

Abscesses may form around varicose vessels and burst on to the surface leading to chronic sinus formation.

Varicose vessels may become inextricably mingled with local enlarged lymphatic glands, forming an irregular mass of tissue which is sometimes known as varicose glands. The glands remain discrete except after necrosis following secondary infection, when they may become matted together.

*Lymph scrotum.* The lymph drainage of the scrotal area is often obstructed early in bancroftian filariasis, usually in association with enlarged inguinal glands. The skin and subcutaneous tissues become swollen and oedematous, the lymphatic vessels dilated and tense with fluid. The skin is erythematous and often covered with small vesicles varying from a millimetre to a centimetre in diameter containing clear or milky fluid in which microfilariae are commonly present. The vesicles rupture so that the skin surface is constantly wet with escaping fluid. Secondary infection occurs almost inevitably and small abscesses are formed which discharge pus and eventually form sinuses. The whole scrotal skin may be affected and becomes greatly coarsened and thickened, eventually passing on to elephantiasis.

The onset of lymph scrotum is often accompanied by some fever and general reaction. Hydrocoele is present in the majority of cases. There is usually a history of former acute involvement of the cord and testis.

*Hydrocoele.* In the endemic area, filariasis is the commonest cause of hydrocoele. Gradual effusion of fluid into the cavity of the tunica vaginalis in bancroftian filariasis is a common result of earlier inflammation and obstruction of the lymphatics draining the testicular region. The fluid may be clear or milky; it usually contains microfilariae. There may or may not be a history of one or more acute attacks of orchitis or epididymitis or both and acute episodes may be repeated after the hydrocoele has formed, leading to increase in the size of the tumour.

The condition may be unilateral or bilateral. The regional glands are usually enlarged and there are often concomitant varices of the superficial lymphatics of the scrotal sac and sometimes oedema of the scrotum and lymph scrotum. As in north-west Thailand, hydrocoele may be the only obvious indication of infection.

*Effects of obstruction and varicosity of deep lymphatics.* Ascites, pleural effusion and synovitis may all appear as a result of interference with local lymph drainage.

Obstructed varicose lymph vessels in the abdomen may eventually rupture.

The most striking clinical picture resulting from rupture is chyluria. In this condition, which occurs in bancroftian infections, vessels containing chyle burst through into the urinary tract, their contents escaping into the renal pelvis, the ureters or the bladder. The patient passes a milky mixture of chyle and urine. Albumin is always present. On standing the fluid settles into three layers; an upper thin layer of fat, a deep middle layer of semicoagulated lymph and urine, and a lower usually pink layer of debris and cells, including erythrocytes. Microfilariae are often present.

Chyluria usually develops abruptly. It may be preceded by loin pains and accompanied by fever and some prostration but there may be no accompanying general symptoms. Milky urine is passed for 2 or 3 days at a time. Attacks tend to be recurrent with long quiescent intervals of weeks or years. In rare instances coagulation of the chyle may cause obstruction to urinary flow and retention of urine. The passage of coagula may cause renal colic.

Lymphatics containing lymph and not chyle may also occasionally rupture into the urinary tract, leading to the passage of blood-stained urine containing lymph. This condition has been called lymphuria.

Lymph or chyle may occasionally escape direct into the abdominal cavity giving rise to lymphatic or chylous ascites. In such cases the symptoms at the time of rupture may resemble acute peritonitis. Escape of chyle may also lead to chylocoele, clinically indistinguishable from hydrocoele except that the fluid content is milky.

*Elephantiasis*
In regions of high endemicity the majority of cases of elephantiasis probably arise from filarial infection. The condition is, however, basically the end result of chronic lymphatic obstruction and may arise from causes other than filariasis. It is not always possible to say for certain whether in a given case filarial infection is the cause, but there is often a history of repeated attacks of local lymphangitis and adenitis interspersed with remissions of variable length and the gradual advance of the tissue lesion to fully developed elephantiasis. In some cases there is no such history, the development being continuous without any particular localizing incidents. In the great majority of cases, however, there is a clear history of long exposure to infection. The apparent necessity for frequent reinfection in the production of elephantiasis probably explains the age incidence of the condition, which develops late in the disease in young adults and is rare in children.

In some cases elephantiasis may appear or develop during a period in which the more active inflammatory or obstructive phases of the disease are going on in the same anatomical region or elsewhere in the body. In most cases, however, the full development is met after the signs of active filariasis have ceased.

The prevalence of elephantiasis varies widely in endemic regions. In some regions, such as Samoa, the condition is exceedingly common; in others, such as certain areas of China, it is rare.

The distribution of the lesion in the body is also very variable and depends to some extent on the geographical locality and the type of infecting filaria.

In bancroftian infections one or both of the lower extremities with or without the scrotum are most commonly involved. Elephantiasis in the leg is most frequently seen below the knee but the whole limb is often involved. The upper extremities, the breasts, the labia, may also be affected. In malayan infections the legs are most commonly involved; the arms are involved sometimes in some regions and scrotal involvement and hydrocoele are very rare.

The part played by secondary infection or repeated local trauma in the development of elephantiasis is uncertain. On the whole, these factors are probably of minor importance.

The regional lymph glands are usually involved, the inguinal and femoral glands in elephantiasis of the legs and scrotum, the axillary and epitrochlear in elephantiasis of the arms. The glands are large, firm, and discrete except where abscess has occurred. When the arm is involved one or more of the axillary glands are often enlarged enormously in the very early stages and serve as a useful diagnostic indication.

Elephantiasis arises as a thickening of both the skin and the underlying tissues; its progress can perhaps best be followed by a specific example, say, in the leg.

The femoral and inguinal glands are probably enlarged after a series of previous attacks of adenitis. There may be varices and obstructive lesions in the lymphatics, for example in the femoral region. Oedema of the lower half of the limb may come on slowly and gradually spread from the foot and ankle eventually up to the thigh. At first the oedema is soft but, as time goes on, in the course of months or years, the character changes and it becomes hard. The skin epithelium hypertrophies and in places wart-like thickenings appear. The subcutaneous tissue changes in structure. There is oedema, increase in number and dilatation of lymphatic vessels, sometimes local varices. All soft tissues tend to increase. The limb becomes noticeably thickened and eventually enormous, the changes developing most rapidly below the knee. At first the muscle hypertrophies; but later it atrophies and is partly replaced by myxomatous fibrous tissue. At this stage the efficiency of the limb suffers and the patient often finds it difficult to get about. As the limb increases in size the skin billows out in irregular folds in the creases of which secondary infection is common.

All stages are met from slight uniform swelling with oedema and thickening of the skin to enormous grotesque enlargements.

Changes in other parts of the body are essentially of the same kind. Scrotal tumours may reach immense proportions in bancroftian infections. Some have been recorded weighing over 200 lb. The penis is not usually affected in scrotal elephantiasis but is completely retracted within the tumour, the urine reaching the surface along a tube of skin pulled out by the hypertrophic mass. The inguinal glands are generally enlarged and discrete and there may be local evidence of lymphatic obstruction, such as varices. The testes are dragged down by the tumour and may be found attached to the under part of the scrotum; the cords are greatly lengthened. In spite of this anatomical strain, however, the testicular function may be unaffected. Many cases have bilateral hydrocoele.

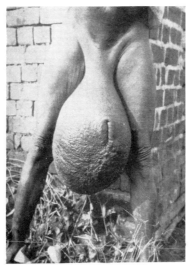

FIG. 6. Bancroftian filariasis.
Elephantiasis of scrotum.
[Courtesy Sir Clement Chesterman]

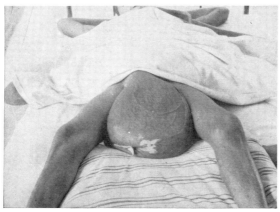

FIG. 7. Scrotal hernia.
Important in the differential diagnosis of elephantiasis.

Other parts of the body may be involved including the penis (usually without involvement of the glans), the labia and breasts, circumscribed areas of skin on the trunk (especially the lower abdominal wall), the neck or the limbs and, occasionally, the tongue and the nose.

*Course and prognosis*
The progress of the disease is slow. It usually takes years for the full development to be reached.

Filariasis is much more likely to progress to elephantiasis in a native of an endemic area than in the infected visitor. In the early stages of the disease removal of the latter from the endemic region will be followed by gradual recession of the signs and symptoms and recovery.

Once elephantiasis has commenced the future development will depend on care and treatment, including the prevention of sepsis. In the early stages the prognosis may be improved by suitable chemotherapeutic measures, which are considerably less effective later.

It is impossible to estimate the prognosis of the asymptomatic infection in which microfilariae are present in the peripheral blood. Some of these cases in young people probably proceed to the advanced disease.

The likely development of elephantiasis in a group of individuals may be assessed to some extent by the characteristics of the disease and the frequency of its appearance in the particular geographical region concerned. In Samoa, for instance, the probability of ultimate elephantiasis is high; in other areas it is low.

CLINICAL DIAGNOSIS

Many infected persons have no clinical signs and the diagnosis can be made only by discovery of microfilariae in the blood or tissue fluid (see later).

Early cases may present with no signs other than enlarged lymph glands which are discrete, usually asymmetrically distributed and may or may not be tender, depending on whether or not the condition is active at the time of examination. Enlarged glands are commonly found in the epitrochlear and axillary regions or in the groin. Diagnosis from other causes of asymmetrical gland involvement is difficult, but careful inquiry may elicit a helpful history of febrile attacks and possibly of acute local adenitis and lymphangitis; microfilariae may be found in the blood.

The differential diagnosis of filarial lymphangitis may be difficult in the absence of a clear history or of microfilariae in the blood. In most cases the general reaction and local signs are less severe than in acute bacterial lymphangitis. The local glands are also less tender than during bacterial infection. The absence of any focus of infection may suggest a wider search. The centrifugal development of the lymphangitis, and focal points of intense tenderness and possibly abscess formation along the course of the inflamed lymph vessel, are suggestive of filariasis.

Acute filarial funiculitis, orchitis, and epididymitis may be indistinguishable from the results of gonococcal infection, which may be coexistent. In uncomplicated filarial inflammation there is no urethral discharge. The history of repeated attacks, the thickened cord, the frequent involvement of local glands, and the development of hydrocoele are all suggestive of filariasis.

In an endemic area varicose superficial and deep lymphatics, especially in the femoral or scrotal region, and hydrocoele should be regarded as filarial in origin unless proved otherwise. By this stage the microfilariae may usually be found in the blood.

Elephantoid tissue changes appearing in an endemic area, especially in native inhabitants, are regarded as being mostly filarial in origin. In some individuals and in non-endemic geographical areas other causes such as secondary malignant deposits in the lymph glands, tuberculosis, and trauma must be sought. In the early stages of elephantiasis, oedema of a limb, especially when unilateral and associated with enlargement of local lymph glands, should be regarded with suspicion.

A moderate eosinophilia develops in the early stages of the disease and may persist into the late stages.

## LABORATORY DIAGNOSIS

The certain diagnosis of filarial infection can be made only by demonstrating the presence of the worm. This is done most easily by finding the microfilariae in the blood. Occasionally, the adults may be found in lymph glands excised for the purpose, or by X-ray when calcified. Biopsy of lymph glands is not a wise procedure, however, since it may further interfere with the already impeded drainage of lymph from the affected area. The identification of adult worms should be left to the expert. Some indication of the species being dealt with may often be obtained from knowledge of the likely breeding grounds of the vectors.

*Microfilariae* are found in the blood in the intermediate stages of the disease. They are absent in the very early and late stages. It is most unusual to find microfilariae in the blood of patients with established elephantiasis. They must be looked for at the right time. If the prevailing worm produces periodic microfilariae, the blood should be examined somewhere about midnight. If the microfilariae are relatively aperiodic, the blood is often best examined in the early afternoon, although microfilariae are usually present throughout the day.

The numbers of microfilariae found in the blood vary enormously from patient to patient and may be very great.

Blood is examined by scrutinizing wet film preparations under a coverslip or, more commonly, by taking six or more thick films as for malaria. Field's

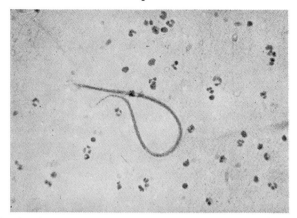

FIG. 8. Microfilaria of *W. bancrofti* in a stained thick blood film taken at night.
[Courtesy Professor W.E.Kershaw]

stain may reveal the microfilariae well enough to make the differentiation of species possible but it is better to stain with haemalum.*

Microfilariae may be distinguished by their appearance and the arrangement of their body nuclei. Expert advice is needed for identification (see Table, p.79).

If microfilariae are not found by examination of thick blood films in a suspected case, various methods of concentration of the blood specimens may

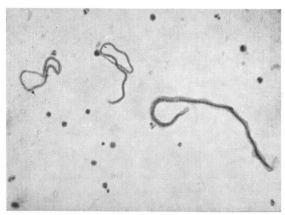

FIG. 9. Microfilaria of *L. loa* and *A. perstans* in stained thick blood film taken during the day.

[Courtesy Professor W.E.Kershaw]

* *Thick blood films*. Films are prepared as for malaria (p. 269) and allowed to dry. They are then dehaemoglobinized by suspending in water for 2–5 minutes. They are again allowed to dry and then fixed by dipping in alcohol. After drying they are stained in hot Mayer's haemalum for 3–5 minutes and washed in water for 1 hour.

be employed. Knott's method consists in taking 1 ml venous blood into 8 ml of 2 per cent formalin solution in distilled water. The mixture is centrifuged for 5 minutes and the deposit examined for dead microfilariae, which may be present in enormous numbers. Bell has proposed a method using blood

## TABLE

### THE DIAGNOSIS OF MICROFILARIAE

| Characteristics | Stained preparations | Periodicity | Diagnosis |
|---|---|---|---|
| **1. Microfilariae present in the blood** | | | |
| *Sheathed and large* | Graceful curves | | |
| | Discrete nuclei; tail tip free of nuclei | 1  Plentiful at night, rare during the day (periodic). | |
| | | 2  Present during day and night (diurnal). | Mf. of *W. bancrofti* |
| | | 3  As 2, with maximum in early evening (subperiodic). | |
| | Irregular, with heavy nuclei | | |
| | 1  Long thin tapering tail; nuclei to tip | Plentiful during the day; rare at night. | Mf. of *L. loa* |
| | 2  Tail long; 2 small round nuclei separated from 2 long spaces from body nuclei | Plentiful at night (periodic) or in evening (subperiodic) | Mf. of *B. malayi* |
| *Unsheathed and small* | Bulbous nucleus at tail Pointed tail with nuclei | Non-periodic | *A. perstans. M. ozzardi* |
| **2. Microfilariae present in the skin** | | | |
| *Unsheathed* | Head spatulate; tail sharply pointed; no nuclei at tip | | Mf. of *O. volvulus* |
| | Head cylindrical; tail curved sharply at tip; nuclei to tip. | | Mf. of *O. streptocerca* |

collected in sequestrine, later haemolysed in dilute teepol and passed through a millipore filter. This technique is suitable for blood stored for 48 hours and is therefore useful in surveys.

Fresh coverslip preparations of blood may also be examined at the same time as the dried, stained specimens. The microfilariae are actively motile and may be seen swimming about agitating the erythrocytes. This form of examination is unreliable and should never be used without stained films.

Microfilariae may be found in the fluid obtained from varices, from hydrocoele sacs and sometimes in ascitic and pleural accumulations of fluid and even in joint fluid during synovitis. They are usually present in the sediment of the milky urine passed during chyluria; their absence from the urine in this complication does not exclude the diagnosis.

### OTHER DIAGNOSTIC METHODS

Acute allergic responses arising during the first few days of a course of diethylcarbamazine are of significant import in the diagnosis of suspected filarial infections.

Complement fixation tests have been devised in which the antigen is made from an alcoholic extract of the dog heart worm *Dirofilaria immitis* or from microfilariae or adults of *W. bancrofti*. A positive reaction is an indication of present or past infection.

Skin sensitivity tests with similar antigens have also been used, and may be helpful in difficult cases, or in late cases of elephantiasis in which microfilariae cannot be found. The antigen is injected intradermally near a control injection of saline and after an interval of 10–15 minutes the resulting wheal is measured and compared with the control. Details for this test vary according to the antigen used and should be consulted before the method is employed. The development of occasional false positives sometimes makes interpretation difficult.

### TREATMENT

The treatment of filariasis is local and general.

If the patient is febrile he should be nursed in bed: in the acute stages he should be taken off all duties. Inflamed parts should be rested as much as possible. A suspensory bandage is necessary in epididymitis and orchitis and in lymph scrotum. The application of heat may exacerbate the condition.

Oedema in a limb should be treated by rest and, in the leg, by elevation and firm bandaging from below upwards.

The oedema in the early stages of elephantiasis in the leg may be relieved by firm bandaging, preferably after a period of rest and elevation. The bandage is started on the foot and continued upwards to the knee or higher. Sorbo rubber strips may be placed against the skin before bandaging. Such treatment is purely symptomatic and helps the patient carry on his work; it does not affect the course of the condition.

Secondary infection through the skin in elephantiasis can be avoided to some extent by keeping the affected part clean by frequent washing and drying. The skin in lymph scrotum is particularly liable to infection and must be carefully protected.

Surgical procedures are helpful in certain conditions, notably hydrocoele, lymph scrotum and elephantiasis of the scrotum. No surgical procedure should be carried out until existing sepsis has been controlled.

Hydrocoele sacs should be removed together with local lymph varices. In operation involving the scrotum care must be taken not to cut the cords or damage the testes, which are usually functional and which are tied down to the posterior aspect of the tumour. It is the common practice to implant them in the medial aspects of the corresponding thighs. Details of surgical procedures must be sought in the appropriate texts.

Chronic discharging sinuses may need radical excision.

The prognosis after surgical removal of the scrotum is usually very favourable. Attempts to remove strips of elephantoid tissue from the legs have not been so successful. Fat embolus and fatal vascular collapse have followed such operations, and there is sometimes considerable difficulty in closing the skin incisions. Elephantoid tissue arising from the trunk may sometimes be removed *in toto* by section of the pedicle.

Chyluria does not usually require treatment other than rest.

A very important aspect of treatment, especially in visitors to endemic areas (such as service personnel) who have become infected after relatively short exposure, is the psychological handling of the case. Such patients should be assured that the likelihood of elephantiasis, sterility or impotence is remote.

*Chemotherapy*

Antibiotics are helpful only for the relief of secondary infections. Temporary diminution in numbers of microfilariae in the blood stream may result from the use of a number of drugs, including certain trivalent and pentavalent antimonials, which are believed to kill some of the adults. Organic arsenicals of various kinds have also been tried with poor or equivocal results.

*Diethylcarbamazine.* The most active drug available is diethylcarbamazine citrate. During treatment the microfilariae disappear from the blood-stream in a matter of days.

Allergic effects resulting from the rapid destruction of microfilariae and the consequent release of antigen may be severe. In some bancroftian infections and in most malayan infections, there is a febrile reaction during the first 3 or 4 days of therapy. There may be local inflammatory reactions in the cord and testis, and generalized urticaria and oedema, especially of the face. These reactions seldom last for longer than a few days during which the treatment should not be suspended. Relief is obtained by the use of antihistamine drugs such as Phenergan in standard doses. It is usual to give such drugs daily for the first 4 or 5 days of diethylcarbamazine therapy.

The long-term results of treatment with diethylcarbamazine are good. Since it has apparently little action on the adult except in very large dosage, control of a given infection will probably require repeated therapy at intervals of about a year.

*Dosage.* 2 mg per kg body weight diethylcarbamazine citrate given orally thrice daily for 21 days. Dosages for children are in proportion to body weight.

Because of allergic effects the dose on the first 2–3 days is often limited to a total of 2 mg per kg body weight. The dose is doubled on the fourth day and the full dose is given on the fifth day and thereafter.

## CONTROL

The control of filariasis is largely an entomological matter.

The use of diethylcarbamazine as a prophylactic in populations in endemic areas in the hope of reducing the transmission rate by controlling the human reservoir has been successfully employed in some endemic areas.

Mass campaigns should be preceded by health education including a warning about possible side-effects, especially fever. A single dose of 4–6 mg per kg body weight, given once weekly for 12–24 weeks is effective in *W. bancrofti* infections. The same dose given for 6–8 weeks is adequate in *B. malayi* infections. Febrile reactions are common in the early stages of dosage, especially *B. malayi* infections, and may lead to some opposition to completion of therapy. Health education is thus very important. It is also important to remember that in some areas *B. malayi* infection may occur in animal hosts, thus making control by human therapy alone more difficult.

## ONCHOCERCIASIS

### DEFINITION

The so-called blinding filarial disease is caused by infection with *Onchocerca volvulus* transmitted by black flies of the family *Simulidae*. It is characterized by the development of subcutaneous nodules, pruriginous and other skin changes and ocular lesions which may lead to blindness.

### GEOGRAPHICAL DISTRIBUTION

Onchocerciasis occurs in localized areas of Central and South America including Oaxaca and Chiapas states in Mexico, also in Guatemala, several States in Venezuela, and in a coastal zone of Columbia. It is also found in aboriginal Amerindians in Surinam. It occurs in many parts of Africa between 15° N and 13° S latitudes, including Kenya, Uganda, Tanzania, Zimbabwe-Rhodesia, Malawi, the Sudan, Ethiopia, Senegal, Liberia, Upper Volta, Ghana, Nigeria, the Cameroun Republic, and Zaïre; it is also present in the Yemen. It does not occur in corresponding latitudes of Asia, Indonesia or Australasia.

### AETIOLOGY
#### Causative agent
*O. volvulus* is a nematode belonging to the superfamily Filarioidea. It is related to other filarial worms which infect animals including cattle and horses.

Man is the true host and usual reservoir of the infection. Recent evidence indicates that the chimpanzee may also become infected and could act as a reservoir.

Certain species of fly of the genus *Simulium* are the intermediate hosts.

The infective larvae introduced by the fly develop very slowly in the human host; a period of a year or more often being necessary before maturity is reached.

In man the adults and microfilariae are found.

*O. volvulus* is a filiform white worm with characteristic annular thickening of the cuticle. The females may measure over 50 cm in length and are much longer than the males. Females are ovoviviparous: the uteri of the gravid female are filled with eggs containing larvae in all stages of development.

Adult worms are present in the subcutaneous nodules which form a characteristic feature of the condition. They may also very occasionally be found free in the tissue spaces of the host, especially in dense fibrotic tissue.

Most nodules contain several worms of both sexes coiled up together in an intricate tangle lying in cystic spaces which are incompletely lined with degenerate endothelium.

Worms live for years within the nodules. After death they are frequently calcified.

The unsheathed microfilariae vary greatly in size (150–350 μm). They have slightly bulbous heads and tapered tails. The nuclear column does not reach into the head or the tail. They are found in the nodules near the gravid females, in tissue spaces just beneath the skin epithelium, especially over the nodules, and often in the conjunctiva. They may be found in the skin of any part of the body and occasionally in lymphatic vessels and lymph glands.

The microfilariae are actively motile and migrate beneath the skin. They are believed to live for as long as 2 years in the human host.

## The vector

*Simulium*, often called the buffalo gnat, measures about 3–4 mm long. Only the females transmit the worm.

The most important species known to transmit the infection are *S. damnosum* (West Africa), *S. naevi* (East Africa) and *S. ochraceum, S. metallicum, S. callidum*, and *S. exiguum* (America).

The vector is a voracious biter and causes severe local reactions which are itchy and irritating and may bleed. The nuisance is very considerable and may be sufficient to make some areas very nearly uninhabitable.

## Development in the fly

Microfilariae are ingested during a blood feed. Those which escape from the insect's stomach into its tissues within 24 hours develop in the thoracic muscles and after a series of ecdyses become converted into infective larvae which reach the proboscis and enter the human host during the insect's bite.

The development in the fly takes about a fortnight. It requires suitable conditions, including the right range of external temperature (about 10–30° C).

*Transmission*

Recent work indicates that the fly may become infected after biting skin areas involved in early or well-developed lesions, but not in late 'burnt-out' lesions in which the few remaining larvae are too deep in the corium to be reached by the fly, which is a shallow biter.

The factors governing the infectivity of *Simulium* are not clearly understood. The degree of infectivity of flies and the rate of transmission vary sharply from area to area. In most endemic areas where the infected human host is exposed to biting, the infectivity rate in the flies is high. Occasionally, however, it has been found that the usual vector is present and apparently uninfected whereas a less common species is heavily infected.

On the whole, however, transmission of the disease occurs where the common vectors and infective human hosts are present simultaneously. The distribution of the disease is thus largely controlled by the ecology of the fly. Transmission occurs most commonly in moderately high rocky undulating country where there are fast-moving streams.

*Simulium* spp. require hot moist shady conditions for breeding. The larvae become attached to stones or vegetation or sometimes crustaceae in fast-running, well-aerated water and are thus especially frequent during rainy seasons, often in streams running over rocks which may be dry and exposed in the dry seasons.

Details of breeding depend on the locality.

In Africa, the fly practically disappears in the dry season, reappearing suddenly with the rains. Breeding is greatest in the wet seasons. Larvae are found in small, rapidly running streams in the vicinity of large rivers in undulating country usually above 300–450 m. The adults rest in shade under leaves or in grass very near the breeding grounds. They seldom fly more than a few feet from the stream in dry and sunny weather but may wander several hundred feet in cloudy moist conditions. They have been found to fly miles along the river beds in the dry season. If disturbed they bite at any time of day, especially in the afternoon. Biting occurs most frequently on the legs below the knee. Fishermen and others with occupations associated with the breeding streams are thus particularly liable to infection. Local reactions to the bite are vigorous.

In America breeding continues on a large scale the whole year round in damp virgin forest lying between 600–1500 m above sea level. It is maximal during the rains, i.e. between September and February. Similar conditions to those in Africa are required, including fast-running, well-aerated streams. The adult flies leave the forests for the local coffee plantations where they shelter in the shade of leaves or in the grass. Biting is much more frequent on the upper part of the body in these conditions than it is in Africa.

## General

Infection occurs at any age. Nodules have been observed in children under the age of 1 year, but begin to appear more commonly in children of 3 years or more, and in adults. The appearance of the signs of infection is generally very slow, in keeping with the maturation of the worm in the human host.

Either sex may be infected. The relative incidence of lesions in the sexes is largely a matter of chance exposure to infective flies. For instance, in villages set some way from streams and rivers to which the men go daily for fishing, the incidence is much greater in men than women.

There is no racial resistance to infection. The disease is much commoner in the local populations of infective areas than in visitors, but the latter may become infected, especially after long-continued exposure.

Intensity of infection is the chief factor in deciding the development of the clinical syndrome. It is measured by counting the number of viable microfilariae observed per mg of skin removed from appropriate parts of the body.

### PATHOLOGY

The lesions of onchocerciasis include the nodules, certain skin changes and occular changes. The nodules arise directly from the presence of the adult worms. Opinion is divided concerning the pathogenesis of other lesions, but it is generally agreed that microfilariae, especially when dead, play an important role in them. There is also an allergic factor.

## Nodules

Nodules may contain living or dead adults. In the development stages of the tumour the worms are always alive.

Nodules develop in subcutaneous tissue, especially near bony structures. They consist essentially of a fibrous capsule within which lies a mass of coiled worms of both sexes surrounded by an avascular fibrous inflammatory tissue of varying degrees of cellularity. The infiltrating cells are usually lymphocytes and plasma cells; occasionally epithelioid or giant cells may be present. There are large numbers of eosinophils. Polymorphs are present in large numbers only after heavy secondary infection has taken place.

On section the tumour is usually whitish yellow and contains a central hard spongy mass consisting of cellular fibrous tissue honeycombed with sections of worms, together with eggs and microfilariae. Occasionally the central mass may be soft and pultaceous; in late lesions the nodule becomes a mass of fibrous tissue in which the dead worms may be calcified. The worms appear to be lying free inside endothelial-lined spaces which are presumed to be lymphatic.

The skin over the nodules usually contains numbers of active microfilariae, the numbers falling as the distance from the tumour increases. There may be no other epidermal change, but occasionally there is some oedema and slight general and perivascular infiltration with lymphocytes, plasma cells, and eosinophils.

*Skin lesions*

In many parts of the body the microfilariae may be found immediately beneath the skin epithelium, without any local reaction in the tissues. In other areas there may be some thickening of the epithelial layers, especially the horny layer, associated with reduction in numbers of sweat and sebaceous glands. A mild degree of cellular infiltration of the subdermal tissues and some perivascular infiltration of local vessels is common, together with some congestion and dilatation of vessels and lymphatics. There may be some oedema. Acute inflammatory changes may arise from secondary infection subsequent to pruritus and scratching.

Changes in the skin are usually associated with the presence of microfilariae but these are not always present; especially in lesions which are essentially allergic in origin. Reactions to filarial antigens are vigorous in individuals subject to pruriginous changes in the skin.

The distribution of lesions and microfilariae in the body in a given case depends on the intensity of the infection and possibly on the site of the original biting. In Africa serial skin snips taken from selected areas have shown that lesions and microfilariae are concentrated in the region of the calf and hip and to a lesser degree in the thighs and legs. The upper parts of the body are affected only in relatively heavy infections. The distribution in American onchocerciasis is the reverse of this, the upper half of the body including the eyes being most affected.

*Ocular lesions*

Microfilariae have been found in most parts of the eye except the lens. In some regions they are particularly common in the cornea and uveal tract. Corneal opacities may cause some blurring of vision and blindness may result from glaucoma caused by changes in the anterior chamber or from choroidoretinal degeneration, secondary cataract and optic atrophy. They have been reported in the retina only very rarely.

The conjunctiva often contains large numbers of active microfilariae, usually with little or no tissue reaction. After some time inflammatory infiltration develops (probably about dead microfilariae) and the whole tissue thickens and becomes irregularly pigmented.

Living microfilariae do not apparently damage the cornea. Opacities develop around dead microfilariae and consist of lymphocytes and plasma cells grouped round the body of the larva which lies stretched out horizontally. These areas of reaction tend to clear spontaneously in the early stages but later may become permanent and confluent. The lesions in the cornea develop in the substantia propria between Bowman's and Descemet's membranes. The epithelium is unaffected until the late stages during which there may be some degenerative changes and accompanying vascularization. Ulceration results only from secondary sepsis. There may be considerable folding and some pigmentation of Descemet's membrane.

The anterior chamber often contains large numbers of living motile microfilariae, which are sometimes linked end to end in roughly star-shaped fashion. A brownish mass of dead microfilariae slowly deposits at the bottom of the chamber, engendering a mild inflammatory reaction. The obstruction caused by this mass sometimes leads to glaucoma. Distortion of the pupil arises from involvement of the iris in the inflammatory processes proceeding in the anterior chamber. There is generalized loss of iris pigment which tends to clump and become adsorbed on Descemet's membrane and in the mass in the anterior chamber. The ciliary body undergoes a similar low grade inflammation; microfilariae are sometimes present in large numbers. The cyclitis produced may give rise to secondary cataract and glaucoma. Microfilariae occasionally appear in the vitreous which, however, normally remains clear.

Certain changes in the retina, including narrowing of the vessels, irregular clumping of pigment, atrophic choroiditis and sometimes optic atrophy with complete loss of vision, are widely believed to result from onchocercal infection, but there is still some division of opinion as to their origin. It has been suggested that they may be congenital and unrelated to the infection but the general consensus is that they are probably caused by microfilariae.

CLINICAL PICTURE

Onchocerciasis develops slowly as the worms mature. The period of time necessary for the full maturity of the adult is not certainly known but nodules have been reported in children less than 1 year old. In most cases, however, the period is considerably longer. It is uncommon to find nodules in children before the age of 3 years. After this they become increasingly more frequent.

Cases in the indigenous population are nearly always seen in the late stages. The early stages of the disease are more often seen in visitors. The latter may exhibit occasional fever and transient urticarial pruriginous skin reactions limited to areas of the face and trunk. These lesions resolve with the appearance of the more permanent signs of infection.

The commonest first indication of infection is probably the development of subcutaneous nodules, followed by the appearance of skin lesions. In some regions, however, the latter appear and may become extensive before, or sometimes in the absence of, palpable nodules.

Eye lesions appear late, usually in adults with a long history of nodular or skin lesions. They may develop without obvious intervening nodular or skin stages. They are rare in non-indigenous cases.

*Nodules*

Nodules first appear as small tumours beneath the skin, gradually developing to full size over the course of 3 or 4 years. They vary greatly in size. Some may be as small as 2 or 3 mm across, others as much as 60 mm. Some are too deeply situated for palpation.

The nodules are firm and not tender. In the quiescent stage the skin moves freely over them. In some areas they are loosely attached to the bone below, especially on the skull, where they may be bound to the periosteum and in the course of time come to lie in a shallow depression.

The nodules are usually obvious, raised above the general surface of the skin and sometimes pedunculated, especially in the groin or near joints.

They tend to remain quiescent for years and normally cause the patient little trouble except for discomfort from pressure over bones, such as the trochanters, or when they become secondarily infected. Occasionally, however, there may be a mild inflammatory episode, lasting a few days in which the tumour enlarges and becomes tender and the overlying skin becomes erythematous and oedematous. These inflammatory changes are most often seen in tumours in the neighbourhood of large joints.

The number of nodules varies enormously from patient to patient and from region to region. In the individual there may be only one, or many of varying sizes. In one district it may be common to find multiple nodules, in another none or only a few. In parts of West Africa, for instance, the number

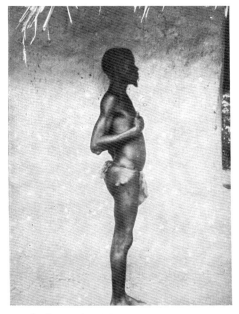

FIG. 10. Onchocercal nodules over trochanters and elbows.

in a given patient varies from one to twenty; in certain areas of East Africa it is common to find thirty or more, sometimes over 100; in America there are usually only a few. In some areas it is common to find extensive skin lesions with few or no nodules.

The distribution on the body is also uneven. In Mexico and Guatemala nodules are found almost always in the head, particularly in the scalp, and there are few on the trunk. In many parts of Africa, they are rarely found on the head and are commonest on the trunk, in the lateral intercostal spaces, in the axillae, in the pelvic region or in association with joints, especially the elbow and knee. In some areas in East Africa they are found commonly on the head and also on the trunk.

There is no good explanation of the location of the tumours. It is believed that some arise at points where there is a confluence of lymphatic vessels, or where some obstruction to lymphatic flow arises as a result of pressure, for example, from head loads. It has been noted that the common sites in Africans, such as the trochanteric regions, are often those habitually subjected to pressure or trauma.

Where the tumours are multiple they often appear in circumscribed groups of half a dozen or more scattered unevenly over the trunk. Lesions on the scalp often occur in groups of two or three.

*Skin lesions*

The appearance of nodules is usually followed, occasionally preceded, by the changes in the skin which develop insidiously and may become very disturbing to the patient.

In Africans the commonest of these is a pruriginous condition commonly called 'craw craw' (a general term for irritating skin lesions) which involves irregular wide areas of skin, especially on the trunk in the pelvic region, over the trochanters, thighs and shins, and to a lesser extent, the arms and shoulders. The skin becomes slightly raised, thickened, infiltrated, occasionally oedematous and sometimes darker than the surrounding skin. There may be desquamation of the horny layers. These areas are intensely itchy and may cause insomnia; secondary infection often arises from constant scratching. Other changes in the skin include local painless oedema and thickening and wrinkling of the skin giving an appearance sometimes described as lizard or elephant skin.

Microfilariae are usually present in the superficial layers of the corium in early lesions and deeper in later, more developed lesions. Old lesions are often referred to as 'burnt out'. In them the skin is thin and depigmented in patches. The elasticity is gone and the microfilariae are found only in the deep layers of the corium. This type of lesion is no longer infective to the fly.

American onchocerciasis gives rise to somewhat similar changes in the skin which have been given special names from time to time. The distribution of lesions and microfilariae is from above downwards, unlike the African form

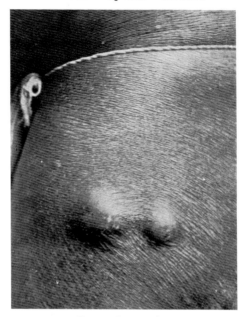

FIG. 11. Same patient.
Note nodules on buttock and changes in the skin texture.
[Courtesy of *Annals of Tropical Medicine and Parasitology*, Liverpool. School of Tropical Medicine, Photograph by Professor D.B.Blacklock]

of the disease. Thus, the most advanced lesions and the nodules are found on the head, neck, shoulders and upper arms, and trunk. Hard oedema of the neck and face, including the eyelids and sometimes the ears, has often been described. This oedema is accompanied by some lymphocytic infiltration and in the early stages may give the skin a hard glossy appearance. Urticaria is sometimes also present. In white skins a greenish tinge has been observed in the affected skin, giving rise to the local name of *mal morado*. These lesions are often extremely itchy and frequently infected from scratching.

*Coast erysipelas* has been described as a complication of American onchocerciasis but is now considered to be primarily bacterial in origin. The patient suffers from hard oedema of the face, sometimes involving the lips and eyelids. The skin is tense, oedematous and painful and there is a severe general reaction with high fever. Similar lesions have been described on the limbs.

It is often difficult to distinguish onchocercal skin lesions from the effects of secondary infection, the presence of infestations such as scabies, or the effects of food deficiencies. Nevertheless, there is ample evidence to indicate that the pruriginous and xerodermatous lesions described above are related to the worm infection.

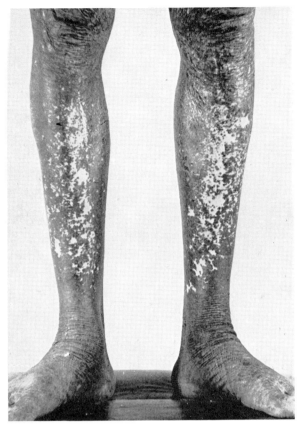

FIG. 12. Pretibial atrophy of skin and depigmentation in late ('burn-out') onchocerciasis.
[Courtesy Professor H.M.Gilles]

*Ocular lesions*
The incidence of eye lesions in endemic onchocerciasis varies considerably. In Mexico and Guatemala it is high. In some areas 20 per cent of infected individuals develop eye lesions and of these from 5 to 10 per cent may become totally blind. Similar high incidence is reported in some parts of Africa, but in others the incidence of eye lesions is low and that of blindness very small. The latter is particularly so in districts of Sierra Leone, for example, in which nodules are rarely found in the head and eye lesions are uncommon. In Ghana the incidence of eye lesions varies. In some areas in the north along the Volta River it is 10–20 per cent of those infected, sometimes with a high blindness rate. In such areas the disease has received the evil name of 'river blindness'.

In general, ocular changes appear most commonly in individuals with nodules on the head, but they may occur in cases with nodules elsewhere or without obvious nodules.

In the ordinary course of events ocular lesions develop late. An interval of years usually elapses between the appearance of the first nodules and the beginning of changes in the eyes. This interval is believed to be controlled to some extent by the age and general condition of the patient and the presence or absence of nodules near the eyes.

The more advanced eye lesions are commonly found in middle-aged or older individuals. They have occasionally been reported in children under 5 years of age.

The development of ocular lesions in African onchocerciasis may follow a steadily progressive pattern, the early stages of which are so mild as to be often overlooked. In the American disease the onset may be more rapid and is accompanied by local pain which is persistent during the hours of sunlight. There is first a mild chronic conjunctivitis subject to exacerbations with gradual thickening and some pigmentation of the conjunctiva with little or no infection. Corneal opacities gradually form and photophobia develops. At this stage there may be oedema of the eyelids accompanied by more generalized oedema of the face as described above. Some degree of conjunctival vascular engorgement may appear. Vascularization of the conjunctiva such as is seen in infective conjunctivitis is not, however, a feature of the condition except in the late stages. Lesions of the anterior chamber, iris and ciliary body may continue to develop insidiously, with very little pain or discomfort but with increasing deficiency of vision. In the course of 5–10 years blindness may result, especially in the presence of secondary infection or trachoma, from opacity, secondary cataract or glaucoma. Uncomplicated anterior eye lesions probably do not often lead to blindness.

In many cases of onchocerciasis, even when there are no nodules in the head, microfilariae are present in considerable numbers in the conjunctiva. Changes similar to those in the skin may or may not be present in the early stages, but as the condition develops, mild cellular infiltration of the superficial tissues occurs and there may be some thickening and pigmentation of the epithelium.

Some degree of involvement of the cornea is nearly always present in cases in which the eyes are affected. An avascular interstitial keratitis develops, affecting mainly the interpalpebral area especially on the nasal side but often involving also the pupillary area. The opacities develop as tiny, rounded grey areas with ill-defined margins; many may develop and ultimately become confluent, producing a characteristic 'frosted glass' appearance. Even at this stage there is very little vascularization unless secondary infection is present. Pannus, when present, usually develops on the inferior segment in contrast to that in trachoma. The cornea does not ulcerate in the absence of infection.

With a slit lamp microfilariae may often be seen in the aqueous, sometimes singly, sometimes in groups. Dead microfilariae may accumulate in the course of time in the bottom of the anterior chamber to form a brown-grey mass which later becomes involved in progressive slow inflammatory changes which include the iris. The most characteristic early change in the latter is generalized loss of pigment, especially from the inner margin of the iris producing the so-called spongy 'pumice-stone' effect. Pigment occurs in scattered clumps in the iris, in spots on the corneal endothelium or on the adjacent lens surface. Pigment may also be mixed with the mass of dead microfilariae and inflammatory tissue involving the floor of the chamber. The iris becomes involved in the inflammatory processes and may be pulled and distorted giving the pupil the appearance of an inverted pear with the apex pointing nasally and medially. The most striking points about changes in the iris are the absence of acute general inflammation and the peculiar lack of severe symptoms. Similar changes in American onchocerciasis have occasionally been associated with intense pain, which may arise from complications, including glaucoma. Cyclitis of a similar mild asymptomatic type commonly follows the iritis and leads to serious complications, particularly secondary cataract.

Glaucoma, with ultimate optic atrophy, may result from either cyclitis or obstruction in the anterior chamber arising from the inflammatory changes described above. It eventually leads to blindness.

The lens does not harbour microfilariae. Nevertheless, cataract is common, presumably following degenerative changes in the ciliary body. Microfilariae have been seen in the vitreous and may cause some opacities. It is not known how significant these are.

In some geographical areas changes in the fundus have been observed in individuals with heavy infections or with extensive 'burnt-out' skin lesions.

Microfilariae have not been identified in the living retina, but have been observed occasionally in enucleated eyes.

The retina may show one or more areas of degenerative changes which may extend to the disc margin and are roughly circular and fairly well demarcated from the normal area. Within these lesions the retina is abnormally transparent and the pigment is collected centrally in a few large masses; the background has been described as resembling 'cracked sun-baked mud'. Small aggregations of pigment lying over the vessels may be present in the otherwise normal retinal fields. There is commonly atrophic choroiditis. The choroidoretinal changes are accompanied by some degree of optic nerve atrophy, with well-defined disc margins. They are a common cause of blindness.

Retinal changes may be associated with lesions in the anterior eye. It is important to note, however, that in some regions it is common to find cases with extensive retinal damage and little or no change in the rest of the eye beyond minor lesions in the iris or cornea. Cases of the latter type may have no palpable subcutaneous nodules, but there are nearly always extensive skin changes.

Individuals with well-developed retinal changes are usually completely blind. There remains some doubt about the cause of these retinal lesions (see above, p.86).

*Other complications*

Moderate degrees of elephantiasis may develop occasionally in onchocercal infections. The oedematous skin changes are less pronounced than in the other filarioid infections, and appear most commonly in the skin of the groin, the scrotum and in the leg below the knee. Lymph scrotum and hydrocoele have been reported in infected individuals; the hydrocoele fluid may contain identifiable microfilariae. In such cases the local lymph glands may be enlarged.

There is normally a considerable eosinophilia in established cases. Occasional, very high counts of eosinophils have been recorded.

*Course and prognosis*

Onchocerciasis is a progressive condition which causes little harm to the patient unless the eyes are involved. In the latter event the prognosis for vision may be unfavourable.

### DIAGNOSIS

It may be difficult clinically to distinguish between an onchocercal nodule and a fibroma, lipoma or enlarged lymph gland. Nodules may sometimes be mistaken for the juxta-articular nodules of yaws.

Diagnosis is made by excision for histological examination and identification of the worm, or by aspirating fluid from the nodule and identifying the microfilariae and eggs. Fluid aspirated from a nodule will usually contain microfilariae but their absence is not absolute evidence of a negative diagnosis, since a tumour may be completely fibrosed or occasionally carry worms of only one sex or even only one worm.

Microfilariae should also be identified by examination of skin or conjunctival snips. They may be found most easily in samples of skin taken from the region of a nodule. The skin is lifted (by inserting a needle beneath it or squeezing it firmly between the finger and thumb of one hand) and cleaned with alcohol; a fine shaving is then removed with a razor blade without bleeding. The specimen is teased out gently on a slide in a drop of physiological saline and it is then covered with a coverslip, slight pressure upon which will often result in the appearing of free swimming larvae at the edges of the preparation. Samples of bulbar conjunctiva are removed under local anaesthesia with a pair of fine scissors and treated in the same way as skin snips. Stitching of the conjunctiva is unnecessary for repair.

In most cases of ocular onchocerciasis microfilariae are to be found in large numbers in the bulbar conjunctiva. A slit lamp is necessary to identify them in the anterior chamber of the eye. They are best looked for in the inferior medial quadrant.

Differentiation of the microfilariae from others sometimes found in the skin requires stained preparations (see p. 79).

### Other diagnostic methods

Intradermal injection of 0.1 ml of an antigen prepared from *D. immitis* is followed by an immediate wheal reaction in 15–30 minutes in individuals who are or have been infected. This is useful in surveys. Complement fixation tests using this antigen or one made from adult *Onchocerca* are also useful. Indirect fluorescent antibody tests are unreliable, but the soluble antigen fluorescent antibody test, using lipid-free *D. immitis* antigen is sensitive and specific, and can be used in surveys with dried blood specimens.

### TREATMENT

### Surgical excision of the nodules

Where it is practicable an attempt may be made to remove all identifiable nodules. Successful excision of nodules eliminates at any rate the great bulk of adult worms and may eventually lead to improvement in skin and ocular lesions or at least to the retardation of the progress of the latter.

### Chemotherapy

Chemotherapeutic measures may be successful in removing the microfilariae and sometimes the adults, but may be hazardous if active eye lesions are present, since severe allergic reactions causing exacerbation of signs may follow treatment.

Two drugs are at present used with some success, i.e. suramin (Antrypol) and diethylcarbamazine.

(i) *Suramin.* This drug is also used in the treatment of trypanosomiasis (see p. 463). It causes the slow disappearance of microfilariae from the skin and kills the adult worms in the nodules.

*Dosage.* For an adult, an initial dose of 0.1 g, followed by 1.0 g intra-venously repeated once every 5–7 days for 5 or 6 doses.

The initial dose of suramin is given to test for possible idiosyncrasy to the drug, indicated in the first instance by the appearance of proteinuria and casts. The urine must be regularly examined throughout treatment, which should be stopped if albumin, blood, or casts appear.

(ii) *Diethylcarbamazine citrate.* The chief action of this drug is on the microfilariae. It is much more rapid than suramin in its action. It is not very effective in killing the adults, but these may disappear after repeated courses of treatment.

*Dosage.* Where there is no ocular involvement a dose of 3 mg per kg body weight daily is given in three divided doses for 2 days; this dose is doubled for the next 2 days; trebled for the following 2 days; and quadrupled for the next 2 days. The dosage reached at this point (12 mg per kg body weight) is continued for 15 days.

When the eyes are involved, the same technique of dosage is used, starting at 0.5 mg per kg body weight.

*Allergic effects.* Both suramin and diethylcarbamazine may be followed by unpleasant effects, including burning and redness of the eyes, pruritus, hard oedema of the face and ears, and sometimes of the limbs, and slight fever. The reactions are more severe with diethylcarbamazine. Antihistamine drugs often relieve these reactions, and should be given as a routine for the first 5 days of treatment.

In severe allergic reactions in individuals in whom corticosteroids are not contraindicated, beta methazone 1.0 mg 8-hourly for 2 days, followed by 0.5 mg 8-hourly for 2 days, then 0.25 mg 8-hourly for 2 days will greatly modify the response without interfering with the activity of the diethylcarbamazine on the microfilariae.

In the treatment of severe irido-cyclitis or choroidoretinitis, the use of diethylcarbamazine may be combined with prednisolone 5 mg three times a day for 5 days then twice daily for 4 days and once daily for 3 days. Severe ocular allergic lesions can be relieved by local instillation of 1 per cent cortisone acetate, 3 drops daily, with atropine 1 per cent thrice daily.

### Prophylaxis

The control of the vector is a difficult entomological problem which has its own special aspects in different localities. The elimination of *Simulium* flies is the ultimate objective.

Protection against biting is afforded in some degree by means of protective clothing designed to protect the lower legs and by use of repellents.

Mass treatment of selected groups in highly endemic areas where there is considerable incidence of blindness is reasonably successful. Small weekly doses of diethylcarbamazine (50–200 mg) are given to reduce the microfilarial concentrations in the skin and so the local clinical effects. This can be continued over long periods. It does not affect the fecund adult female which may remain alive for 10–15 years. Reactions occur following the first three or four doses, then disappear. After some years the treated individuals are for practical purposes no longer infective to *Similium*, thus depressing transmission.

## LOIASIS

### DEFINITION

Loiasis is caused by infection with the filarial worm *Loa loa*; it is transmitted by large tabanid species of *Chrysops* flies (known locally as 'mango' or 'softly-softly' flies). The condition is confined to certain regions of tropical Africa and characterized clinically by fugitive or 'Calabar' subcutaneous swellings.

Loiasis is confined to equatorial rain forests and their fringes across a narrow band of territory stretching roughly from latitude 10° N to 5° S from the shores of the Gulf of Guinea to the Great Lakes.

Within this area the distribution is very irregular. Areas of intense infection occur in parts of south-eastern Nigeria, the Cameroun Republic, Gabon, Zaïre, and the Central African Empire.

*The causative agent*

Loiasis results from infection with *L. loa*, a filarial worm the adults of which are shorter and thicker than *W. bancrofti* and exhibit rounded bosses on an otherwise smooth cuticle. The female measures up to 70 mm, i.e. about twice the length of the male. The uterus is usually filled with masses of eggs containing embryos in all stages of development.

Both sexes are found in man in the connective tissues. They are found singly, never *in copula*. Maturation in the host tissues takes 6–12 months in most cases.

Little is known of the history of the worm in the human host. It is not known where fertilization and larviposition take place.

The adults wander about the tissues, usually in the soft tissue planes and cause little direct reaction on the part of the host. From time to time they appear beneath the skin in various parts of the body, especially where the connective tissue is loosely knit.

For practical purposes man may be regarded as the only reservoir. It is possible that in some regions monkeys may act as reservoirs.

Most subjects in whom adults have been identified will be found to carry microfilariae also, but there are some in whom the latter cannot be found even after the most exhaustive search. It is not known whether in these individuals there has been unisexual infection or failure of fertilization or whether larviposition has occurred in some reservoir organ and the numbers in the blood are too small for detection.

The actively motile microfilariae are commonly present in the blood. They are sheathed and vary in size considerably, the largest being about the same size as those of *W. bancrofti* (for identification, see p. 79).

Microfilariae are rarely found elsewhere than in the blood or within gravid females. They have occasionally been recovered from lymphatic glands. They are found in greater numbers during the day than during the night. There is great variation, however, in this diurnal periodicity not only from patient to patient, but in the same patient from time to time. They are commonly in greatest concentration about midday.

*The vector*
The distribution of the genus *Chrysops* is considerably wider than that of the disease. The species responsible for transmission, however, are those found only within and at the edge of the equatorial rain forest, namely *C. silacea, C. dimidiata* and *C. distinctipennis*. Only females are concerned in transmission.

Infective microfilariae are ingested by *Chrysops* while feeding on the human host. The larvae pass from the stomach of the insect to the thoracic muscles and eventually present in the proboscis as the infective form by the tenth to twelfth day after feeding. The flies are usually free of infective forms by the seventeenth day.

*Chrysops* breeds in densely shaded, slowly running streams or stagnant pools where the bottom is sandy but covered by mud and decaying vegetation. The adults normally live high in the canopy of the forests but are attracted by movement in open spaces especially when the latter are on high ground roughly level with the canopy, or in rubber plantations in which there is no cover crop. In such situations adults may be found in abundance. They bite freely in shade chiefly between 08.00 and 17.00, but not in darkness or in direct sunlight. There is some evidence that the flies prefer to bite dark skin. They bite freely on the bare skin and can penetrate loose-knit clothing.

There is sometimes a severe local reaction to the bite, but this is of very irregular occurrence and though it has been suggested that the development or otherwise of local reactions depends largely on whether infective larvae are introduced at the bite, it may depend on the previous sensitization of the patient to the bite of the fly.

The mode of entry of the infective larvae during the bite of the fly is not known. It is most likely that they are introduced through the wound made during feeding.

*General*
All races seem to be susceptible to loiasis. The condition appears more commonly in adults than in children, possibly because of the slow maturation of the worms. Males are more commonly infected than females in some areas, probably owing to differences in occupation. In highly endemic regions practically the whole adult population is infected.

### PATHOLOGY

Adult worms apparently circulate freely in the connective tissue without usually causing local tissue reactions. They may, for instance, be found accidentally during surgical operation, sometimes in considerable numbers.

The Calabar swelling consists mainly of oedematous tissue in which the adult worm may or may not be present. In the more persistent swellings there may be some lymphocytic infiltration of the connective and perivascular tissues. The origin of these swellings is not understood. Many authorities regard them as local sensitivity responses to the recent presence of the adult worm which may have been injured by trauma. Similar tumours have been produced by the injection of antigens made from the filarial worm of the dog into the subcutaneous tissues of known sufferers from loiasis and bancroftian filariasis.

### CLINICAL PICTURE

In many subjects infected with *Loa loa* pathogenic signs and symptoms may never appear or may be so trivial as to escape notice. In others the reactions to the infection may be severe, painful, and temporarily crippling. There is frequently an additional psychological factor which may assume considerable importance and lead to invalidism.

It is not clear what determines the individual reaction to the infection; the intensity of the original infection or repeated reinfections may be significant and it is possible that some have a peculiar susceptibility to light infections.

The eosinophil count is usually high in loiasis; counts as high as 80 per cent have been recorded. It varies greatly from time to time in the individual.

In some early cases irregular local erythematous patches may appear almost anywhere on the body; these are sometimes followed by local relatively persistent oedematous swellings, and allergic papular dermatitis or urticaria. The lesions are commonly pruritic.

The clinical effects are mainly related to the appearance of the characteristic Calabar swellings or to the constant migration of the adult worms. The microfilariae in the blood are not believed to be concerned in the clinical picture.

### Calabar swellings

These may appear as early as 3 months after infection; they more commonly develop after a year or more and may reappear from time to time for many years. It is common to find only one swelling at any one time but there may occasionally be two or three.

The swellings are essentially caused by the development of localized subcutaneous oedema. The onset may be preceded for an hour or two by sharp local pain and itching after which the swelling appears and diffuses rapidly, usually becoming several inches across. It remains this size for several days and subsides slowly. Occasionally a tumour may last a week or several weeks, particularly in areas exposed to frequent trauma. Individual tumours usually arise and subside in the same anatomical area but occasionally they migrate slowly, moving several inches before completely disappearing. In some individuals the swellings tend to recur in particular parts of the body, especially near certain joints such as the wrist or knee. In others the appearance of the tumours both in time and position seems to be entirely fortuitous, although there is often a history of some mild local trauma shortly beforehand.

The patient may suffer from Calabar swellings at infrequent intervals or there may be bursts of them, as many as six or seven following one another inside a month.

The swellings may appear anywhere on the body, but are especially common in areas open to trauma, including the orbit, the lower limbs and the arms. The skin over the tumour is not much affected by oedema as a rule; it may be a little reddened and is frequently very itchy and hyperaesthetic. Sometimes the Calabar swelling may be preceded by a localized macular or urticarial rash over or near the area subsequently swollen.

The tumour may cause great pain and discomfort especially if it appears in regions in which the subcutaneous tissue is firm. Where the latter is loose and free there may be little or no discomfort. Trauma in the region of the tumour often results in transient severe dragging pain.

The most serious effects occur in the region of large joints, especially about the ankles and knees or wrists. Calabar swellings in these areas are usually tense and painful and some involuntary immobilization results which may temporarily incapacitate the patient. The swellings tend to persist around joints for longer than in other areas because of trauma produced by attempts at movement and may sometimes last for weeks, during which the patient suffers severe pain and inconvenience. Irritating pruritus over the affected area is often an important factor in promoting a thoroughly bad psychological reaction to the condition. The latter is of considerable economic and social importance particularly in endemic districts in which work has to be carried on by labour imported from relatively free areas.

Swellings, especially in the eyelids, sometimes follow rapidly on the appearance of an adult worm in the local subcutaneous tissues. A blow over the region occupied by an adult may also be followed by a local swelling. In most instances, however, there is no evidence of the presence of the adult worm at the time of onset of the tumour.

Calabar swellings are not commonly accompanied by any general reaction.

*Effects of migration of adults*
Adult worms are observed from time to time moving actively in the subcutaneous tissues, especially in areas in which the tissues are loose, for example, the breast, the frenum of the tongue, the eyelids, conjunctiva, penis, and scrotum. In these areas the worm can often be seen very clearly beneath the skin, moving rapidly with an undulant movement until finally disappearing into the deeper tissues. Local reaction, apart from some slight stinging feelings and sometimes very disturbing local pruritus, is usually minimal except in the eye. Worms may sometimes be attracted to the surface by heat and are said to

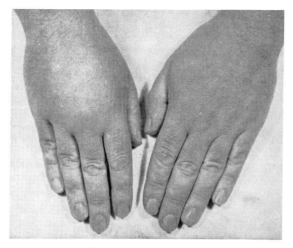

Fig. 13. Calabar swelling.
[Courtesy Professor W.E.Kershaw]

move away from cold. In temperate climates the adults tend to appear more frequently in the warmer weather.

The movement of the worm across the conjunctiva results in one of the most irritating and characteristic features of the condition. The eye feels as though there were a foreign body on the conjunctiva; there is considerable irritation and itching. Within a few minutes the worm appears beneath the conjunctiva, usually in the lower half. It crosses the eye at the rate of about an inch every two or three minutes and may be followed by rapidly developing conjunctival oedema and vascular congestion. The eyelid becomes oedematous and lachrymation is severe. Pain and local irritation are sometimes intense. The swelling of the lids and conjunctiva lasts several days before subsiding completely. The episode has been described as a feeling of being 'kicked in the eye'.

The clinical manifestations of loiasis are usually limited to those described above, namely the Calabar swelling and the occasional reaction to the subcutaneous wanderings of the adult worms and eosinophilia. In some cases temporary diffuse oedema of a part or the whole of a limb may develop and last for a few days to a fortnight or longer; such oedema, particularly involving the hand and wrist or the forearm, is commonly seen in some districts. It may occur in association with an obvious Calabar swelling, but often arises spontaneously. Elephantiasis occasionally results from loiasis.

Other effects reported have included generalized urticaria and oedema in the region of the wandering adult.

### DIAGNOSIS

In individuals exposed to infection the appearance of transient subcutaneous swellings is usually diagnostic. Months or years may elapse between the first appearance of the swellings and the discovery of the adult worm in the eye or microfilariae in the blood. Adults may sometimes be observed beneath the skin years before microfilariae appear in the blood. In light infections the microfilariae may be present in numbers too small for detection by ordinary methods; in others it is possible that larviposition may be confined to reservoir organs in the body without any spill over into the blood stream.

The absence of microfilariae from the blood is therefore not necessarily of great diagnostic significance.

Nevertheless in many cases microfilariae are found in the peripheral blood. They should be looked for during the day, preferably round midday; they are often present throughout the 24 hours. The numbers of microfilariae vary in some cases from hour to hour. There may be many, easily identified in a single thick blood film; on the other hand they may have to be searched for assiduously through many films. They may be seen moving freely amongst the corpuscles in wet preparations in which a drop of blood has been covered by a coverslip. For diagnostic purposes, however, dried stained thick blood films are required. The technique is the same as that required for the detection of other microfilariae (see p. 79).

The adult worms can be seen clearly as they wriggle beneath the conjunctiva. When they are present there is no doubt about the diagnosis.

Differential diagnosis of Calabar swelling from the transient oedemas of trypanosomiasis and of other filarial infections may occasionally be difficult, but the history of repeated swellings and the search for the causative agent should settle the question.

In persons with Calabar swellings but no microfilariae in the blood the presence of the very high eosinophilia is a constant and valuable diagnostic sign. A history of exposure on an endemic area is essential for diagnosis.

Skin sensitivity tests using antigen prepared from *Dirofilaria* or from adult *Loa* may be useful in diagnosis. The same antigens can be used for the detection of complement-fixing antibodies in the serum which are present and detectable in early cases before the appearance of microfilarias in the blood.

### TREATMENT

Diethylcarbamazine has considerable effect on the microfilariae and less on the adults. The immediate results of therapy have been promising. During treatment the microfilariae have been observed to disappear from the peripheral blood within a few days and in some instances dead adults have been removed from subcutaneous tissues. Calabar swellings may, however, recur after some months.

The allergic reactions to treatment may be violent, and include generalized urticaria and local irritation and oedema in the region of adult worms. There may be an associated fever and it may be necessary to interrupt treatment until the effects have subsided. There may be a febrile reaction only.

*Dosage.* A small dose (1 mg per kg body weight for an adult) should be given after a meal over the first few days, especially in areas where onchocerciasis may also exist.

The daily dosage is increased to 4 mg per kg over the next 2 days. The following day the dose is doubled (amounting to about 200 mg twice daily); the dose is given thrice daily on the next day (12 mg per kg body weight: maximum single dosage 200 mg). This dosage is continued for 3 weeks. It may be necessary to repeat after 2–3 months.

Children are given doses in proportion to their body weight.

Antihistamine drugs should be given for the first 5 days of treatment.

## Local treatment

Adult worms should be aseptically removed if possible when they appear in the conjunctiva. Damage to the worm or incomplete removal may result in several local reactions of oedema and intense pain and sometimes secondary sepsis.

Antihistaminic drugs have some effect locally and may relieve itching and swelling after oral administration.

The incapacitating effects of lesions near joints can be relieved only by rest. If this is impossible, swellings may persist for weeks.

## Prophylaxis

Entomological control is successful in some areas. Chemoprophylaxis is recommended, using diethylcarbamazine 200 mg twice daily for 3 days once each month for adults; for children the dose is reduced in proportion to weight.

## DRACONTIASIS

### DEFINITION

Infection with the nematode *Dracunculus medinensis* or guinea worm.

### GEOGRAPHICAL DISTRIBUTION

Dracontiasis is found scattered over West, Central and East Africa; in the Sudan, Egypt, Arabia, Iran, Afghanistan, Turkey, southern Russia, western, central and southern India, Burma, the Caribbean Islands, and northern South America.

In these areas the distribution is patchy. The local incidence may be very high.

Dracontiasis results from infection with the nematode worm, *D. medinensis*. The clinical effects are produced solely by female worms. The male has not been observed in the human host.

The gravid female is enormous compared with the male, measuring a metre or more in length in contrast to 30 or 40 mm in the male. The cuticle is smooth, the anterior end bluntly rounded, and the body when mature is largely filled with the uterus.

The female matures in the connective tissue of the host. The gravid worm eventually reaches the surface of the host's body. The host skin ulcerates near the head of the worm and enormous numbers of free-swimming larvae are ejected through prolapsed portions of the uterus whenever the lesion comes into contact with water. Larvae do not appear in the host except within the uterus of the worm.

The male worm has been identified in laboratory infections of monkeys and dogs. It is believed to be absorbed shortly after impregnating the female. Some authors hold that the female does not always require fertilization in order to produce viable larvae.

The intermediate host is the crustacean *Cyclops* which becomes infected by the free-swimming larvae liberated by the adult worm. These larvae will survive and remain infective for up to 6 days in clean water and for as long as 3 weeks in dirty water or liquid mud. After ingestion by the intermediate host the larvae become infective to man in 10–12 days, provided the water is suitably warm.

*Transmission*

The human host becomes infected by swallowing water containing infected cyclops. The infective larvae are freed unharmed in the gastric juice and escape through the small intestinal wall. Subsequent development takes place in the connective tissues. Full maturity is reached in about a year.

Cyclops abounds in standing dirty water, particularly in puddles, ponds, wells, borrow pits, and tanks. Infection is especially likely under circumstances in which the same supply of water is used for drinking and washing. Step wells are notorious examples of such infective localities.

Dracontiasis is rare before the age of 4. After this the incidence steadily increases, to become highest in the young adult.

The incidence is seasonal in many areas especially in India. Infection with a single worm is usual, but multiple infection is not uncommon. There is no racial or other immunity and reinfection is frequent, even in the already infected subjects.

The worm gives rise to no clinical signs until near the point of discharge of larvae. The active stage of the infection is accompanied by both general and local signs and symptoms.

A few hours before the appearance of the worm at the surface of the skin there may develop some local erythema and tenderness over the area in which the pointing is to take place. In some cases there may be general effects sometimes of a severe nature, but in the majority the local lesion tends to develop without any general reaction.

In severe cases there may be generalized pruritus sometimes accompanied by scattered urticaria. There may be nausea, vomiting and watery diarrhoea. In some cases dyspnoea may appear and lead to attacks resembling asthma. These general reactions vary greatly in intensity and incidence from patient to patient and locality to locality. They subside as a rule by the time the local lesion has ruptured and the ejection of larvae has commenced.

*Local changes*
The gravid female presents somewhere in the legs or feet in over 90 per cent of all cases. It may appear elsewhere, especially in the back, the arms, and scrotum. It has been reported in the orbit. It may often be visible or palpable for its whole length in the subcutaneous tissues.

The patient complains of deep-seated stinging pain in the site in which the worm is reaching the surface. A papule or group of papules (which later coalesce) forms rapidly and enlarges over the course of 1 or 2 days becoming slowly more indurated. The central region becomes raised and eventually forms a vesicle which soon ruptures, leaving a superficial ulcer large enough to admit a probe. The head of the worm is often visible within this ulcer.

If the ulcerated lesion is douched with water a drop of milky fluid wells up in a few seconds. After an interval of about an hour further douching will have the same effect. This fluid contains myriads of active larvae ejected from the uterus in response to the stimulus of water.

Discharge of larvae will continue intermittently whenever the affected part is exposed to water until the worm has discharged its full load of larvae, which may take anything up to 3 weeks. The tissues about the presenting head of the worm become indurated, oedematous, reddened, and very tender. These reactions, which may involve wide areas around the worm, are probably allergic. Even in the absence of secondary infection walking may be very difficult and the patient is compelled to give up his work.

In the case not complicated by secondary infection the local lesion will heal completely about 4 to 6 weeks after its appearance.

Secondary infection is, however, the rule and may lead to serious and unpleasant complications.

Occasionally worms never fully mature or may die before they reach the surface. Under these circumstances they are absorbed completely or partly calcified, sometimes leaving a cord-like mass palpable beneath the skin; they

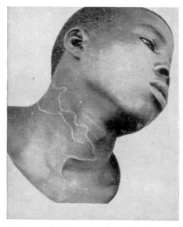
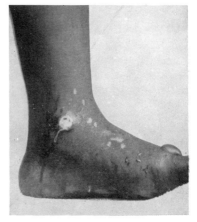

FIG. 14. Adult worm in subcutaneous tissues.

FIG. 15. Portion of worm extruding from ulcerated papule on ankle. Bleb from second worm over big toe.

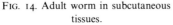

[Photograph by Dr E.C.Smith]

may also become secondarily infected and lead to abscess formation so that the first indication of the infestation may be the discovery of fragments of the worm in the abscess contents.

Gravid females which have not yet presented at the surface are occasionally ruptured accidentally and give rise to aseptic abscesses which are frequently severe and sometimes accompanied by general symptoms.

Abscesses in relation to the worms are nearly always the result of secondary infection. Such infections may involve deep structures including tendons, the periosteum, and bones, and may be accompanied by severe or even fatal septicaemia.

In some areas a large proportion of patients (in some parts of India, over 20 per cent) suffer from joint lesions, varying from painful reddened swellings to advanced pyogenic infections with later fixation and deformity. The majority of such lesions occur in the ankles and knees. Changes in joints are believed to occur occasionally without secondary infection.

The peripheral blood usually shows an increase in eosinophils which may constitute up to 10 per cent of the total leucocytes.

*Course and prognosis*

In the absence of secondary infection the worm will continue to discharge larvae if brought into intermittent contact with water. The incident is over when the uterus is finally emptied and the worm either withdraws and is absorbed or becomes extruded to the surface. This may take several weeks. Full healing of the ulcerated area may be expected in about 4 to 6 weeks from the onset.

Rapid healing also occurs if the worm is artificially removed without damage. Serious effects are produced if it is broken during removal. After such rupture and retraction local sensitivity reactions and secondary infection in the region of the broken area are almost inevitable.

The most serious consequences arise as the result of secondary infection. This includes tetanus.

### DIAGNOSIS

Patients are usually fully alive to their condition from their own experience. The development of the local lesion is characteristic. The head of the worm can sometimes be identified in the uncomplicated local lesions. Fragments may be recovered from contents of abscesses. Larvae may be seen in fluid exuded after douching the papule with warm water.

Intradermal tests with antigens made from adult *D. medinensis* have given equivocal results.

### TREATMENT

The patient should be rested. If possible the affected part should be elevated.

The local lesion should be kept as clean as possible and secondary infection dealt with by standard methods. General septicaemia requires antibiotics.

*Niridazole* (Ambilhar) is remarkably effective and rapidly produces cure. The drug is given orally in two divided doses, totalling 25 mg per kg body weight daily for 7–10 days.

Pain, tenderness and swelling are quickly relieved. The worms emerge or are easily removed. No ill effects result from rupture of the worm. The immobilized patient can return rapidly to work. Side effects are negligible.

*Thiabendazole* is also active, given orally in doses of 50 mg per kg body weight, daily for 2 days.

*Metronidazole (Flagyl)*, 25 mg per kg body weight for 10 days, is also effective but the longer treatment makes it less acceptable to the patient.

It is believed that these compounds primarily act as anti-inflammatory agents, reducing local inflammation and oedema, thus making the emergence of the worm easier. Experimentally they do not kill non-emergent worms in monkeys.

Antibiotics such as tetracycline in the usual doses should be given during the specific treatment in order to deal with secondary infection.

Where drugs are not available the time-honoured method of extraction probably gives the best results. The local lesion is continuously treated with wet compresses until the discharge of embryos stops, which may take 1 or 2 days. The head of the worm is then identified and tethered with a fine thread which is tied to a small stick about which the worm is gently wound, a little each day, until it is finally withdrawn. The process of extraction may take a fortnight or more. Care must be taken not to rupture the worm since this accident is almost always followed by sepsis at the point of the break leading to abscess, cellulitis or generalized septicaemia. The stick and rolled worm should be kept covered by a sterile dressing and the whole region should be kept clean and as aseptic as possible.

Involvement of joints requires especial care. It may be necessary to aspirate and immobilize. Expert advice is called for.

### Control

The successful control of dracontiasis is achieved by providing adequately protected water supplies, and the erection of infection-proof wells. Insecticides such as DDT may be useful for controlling cyclops but carry their own risks of poisoning. The cyclops may also be controlled by the introduction of fish.

## OTHER FILARIAL INFECTIONS

### Dipetalonema perstans

Infection occurs in West, Central and East Africa, northern South America, Brazil, northern Argentina and Trinidad.

The adults live in the body cavities. The unsheathed microfilariae are found in the blood; there is no periodicity.

There are usually no clinical manifestations. Occasionally eosinophilia, subcutaneous swellings resembling Calabar swellings, patchy skin oedema and pruritus, fever, lymphadenopathy, and joint and bone pains have been attributed to it. Relief is obtained by the usual doses of diethylcarbamazine.

Neurological and psychological disturbances have also been accredited to *perstans* infection. Microfilariae resembling those of *A. perstans* have been found in the cerebrospinal fluid. In one case the patient complained of headache, dizziness, vomiting, and other cerebral signs and became stuporose. The cerebrospinal fluid was under pressure and contained numerous microfilariae; the cell count was raised. The possibility of co-existing occult infections with other filarial worms makes the interpretation of such cases difficult. Metrifonate in fortnightly doses of 10 mg per kg body weight for four successive doses is said to be effective and without serious side effects.

### Dipetalonema streptocerca

Infection with *D. streptocerca* occurs in rain forests of West Africa from Ghana to Zaïre. The vector is *Culicoides* spp. Adults occur in subcutaneous tissue, commonly in the shoulder girdle and upper arms. The small unsheathed larvae are found immediately beneath the epithelium of the skin on the upper trunk and arms and can be identified in skin snips, as in onchocerciasis. The infection rarely causes clinical signs but acute intensely itchy erythematous eruption of the arms and trunk has been recorded and it is believed that the infection may occasionally lead to elephantiasis. The rash responds to diethylcarbamazine in the usual dosage.

## Mansonella ozzardi

This infection is found in the north coast of South America, northern Argentina, the Amazon valley and some states of Central America and the Caribbean Islands. The vector is *Culicoides* spp. The adults are found in fat tissue beneath the peritoneum and in other body cavities. The non-periodic unsheathed larvae occur in the peripheral blood. Inguinal adenitis, erythematous skin rashes, skin oedema, joint pains, severe headache, and high eosinophilia have been attributed to the infection. Conflicting reports have been given of the action of diethylcarbamazine, but the consensus is that it is not effective.

## TROPICAL EOSINOPHILIA

### DEFINITION

Tropical pulmonary eosinophilia; eosinophilic lung; tropical eosinophilic asthma. An inclusive term for a condition of high eosinophilia associated with loss of weight, pulmonary symptoms sometimes resembling asthma or tuberculosis and with characteristic radiographic pulmonary changes. The syndrome is regarded usually as the result of filarial infection.

### DISTRIBUTION

The disease occurs most commonly in India, Pakistan, Bangladesh, and Sri Lanka. It also occurs in tropical Africa, the West Indies, northern South America, China, Burma, Thailand, Malaysia, and Indonesia. Isolated cases have been reported from Korea and Australia.

### AETIOLOGY

It is now generally agreed that filarial infection is responsible for most cases. The worm concerned is usually unadapted to man but human filariasis including *B. malayi* (experimentally) may cause the syndrome. Helminth infections other than filariasis are occasionally responsible; *Toxocara canis* produces a similar clinical picture in man.

### PATHOLOGY

The classical effects arise from allergic and granulomatous response to the presence of the worm larvae. Information obtained from a few autopsies and from biopsies of lung and liver indicate that the characteristic lesion is a granuloma made up of necrotic eosinophilic material or microfilariae or other larvae surrounded by epithelioid cells, lymphocytes, eosinophils, giant cells, and macrophages. Lesions are scattered in the lung substance, the liver and sometimes the lymph glands.

The only change in the blood cells is in the leucocytes. There is a great increase in absolute numbers of eosinophils. Other white cells are not affected. Details are discussed below. The erythrocyte sedimentation rate (ESR) is increased in the acute condition and restored after treatment. Sternal marrow smears often show an increase in eosinophil elements which decrease slowly after treatment.

Smears of sputum show epithelial cells and eosinophils in clumps. The bacterial content is mixed and not specific. Blood may be present. Larvae of nematodes are found only exceptionally.

### CLINICAL PICTURE

The importance of diagnosing tropical eosinophilia lies in its sometimes severly incapacitating effects, in the possibility of early relief by chemotherapy and in the frequent confusion between it and pulmonary tuberculosis, bronchial asthma and bronchiectasis.

The clinical picture is essentially that of a sustained sensitivity reaction in which pulmonary signs and symptoms usually but not invariably predominate.

#### Clinical history

In the fully developed syndrome the commonest complaint is coughing, which appears in paroxysms and is worse at night. Occasionally the patient may present with acute respiratory distress resembling asthma or even bronchopneumonia.

Paroxysms may be of considerable violence, lasting a few minutes to half an hour, often repeating several times during the night. The patient is forced to sit up and his sleep is badly disturbed.

There is considerable breathlessness after coughing and frequently a feeling of suffocation, accompanied by rapid panting respiration. In many patients the breathing resembles that in asthma but bronchial spasm is not always present and the dyspnoea is not always expiratory in type. In some, however, there is true bronchospasm leading to asthma. *Status asthmaticus* has been reported.

Coughing is followed by expectoration of mucoid or mucopurulent sputum sometimes in considerable quantities. The sputum is often streaked with blood and occasionally small haemoptyses may occur and continue for several days.

In some cases there may be no cough or other respiratory signs, the chief complaint being progressive fatigue, loss of weight, and sometimes abdominal discomfort.

### Chest signs

In about a quarter of cases there may be no obvious signs even when the clinical picture is severe. Scattered sibilant or sonorous rhonchi may be heard over both lungs; there may be coarse basal crepitations. Adventitious sounds are rarely heard in the apices. The expiratory sound is usually prolonged. Signs of emphysema are common.

### Pulmonary radiographs

In the active stage the hilar shadows are usually enlarged irregularly, with blurred outlines. The lung fields are commonly crossed more or less transversely by fine irregular branching striations which are most evident in the mid and basal zones.

Mottling is present in most cases at some stage. It is most prominent in the basal zone or mid zones. The mottled shadows appear as discrete soft, rounded, ill-defined spots varying from pin-head size to 3 cm across. They closely resemble the shadows of miliary tuberculosis but are not so sharply marked out and are much more regionally distributed.

The radiological patterns are frequently bilateral and basal. Occasionally they may be unilateral and may occupy the infraclavicular lung fields, closely resembling tuberculosis.

The radiological shadows disappear quickly on treatment, i.e. usually within a month. They commonly reappear in relapses.

The appearance of these shadows is irregular during the disease. It is not always possible to correlate them with either the prevailing degree of eosinophilia or the clinical respiratory picture. They are more marked in early cases. There may be shadows of large consolidations in rare cases, and sometimes thickening of the pleura, especially at the bases.

### Other signs

About one case in four develops abdominal signs and symptoms, including anorexia, discomfort over the liver area, vague abdominal pains, and diarrhoea. These are occasionally the only clinical manifestations.

Various kinds of skin lesions have been reported, including patchy erythema, erythema nodosum and urticarial rashes. Occasionally there may be generalized enlargement of lymph glands.

#### THE BLOOD

*White cell count.* The white count is invariably raised, due to a great increase in mature eosinophils. The latter constitute 25–90 per cent of the total cells. The other cells are present in normal numbers.

Total white counts range between 10,000 and 100,000 cells per mm³.

In a given case the white count and the percentage of eosinophils fluctuates from time to time but it is an essential criterion of the diagnosis that the latter should always be of the order of 20 per cent or more.

*ESR.* This is increased in most cases. The actual figure varies from patient to patient and from time to time in the same patient. It is often of the order of 20–60 mm per hour. The rate returns slowly towards normal after treatment or spontaneous recovery.

## COURSE AND PROGNOSIS

The disease is rarely fatal. It may last for years with alternating periods of remission and exacerbation. As a rule the development of symptoms is gradual, and the full picture is not achieved for months or years. Occasionally it may be rapid.

Spontaneous recovery occurs as a rule after a few months or years. Recurrences are rare after more than 2 years of quiescence.

Response to treatment is usually excellent.

## DIAGNOSIS

Clinical diagnosis is often difficult. The eosinophil count is usually conclusive. The total number of eosinophils per mm³ should exceed 2000. The total white count should not be less than 10,000 cells per mm³.

Tropical eosinophilia must be differentiated from other allergic states, such as bronchial asthma and Loeffler's syndrome in ascariasis and from other causes of high eosinophilia, including eosinophilic leukaemia and Hodgkin's disease. Examination of the sputum is essential. In tropical eosinophilia, eosinophils and epithelial cells occur in clumps and the sputum is usually streaked with blood. Bacteria are mixed and not specific.

The lung signs may be easily confused with those of tuberculosis. Points of distinction are the presence of fine crepitations in the apices in tuberculosis and the tendency for eosinophilic lesions to affect the bases and leave the apices clear. The chief criteria, however, are the absence of *Mycobacterium tuberculosis* in the sputum, the blood picture and response to therapy.

The radiographic picture often superficially resembles chronic bronchitis and sometimes bronchiectasis. Here again the blood picture and clinical history are helpful.

In allergic bronchial asthma and allied conditions the patient complains of expiratory dyspnoea and coughs after relief. In the eosinophilic case there is often no expiratory difficulty and the cough occurs during the paroxysms. Where eosinophilia occurs in bronchial asthma, hay fever, etc., it is never of the order seen in tropical eosinophilia cases. The same is largely true of parasitic infections, which should be distinguished by discovery of the causative agent.

The complement fixation test for filariasis, using antigen prepared from *Dirofilaria,* is positive in most but not all cases resulting from filarial infection. A positive test or a positive skin reaction following intradermal injection of the filarial antigen are useful indications of the agent concerned and of the likely success of treatment with diethylcarbamazine. Allergic response in the first few days of such treatment is also an indication of filarial infection. Specific antigens for other worm infections such as *T. canis,* when causing visceral larva migrans, may be used for skin reactions or complement fixation tests to decide the diagnosis.

### TREATMENT

In cases in which filariasis or other helminth infection is suspected or confirmed diethylcarbamazine in doses of 6 mg per kg body weight twice or thrice daily for 5 days given after meals has dramatic results. Exacerbation of allergic signs accompanied by fever frequently occurs during the first 4 or 5 days of treatment, during which the dose of the drug should gradually be built up to the full course and antihistamine drugs should be given. Relapses require similar treatment.

Cases which do not react favourably to diethylcarbamazine may do so to arsenical compounds, for example, novarsenobillon 300–450 mg given intravenously, the dose repeated at weekly intervals for 6–8 weeks, or to chlortetracycline in the usual doses. Arsenical treatment is now rarely used.

Symptomatic treatment of bronchial spasm with adrenaline or aminophylline is sometimes indicated.

### *Effect of treatment*

With successful treatment, there is an immediate fall of total white cell count largely due to reduction of eosinophil numbers which come to normal levels in the course of 4 to 6 weeks. After treatment the white cell count is usually 10,000–15,000 per mm$^3$, eosinophils 5–10 per cent.

The radiographic pattern responds dramatically, often disappearing within a month. This remarkable effect is of considerable diagnostic importance, serving to distinguish the radiological lesions of eosinophilia from that of all other conditions.

Relapses with return of eosinophilia and radiographic pattern may occur after a full course of treatment and demand a further full course. About 10 per cent of cases relapse, usually within 2 years of treatment. Further therapy is required.

# 8

# FUNGAL INFECTIONS

Fungi pathogenic to man cause diseases known as mycoses. These may affect the skin or mucous membranes, the cutaneous and subcutaneous tissues or the deep tissues and organs.

## DERMATOMYCOSES

### DEFINITION

Ringworm infections. Fungus infections of the skin, nails and hair caused by a group of closely related fungi, belonging to the genera *Microsporum, Trichophyton* and *Epidermophyton.*

### AETIOLOGY

Fungal skin infections have a world-wide distribution. They are particularly common and severe in hot, moist climates. The fungi concerned infect keratinized tissues and only rarely involve the subcutaneous tissues; they never cause systemic lesions.

In the affected tissue they appear as branching mycelial filaments and arthrospores. They grow well on Sabouraud's medium after a fortnight at room temperature. The fungi may be primarily animal infections transmitted accidentally to man or primarily human infections. Certain parts of the body are particularly prone to infection from any of the three genera of fungi. Clinical classification of fungal skin lesions is thus best based on anatomical distribution.

Men are more commonly affected than women.

The infections are spread by contact with active lesions, with infected hair, skin debris and peelings, especially in clothing, towels, and floor coverings.

Generalized cutaneous eruptions, resulting from sensitivity reactions, may occur. These are known as 'dermatophytids' or simply 'ids'.

### CLINICAL PICTURE

1. *Tinea pedis*

Fungal infection of the feet. Athlete's foot: foot rot: ringworm of the feet: epidermophytosis. This is probably the most widespread of all fungal infections. It may occur also on the hands. It is practically impossible to escape in the tropics. The lesions are at their worst in the hot, moist seasons and improve in the cooler weather. They are more severe in individuals who are constantly on their feet, especially if sweating freely and wearing badly ventilated boots or shoes. Infection is spread by contact of bare feet with communal bathroom floors, towels, etc.

The lesions begin most commonly between toes, especially between the fourth and fifth. They start as itchy erythematous areas over which vesicles appear and rupture. The affected skin rapidly becomes white and oedematous; the uppermost layers separate and peeling and cracking occurs, revealing a reddened hyperaemic thinly epithelialized base, which may ulcerate, crack, and bleed. The dead, sodden epithelium exfoliates and is replaced by new layers which in turn undergo the same process. The acute lesions are tender, painful, and smelly.

The dorsum of the foot and the plantar skin may eventually be involved.

Secondary infection is almost always present and pustules may form with oedema of the surrounding tissues. Sometimes there may be rapidly developing cellulitis, lymphangitis with adenitis, and generalized septicaemia.

In long-standing cases the lesions become papulosquamous and hyperkeratotic with considerable scaling on a thickened, sometimes mildly erythematous background. Vesicles and pustules are absent except for occasional exacerbations of the lesions between the toes. These changes in the skin appear most commonly on the plantar surface across the arch proximal to the toes, along the sides of the foot and on the heel. Such lesions seldom cause discomfort and may be unnoticed. Their development may, however, be associated with exacerbations of the original lesions between the toes.

The activity of the latter varies considerably from time to time. The epidermis between the toes is usually swollen, white, sodden, and macerated. From time to time the dead, smelly epithelium peels away revealing the moist, reddened base. Painful fissuring, especially in the web of the toes, is common. Sweating between the toes is usually excessive especially when the patient is wearing leather shoes.

After the subsidence of the acute phase the infection tends to persist for many years unless adequately treated, exacerbations occurring from time to time, especially during the hot season.

*Diagnosis.* This is made by clinical inspection and examination of scrapings from active lesions macerated in 10–20 per cent potassium hydroxide solution which will reveal mycelia or spores (see p. 120).

*Treatment.* The infection responds well to treatment. Mild lesions will heal in a few days. Weeks may be needed in more chronic cases. A few cases may be very refractory and reinfection from previously infected shoes, socks, floors, etc., is common.

Treatment of the immediate lesions must be combined with manoeuvres designed to minimize the chances of reinfection.

*Local treatment.* In acute lesions, preliminary local treatment designed to reduce secondary infection is the first step. The toes should be kept apart by gauze or cotton wool and dusted with aseptic powder between treatments, which should be carried out once or twice a day.

The foot should be bathed in warm permanganate solution (1 in 4000) or other antiseptic solutions and thoroughly dried. As much as possible of the dead epithelium between the toes and elsewhere should be removed with a rough towel. The affected area may then be painted with Castellani's paint or alcoholic gentian violet solution. There are now many efficient and less painful proprietary fungicides. On the whole, a watery or alcoholic vehicle is preferable to an oily one, since the latter, as it melts, may sometimes carry infected material to the adjacent epithelium.

*Oral treatment* with the antibiotic Griseofulvin is usually very successful. The adult dose is 0.5–1.0 g daily for 3–4 weeks or longer. The dosage for children is based on 15 mg per kg body weight up to the adult dose. Side effects are mild and uncommon. Skin rashes and fall of leucocyte count have been recorded.

Over-vigorous treatment should be avoided as it may be followed by exacerbations of local lesions or the appearance of generalized dermatophytids.

Hyperkeratotic scaling lesions are best treated with keratolytic ointments, such as Castellani's paint. Treatment should be continued for some time after local lesions have apparently healed.

*Preventive measures* include frequent changes of socks, which should be boiled during washing, and attempts to keep the feet dry, including limitation of exercise and the use of well-ventilated and easily sterilized sandals instead of shoes. The use of personal towels only and the avoidance of walking barefoot in likely infective places such as floors and baths are very important. The feet, especially the interdigital spaces, should be dusted at frequent intervals with aseptic powder, containing 10–15 per cent calcium propionate.

### 2. *Tinea unguium*

Fungus infection of the nails usually occurs in individuals already infected with fungus elsewhere, particularly in the hands and feet. The infection develops slowly and is chronic and often extremely resistant to treatment. The toe nails are more frequently affected than finger nails.

The affected nails are discoloured, thickened and friable. The distal edges tear easily and large portions may flake off, revealing cheesy epithelial detritus beneath. The surface of the nails is dull, pitted, and scored. The skin at the edges of the nails is often involved and shows active inflammatory reactions from time to time.

*Diagnosis.* (See p. 120.)

*Treatment.* The combination of oral Griseofulvin and local treatment is usually effective. The response to local treatment is poor and there is no tendency to spontaneous recovery. As much as possible of the affected nail and underlying detritus should be removed. The nail should be filed daily to paper thinness and the part immersed in permanganate solution (1 in 4000) for half an hour each day. After thorough drying, sulphur or salicyclic ointments should be rubbed in gently. Surgical evulsion or X-ray therapy may be necessary.

### 3. *Tinea cruris*

Dhobie itch: groin or body ringworm. Tinea cruris is found in the groin, crutch, perineum, or perineal regions. Similar lesions may appear in other areas, including the axillae and the folds beneath the breasts. It may be caused by several fungi. It commonly appears first on the inner aspects of the thighs and spreads rapidly to the perineum or scrotum and anal cleft. The lesions may eventually involve large areas of skin, which become reddened, rough, and scaling. The advancing serpiginous edge is sharply defined, often raised, and may be papular or pustular. The older lesions are flat, scaly, and often brownish and discoloured in white skins.

The lesion is intensely itchy and irritating and involuntary scratching commonly leads to secondary infection. It may be so painful and uncomfortable as to interfere with walking, the patient proceeding on a broad base with legs well apart.

*Diagnosis* is usually obvious from inspection. Scrapings reveal fungal mycelia and spores (see p. 120).

*Treatment.* Griseofulvin orally combined with local treatment is usually effective. The lesions should be cleaned with soap and water.

In the acute stage permanganate baths should be given twice a day, followed after thorough drying by aqueous gentian violet solution (1 per cent) and calamine lotion. In more chronic cases Castellani's paint, or 4 per cent gentian violet in 10 per cent alcohol, followed by 10–15 per cent calcium

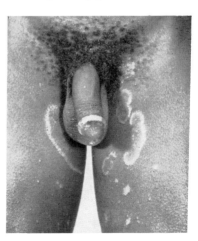

Fig. 16. Tinea cruris.

propionate dusting powder will usually promote healing in a few weeks. Tincture of iodine is an old remedy which is effective but severe and should be used only under medical supervision. If any treatment excites an acute exacerbation it should be temporarily stopped. As in *Tinea pedis* infections, many proprietary compounds are successful and more easily tolerated.

Treatment should be continued for at least 1 week after the disappearance of the lesions.

Local treatment should always be combined with precautions against reinfection which should include frequent changes of light underwear which will stand boiling.

### 4. *Tinea corporis*
Tinea circinata: body ringworm. Small, well-defined annular erythematous papulosquamous lesions, varying in size from 0.5 to 5 cm wide, appear on any part of the body. They may be single or multiple and may coalesce to cover areas of skin several inches across. The central region is reddish and scaling; the advancing edge is elevated, vesicular, and sometimes pustular. Old standing lesions may show thickening of the skin and hyperkeratosis. The intervening skin is normal.

The infection may be acquired from animals. It is commoner in children than adults.

*Treatment.* Griseofulvin is effective. The lesions are cleaned with soap and water twice daily. After drying, ammoniated mercury ointment (5 per cent) or sulphur-salicylic ointment (each 3 per cent) is rubbed in thoroughly. Tincture of iodine may also be used. Many modern proprietary compounds are successful.

### 5. *Tinea imbricata*
Scaly ringworm. This condition is seen particularly in south China, Sri Lanka, South Africa, South and Central America, and the South Pacific Islands. The lesions may be widespread over the body and are composed essentially of superficial, slightly elevated, closely set concentric rings of dry scaling skin which coalesce to form serpiginous patterns. Diffuse eruptions in chronic cases have the appearance of ichthyosis. Diagnosis is obvious on inspection.

*Treatment.* Whitfield's ointment and Castellani's paint or 10 per cent chrysarobin ointment are indicated twice daily. Response to local treatment is slow and poor. Griseofulvin orally is indicated.

### 6. *Pityriasis versicolor*
Tinea versicolor. A superficial fungal infection commonly seen in poorer sections of the populations of many tropical areas. The most superficial layers of the skin are involved. There is little inflammation but considerable furfuraceous scaling. In light skins the skin pigment in the lesion is deepened; in dark skins it is lightened. The lesions occur as macules which vary in size from

about a millimetre to several centimetres across and frequently coalesce. They are most commonly seen on the neck, shoulders and outer aspects of the arms. They are rarely found on the abdomen.

Superficial lesions with a white powdery scaly surface occurring in the common areas of distribution are diagnostic. The mycelia and characteristic grape-like clusters of spores may be discovered on examination of scrapings from the lesions.

*Treatment.* Cleansing with soap and water, followed by any mild fungicidal application, is usually rapidly successful.

### 7. Infections of the hair and scalp

Hair included in an area infected with fungus will often undergo changes, becoming lustreless and brittle. Areas of alopecia are common when fungus infection occurs in the scalp.

Infections around the beard hairs may lead to an appearance very similar to pyogenic sycosis barbae. Diagnosis is made by discovery of the causative organism. Treatment consists in shaving daily and the application of permanganate or other antiseptic solutions, removal of infected hairs, and the use of 5 per cent ammoniated mercury ointment or 10 per cent sodium propionate in alcohol. X-ray therapy for depilation may be required in resistant cases.

### Tinea capitis

A fungal infection of the scalp which occurs in childhood and disappears after puberty. It begins as an erythematous papule through which passes a hair. The papules spread peripherally and coalesce. The hair becomes very brittle, splits and can be easily pulled out. Scattered patches of alopecia develop. Itching is intense and leads by scratching to secondary infection.

The infection is highly contagious. It occurs most commonly in poorer classes living in overcrowded conditions. It may be spread originally from cats and dogs.

*Treatment* is usually rapidly effective. Griseofulvin should be given in the usual doses. Scales and crusts should be removed daily in soap and water. Infected areas should be covered with compresses of permanganate solution (1 in 4000) for half an hour. The head is then thoroughly dried and ammoniated mercury or sulphur-salicylic (3 per cent each) ointment rubbed in. Resistant cases are common and may need X-ray therapy.

### Tinea favosa

A fungus infection usually limited to the scalp but occasionally involving the skin and nails. It is found in filthy conditions, particularly in the Middle east.

The lesions are characteristically yellowish and have cup-shaped crusts which emit a peculiar 'mousy' odour. Beneath the crusts are depressed moist red areas. Hair in the infected area is soon lost. In untreated cases the condition may involve the whole scalp and lead to scarring and baldness.

*Treatment.* Removal of infected hairs by depilation and the application of fungicidal ointments. The results are slow but satisfactory except for scarring. Lesions due to *T. favosa* unlike those caused by *T. capitis* do not resolve with puberty. Griseofulvin should be given in the usual doses.

### 8. *Dermatophytids*

Generalized secondary sensitivity eruptions may occur in subjects infected locally with fungi. A primary lesion containing the fungus is usually present, often in the feet. Fungi are not commonly found in the secondary lesions.

These lesions are known as dermatophytids, trichophytids, or 'ids'. They usually appear during an exacerbation of the original focus of infection following trauma or overtreatment.

The fingers and hands are most commonly involved but the 'id' may be widespread over the whole body.

The commonest manifestation is the appearance of groups of tiny deep vesicles filled with clear or cloudy fluid and lying along the fingers or in the palm of the hand (so-called cheiropompholyx) or of larger superficial vesicles or scaling areas. The lesions itch intensely and scratching may lead to secondary infection with pus formation. The vesicles usually subside without bursting and are often succeeded by areas of scaling.

Occasionally there may be a generalized and itchy follicular papulovesicular eruption scattered over the back, buttocks, thighs, and palms.

*Treatment.* The reaction subsides as a rule upon treatment of the primary focus. Overtreatment of the latter may exaggerate it.

Local treatment of secondary infection is necessary.

The administration of Griseofulvin is sometimes effective; on occasion it may exacerbate the condition.

### DIAGNOSIS OF THE SKIN FUNGI

Many dermatomycotic infections may be diagnosed as such by clinical inspection. The presence of fungi may be confirmed by the method described below. Detailed mycological identification of the offending fungus is a highly technical procedure.

### *Examination of epithelial scrapings and debris*

Scales and epithelial debris should be scraped with a knife from the advancing edge of the active lesion. They should be placed on a slide and mixed or macerated with a solution of 10–20 per cent potassium hydroxide. A coverslip is placed over the preparation and the slide is gently warmed. The unstained material should be examined microscopically for hyphae and spores with the 16 or 8 mm objective, with the light cut down by partial closure of the diaphragm.

For further mycological investigation the material should be scraped on to a clean slide covered with another slide and wrapped in paper or gauze for transport to a laboratory for attempted culture.

## TISSUE INFECTIONS

Mycotic infections of tissue other than skin are acquired as a result of the introduction of the agent into the tissues, usually by trauma, or following inhalation of spores.

### ACTINOMYCOSIS

Infection with *Actinomycetes*, an organism possessing many of the properties of bacteria is still regarded conventionally as lying within the range of mycological agents. It causes several clinical forms of disease, including cervicofacial, dermal, abdominal and pulmonary. The lesions produced are usually suppurative and may communicate with the surface by sinuses, exuding pus-containing granules which under the microscope show meshed filaments and radial clubbed striations.

The infection commonly causes sarcoma-like, tender, firm swellings of the jaw, often along the angle, and the neck. There are usually areas of softening, in which abscesses form, giving rise to multiple sinuses. Similar swellings may occur in the subcutaneous tissues in any part of the body, either alone or in association with sinus formation from deeper lesions. These dermal lesions also form sinuses and may discharge characteristic yellow 'sulphur' granules.

Unilateral or bilateral lesions may develop slowly in the lungs, usually in the bases, producing a syndrome resembling pulmonary tuberculosis or neoplasm, with irregular remittent fever, cough, and sometimes haemoptysis. In the later stages there is wasting with fever and purulent expectoration. The pleural cavity is invaded and the periosteum of the rib cage may be involved. The lesion may penetrate through sinuses to the surface.

In the abdomen lesions occur most commonly in the caecum and appendix. There is commonly a slow-growing mass in the right iliac fossa, with local pain and tenderness, and general signs including fever. The infection tends to spread to the peritoneum, sometimes to the liver and to the abdominal wall; the latter may produce sinuses which penetrate to the surface.

Diagnosis is made by examination of pus or other material obtained on biopsy. The characteristic branching filaments and granules are diagnostic. Culture is difficult, but is the only certain way of identifying the agent.

### MYCETOMA

*Mycetoma pedis*, or Madura foot, is a condition due to infection of tissue with fungal organisms belonging to species of several genera of the true fungi

Maduromycetes (*Nocardia asteroides, Streptomyces madurae*) and the Actino-mycetes (*Madurella mycetomii*). These organisms are normally free-living saprophytes. On establishment in man they cause a localized and chronic progressive granulomatosis, commonly in the foot, with ultimate destruction of the affected tissues and the formation of numerous discharging sinuses.

Cases of mycetoma pedis have been reported widely throughout the tropical and subtropical parts of all the continents. They are most prevalent in the tropics.

The causative organisms are found in soil and on rotting wood and vegetation. Puncture of the skin of man results in the introduction of the organism, which can establish itself and multiply locally in the human tissues, destroying them in the process. The infection does not spread from one patient to another. According to the species, the discharges produced contain small granules coloured red, yellow, black, or grey; the granules may be seen in the discharge from multiple sinuses in the affected part and colour the tissues around the sinuses, giving rise to so-called black or white Madura foot.

Mycetoma is a localized and not a systemic disease. A common first indication of its presence is the appearance of a small rounded painless

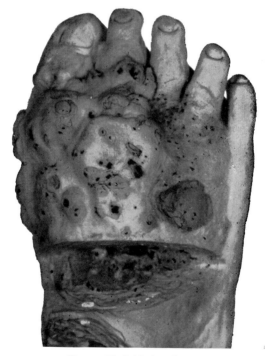

FIG. 17. Black Madura foot.

[By courtesy of *British Encyclopaedia of Medical Practice,* Butterworth & Co. (Publishers) Ltd., London.]

swelling, usually on the dorsum or on the sole of the foot, more rarely on the hands and face. The swelling enlarges peripherally over many months or years until there is an irregular rounded mass extending throughout the tissues of the affected part. At any time during this development, but commonly within 3 months, sinuses develop from the deeper parts of the lesion through the skin to the exterior. From these exudes a viscid, oily, foul-smelling discharge containing amorphous necrotic material and visible mycelial granules; these granules may be hard or soft and coloured according to the species of fungus responsible. Superimposed bacterial infection may cause the discharge from some sinuses to be purulent; as a rule the discharge is not great in amount and contains few pus cells.

By the time the whole of the foot is involved a large tumour is formed riddled with areas of necrosis and abscess formation; these communicate with each other and to the exterior by innumerable sinuses. The foot becomes club-shaped and useless, but is painless unless secondarily infected. The lymphatic channels and glands draining the area are unaffected, except when there is gross secondary bacterial infection.

The inconvenience caused by the useless swollen foot, and the consequences of secondary bacterial infection, greatly debilitate the patient.

In cases of superficial implantation of an infection with less infiltrative species of fungi, for example on the dorsum of the foot, there may be a localized increasing swelling resembling a ganglion, without deeper invasion of the tissues or fistulation.

There is no invariably succesful specific drug treatment. Surgical extirpation of the whole of the fungus-infected tissues is the only certain cure. In practice this usually means amputation through healthy tissue. Before resorting to this drastic procedure drugs should be given over long periods. *Diaminodiphenyl sulphone* (DDS), the staple of chemotherapy in leprosy, is fungiostatic and is sometimes useful in high doses (100–200 mg daily for 1–2 years). It is given by local infiltration, or by irrigation into the sinuses, and concurrently by mouth; temporary clinical improvement may also come from penicillin or broad-spectrum antibiotics, especially the tetracyclines, streptomycin or both, which also deal with local secondary infections.

### OTHER FUNGAL TISSUE INFECTIONS

Many other fungal infections occur. These are often of world-wide distribution, but are more common in the tropics or subtropics, sometimes in special regions. Some are discussed below.

*Skin and subcutaneous tissues*
    *Chromoblastomycosis* (verrucous dermatitis) is a chronic infection of the skin and subcutaneous tissue caused by three pigmented fungi, and characterized by warty lesions, usually in the legs, which may encrust and ulcerate.

The lesion begins as a papule at the site of introduction (an injury) and extends slowly as a granuloma develops containing micro-abscesses, in which the brown, thick-walled cells of the fungus may be found. Satellite lesions are common. Diagnosis is made by finding the fungal cells in biopsy or skin scrapings. Surgical removal is required.

*Rhinosporidiosis* (caused by infection with *Rhinosporidium seeberi*, which has not yet been cultured) develops as localized chronic granulomatous lesions usually in the nose, eyes, ears, and larynx and occasionally the vagina, rectum, and penis, appearing first as soft pink polyps, which become irregularly covered with grey areas of fungal cells containing spores. These lesions develop very slowly in the mucosa, to form vascular pedunculated polyps which give rise to obstruction of the nasal passages, the lachrymal ducts or pharynx, and may resemble mucocutaneous leishmaniasis.

Lesions in the genital organs and rectum (usually in males) resemble condylomata. Diagnosis depends on identifying in biopsy material the fungal cells containing the spores. Surgical excision of early lesions is sometimes successful. Later lesions may be cauterized.

*Phycomycosis* is a subcutaneous infection (with the fungus *Basidiobolus ranarum*) which develops as a slowly spreading rubbery subcutaneous induration which does not ulcerate. It occurs in West Africa, notably Ghana and Nigeria, and has been reported in parts of East Africa and India. The mode of infection is unknown. The lesions are caused by chronic inflammatory reaction associated with the broad fungal hyphae; there are numerous eosinophils and eosinophilic debris about the fungus. They may occur anywhere on the body, particularly on the limbs. The disease appears to be self-limited; it may respond to iodide therapy.

DEEP TISSUES

Certain fungus infections are primarily of respiratory origin. They may involve the lungs and metastasize to other tissues.

*Nocardiosis* may cause single pulmonary lesions or involve both lungs, producing irregular pneumonitis, sometimes with cavitation resembling tuberculosis. Extension to the chest wall may occur as in actinomycosis, but with less extension to contiguous tissues and less formation of sinuses; pus does not commonly contain 'sulphur' granules, as in actinomycosis. Dissemination may lead to granuloma and abscess formation in the brain, spleen, liver and other organs. Diagnosis is made by finding the long branching filaments of *N. asteroides* in sputum or pus. These are lightly acid fast and may be confused with *Mycobacteria*. The infection responds slowly to sulphonamides and streptomycin.

*Histoplasmosis* is caused by the fungus *Histoplasma capsulatum* and usually begins as a mild pulmonary lesion which may remain inapparent or occasionally extend as pneumonitis with cavitation resembling tuberculosis.

The infection is acquired by inhaling dust containing spores. Granulomata are produced in which the macrophage cells contain the very small 'yeast bodies' which are easily mistaken for *Leishmania*. There is widespread reticuloendothelial dissemination commonly with hepatosplenomegaly and mucocutaneous ulcerating lesions which closely resemble those of mucocutaneous leishmaniasis. In diagnosis a positive skin sensitivity reaction, using *histoplasmin* antigen, indicates past or present infection. In smears of biopsy material the presence of the small 'yeast' cells, usually intracellular, indicates the diagnosis which can be confirmed by culture. Amphotericin B has been used for treatment in doses of 0.1 rising to 1 mg per kg body weight intravenously in solution in 5 per cent glucose on alternate days for periods of 45–70 days. This drug is toxic (see p. 184).

South American *Blastomycosis* caused by a diphasic fungus, *Paracoccidiodes braziliensis,* produces chronic granulomatous lesions in the mucous membranes of the mouth and nose with local lymphatic node invasion and often considerable enlargement and metastasis to other tissues. The disease, which is fatal if not treated, occurs in South and Central America where the organism is found in the soil. The portal of entry is usually the mouth or nose and respiratory tract, sometimes the perianal region in areas where leaves are used for toilet following defaecation. The early lesions appear at the mucocutaneous junctions of the mouth, nose and conjunctivae, sometimes the anus. They form growing granulomata which eventually ulcerate. A common clinical picture is one of swollen bleeding ulcerated gums and loosened teeth, oedema and ulceration of the lips and pharynx. The lesions may closely resemble those of mucocutaneous leishmaniasis. There is frequently enlargement of the local lymph glands; in children involvement of abdominal glands may occur with signs suggestive of abdominal tuberculosis. Enlarged hilar glands and granulomata in the lungs may also suggest tuberculosis. Adrenal function may be disturbed, leading to a picture resembling Addison's disease. Secondary skin lesions may occur. The 'yeast' cells can be found in pus and biopsy material taken from lesions. Amphotericin B is the most effective drug for therapy. Relapses are common.

*Aspergillosis* is a fungus infection which does not occur primarily but is sometimes superimposed on other infections or lesions, notably in the lungs, especially in bronchitis, tuberculosis, and asthmatic patients. The sputum is commonly purulent, with many eosinophils; the fungus can be cultured from it. Amphotericin B administered intravenously is the treatment of choice.

# 9

# THE HAEMOGLOBINOPATHIES AND GLUCOSE-6-PHOSPHATE DEHYDROGENASE DEFICIENCY

## (Contributed by H.M.Gilles)

### INTRODUCTION

Certain hereditary anaemias are associated with abnormalities of haemoglobin. This group of anaemias includes thalassaemia and certain diseases, of which sickle cell anaemia (or sicklaemia) is a notable example, in which the protein fraction of the haemoglobin molecule differs from that of normal haemoglobin.

Electrophoretic separation of haemoglobins has identified many forms, each of which has been labelled by a capital alphabetical letter. Thus, normal adult haemoglobin is called Haemoglobin A; foetal haemoglobin, Haemoglobin F; sickle haemoglobin, Haemoglobin S; and the letters, C, D, E, H, I, J, L, M, N, and others have been allotted.

The synthesis of each abnormal haemoglobin is controlled by a specific gene which is usually an allele of the gene responsible for the production of normal haemoglobin. The genes are transmitted as Mendelian dominants. Thus, for each haemoglobin there are two possible inherited combinations. For instance, a child receiving the Haemoglobin S gene from both parents is in the homozygous state, SS. A child receiving the S gene from one parent only is heterozygous, AS.

Each haemoglobin is associated either with a homozygous 'disease' or a heterozygous 'trait'. The disease is always more serious clinically than the trait. The heterozygous trait of one haemoglobin may also be associated in the same individual with the heterozygous trait of another; such combinations may sometimes produce severe clinical effects, for example, SC.

There is evidence that the possession of the sickle gene affords protection against *P. falciparum* malaria. This may explain the very high incidence of this gene in some areas of Africa.

In the normal subject the haemoglobin is mostly in the form of Haemoglobin A, with small fractions of $A_2$; the remainder is Haemoglobin F, the alkali-resistant foetal haemoglobin. At birth about 80 per cent of haemoglobin is F; at 6 months only 5 per cent; in adult life not more than 2.5 per cent.

In the haemoglobinopathies all the pigment may be abnormal (in the form of one abnormal haemoglobin, for example, homozygous SS, or sometimes in more than one form, for example SC) or a mixture of normal and abnormal, for example AS.

The more important clinical conditions are described below.

## SICKLE CELL ANAEMIA OR HAEMOGLOBIN S DISEASE

Sickle cell anaemia occurs in the homozygous state SS in which the haemoglobin is nearly all Haemoglobin S, the remainder being F. In the homozygous individual there is no Haemoglobin A.

### PATHOLOGY

Relatively slight reduction in oxygen tension causes Haemoglobin S to crystallize, so contorting the erythrocyte into the characteristic sickle shape. The sickling leads to intravascular stasis and occlusion, increasing blood viscosity, and varying degrees of local ischaemia and anoxia, associated with infarction, thrombosis, degeneration, necrosis, and haemorrhage. Intravascular haemolysis occurs, together with active erythrophagocytosis and impedance of local circulation resulting from the sickling, thrombosis, and embolism. These processes may proceed in any organ.

The changes found in the organs are basically due to these pathogenic processes, the final pattern being determined by the functional and anatomical

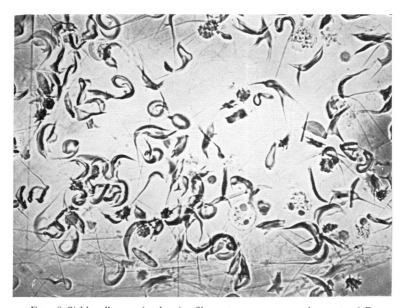

FIG. 18. Sickle cell anaemia, showing filamentous processes, 12 hours at 37° C.

damage achieved. Thus, infarcts in local areas of tissues, haemorrhage, necrosis and sometimes ultimate fibrosis can occur in any part of the body, including the spleen, liver, kidney, bone marrow, bone, gastro-intestinal tract, and the brain.

In most parts of rural Africa homozygotes seldom live beyond the early years of life. In those that survive to later years, the intermittent impairment of tissue blood flow results in some organs in the gradual replacement of the parenchyma by fibrous tissue. The spleen, for instance, is enlarged and congested in early life, with the pulp packed with sickled cells and the sinuses compressed to 'tiny chinks in a sea of red blood cells'. The Malpighian corpuscles are compressed and inconspicuous, and there are scattered areas of peri-follicular haemorrhages; later, following infarct, necrosis and fibrosis, the organ becomes smaller and the architecture is lost and replaced by dense bundles of fibrous tissue enmeshed in which are areas of iron-containing brown pigment, sometimes enclosed within a giant-cell reaction. The small 'siderofibrotic' spleen seen in these cases is unique to sickle cell anaemia. It may ultimately be much smaller than normal.

The liver is usually large and congested even in adults, with cellular infiltration of the portal tracts and scattered centrilobular and focal necrosis of the parenchymal cells. The sinusoids are congested and dilated and may contain sickled erythrocytes enmeshed in a fine fibrin network. Erythrophago-cytosis by the Kupffer cells is prominent.

Emboli may affect the pulmonary vessels and commonly involve the bones, especially the head of the femur (causing focal necrosis), other long bones and the bones of the skull. In the latter, changes commonly develop due to the intensely vascular marrow hyperplasia. The medullary area between the tables is widened and a combination of cortical thinning, erosion and new bone formation leads to extensive bossing which gives a characteristic look to the head and the 'hair-on-end' X-ray shadow.

Except during aplastic crises, the bone marrow exhibits active normoblas-tic erythropoietic hyperplasia. Nucleated erythrocytes and reticulocytes are common in the peripheral blood.

The blood is similar in appearance to that in other haemolytic orthochro-mic anaemias. Sickling occurs rapidly in blood on removal from the body. The sickled cells adopt bizarre crescentic shapes with long filamentous processes, which are rarely seen in the trait. There is marked decrease in osmotic fragility. The sedimentation rate is raised but is usually less than would be anticipated from the anaemia.

The plasma bilirubin is increased, but frank jaundice is not always present. Other chemical changes in the blood are dependent on the prevailing damage to organ function.

Most of the haemoglobin is Haemoglobin S. Haemoglobin F may comprise as much as 30 per cent but in older children and adults its concentration falls to about 5 per cent.

CLINICAL PICTURE

Sickle cell anaemia usually becomes clinically evident about the third to sixth month of life, starting mildly but evolving rapidly. In rural areas of Africa mortality is still very high in the first 3 years, but in the West Indies and in Saudi Arabia prolonged survival in SS disease is common. In Saudi Arabia the disease is rendered benign because of the ability in the oasis Arabs to produce large amounts of foetal haemoglobin.

In infants and young children the initial anaemia is not very severe. Between 6 months and 2 years of age, however, it becomes progressively worse. Crises during which the haemoglobin drops sharply to 2–5 g per cent are common, especially in the second 6 months of life and may be fatal. These episodes are usually accompanied by fever, which is seldom high. Mild jaundice is common, with discoloration of the sclerae and deeply coloured urine.

The spleen becomes moderately enlarged and palpable and the liver less so. Great enlargement of these organs is rare at this stage but there is usually further increase in size during the haemolytic crisis associated with local tenderness.

Acute painful swellings of the bones of the hands and feet or of the limbs occur at intervals. In relevant areas in the tropics it is a good maxim to regard 'rheumatism' in an anaemic African child as due to sickle cell disease until the contrary is proved.

Those who survive beyond the age of 2 usually live on for some years in indifferent health. The child is more often ill than well, with a history of frequent bouts of fever or painful bones or joints. Haemolytic crises occur at intervals and may be fatal. A moderate degree of anaemia, for example 9–10 g haemoglobin per cent, persists in between the crises. Occasional episodes of mild jaundice may occur; some children remain persistently jaundiced. Haemolytic crises may be accompanied by very severe jaundice. Splenomegaly is not usually marked, although in some cases it may be notable and persistent and give rise to the syndrome of hypersplenism. Indeed, as the child gets older, the spleen may recede until it is no longer palpable. The liver may remain palpable. During crises there may be pain and tenderness over these organs. Limb pains, especially in the hands and feet, are persistent and may be incapacitating. From time to time acute exacerbations with local swellings over bones or joints may occur. Chronic leg ulceration is the greatest single determinant of morbidity in SS disease in Jamaica, increasing with age to affect 75 per cent of patients. Radiological evidence of gall-stones is found in 28 per cent of adult patients.

Death follows a haemolytic crisis or may result from intercurrent infection.

Adolescent children and young adults may be found to have homozygous sickle anaemia. They usually present a long history of poor health and repeated crises, but occasionally there may be no obvious history of previous attacks.

At this stage the appearance is usually that of a thin underdeveloped asthenic individual with long thin limbs, delicate hands and feet, and poorly developed secondary sexual characters. Limb pains are often very severe. Transient arthropathies occur in some patients, making the picture (apart from the anaemia) not unlike that of acute rheumatism.

Haemolytic crises occur, but are less common and tend to be less severe than those in earlier age groups. In between crises, the anaemia remains at a moderate level, the haemoglobin concentration falling considerably during the crises and returning to its previous level, but not to normal, after recovery from the haemolytic attack.

Mild jaundice is common and may be constant. The spleen may or may not be palpable; occasionally it may be considerably enlarged especially in individuals who are suffering from frequent or severe haemolytic crises.

In rural Africa, where very few individuals survive to the third decade of life, the disease becomes less severe with increasing age.

Certain points need emphasis.

The common blood picture is that of a normocytic or slightly macrocytic orthochromic anaemia, with a haemoglobin concentration of 5–8 g per 100 ml. The thin film shows a great increase in nucleated erythrocytes, polychromasia associated with up to 20 per cent reticulocytosis and, in certain cases, some macrocytes. Sickle cells are commonly seen in the film as elongate, slightly curved, 'cigar'-shaped cells. 'Target' cells are usually present in variable numbers.

There is frequently a mild leucocytosis of up to 20,000 cells or more per mm$^3$, with a shift to the left in the neutrophils.

The bone marrow shows a very active normoblastic erythropoiesis. Sickled cells are common. In some cases megaloblastic erythropoiesis also occurs, associated with folic acid deficiency.

Haemolytic crises with precipitate fall in haemoglobin concentration occur in practically all cases. The erythrocyte count drops to low figures, for example 1.0–2.0 million cells per mm$^3$, and there is nearly always evidence of intense bone marrow activity, resulting in the appearance of many reticulocytes and nucleated cells in the peripheral blood. Crises occur more frequently in infants in whom they may be the earliest clinical sign. They vary in severity but may be fatal at any age. Crises are accompanied by fever and some degree of jaundice, which may become severe with bilirubin in the urine and deviation of standard liver function tests. The liver and spleen may enlarge during the crisis and become painful and tender. Severe exacerbations of bone and joint pains are common.

Bone changes are common and repeated in infants. They become less frequent in older children and adults. Clinically there is local swelling, heat and oedema over the affected part, appearing rapidly, reaching a maximum in a week or so and usually subsiding without treatment in a few weeks, some-times with residual thickening and tenderness, sometimes with complete resolution. In the active stage there is fever and very severe local pain. Common sites affected are one or more of the metacarpals or metatarsals, or the fingers. The long bones, especially radius and ulna, the tibia, and the fibula, are more often involved in older children. The affected bones show increase in periosteal bone and rarefaction of the medulla: in older children permanent irregularities of periosteal bone are common. Necrosis may occur, for instance in the head of the femur or in the acetabulum. Spontaneous fractures may occur and coarsening of the trabeculae, thinning of the cortex and lines of arrested bony growth are often seen. It is thought that these changes arise from thrombosis of the local vessels and associated necrosis of areas of bone. When suppuration occurs *Salmonella* organisms are often

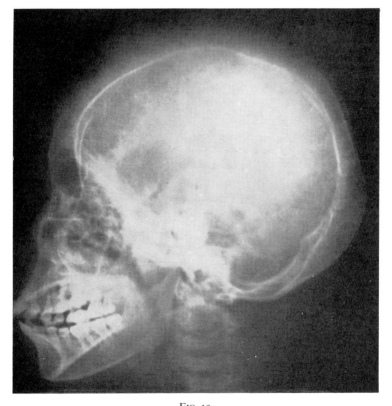

FIG. 19

Skull changes in thalassaemia: Haemoglobin E disease.

The inner table is relatively unaffected. The outer table is expanded. Note the 'hair-on-end' effect.

[Courtesy of Dr Na-Nakorn, Sirriraj Hospital, Bangkok]

recovered from the pus; there is good evidence that patients with sickle cell anaemia are liable to salmonella osteitis. Pneumococcal septicaemia and renal failure are other serious complications. In Jamaica, a syndrome of sudden splenic enlargement, a fall in total haemoglobin level, and peripheral circulatory failure—acute splenic sequestration—is a common and serious manifestation of early life in SS disease.

Characteristic changes are seen in the skull bones. 'Bossing' of the bones, especially the frontal temporal and occipital, is common by the age of 12–18 months. The outer table is thinned; there is gross widening of the bones, the medullary space being filled with fine vertical bony spicules, giving a 'hair-on-end' appearance. The inner table is unaffected. Comparable changes may occur in vertebrae. The changes are believed to be due to the increased vascularity of the over-active bone marrow. Protrusion of the jaw and teeth sometimes occurs, and limb girdle-tattoo is common in adult sickle-cell disease in Ghana.

Changes in joints also occur, especially in adolescents, in whom there may be small effusions and associated periarticular inflammatory reactions.

Cardiac dilatation may occur, usually after the age of infancy. Chronic cardiac failure sometimes occurs in cases with persistent severe anaemia. Acute circulatory collapse may develop during a haemolytic crisis. Unilateral or bilateral haematuria also occurs.

In some regions, for instance in West Africa, older cases sometimes complain of severe upper abdominal pain, with vomiting, low fever, and hepatic and splenic tenderness. This syndrome probably results from vascular abdominal crises. It occurs also in double heterozygous sickle states, for example SC disease.

*The presentation of an acute abdomen in an anaemic child in the relevant tropics should bring to mind the possibility of sickle cell disease and laparotomy should not be undertaken until this possibility has been excluded.*

'Sickling crises' which have also been reported in adults in West Africa, in which the spleen enlarges suddenly with violent local pain and tenderness, may also occur in mixed S haemoglobinopathies.

Coma, convulsions, retinal haemorrhages, and various sudden neurological pictures including hemiplegia have been reported in sickle anaemia. Involvement of the nervous system is, however, relatively uncommon.

## SICKLE CELL TRAIT

The sickle cell trait occurs in the heterozygote, in whom half or less of the circulating haemoglobin is Haemoglobin S, the rest being normal Haemoglobin A.

In most individuals, sickling does not commonly take place in the blood *in vivo*, but it may be demonstrated *in vitro*. Under suitable hypoxic conditions, for instance during flight at high altitudes, some intravascular sickling with its concomitant pathological effects may occur if a relatively high proportion of the haemoglobin is Haemoglobin S. Unilateral haematuria and microinfarcts in the pulmonary and cerebral vessels have been reported. Under such circumstances it may initially be difficult clinically to distinguish between a heterozygote and a homozygote with sickle cell disease, but as a rule the former lives a normal life unaffected by his abnormal haemoglobin, unless some other heterozygous gene is also present (see below).

The sickle cell trait protects the individual against the lethal effects of *P. falciparum* malaria and thus confers an advantage which is reflected in malaria endemic areas by a high incidence of the gene in the population. It has been shown that parasitization of an A/S erythrocyte by *P. falciparum* increases substantially its probability to sickle (possibly due to loss of potassium ions from the cells) and it has been suggested that parasitized cells, once sickled, will be removed more effectively from the circulation by phagocytosis, thus providing a mechanism whereby A/S heterozygotes are at a selective advantage against falciparum malaria.

## HETEROZYGOUS HAEMOGLOBIN S 'DISEASES'

The homozygous disease (sickle cell anaemia) has been described above. The heterozygous trait may also become clinically important in individuals who

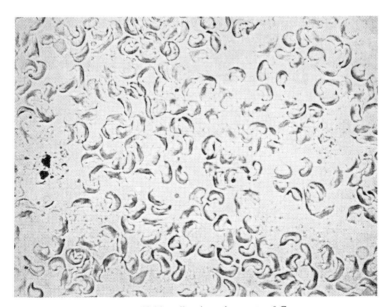

FIG. 20. Sickle-cell trait, 30 hours at 37° C.

[Courtesy of *Transactions of the Royal Society of Tropical Medicine and Hygiene*, London and Dr H.Foy]

are heterozygous to other abnormal haemoglobin genes. The combinations of Haemoglobin S: $\beta$ Thalassaemia and Haemoglobin S: Haemoglobin C are the most important of these conditions. For instance, the pathological processes and the clinical picture of SC disease are similar in some respects to those in SS anaemia; except that they are milder and, in the former, iron deposition in the tissues is minimal, suggesting a less potent haemolysis.

Arthralgia, especially of the shoulder and hips, is one of the commonest presentations of SC disease. Occasionally unilateral renal haematuria occurs. Vitreous haemorrhage is common. The most serious manifestations of SC disease are seen in pregnancy where sudden fatal haemolytic crises may occur. SC disease in pregnancy is commonly associated with folic acid deficiency.

*Diagnosis of conditions associated with Haemoglobin S*
Diagnosis of sickle cell anaemia is made by a study of the familial, racial, and geographical history of the patient and the clinical examination, by discovering evidence of the haemolytic anaemia, by the demonstration of sickling and by analysis of the prevailing haemoglobins. Sickle cell anaemia can now be diagnosed at birth by appropriate laboratory techniques.

The presence of a haemolytic anaemia is determined by examination of thin blood films and marrow smears. The thin film reveals the characteristic picture described above. The marrow shows active erythropoiesis.

The clinical picture of the anaemic retarded child, especially when suffering from chronic joint or bone pains, is highly suggestive in appropriate geographical areas. The possibility of Haemoglobin S disease or SC disease must be excluded in Africans complaining of 'rheumatism', presenting with osteomyelitis or with acute abdominal signs.

Sickling is rapid in sickle anaemia. Most cells are involved. The sickled cells are thin and crescentic with filamentous 'tails'; in the trait only a proportion of cells sickle, sickling is slow and the sickled cells are blunt and leaf-shaped.

Methods of demonstrating sickling are as follows:

*Reducing agent*
Make up a 2.0 per cent solution of sodium metabisulphite in freshly distilled water. Take up a small volume of the solution in a Pasteur pipette and suck in about one-sixth of the volume of blood. Blow on to a clean slide, mix thoroughly, and cover with a coverslip. Examine for sickling under 8 mm objective. Sickling will show in 3–15 minutes. If there is none after 30 minutes the test is probably negative.

The above rapid method gives quick results in both asymptomatic trait and sickle cell anaemia. In the slow technique described below, blood from sickle cell anaemia usually shows sickling long before blood from a carrier of the trait.

*Moist stasis technique*

A drop of blood (usually from a finger which has been congested for a few minutes) is picked up on the under surface of a clean coverslip which is placed on a clean slide. The coverslip is ringed with petroleum jelly and the preparation is examined microscopically after 48–72 hours. Cells from cases of sickle cell anaemia often begin sickling at once in such a preparation. Cells from carriers of sickle cell trait change only slowly.

In vivo *sickling*

Blood is withdrawn into a syringe containing oil and is injected into isotonic formol saline, also under oil. The erythrocytes are regarded as being fixed in the shape in which they were circulating.

*Identifying haemoglobins.* Examination of the haemoglobins is made by some form of electrophoresis, which is a purely laboratory procedure. The quantity of Haemoglobin F present can be estimated by various methods of alkali denaturation.

In sickle cell anaemia Haemoglobin S represents the bulk of pigment present, the residue being Haemoglobin F. There is no normal Haemoglobin A.

In sickle cell trait Haemoglobin S usually makes up about 50 per cent of the total haemoglobin, Haemoglobin A accounting for the remainder.

'Mixtures' of abnormal haemoglobins, such as the double heterozygous states of SC, etc., can be distinguished only by complicated electrophoretic techniques; the 'S' moiety can of course be demonstrated by ordinary methods of determining sickling.

TREATMENT

There is no specific treatment of sickle cell anaemia or the double heterozygous sickle cell 'diseases'.

Blood transfusion, with the usual precautions of cross-matching, is of great but temporary benefit during a haemolytic crisis.

Splenectomy is only useful if there is evidence of 'hypersplenism' and when no response in spleen size occurs with antimalarial therapy.

The patient should be put on to regular malarial suppression, for example, pyrimethamine 25 mg once weekly. It has been found that on such a regime the spleen reduces in size and crises are less frequent and milder. In addition, a maintenance dose of folic acid 5 mg daily is given, since many patients have some degree of deficiency. Where there is any suspicion of infection, such as local tenderness in bones or joints, a course of a wide-spectrum antibiotic, usually chloramphenicol 125 mg 6-hourly, should be given for 1–2 weeks. Because of the predisposition to salmonella infection, chloramphenicol is also indicated when there is patent osteitis or osteomyelitis.

Various agents–intravenous magnesium sulphate, plasma expanders, urea, heparin, arvin—have all been used for the treatment of sickle cell crises but conclusive evidence of their efficacy in controlled clinical trials has yet to be obtained.

Haemolytic crises in SC disease in pregnancy usually require exchange transfusion, blood transfusion coupled with large doses of intravenous frusamide or ethacrynic acid. The patient should in any case be placed on malarial suppressive therapy, for example pyrimethamine 25 mg once a week, and given orally a maintenance dose of folic acid, 5 mg daily.

Analgesics and vasodilators, for example priscoline, are useful in relieving the severe pain associated with sickle cell crises. Genetic counselling and family planning are currently being encouraged in areas where the incidence of the abnormal haemoglobinopathies is high.


## OTHER ABNORMAL HAEMOGLOBINS

Homozygotes exhibit the 'disease', i.e. CC, EE, etc. Most of these are clinically insignificant and may be discovered by accident. Haemoglobin C disease, for instance, is characterized by a mild haemolytic anaemia, an increased number of target cells visible in stained blood films, some decreased erythrocytic osmotic fragility, and pronounced enlargement of the spleen. There are no serious occlusive or embolic phenomena, such as are characteristic of SS disease (sickle cell anaemia).

Heterozygotes exhibit the 'traits' and are important only in combination with certain other heterozygous genes, notably those of Haemoglobin S or Thalassaemia.


## THALASSAEMIA SYNDROMES

The term 'Thalassaemia' includes a group of clinical conditions arising from inherited defects in haemoglobin synthesis. The main feature is defective synthesis of normal Haemoglobin A. The reduction in Haemoglobin A may be accompanied by persistence of synthesis of foetal haemoglobin (Haemoglobin F), increase in amounts of Haemoglobin $A_2$, and sometimes the presence of small amounts of Haemoglobin H or Haemoglobin Bart's. When thalassaemia coexists with other abnormal haemoglobins, notably Haemoglobin S and Haemoglobin E, the proportion of normal to abnormal haemoglobins in the subject may be disturbed. Several forms of thalassaemia exist, the most important being the common $\beta$ Thalassaemia in which the genetic defect is thought to be in the synthesis of the $\beta$ chain of haemoglobin and $\alpha$ Thalassaemia, in which the defect is in the $\alpha$ chain.

Homozygous $\beta$ Thalassaemia (Thalassaemia major, Cooley's anaemia) usually discloses itself in the first years of life. The disease may run a fulminating course in infancy or become chronic, lasting into childhood. Some cases are mild and continue into adult life. The patient is retarded mentally and physically. He fails to gain weight normally and becomes progressively anaemic, suffering from bone and joint pains and irregular bouts of fever. The skin is pale with patchy pigmentation. The spleen and liver enlarge considerably and there is chronic mild jaundice. As time goes on the facies become mongoloid as the bone changes progress, with dilation of the diploic spaces and subperiosteal laying down of new bone, usually giving a typical 'hair-on-end' appearance (see Fig. 19). The cortex of long bones and bones of the hands and feet becomes thinned and rarefied and pathological fractures are common.

Anaemia is severe. There is pronounced aniso-poikilocytosis and the erythrocytes are markedly hypochromic. Target cells are usually common. There are many nucleated red cells in the peripheral blood, some with pyknotic nuclear changes. Reticulocytes are moderately increased. Cytoplasmic inclusion bodies may be found in both the nucleated red cells and reticulocytes. Erythrocytic osmotic fragility is notably decreased. The erythrocyte half-life varies widely, suggesting that some cells (probably those containing predominantly Haemoglobin A) are rapidly destroyed, others not.

The bone marrow is hyperplastic and extramedullary haemopoiesis may develop. Iron turnover is abnormal and siderotic deposits occur in the liver which may become diffusely cirrhotic. Folic acid deficiency is common.

Patients are susceptible to infections and many die young. In those who survive to the second decade, siderosis of the myocardium may result in death from congestive heart failure.

Repeated transfusion and the use of antibiotics enable many patients to survive for years, usually without normal sexual development.

Some patients, with the same pattern of haemoglobins, show little or no clinical effects.

Heterozygous states of $\beta$ Thalassaemia (Thalassaemia minor) may vary from chronic anaemia, mild chronic jaundice, splenomegaly, and bone changes similar to, but milder than, those seen in the homozygous state (Thalassaemia major) to mild anaemia. Most frequently, however, the heterozygote shows no clinical effects and presents with minor blood changes which include a moderately raised erythrocyte count, low MCH and MCV, diminished erythrocyte saline fragility, normal erythrocyte half-life survival time, hypochromic micro-poikilocytosis with target cells, some increase in Haemoglobin $A_2$ and sometimes in Haemoglobin F.

There is a tendency to gallstone formation and chronic leg ulceration. Thalassaemia minor may evoke serious folic acid deficiency anaemia during pregnancy.

In patients heterozygous for both $\beta$ Thalassaemia and Haemoglobin S the clinical findings vary from a state closely resembling sickle cell anaemia to one with practically no overt signs. In the former there is usually little or no

Haemoglobin A; in the milder cases there may be as much as 35 per cent. Severe cases show marked anaemia with reticulocytosis, hypochromic and microcytic erythrocytes and many target cells. Sickling is easily demonstrable. Milder forms may have little or no anaemia. In all, MCV and MCH are low and osmotic fragility is reduced.

The clinical pictures seen in Haemoglobin C–Thalassaemia vary from moderate anaemia with splenomegaly and features of Thalassaemia major to mild anaemia developing in pregnancy or no symptoms at all.

Haemoglobin E–Thalassaemia usually appears in early childhood as anaemia with hepatosplenomegaly, mental and physical retardation, and subsequent failure of secondary sexual development.

The bone changes and haematological findings are similar to those in Thalassaemia major and the course of the condition is much the same.

Homozygous $\alpha$ Thalassaemia is regarded as incompatible with foetal survival. Stillborn infants suspected of being homozygotes (so far, all Chinese) have hydrops, ascites, and hepatic enlargement, peripheral blood smears show the picture of erythroblastosis foetalis, while paper electrophoresis reveals high concentrations of Haemoglobin Bart's.

The heterozygous $\alpha$ Thalassaemia state is most easily discovered in the neonatal period, when there is a rapid change-over from foetal to adult haemoglobin. In the infant it is characterized by increased levels of Haemoglobin H and in the adult by mild anaemia, decreased erythrocyte osmotic fragility, normal levels of Haemoglobins A and F, and traces of Haemoglobin Bart's or H. Heterozygous $\alpha$ Thalassaemia does not react with heterozygous Haemoglobins S or C.

The interaction of the heterozygous $\alpha$ Thalassaemia gene with an unidentified second heterozygous gene is believed to give rise to Haemoglobin H disease, a thalassaemia-like clinical condition of world-wide distribution in which there is some hypochromic microcytic anaemia, the erythrocyte inclusion bodies characteristic of Haemoglobin H, and moderately raised serum bilirubin. Haemoglobin H can be demonstrated electrophoretically.

### MANAGEMENT OF THALASSAEMIA SYNDROMES

As in SS disease, prompt treatment of infections by antibiotics has greatly improved the prognosis in the child. Anaemia is usually controlled by transfusion, keeping the haemoglobin level at about 7 g per cent. Excessive transfusion leads to exacerbation of siderosis. *Iron is contra-indicated,* but a maintenance dose of folic acid 5 mg daily should be given, especially in times of stress, such as pregnancy.

In cases in which the half-life of the erythrocyte is low and in cases in which the organ is very large, splenectomy is required.

Various chelating agents (including trisodiumdiethylene-triamine-penta-acetate (DTPA) and desferrioxamine) have been used to increase iron excretion and so minimize or reduce the iron deposition in the tissues, particularly the myocardium.

Clinical effects arising from coexistent Haemoglobin S are treated as described above.

Splenectomy has proved successful in cases of Haemoglobin H disease.

## GLUCOSE-6-PHOSPHATE DEHYDROGENASE DEFICIENCY

Glucose-6-phosphate dehydrogenase (G-6-Pd) deficiency of the red cell has now been demonstrated to occur in many parts of the tropics and subtropics. The incidence of the trait is very low in Caucasian people apart from those living in the Mediterranean basin. This red cell enzyme defect is apparently harmless unless the red cells are challenged in some way, most usually by the administration of one of a large group of drugs.

### GENETICS AND TYPES OF G-6-PD DEFICIENCY

It was assumed early in the study of G-6-Pd deficiency that a red cell abnormality with marked differences in radical incidence would be genetically transmitted. It has, in fact, been shown that G-6-Pd deficiency is inherited as a sex-linked trait, with full expression in male hemizygotes and female homozygotes and with variable expression in female heterozygotes.

Many different types of G-6-Pd deficiency have now been identified. The two most important are (1) the 'Negro' type of G-6-Pd deficiency characterized by a rapid (A) band on starch gel electrophoresis and (2) the 'Mediterranean' type of G-6-Pd deficiency which is more severe and characterized by a slow (B) band. A fall with age in the frequency of G-6-Pd deficiency occurs.

### CLINICAL ASPECTS

*Haemolytic anaemia*

Primaquine was the first drug to be incriminated in the production of haemolytic anaemia in enzyme-deficient subjects, and since then the list of harmful substances has increased rapidly. The more common ones are: 8-aminoquinolines (primaquine, pamaquine, pentaquine); aniline derivatives (sulphonamides, phenacetin, phenylhydrazine); nitrofurans (nitrofurazone, nitrofurantoin); sulphones; vitamin K analogues; naphthalene (mothballs); probenecid (benemid); dimercaprol (BAL); para-amino-salicyclic acid cotrimorazole. Several drugs have only been associated with haemolysis in Causasian populations and there is evidence that dosage levels play an important role in determining the degree of haemolysis.

It appears that young red cells are insensitive to the haemolytic actions of drugs, while older cells are highly sensitive. Haemolysis usually begins the third day after drug administration and continues for about 1 week, after which the 'haemolytic phase' terminates spontaneously and the 'recovery phase' begins, the blood picture returning to normal. Readministration of a haemolytic drug a few weeks later will, however, produce a new haemolytic episode. Because young red cells in Mediterranean subjects contain very little enzyme, haemolysis does not appear to be self-limited. Occasionally complete absence of G-6-Pd activity may also occur in the African negro.

Fava beans can also produce haemolytic anaemia in enzyme-deficient subjects. The haemolysis is usually much more rapid and may be immediate and fulminant after fava pollen inhalation.

Apart from susceptibility to drugs and Fava beans, there is reason to suppose that enzyme-deficient cells may haemolyse more readily than normal red cells under the stress of infection—whether bacterial, for example umbilical sepsis, typhoid fever; viral, for example infective hepatitis; or parasitic (falciparum malaria). A high frequency of G-6-Pd deficiency in patients with typhoid fever and viral hepatitis has been noted. Acute reversible renal failure precipitated by anaemia and urinary tract infection has been described in G-6-Pd patients.

*Neonatal jaundice*
In the neonate with susceptible red cells, haemolysis, leading to severe jaundice and kernicterus, can occur in the first few days of life in the absence of any precipitating agent. Neonatal jaundice is more common in the 'Mediterranean' variety of G-6-Pd deficiency, but also occurs in Chinese and Negro infants after exposure of the child or mother to certain drugs and, at times, even in the absence of exposure to such agents. The jaundice usually reaches a maximum between the third and fifth days, but sometimes does not do so until the second week of life. It has been shown that in Negro G-6-Pd deficient children vitamin K analogues given routinely (1 mg) to prevent haemorrhagic disease of the newborn do not increase the frequency and severity of neonatal jaundice.

*G-6-Pd and malaria*
It has been postulated that, like the sickle trait, G-6-Pd deficiency protects against mortality from falciparum malaria. The evidence to date in favour of the malarial protection hypothesis outweighs that against it and it has recently been shown that in blood from female children with acute falciparum malaria the parasite rate was 2 to 80 times higher in normal than in deficient erythrocytes.

DIAGNOSIS

In areas of the world where the enzyme deficiency occurs, it is important to consider the haemolytic effect of this red cell defect when assessing the cause of individual cases of haemolytic anaemia with or without haemoglobinuria, and in the differential diagnosis of neonatal hyperbilirubinaemia.

Qualitative as well as quantitative tests for the enzyme deficiency can be carried out at present only in laboratories with special facilities.

An attempt should be made to elicit an adequate history with particular reference to drugs taken.

### TREATMENT

There is no specific treatment for glucose-6-phosphate dehydrogenase deficiency.

Blood transfusion, with the usual precautions of cross-matching, is essential if the haemolysis has been very severe.

Potentially haemolytic drugs should be avoided in G-6-Pd deficient subjects and the need for such a drug should be weighed against its possible ill effects in such patients. In this context it is important to remember that haemolytic episodes seem to occur less frequently and in a less severe form in Negro populations. The haemolytic phase is self-limiting in these of cases and will not recur unless readministration of the drug takes place after an interval of a few weeks. Mitigation of the haemolytic effect of primaquine can be achieved by weekly instead of daily administration of the drug.

Exchange transfusion may be needed to prevent kernicterus in neonates.

# 10

# CLINICAL EFFECTS OF EXPOSURE TO HEAT AND LIGHT

## EFFECTS OF EXPOSURE TO HEAT

The effects of heat on the body arise from interference with the heat controlling mechanisms or from disturbances in the electrolyte–water balance and cardiovascular system, or both.

In the former category are the syndromes of heat hyperpyrexia and thermogenic anhidrosis; in the latter, heat exhaustion. These syndromes may appear as distinct entities or be associated. In the account given below they are treated separately.

Psychological effects of exposure to the living conditions imposed by heat must also be included.

### PHYSIOLOGICAL PRINCIPLES

A short account of the physiological control of body temperature, electrolyte–water balance and the cardiovascular system on exposure to heat is necessary in order to understand the pathogenesis of these conditions and the principles of treatment.

*Body temperature*
At any given moment the temperature of the body is determined by the balance that exists between heat production and heat loss. In cold or temperate climates, metabolic production of heat is dissipated from the body surface by the physical mechanisms of radiation, convection, and (rarely) conduction. Loss is reduced autonomically by peripheral vasoconstriction and artificially by protective clothing. The variations in the blood flow through the skin are regulated by central and local reflexes initiated by temperature changes in skin nerve end-organs and in blood flowing through the hypothalamic areas of the brain.

*Sweating*
In ambient temperatures above body heat, radiation and convection are towards the body and the only methods of heat loss are by evaporation of sweat and (to a much smaller extent) by insensible perspiration through skin and lungs. If the maximum heat loss from the body by these mechanisms fails

to balance heat gain from radiation and metabolism, body temperature rises. Radiation heat gain may be reduced artificially by protective clothing, but this interferes with evaporation of sweat at skin level.

Sweat is secreted by glands which are under autonomic control. It is essentially a hypotonic saline solution. Its salt content is of secondary importance except when sweating is excessive. Its primary function is to provide water for surface evaporation and cooling. Sweating may be initiated by increase in temperature of the skin end-organs but the principal stimulus is a rise of temperature of the blood passing through the hypothalamic centres. Heating of these centres causes panting and sweating; destruction is followed by inhibition of sweating and an uncontrolled rise of body temperature on exposure to heat.

The rate of sweating depends on the external temperature and the length of exposure to it. Short exposure to high temperatures brings about very high rates of sweating which cannot be maintained for long; as exposure continues, the sweating rate falls off. Certain drugs including atropine considerably depress sweating.

The evaporation of sweat is more efficient in hot dry than in hot moist climates. It is facilitated by movement of air at the body surface. About one-third of the amount of sweat secreted is usually evaporated on the skin; the rest escapes as drops or by soaking into the clothes.

Continuous exposure to heat results in acclimatization, effective sweating beginning at a lower body temperature than on first exposure, and the rate of secretion at a given temperature increasing.

*Water–salt balance*
The normal balance may be upset in hot climates by the development of deficiencies of water, salt, or both, brought about by inadequate intake, excessive loss, or both. Water balance in a hot environment is discussed below.

The average healthy individual in a hot climate secretes about 500–700 ml of urine per day. Except in extreme dehydration the daily volume does not fall below 300 ml.

For practical purposes, the only electrolyte of consequence in exposure to heat is sodium chloride. The concentration of salt in the sweat of a healthy subject in a temperate climate varies from 0.1 to 0.3 g per cent. After continuous exposure to heat, especially where there is slight deficiency in intake, the salt content of sweat may fall.

Salt deficiency in heat exposure usually results from excessive loss in the sweat; it may be aggravated by diarrhoea and vomiting. When severe, it leads to secondary dehydration. The loss of salt can be adjusted in heavy working conditions by an intake of 10–25 g per day; the smaller amount suffices in the normal adult not sweating unduly.

Salt loss is limited to some extent by reduction in the output in the urine. Where salt loss is severe, the electrolyte may be undetectable in the urine.

*Cardiovascular system*

Mention has already been made of the changes which occur in skin circulation on exposure to heat. In addition there is a slight increase in blood volume following readjustment of water balance between the tissue cells and extra-cellular fluid.

On first exposure the pulse rate rises. As the subject becomes accustomed to heat the rate falls and cardiac output increases to allow for the changes in peripheral circulation. When the subject is lying down there is at first a small increase in cardiac output, which falls considerably when the posture is suddenly changed to standing, with a corresponding rise in pulse rate and fall of blood pressure. As the subject becomes acclimatized to heat these pheno-mena become less apparent. These orthostatic variations in the circulation are useful to the physician as an indication of the state of cardiovascular acclima-tization. For instance, in heat exhaustion the change in posture from lying to standing may provoke such violent circulatory changes that syncope results.

After exposure to very high temperatures or in an individual in whom the body temperature is very high, the compensatory changes occurring in blood volume and circulation may be inadequate and shock may develop, accom-panied by acute fall in effective blood volume and in blood pressures. Vascular collapse most commonly occurs in heat exhaustion. It may be accompanied or succeeded by renal or hepatic failure.

## HYPERPYREXIA AND HEAT STROKE

### DEFINITION

A great rise of body temperature accompanied by general symptoms after exposure to intense heat. When the temperature reaches or exceeds $41°$ C the condition is arbitrarily referred to as 'hyperpyrexia' and a syndrome develops which may end fatally. The clinical picture originates from failure to control the body temperature consequent on inhibition of sweating; it may be compli-cated by coexistent electrolyte–water imbalance and by shock.

### AETIOLOGY

The appearance of heat hyperpyrexia is independent of exposure to direct sunlight. Exposure to heat must be continuous for some hours at least. Short exposures even to very high temperatures, such as those endured by stokers, seldom initiate the syndrome.

Hyperpyrexia appears most frequently in unacclimatized subjects or in individuals, for example miners, who have lost their acclimatization by leaving the hot environment for some time. It appears in either sex, at any age, although it is probably more common in the elderly than the young, other things being equal.

No race is immune. Given the right circumstances it will occur equally readily in the visitor to the tropics or the indigenous population.

Certain predisposing factors are important. Anything that interferes with the evaporation or production of sweat may precipitate the syndrome. For instance, excessive clothing, lack of air movement, or enclosure in a confined space may prevent evaporation of sweat and so limit heat loss. Extreme dehydration may lower the production of sweat below the amount required to control heat loss by evaporation. Acute febrile illnesses, particularly malaria and pneumonia, may also induce the onset by inhibition of sweating during the fever.

Overproduction of heat is sometimes important. Metabolism may be unduly excited by excessive protein intake or by the overactivity of endocrine glands, especially the thyroid. More commonly, excessive muscular exercise is responsible; this may be induced by overindulgence in alcohol.

A history of previous attacks of hyperpyrexia is unusual.

### PATHOGENESIS AND PATHOLOGY

The essential pathogenic factor in the establishment of the syndrome is inhibition of sweating. The cause is unknown.

The morbid anatomical and histological changes found in the body after death depend largely upon whether the predominant clinical feature was the hyperpyrexia or vascular failure. In either case, rigor mortis is rapid and the cadaver blood is fluid. In cases which have been predominantly hyperpyrexial the brain is congested and the lesions therein are primarily neuronal, the pattern being degeneration and ultimately necrosis of nerve cells and replacement with glial tissue. In rapidly fatal cases the neuronal degenerative changes predominate but in cases which have survived for some days there is considerable infiltration of the degenerate regions with glial cells. Cases complicated by shock show congestion of the small vessels of the brain and minute haemorrhages into the brain substance. In hyperpyrexial cases neuronal changes are most pronounced in the cerebellum and to a smaller extent in the cerebral cortex; in shock the cerebellum is often unaffected and the lesions are mainly in the deeper layers of the cortex and the basal nuclei. Pathological changes in organs other than the brain depend mainly on the existence or otherwise of vascular failure. In cases which survive long enough and in which vascular failure has been prominent, centrilobular necrosis of the liver may occur and there may be renal changes similar to those of anuric renal anoxia with damage to the tubular epithelium and medullary congestion accompanied by ischaemic glomeruli. In shocked cases petechial haemorrhages occur in most tissues including the mucous membrane of the upper small intestine, and the endocardium, peritoneum, and pleura.

### CLINICAL PICTURE

The onset is abrupt and occasionally dramatic and totally unexpected (the so-called 'flash' hyperpyrexia). In a few cases there are well defined prodromal symptoms which appear and develop several days before the onset.

Patients in whom the onset is rapid are frequently admitted in a state of delirium or coma and on recovery may be unable to give a clear history. Where the onset is more gradual, however, there is usually a history of headache, drowsiness, restlessness, and mental confusion, often accompanied by progressive dizziness and sometimes an unsteady gait. Anorexia, nausea, and vomiting are common. There may be difficulty in speech and swallowing. Intense thirst is common leading to heavy consumption of fluids with polyuria and frequency (defined in a hot climate as 2 litres or more of urine and micturition more than four times in the day).

The patient may have observed a reduction of sweating during exercise, especially on the trunk.

By the time he is examined he is often in delirium or deep coma. If still conscious, he is restless, anxious and confused.

*The oral temperature is very high.* It may exceed 43.5° C. The rectal temperature is about one degree higher.

*The skin is dry and flushed.* There may be some cyanosis of the extremities. The dryness of the skin indicates the pathogenesis of the syndrome, i.e. inhibition of sweating.

The pulse rate is fast; frequently over 130 beats per minute. There may be soft systolic cardiac murmurs and transient electrocardiographic evidence of myocardial dysfunction. The blood pressure is not grossly affected unless shock has appeared.

The respiratory rate is high (30 or more respirations per minute). Breathing is shallow but not panting. In the late stages especially in coma it may be stertorous or intermittent. Breath sounds are prolonged, but unless collapse is imminent and lung oedema has appeared there are no adventitious sounds. Alkalotic tetany has been described.

*Central nervous symptoms are pronounced and usually manifest from the onset.* Mental changes and coma have already been mentioned. In rapidly progressive cases, delirium or coma, when present at the onset, tend to persist to the end. If the patient survives for some days before a fatal issue, early coma may temporarily regress and return terminally. In the majority of treated cases, coma and delirium disappear quickly as the body temperature falls. Incontinence of urine and faeces is common in comatose cases.

Convulsions, sometimes resembling Jacksonian epilepsy, and muscular twitchings, especially in the limbs, are common in the acute stages. The neurological physical signs are, however, irregular and vary from patient to patient and from time to time in the same patient. They are most obvious in subjects in whom high fever is the predominant feature.

The presence of salt deficiency in some cases has caused considerable confusion in the description of the syndrome. In the illness heat hyperpyrexia such phenomena are of secondary and not primary pathogenic significance.

The urinary volume and constituents depend on the clinical state. If salt deficiency already exists the volume is small and there may be little or no excretion of salt. There may be some polyuria due to water diuresis initiated by drinking before the onset of hyperpyrexia.

The blood shows no special features other than those associated with complications. The blood urea nitrogen is usually a little raised; occasionally in patients with very high fever the total blood non-protein nitrogen may rise without a corresponding rise in urea nitrogen.

Total blood and plasma chloride concentrations may be within normal limits; they are low if salt deficiency is present.

Without treatment the severe case will die. Death occurs either from the direct effects of the high body temperature or from shock.

The commonest complication is medical shock which may occur at any stage. At first the effects of such vascular collapse are reversible but in a short time irreversible changes occur, particularly in the brain, liver, and kidneys. The onset of shock is shown by notable changes in the patient's appearance. The temperature falls rapidly, often to below normal. The skin becomes pale, cold, slightly cyanosed, and often moist with sweat. Respiration is rapid and shallow. The blood pressures fall. At first, the diastolic pressure drops more slowly than the systolic, so that the pulse pressure is reduced. Ultimately the diastolic pressure may become unmeasurable. The circulating blood volume is acutely reduced, with corresponding haemoconcentration indicated by rising erythrocyte count and haemoglobin concentration. The conscious patient may become restless, irritable, and anxious; coma or stupor may develop. Watery diarrhoea is common and there may be incontinence.

Acute renal failure with anuria and uraemia may develop in cases complicated by shock. Sometimes evidence of liver dysfunction develops. The liver becomes palpable and tender and there may be epigastric discomfort, nausea, bilious vomiting and diarrhoea, and sometimes hiccup. Mild jaundice occasionally develops and bile pigments may appear in the urine and faeces. The vomit and stools in this stage often contain fresh or altered blood. Petechial haemorrhages may appear in the skin and mucous membranes. Signs of pulmonary oedema may develop terminally.

*Prognosis*
With prompt treatment the mortality is low. Death occurs in 24 hours in most fatal cases; some may survive for as long as 12 days. Early death results largely

from the high fever; later deaths from shock. The prognosis in an individual subject is determined by the length of illness, height, and duration of the fever and the presence or absence of shock. Shocked cases or those with very acute onset and rapidly developing coma have the poorest prognosis.

With adequate treatment the recovery should be rapid (i.e. a matter of a few days) and permanent. In some patients, however, unpleasant sequelae develop, including changes in personality, persistent and irritating amnesia, severe headaches, and signs of cerebellar dysfunction.

### DIAGNOSIS

There must be evidence of exposure to intense heat. There is often a history of predisposing causes. Clinical diagnosis can be made from the triad: the high fever, the flushed dry skin and the central nervous system signs. Other causes of fever must be excluded, *especially falciparum malaria in which hyperpyrexia may occur as a complication. The blood must always be examined for malaria parasites.*

This is essential in an endemic region and also in individuals, such as seamen, who may have been exposed to falciparum malaria elsewhere before the onset of presumed heat hyperpyrexia in a hot area.

The same applies to the visitor to falciparum malaria endemic areas which are also often very hot. The modern, enormous growth of tourism makes this point especially important, since areas such as West and East Africa are now included in so-called 'package tours' for holiday-makers. Information about dealing with exposure to heat and malaria is seldom given to the traveller. It might be said that the coffin is sometimes included in the package.

### TREATMENT

Treatment is designed to lower the temperature and promote sweating. For the immediate reduction of the temperature any available method of cooling should be used.

The body temperature is best reduced by bathing or spraying the skin surface with chilled water, in a good stream of dry air. Cooling is achieved in this method by convection and evaporation. Immersion in an ice-water bath may be effective, although cooling is then by conduction only. In the absence of chilled water, ice and motor driven fans, the patient should be bathed with water at ordinary temperatures, or wrapped in a wet sheet, and fanned vigorously. Chlorpromazine is useful in promoting peripheral vasodilation, abolishing shivering, and controlling restlessness or convulsions; it is customary to give 25 or 50 mg intravenously at the outset of cooling. The temperature must be recorded every few minutes while cooling is applied. It usually falls rapidly after the start of treatment. When it has fallen to about 39° C, active treatment should be stopped, otherwise the patient may collapse. The temperature usually continues to fall to normal or below without further treatment. Secondary rises of temperature may occur within the next few hours or even days. These may require treatment on the same lines. In most cases natural sweating is restored after the first treatment. In more severe cases the re-establishment of sweating is slower and treatment may have to be repeated.

Complications are treated as they appear. Shock and dehydration need parenteral fluid therapy (see pp. 60, 280). Intravenous infusion is not otherwise indicated.

Sequelae are often resistant to treatment. These include personality changes and neurological signs, such as involvement of the cranial nerves or hemiplegia, which tend to persist. Persistent headache is common but usually clears up after weeks or months; it may be relieved in some patients by nicotinic amide.

## HEAT SYNCOPE

Also called heat collapse and exercise-induced heat exhaustion, this syndrome is a state of syncope or subjective giddiness and intense fatigue arising from hypotension and cerebral anoxia. It is not primarily related to the state of water or salt depletion in the subject, but arises from incomplete acclimitization to heat, which leads to peripheral vasodilation and venous pooling of blood and to hypotension. The lack of acclimatization of the cardiovascular system can be demonstrated by the very rapid heart rate induced by moderate exercise and the slow return of the rate to normal subsequently.

The symptoms commonly develop in the first few days of exposure to heat. Residents in hot climates are not affected except after strenuous exercise or sudden change in ambient temperature or humidity.

The patient feels restless, light-headed, and dizzy. He is forced to sit or lie down and may faint. He often feels nauseated, with epigastric discomfort, sometimes an intense desire to defaecate. Frequent yawning is common. The skin is pale and clammy, especially on the face, in the axillae and hands. The pulse rate is at first fast and then slow after recovery from syncope. Complete recovery can be expected after a few hours' rest in cool surroundings.

## HEAT EXHAUSTION

### PREDOMINANT SALT DEPLETION

This syndrome is most frequently seen in hot conditions, especially in association with heavy manual labour. Sweating is not inhibited and heat loss is thus not affected. The body temperature is seldom elevated much above normal.

Disturbances of body salt–water balance and of the cardiovascular system are always present. The most severe cases are dehydrated and shocked.

### AETIOLOGY

Heat exhaustion occurs commonly during the hottest time of the year. It appears in visitors and local inhabitants of all ages and in either sex. The most important predisposing factor is heavy and prolonged sweating, with failure to replace water and salt.

Coexistent febrile illnesses, especially malaria, are also important as are gastrointestinal disturbances involving diarrhoea and vomiting.

### CLINICAL PICTURE

There is usually a prodromal period lasting several days during which the patient notices progressive headache and anorexia, often associated with nausea and mild vomiting. Fleeting muscle cramps occur, especially in the calf and foot. Giddiness and unsteadiness of gait may develop early. Sweating is free in all parts of the body. The urinary output is commonly low.

Visual and aural disturbances, such as 'spots in front of the eyes' and 'ringing' in the ears may occur. In miners and other manual workers a frequent history is: 'I felt giddy, and took a big drink of water, after which I promptly vomited and felt cramps in my limbs.'

The seriously affected patient nearly always vomits. Muscular cramps are more common in patients who are vomiting. Tremendous losses of fluid and salt occur during heavy work and will usually indicate the likelihood of direct dual deficiency.

On examination the patient is extremely exhausted. In serious cases he may be restless and anxious or lightly comatose. Central nervous system signs are, however, much less prominent than in heat hyperpyrexia. They are usually of short duration and respond readily to treatment.

The oral temperature may be normal or subnormal, or slightly raised.

The skin is cold, moist, pale and inelastic. The facies are pinched, the eyes sunken, the malar bones prominent. Sweating may be profuse.

In comatose cases the respiration may be deep and stertorous. Where vascular failure has developed there may be evidence of pulmonary oedema.

Most patients vomit frequently. The vomiting is not always accompanied by nausea and may be intractable. It is often followed by muscular cramps, which may be fleeting or severe and occur most commonly in the legs, arms, and abdominal muscles. Occasionally there may be tetanic carpopedal spasm.

The pulse rate is nearly always fast; very occasionally there may be noticeable bradycardia.

In mild cases the systolic pressure may fall to below 90 mmHg but the pulse pressure is low, since the diastolic pressure tends to remain high at first in relation to the systolic. Sudden change of posture from lying to standing may have a profound effect; the pulse races, the blood pressure falls and the patient may faint.

In severe cases vascular failure appears. The pulse rate rises, sometimes to 150 or more beats per minute. Both systolic and diastolic blood pressures fall. The pulse may be imperceptible at the wrist. The circulating blood volume is grossly reduced; the viscosity of the blood increases and the haemoglobin concentration and the red cell count temporarily rise.

*Urine*

The urinary volume is reduced to less than 300 ml per day. When shock has appeared, the renal anoxia syndrome may develop. The urine may contain albumin and hyaline and granular tubular casts. It is unconcentrated; chloride is present in low concentration or is absent.

*Blood*

The whole blood and plasma chloride and sodium concentrations are low, especially if vomiting is, or has been, severe. The blood urea nitrogen concentration is high, of the order of 100 mg per cent, even in cases without obvious renal dysfunction; it rises much higher if anuric uraemia develops.

*Prognosis*

Uncomplicated and correctly treated cases recover very rapidly. Shock considerably worsens the prognosis, although it usually responds to treatment. The outlook is bad in anuric cases.

Relapses are uncommon if the salt–water balance is maintained and acclimatization re-established. There is no indication for removal of the patient from the hot environment.

### DIAGNOSIS

This history of exposure to heat, especially under working conditions, and the circumstances of the onset are usually diagnostic. In severely affected patients other causes of vascular collapse must be excluded. *In all cases the blood must be examined to exclude malaria, especially falciparum.* The presence of malarial or other infection does not affect the treatment required for adjustment of the electrolyte balance and plasma volume. There is often no detectable chloride in the urine; in any case the chloride content is extremely low. Reduction of chloride and sodium levels in the blood will place the diagnosis beyond reasonable doubt.

### TREATMENT

The aim of treatment is to restore the electrolyte–water balance and the blood volume where necessary.

The patient should be treated in bed. An input–output fluid balance account should be kept. The volume of each specimen of urine passed should be recorded. Most cases can be treated orally.

Mild cases are given orally up to 5 or 6 litres of fluid, and a total of 25–40 g salt (including the salt in the diet) in the first 24 hours. It can be administered in capsules or in foods such as soup. Water must be given as well as salt.

In severely dehydrated and shocked cases or in those with intractable vomiting, fluid must be given parenterally.

An initial 0.5 litre of plasma given in 30 minutes is required in shocked patients.

If dehydration is severe, the first litre of isotonic saline should be administered in about a quarter of an hour, and followed by a further litre in half an hour. Infusion thereafter should be slower, i.e. at the rate of 0.5 litre every 4 hours by drip. Not more than 5 litres need be given in the first 24 hours unless fluid continues to be lost by diarrhoea or vomiting, in which case, as in cholera, the amount of extra infusion should match the amount of fluid lost. It is seldom necessary to continue parenteral treatment longer than 24 hours.

A check should be kept on the urinary chloride concentration during parenteral treatment. 'Hypotonic' saline (one part isotonic saline plus two parts isotonic glucose) should be substituted for isotonic when the chloride concentration begins to rise.

In severe cases the replacement of potassium is important. Ten mEq may be added to each litre of infused fluid after administration of the first litre of saline, provided the rate of administration does not exceed 200 ml per hour. If oral administration is possible, the patient should be given up to 10 g potassium chloride in the first 24 hours.

Response to treatment is usually rapid, even in the severely dehydrated individual. The mildly affected patient may be fit to return to work in a few days.

## PREDOMINANT WATER DEPLETION

During the working period of the day, the water intake of the average individual in hot climates fails to keep pace with losses in sweat and insensible perspiration. The deficit which results, so-called 'voluntary dehydration', is usually made good in evening and leisure hours, if fluid is available. In these circumstances, primary water deficiency of clinical significance rarely occurs. Thirst is an inconstant and often inadequate signal of moderate water deficiency and fluid intake may be influenced by habit.

Headache, giddiness, fatigue, oliguria, and slight elevation of the body temperature are features of mild water deficiency arising when water intake is inadequate for unaccustomed and high levels of activity and sweating. More severe features, attendant upon haemoconcentration and vascular collapse, occur generally only in abnormal circumstances.

Primary water depletion is diagnosed readily by the clinical signs common to all forms of dehydration.

In severe cases, as seen in men stranded in the desert without water, the earliest symptom is thirst, which rapidly intensifies, until the patient becomes obsessed. The mouth and tongue become dry, swallowing becomes difficult, and there is increasing weakness and loss of weight. Mental judgment is impaired and restlessness and hysteria are common. The patient becomes giddy and movements are uncoordinated. Delirium, coma, and death follow unless there is rapid rehydration. Survival time depends on the ambient temperature and the activity of the subject. Marching waterless across hot deserts may cause death within 24 hours. Sweating diminishes rapidly. The output of urine falls, but the urine is highly concentrated and contains measurable amounts of sodium chloride. There may be terminal renal failure with anuria with or without oligaemic shock. Plasma sodium and chloride concentrations are normal or raised. The body temperature rises, sometimes suddenly, and hyperpyrexia may develop.

The diagnosis of severe water depletion is usually indicated by the circumstances in which the patient has been exposed. Points of distinction between water depletion and salt–water depletion include, in the former, the intense thirst, absence of muscle cramps and often of vomiting, diminution of sweating, measurable chloride content of the urine, and the predisposition to heat stroke. It should be noted that elements of both forms of depletion may exist in the same patient.

Treatment consists of rest in the cool and oral administration of cool fluid, up to 8 litres in 24 hours. Salt intake should be normal; there is no indication for forcing salt.

Intravenous fluid replacement is needed in the worst cases, using isotonic saline or 5 per cent glucose solution, 4 litres or more in the first 24 hours. Oral fluids should be substituted as soon as possible. Hyperpyrexia and pyrexia should be treated as described above.

## ANHIDROTIC HEAT EXHAUSTION

### DEFINITION

Thermogenic anhidrosis, tropical anhidrotic asthenia. This syndrome was first described in the Second World War. There is some inhibition of sweating, principally on the trunk and limbs, but not on the face and neck. High fever does not develop. There are characteristic skin changes which may appear occasionally without other symptoms. The syndrome may be complicated by water–salt imbalance and cardiovascular disturbances. These are, however, not essential features.

PATHOLOGY

It is not known whether the inhibition of sweating is central or peripheral. The high sweat chloride is regarded by some as an indication of exhaustion of the sweat glands. Others hold that pathological changes found in the glands account for the inhibition of sweating. In any given area of skin, however, relatively few glands are obviously affected. In those affected there is some hyperkeratosis which appears to obstruct the ducts, leading in some to rupture into the surrounding epithelium which becomes disorganized, producing an intradermal vesicle filled with clear fluid. The local lymphatics are dilated and the associated blood vessels congested.

CLINICAL PICTURE

Thermogenic anhidrosis develops after long exposure to high temperatures. The onset is usually gradual. The symptoms are most severe during the hottest part of the day.

*History and Diagnosis*
The patient complains of exhaustion, dyspnoea, and cardiac palpitation after work or exercise. Most patients suffer from anorexia and epigastric discomfort, giddiness, frontal headache, and insomnia. There are frequently subjective feelings of warmth and tightness in the affected skin. The symptoms pass off with rest in cool conditions, but as the syndrome progresses, increasing periods of rest are needed, until finally work becomes impossible. This often gives the impression that the patient is malingering.

The patient usually gives a history of extensive prickly heat, which may have improved considerably some weeks before the syndrome develops. He also often notices that sweating on the body but not on the face progressively diminishes as the syndrome develops. Sometimes this may be preceded by a short period of excessive sweating.

The patient is restless and apprehensive. The oral temperature lies between 37.2 and 39° C. The pulse rate is fast. Respiration is deep and fast; the rate may exceed 40 per minute. In the uncomplicated case the blood pressure is unchanged.

On the limbs and most of the trunk the skin is dry. There may be small isolated islands of sweating. Sweating is free on the face and neck; the palms, soles, axillae, and groin are usually moist. The distribution of sweating is thus similar to that in so-called 'cold sweating'.

The skin eruption or mammillaria is characteristic. It is composed of myriads of tiny greyish papules about 1 mm in diameter, commonly surmounted by vesicles containing clear fluid. These occur only in dry areas of skin, in patches on the trunk, and the upper dorsal aspect of the limbs. Superficially the condition resembles goose flesh but the skin hairs are not involved. It may be mistaken for prickly heat, but there is no erythematous ringing of the papules and there is no itching or prickling. Between the papules and on the rest of the area involved the skin is dry and warm. The lesions commonly develop first on the arms and may spread to the trunk and finally the legs. In some cases the arms, legs, and trunk are involved simultaneously. The papules do not appear on moist areas and are thus found on the head and neck only very exceptionally.

Mammillaria may occur without widespread anhidrosis or symptoms of exhaustion. In such cases, body sweating is nevertheless notably reduced.

Firm oedema of the fingers and arms may occur in some cases and be associated with enlarged discrete axillary or inguinal lymph glands.

Changes in the blood or urine depend on the state of the body water–salt balance.

Polyuria due to water diuresis with dilute urine but with a normal output of salt may occur in cases in which thirst is a prominent feature.

The salt concentration of the sweat is high and frequently exceeds 0.5 per cent.

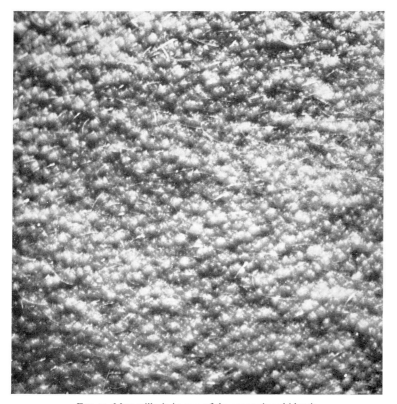

FIG. 21. Mammillaria in case of thermogenic anhidrosis.

[Courtesy of *Transactions of Royal Society of Tropical Medicine and Hygiene*, and Dr R.H.Mole]

*Prognosis*

The uncomplicated condition is not fatal. Recovery occurs with treatment.

## TREATMENT

The only treatment required is rest in cool surroundings. Where there are disturbances of water–chloride balance, these should be controlled by adequate administration of water and salt; parenteral administration is seldom necessary.

There is a rapid response of temperature, respiration, and pulse. The skin changes disappear more slowly and are commonly succeeded by branny desquamation, particularly on the limbs. Enlarged lymph glands and oedema subside slowly. Within a few days there is increasing ability to exercise without reappearance of symptoms. Sweating returns first as a rule on the trunk. At the beginning of treatment, exertion, exposure to heat, or injection of pilocarpine cause a return of symptoms and the peculiar distribution of sweating. Later exposure produces no symptoms and a normal sweating reaction.

Full recovery may be expected in about a fortnight. Relapses are common, especially if treatment is too short. It is advisable to remove the patient from the hot environment if possible.

# PRICKLY HEAT

## DEFINITION

Miliaria rubra. An extremely common and irritating superficial skin eruption distributed widely over the tropics and subtropics.

## AETIOLOGY

The cause is uncertain. Secondary infection with pyogenic organisms and sometimes fungi occurs and affects the progress of the condition, but such infection is not regarded as the primary cause. Pathological changes in the sweat glands suggest that the ducts may become mechanically blocked by soggy, swollen epithelium.

Prickly heat is especially common in hot humid regions where sweating is likely to be heavy and continuous. Infants and children with thin skin, and obese individuals with multiple skin folds are often severely affected. Recent arrivals usually suffer most. Males are affected more commonly than females.

## CLINICAL PICTURE

The lesions develop soon after arrival in the hot humid area. They begin as numerous scattered small papules 1–2 mm in diameter, which soon develop vesicles, containing clear or slightly milky fluid. Each papule may be surrounded by a halo of erythema, or there may be a general erythematous background upon which the papules develop. In some cases the first sign is patchy erythema which appears on heating and goes on cooling. Papules soon appear in large numbers in such areas and develop vesicles.

The lesions are very irritating and the itching and prickling leads to involuntary scratching, followed invariably by secondary infection. In some parts of the body a purulent eczematous lesion may result in this way; in others the papules subside and are replaced by a white powdery desquamation. In chronic cases the affected skin is thickened and erythematous and batches of papules appear and subside at intervals. Itching may persist throughout the condition.

Prickly heat tends to appear in parts of the body where there is close contact with clothes, for example around the waist or on the shoulders. It is common in friction areas, for example on the wrists where the coat or shirt cuff moves over the skin, or in areas where skin is in contact with skin, for instance in skin folds in obese individuals or below the breasts. Its relation to the local production of sweat is not clearly defined. Most of the areas mentioned tend to be moist, but the lesions also commonly occur on the backs of the hands where sweating is minimal.

In infants practically the whole skin may be involved and secondary infection may lead to serious results. It may be necessary to remove the child from the district to some cooler spot.

Prickly heat is at its worst in the hot wet season and may clear completely in the cool. It tends to recur (in the same areas of the body) in a given individual with the advent of the hot season, usually with diminishing severity as the sufferer becomes more used to dealing with it.

In some individuals the general effect is intolerable and psychological reactions are not uncommon. Sleep may be difficult. Unless caused by secondary infection, general reactions such as fever are negligible.

### DIAGNOSIS

Prickly heat can be diagnosed by its appearance and distribution. The groups of small papules, with or without crowning vesicles, surrounded by haloes or background of erythema, are usually unmistakable. In the early stages they may be mistaken for the mammillaria of thermogenic anhidrosis but the latter can be distinguished by the absence of local sweating and erythema.

### TREATMENT

The lesions may be very difficult to deal with in a delicate skin and sometimes the only way out is the removal of the individual to a cooler climate. Recovery in a temperate climate is usually very rapid and complete so long as secondary infection is not severe.

The areas involved should be washed gently with an antiseptic soap. It may be necessary to determine by trial and error which of the latter is suitable, since some may irritate the lesions and cause exacerbations. The soap may be allowed to dry for 20 minutes or so on the lesions. It is then washed off and the area is thoroughly dried and powdered with talc.

Local applications vary in their effects from patient to patient. What is good for one individual is sometimes harmful to another. Some astringent such as mercuric chloride (1 in 2000 in 95 per cent alcohol) is often soothing and effective.

After such applications a bland dusting powder containing zinc oxide or a rapidly drying lotion such as calamine lotion may be applied from time to time during the day.

Pyogenic infections must be treated before the above treatment is applied. Local permanganate baths given for half an hour twice daily and followed by zinc oxide dusting powder may be effective. Antibiotics or sulphonamides may be necessary.

*Prevention*
Local treatment is unsatisfactory without concurrent preventive measures. The subject should avoid high temperatures as much as possible. He should forgo unnecessary exertion or frequent drinking, especially tea, which may enhance sweating. Hot baths should be avoided unless there is ample time for subsequent cooling. The shower is to be preferred to the bath in hot environments, in any case.

Clothing should be loose and designed to avoid pressure or friction. For example, there should not be constrictions at the wrists or waist.

Care must be taken to see that the skin is thoroughly dried after bathing. The frequent use of ordinary alkaline soaps may be harmful. Frequent drying of the skin with handkerchiefs or towels will help keep the lesions under control.

Controlled sunbathing is beneficial, especially for children; sea bathing often exacerbates the condition.

## TROPICAL FATIGUE

Neurotic reactions falling under this heading are advantageously divided into acute and chronic. The relationship of the syndromes to the heat of the environment is not clear. In the tropics, they affect mainly the white immigrants, on whom the sociological and psychological stresses of a small community in untraditional surroundings have an effect which tends to become more pronounced the longer the time spent in the environment and the more unadjusted the individual. Highly motivated individuals are rarely implicated.

### ACUTE HEAT FATIGUE

There is no doubt that human performance of skilled tasks, involving mental concentration, accurate muscular co-ordination, and speedy reaction times deteriorates as ambient temperatures rise. After several weeks or even days of working under such difficulties, some individuals become irritable, disinclined to continue, and even hysterical. They recover only when removed from their environment, to which they are temperamentally unsuited.

### CHRONIC HOT CLIMATE FATIGUE

Tropical deterioration or neurasthenia is probably in no way specific to the 'tropics'—or to the disadvantaged world. In expatriates in Ethiopia, Leithead aptly described the situation as 'outpost' rather than 'tropical'. Numerous minor dissatisfactions inevitable to small communities combine with physical stress imposed by late hours, alcoholic indulgences, boredom (especially in women), inability to sleep well in hot climates and the effects of glare to cause an ill-defined percentage of expatriates to deteriorate in terms of working efficiency and actual physical health. It is not enough to judge such people as unsuitable for life in the tropics and the ecological problems involved deserve further study and research.

## EFFECTS OF EXPOSURE TO LIGHT

### SUNBURN

#### DEFINITION AND AETIOLOGY

Acute solar dermatitis. Sunburn is an acute dermal reaction to exposure to ultra-violet light of wavelength 290–320 nm. Heat plays no direct part in its appearance, although heating may sometimes make the skin more sensitive to ultra-violet light. Reactions identical to sunburn occur after exposure to sources of ultra-violet light or to 'cold' light such as that reflected from snow or water.

The essential aetiological factor is exposure to direct sunlight for sufficient time.

The severity of the reaction depends on many factors especially the duration and intensity of exposure, and the area of skin exposed. Certain areas, including the skin of the back of the trunk and neck and the popliteal regions, are highly susceptible. Skin pigment protects against ultra-violet light: dark or coloured skin burns much less readily than fair. Slow acclimatization to exposure leads to protection from increasing thickness of the horny layers of the epithelium and deepening pigmentation.


CLINICAL PICTURE

Sunburn follows exposure after a symptom-free period of a few minutes to some hours.

The first indication is erythema of the exposed parts accompanied by itching. In mild cases the erythema may be transient, fading in a few hours, followed by complete recovery. In more severe cases the erythema increases and the affected skin becomes oedematous and slightly raised. The edges often follow the pattern of the exposure, and there is frequently a surrounding well-developed arteriolar flare. Vesicles and bullae containing clear fluid rapidly form on the surface.

The burned area is intensely painful and sensitive. There may be intolerable pruritus, especially in the healing stages.

Unless there is secondary infection the inflammatory reaction fades in the course of a few hours or days, depending on its severity. Blisters either rupture or absorb and are followed by desquamation and peeling.

The area involved may show irregular hyper- and hypopigmentation after subsidence of the acute lesion. Areas which were covered by blisters are usually depigmented.

Healing is usually rapid and complete unless there has been secondary infection through ruptured blisters. Such infection may lead to the development of lesions resembling those of impetigo and is capable of causing considerable local damage and scarring.

Areas of skin which have been sunburned are often left with increased sensitivity to ultra-violet light and may burn more easily on re-exposure to sunlight.

Most cases show some general symptoms including headache, malaise, and mild nausea. In several burned patients there may be high continuous fever and considerable prostration with fast pulse and respiration. Nausea and vomiting are common and often severe. Vascular failure, sometimes fatal, may appear in individuals in whom large areas of skin are involved.

The general reaction in mild cases lasts only a few hours. In more severe cases its duration depends on the extent of burning and the development or otherwise of secondary sepsis.

*Prognosis*
There is a tendency to regard sunburn lightly but it must be realized that the general reaction may be very severe and sometimes even fatal. The progress of local lesions depends on the degree of exposure and the development or otherwise of secondary infection. Usually recovery is complete.

## TREATMENT

The burned area should be carefully cleaned with calamine lotion or liquid paraffin. Analgesic or antiseptic ointments and soap are to be avoided. Blisters should be ruptured and the peeling skin removed. Exposed areas should be painted with calamine lotion containing 0.5 per cent crystal violet. Badly involved areas may be temporarily covered with calamine compresses. After the subsidence of the early inflammatory reaction, further application of calamine or zinc oxide plus castor oil ointment is advisable.

Great care should be taken to avoid secondary infection of blistered areas, which may be bathed at intervals with antiseptic solutions such as weak mercuric chloride (1:4000). Local sepsis is treated on general lines.

Local application of antihistaminic agents in the form of unguents is helpful. These drugs may also be administered orally. They may considerably relieve the local pruritus and burning sensations which are often troublesome and may lead to insomnia, especially in the recovery stage.

The sunburn should be treated like a burn from any other cause and protected against injury if necessary by cradling.

General treatment aims at sedation, the control of secondary infection and avoidance of further exposure.

Severely burned patients may be given barbiturates or morphine if they are restless or sleepless. The administration of penicillin or other antibiotics, or of sulphonamides may be necessary in severe secondary infection.

Shock and dehydration must be treated on general lines.

*Prevention of sunburn*
Sunburn can be avoided by limiting direct exposure by the use of sensible clothing, sun unbrellas, etc. Window glass affords considerable protection since it absorbs most of the active wavelengths. Acclimatization may be achieved by graded exposure.

Protection is also provided by the use of chemical screens applied to the skin the form of powders or creams.

Cosmetic face powders and creams have some protective properties but these can be enhanced by the addition of certain chemicals, for example tannic acid (5 per cent), quinine (5 per cent), *p*-aminobenzoic acid, and salol (10 per cent), which selectively absorb the active ultra-violet light.

Creams containing these agents should be applied every 3 or 4 hours during exposure, especially after swimming in salt water.

Certain vegetable oils filter off ultra-violet light but not infra-red waves, which are mainly responsible for the mobilization of skin pigment. They are often used in so-called 'sun-tan' lotions and creams for promoting pigmentation on exposure without undue risk of burning.

The use of creams and lotions containing light-filtering agents may sometimes interfere with sweating and the escape of body heat. Dermal sensitivity to the contents may exist, leading to various unpleasant skin eruptions.

### CHRONIC DERMAL EFFECTS OF SUNLIGHT

The most persistent effects of sunlight on the skin occur in people continuously exposed, as in the tropics, Australia, etc. They include epidermal atrophy, patchy pigmentation varying from a few irregular macules or splashes of brownish discoloration, commonly seen on the sides of the face, to multiple spattering of the exposed areas (freckles). There may also be irregular patches of depigmentation, not uncommon on the face and the backs of the hands.

Solar keratitis is frequently seen in fair-skinned people intermittently exposed over long periods to strong sunlight. Raised wart-like local areas of hyperplastic epithelium with a hard roughened surface appear on the face, forehead, scalp and the dorsum of the hands. These vary in size from a few millimetres to several centimentres and may from time to time recede or hypertrophy but do not disappear. Small, plaque-like, pinkish excoriated scaly lesions of this sort are common on the cheeks and beneath the eyes in the areas where light is concentrated by spectacles.

The lesions of solar dermatitis are often itchy and may become scratched and occasionally bleed and ulcerate. They are exacerbated during exposure in summer and remit in winter. Large or active lesions are refractory to local treatment and should be removed surgically, especially in areas where they are constantly being rubbed or chafed since, after long slow development sometimes lasting years, rodent ulcer and even squamous cell carcinoma may develop in them.

Various polymorphic erythematous and pruriginous eruptions involving the superficial layers of the skin may appear on long-exposed skin, including an itchy papular vesicular eczema and solar urticaria, in the form of non-confluent urticarial wheals particularly common in those recently recovered from acute sunburn.

Apart from the surgical removal of solar keratotic lesions where considered desirable, treatment of these chronic effects of exposure is unsatisfactory. Protection against over-exposure is the best measure in the long run.

### GLARE

Exposure to very bright light for even a short time irrespective of the ambient temperature will produce headache and sometimes dizziness and difficulty in focusing, coming on more rapidly in light-skinned, blue-eyed than in pigmented, brown-eyed people.

Prolonged exposure may lead to changes in the lens, including cataract.

Acute exposure to ultra-violet light causes photophobia, continuous lacrimation and acute severe ciliary pain. As exposure continues there may be blepharospasm and lid oedema, followed by conjunctival vascular congestion. The retina may be damaged by looking into a source of ultra-violet light.

The effects of glare can be controlled or prevented by the use of appropriate dark glasses. The best form of prevention is the avoidance of over-exposure.

# 11

## HOOKWORM INFECTION AND ANAEMIA

### (Contributed by H.M.Gilles)

DEFINITION

Infection with the nematodes *Ancylostoma duodenale* and *Necator americanus* with or without physical signs including hypochromic anaemia.

GEOGRAPHICAL DISTRIBUTION

Hookworm infection is found under insanitary conditions in temperate regions and in hot, damp areas throughout the tropics and subtropics.

The geographical distribution of the two hookworms, *A. duodenale* and *N. americanus* used to be regarded as relatively distinct, the former being more prevalent in the Old World in Europe, the Middle East, etc., and the latter in the New World in America and tropical Africa. During the past few decades both parasites have become widely distributed throughout the tropics and subtropics, and rigid demarcations are no longer tenable. When a parasite is universally distributed it is always difficult to be sure to what extent it is responsible for disease in the community and what significance to attach to its presence in an individual. A variable proportion of any population where hookworm is endemic develops serious disease as a consequence of infection and hookworm anaemia may be considered to represent a breakdown of adaptation.

AETIOLOGY

Hookworms are nematodes belonging to the family *Ancylostomidae*. Man is the natural host and harbours the adults in the small intestine. Eggs are passed in the faeces. Human infection is caused by *A. duodenale* and *N. americanus* which complete their life cycles in man. Infection of the subcutaneous tissues with *A. brasiliense*, the hookworm of dogs and cats, may also occur in man; in this case the worm does not reach maturity.

The adults of *A. duodenale* are small, measuring between 8 and 13 mm. The female is only a little larger than the male. The body is slightly curved and tapered at both ends; the buccal cavity has pointed clawed teeth.

Adults of *N. americanus* are slightly smaller. The worms are fine and tapered; the head in both sexes is bent back in a short reverse curve which makes for easy identification. The buccal cavity contains two chitinous plates. plates.

*Life cycle*

The life histories of *A. duodenale* and *N. americanus* are identical. The adult worms are small (8–13 mm long) and live in the upper part of the small intestine, mainly the jejunum, attaching themselves to villi which are sucked into their buccal cavities.

The egg (about 60 μm) is passed in the faeces containing a segmented ovum. When deposited on warm, moist soil, a larva rapidly develops in the egg and hatches after 1 or 2 days. The newly hatched 'rhabditiform' larva passes through a 7–10 day free-living cycle in the soil, moulting twice, and becoming the sheathed 'filariform' larva which is infective to man. In a suitable environment—warm, damp soil—these larvae can survive several months. Man is infected by the larvae penetrating his skin; they then migrate by way of the venous system to the right ventricle of the heart and to the lungs into the alveoli. From the alveoli the larvae are passively carried upwards to the trachea and larynx into the oesophagus to the stomach and small intestine which they reach 3–5 days after they have penetrated the skin. After a further 4–5 weeks the worms become sexually mature and may live from 1 to 9 years. It has been shown that whereas migrating larvae of *Necator* grow and develop in the lungs, those of *Ancylostoma* do not; they undergo the same early development in the intestinal mucosa. One female *Ancylostoma* produces about 30,000 eggs and one female *Necator* about 9000 eggs per day.

*Epidemiology*

Although man is the only important source of human hookworm infection, the epidemiology of the disease is dependent upon the interaction of three factors—the suitability of the environment for the eggs or larvae; the mode and extent of faecal pollution of the soil; and the mode and extent of contact between infected soil and skin.

Thus, survival of hookworm larvae is favoured in a damp, sandy or friable soil with decaying vegetation and a temperature of 24–32° C. Larvae move very little horizontally but can migrate upwards as much as 3 feet. *A. duodenale* eggs resist desiccation more than those of *Necator*, while the development of hookworm larvae in the eggs and subsequent hatching can be retarded in the absence of oxygen. Insanitary disposal of faeces or the use of human faeces as soil fertilizer are the chief sources of human infection in countries where individuals are bare-footed. Thus, it is to be expected that hookworm infection will have a higher prevalence in agricultural than in town workers—and that in many tropical countries it is an occupational disease of the farming community. Experiments have shown that although necator infection is acquired almost exclusively by the percutaneous route, ancylostoma infection may be contracted either percutaneously or orally—the latter mode of entry gives special point to the reports of contamination of vegetables by these larvae.

Contrary to the general belief, it has been shown that larvae of *A. duo-*

*denale* do not always develop directly to adulthood upon invasion of man. Thus, in West Bengal, India, arrested development appears to be a seasonal phenomenon which results in (a) reduction of egg output wasted in seeding an inhospitable environment and (b) a marked increase in eggs entering the environment just before the monsoon begins. The relationship of some key behavioural and social factors to the levels of hookworm infection by studying the defaecation habits of a population in rural Bengal, India, has been investigated.

*Immunity*

Providing people are equally exposed to hookworm infection, both sexes and all ages are susceptible. In communities in which the parasite has long been endemic, the inhabitants develop a host–parasite balance in which the worm load is limited, thus although the infection rate in some rural areas of the tropics may be 100 per cent only a small proportion develop hookworm anaemia. It is not known whether these heavy infections resulting in anaemia are dependent upon repeated exposure to a high intensity of infection, or whether they represent a failure of immunity. Many workers have reported that in their experience the heaviest worm loads are seen at the ages at which infection is first acquired—whether in infancy, later childhood, or, in the case of newcomers to endemic areas, in adult life. Moreover, there seems to be clinical differences in the reactions of the host to a first infection in contrast to chronic infections—eosinophilia and malabsorption, which are usually features of the former, are often absent in the latter. In dogs, the appearance of immunity coincides with the disappearance of eosinophilia and malabsorption.

There is little direct evidence about the effects of host immunity on hookworm in man. It is felt that the response of the skin to a hookworm larva antigen was both specific and sensitive and thus reliable enough for the screening of infected populations. On the other hand, caution in the interpretation of both positive and negative responses to immediate and delayed hypersensitivity skin reactions is suggested. The results of repeated infections with *Nematospiroides dubius* of a population of mice, reproduced features common to highly endemic human hookworm infection, notably its stability and the occurrence of very heavy infections at first exposure and in a small proportion of repeatedly infected animals. Exposure of mice to heavy infection during the period required for resistance to develop consistently resulted in a heavy worm load and provides a possible explanation for early heavy infections in man.

Gel diffusion precipitation and indirect haemagglutination tests on sera of individuals aged from 6 months to 60 years in a *Necator americanus* endemic area have been carried out. Children younger than 24 months showed either no, or a low, antibody response to hookworm antigen. Adults showed higher and at times very high titres. Some specificity was demonstrated by absorption studies between the haemagglutin response to *N. americanus* and *A. lumbri-coides* and between larval and adult hookworms. On electrophoresis, a change in the location of haemagglutins in the serum was noted in patients with hookworm anaemia as compared to normal blood donors. Good reviews on the immune response to nematode infections have been submitted.

CLINICAL PICTURE

Since there are distinct differences in the reaction of the host to first infection and to chronic infection, these two facets will be dealt with separately.

*First infection*
Infection is first acquired in infancy, later childhood, or in the case of newcomers to endemic areas, in adult life. The site of entrance through the skin of the filariform larvae is often characterized by a dermatitis known as 'ground or coolie itch'. There is intense itching, oedema, and erythema and later a papulo-vesicular eruption which lasts up to 2 weeks. In endemic areas, these symptoms either pass unnoticed or are rare.

The pathogenicity of the migratory stages of hookworm is mild compared with that of *Ascaris,* although pulmonary reactions to ancylostoma infection have been noted. In the stage of migration through the lungs, minute haemorrhages may occur with eosinophilic and leucocytic infiltration but once again these seem rare in the tropics.

In the stages of maturation of the worm and sometimes even before eggs appear in the stools, there is abdominal pain, steatorrhoea or sometimes diarrhoea with blood and mucus and a blood eosinophilia of 30–60 per cent. A subject who had been repeatedly infected with *N. americanus* over a period of 5 years showed a rise in serum IgE from an initial figure of 120 ng per ml to 7359 ng per ml. There was little correlation between skin sensitivity reactions, eosinophil count and serum IgE level. Many workers have reported that, in their experience, the heaviest worm loads are seen at the ages at which infection is first acquired. In many instances, however, a residual innocuous worm load is maintained throughout life resulting in symptomless infections.

*Chronic infection*
The majority of sick patients seen in the tropics are chronically infected, a marked eosinophilia is usually absent and the main pathological features of the disease are due to anaemia and hypoalbuminaemia.

*Clinical features*
The patients with hookworm disease describe these symptoms as having been present for between a few days and 3 years. Most of them—farmers—complain that they are unable to work on their farms and their commonest spontaneous symptoms are lassitude, shortness of breath, swelling of the legs,

loss of their normal skin colour, anorexia, and impotence. Some patients have angina pectoris and many complain of aching in their thighs or calves on walking.

By definition the patients are all severely anaemic, yet the accompanying physical signs vary. The majority of them have an increased pulse pressure, peripheral vasodilatation and a raised venous pressure. These patients are usually relatively well and walk to the clinic with haemoglobin levels as low as 2 g per cent. A minority of patients have a small pulse, collapsed veins, severe oedema, often affecting the face and arms, and ascites. They look very ill, continually feel cold and are hypothermic (36° C).

Koilonychia and retinal haemorrhages are present.

*Skin depigmentation*

In negroid patients, the skin is initally pale but begins to darken again within a few days when they are treated with iron, often before the haemoglobin level has risen. In hypoalbuminaemic patients the depigmentation is much more severe and in its distribution resembles that seen in children with kwashiorkor. There are thus two kinds of depigmentation that can be seen in hookworm anaemia; one is attributable to iron deficiency, is nearly always present and recovery begins before anaemia is corrected; the other accompanies hypoalbuminaemia and improves only slowly with treatment. Changes in the colour and texture of the hair as well as parotid enlargement also occur.

*Anaemia*

The main feature of the established adult infection is the production of anaemia. The pathogenesis of the anaemia caused by hookworm is dependent upon three parameters: (1) the iron content of the human diet; (2) the state of the iron reserves; (3) the intensity and duration of infection. These factors will vary in different tropical countries but must always be taken into account for a proper evaluation of a particular situation. Thus, in Nigeria, where the iron intake is high, 21–30 mg daily, people whose only pathological source of bleeding is hookworm infection show no evidence of iron depletion, as evinced by a low serum iron concentration or an iron-deficiency anaemia, unless they harbour more than 800 worms. Whereas in Mauritius where the total iron content of the food is only between 5–10 mg daily, it was found that even moderate hookworm loads could cause sufficient blood loss to precipitate anaemia (Table 1. p. 168).

In human hookworm infection the loss of red cells into the gut is proportional to the worm load and has variously been reported as between 0.03 and 0.05 ml of blood per worm per day for *N. americanus* and between 0.16 and 0.34 ml for *A. duodenale*. The volume of blood sucked does not alter significantly with the development of anaemia, though the quantity of red cells of course decreases. The concept of persistent bleeding ulcers left behind by migrating worms has little histological support in human infections and

TABLE I

RELATIONSHIP BETWEEN HOOKWORM ANAEMIA,
WORM LOAD AND IRON INTAKE IN VARIOUS PARTS
OF THE WORLD

| Author | Country | Threshold of worm load | Dietary iron mg/day |
|---|---|---|---|
| Carr | Mexico | — | |
| Stott | Mauritius | — | 5–10 |
| Sturrock | Tanzania | 40 | |
| Layrisse and Roche | Venezuela | ♀ 80 | |
| | | ♂ 200 | 12–20 |
| Hill and Andrews | U.S.A. | 200 | |
| Darling *et al* | Fiji | 300 | |
| Gordon | Sierra Leone | 800 | |
| Gilles *et al* | Nigeria | 800 | 30 |

bleeding usually stops immediately after complete worming. These findings are not unexpected when it is considered that there is a complete turnover of the jejunal epithelium every 6–24 hours. Nor is any concrete proof available to date in support of the toxic theory of the causation of hookworm anaemia. It is important to recognize that part of haemoglobin iron which the hookworm ingests and excretes while in the duodenum and upper jejunum is reabsorbed from the gut. This proportion increases as the patient becomes depleted of iron and amounts to between 40 and 60 per cent as measured by double isotope studies.

In some parts of the tropics, for example India and Colombia, there occurs a superadded folic acid megaloblastic anaemia which is often masked by the severe iron-deficiency anaemia and which only becomes overt after a partial haematological response to iron therapy. The pathogenesis of folic acid deficiency in severe hookworm infection may be due to a variety of factors: defective folic acid absorption, deficient folic acid in the diet, and increased demands. The classical anaemia of uncomplicated hookworm disease is, however, a hypochromic microcytic anaemia. The distribution of haemoglobin phenotypes is similar in patients with hookworm anaemia as in the general population (Table 2).

*Hypoalbuminaemia*
In addition to anaemia, loss of protein is another important manifestation of hookworm infection. When hypoalbuminaemia occurs it is due to a combined loss of blood and lymph and the protein loss is well in excess of the red blood cells loss. There is nearly always also a limited capacity for albumin synthesis,

TABLE 2

HAEMATOLOGICAL FINDINGS AND OVA COUNTS IN 183 MALE NIGERIAN
PATIENTS WITH HOOKWORM ANAEMIA

| No. of patients | Haemoglobin (g/100 ml) | Mean cell haemoglobin concentration | Serum iron (μg/100 ml) | Ova/g of faeces | Hb genotype (%) | | |
|---|---|---|---|---|---|---|---|
| | | | | | AA | AS | AC |
| 183 | (Mean) 3.2 | 20 | 20 | $46.10^3$ | 72 | 22 | 6 |
| | (Range) 1.3–6.0 | 17–30 | 4–70 | $22.10^3$– $116.10^3$ | | | |

the latter being brought about by a variety of factors such as anaemia, which affects the liver-cell function; and possibly failure to reabsorb amino acids from the albumin passing into the gut. It has been found that the serum albumin concentration was often low in hookworm anaemia and the severe oedema has been attributed to hypoalbuminaemia rather than to heart failure that may be present. Some workers have found that, in some of their patients, oedema did not respond to mercurial diuretics, even after their anaemia had been corrected, but subsided rapidly when they were wormed. It was suggested that oedema might be due to hypoproteinaemia following loss of plasma proteins in the stools. Hookworm disease can therefore be added to the list of causes leading to a protein-losing enteropathy.

*Gastrointestinal function*
Various types of digestive disorders have been attributed to hookworm disease. They range from epigastric disorders to dirt eating. Duodenitis and peptic ulceration have both been suspected of being the result of hookworm infection. The prevalence of duodenal ulceration in our 183 male patients with hookworm anaemia was similar to that encountered in the general outpatients population of University College, Ibadan. Workers have found that gastric acid secretion was low, both at the basal state and after maximal stimulation with histamine, as compared with normal controls, moreover, fibrogastroscopy did not reveal any gross abnormality. Barium meal X-rays reveal non-specific changes of disordered motor function and any appearances consistent with a diagnosis of duodenitis are unrelated to hookworm disease.

There is some disagreement in published reports about the effects of hookworm on the mucosa of the duodenum and jejunum. The experience of the majority of workers is that uncomplicated hookworm anaemia is generally not associated with gross malabsorption and that intestinal morphology, as determined by peroral mucosal biopsies, is within normal range. No clinical evidence of malabsorption in Jamaican patients could be found nor was there any significant difference in the rate of small-intestinal dioxyribonucleic acid (DNA) loss when compared with normal controls. It is more than likely that some investigators reporting abnormalities have in fact studied patients with hookworm infection and pre-existing intestinal disease, especially when anaemia and the presence of hookworm ova in the stools have been the criteria of selection, without consideration of the number of worms present. It is possible, however, that there may be true differences between patients, depending upon such factors as duration of infection, race, and presence of other parasites, for example strongyloidiasis or giardiasis.

DIAGNOSIS

There are several different techniques available for the diagnosis of hookworm infections—the direct smear which may or may not be quantitated; some form of salt flotation; some form of faecal concentration procedure; and faecal culture (coproculture) for species diagnosis. These have been thoroughly and critically reviewed. The ordinary direct saline smear is an examination of 2–3 mg of faeces; quantitative approaches to this examination have been made frequently, notably by Beaver, but provide no more than a rough estimate of worm burden because of the inherent insensitivity of the technique. Another form of direct smear, the cellophane-thick smear or Kato technique, samples 50–60 mg of faeces, is simple to perform, of wide application and gives better quantitative estimates of egg output and hence worm load.

While brine flotation (with sodium chloride, magnesium sulphate, or zinc sulphate) uses 1 g of faeces and is sensitive for nematode egg recovery, sub-sampling from the surface is unreliable for quantitative estimates and trematode eggs shrink; it is essentially a variant of a concentration method. Lane's direct centrifugal flotation (DCF) modification gives quantitative estimates but has the disadvantage of requiring special centrifuge buckets.

The various types of formalin-ether or acid-ether techniques are all concentration methods and the purpose is to recover small numbers of eggs.

Stoll's dilution egg-counting technique, probably more widely used than any other, uses 4 g faeces. It depends essentially on the formulation of a homogeneous suspension of eggs in the diluent with examination of sub-samples representing 5 or 10 mg of faeces. It has the advantage that numerous replicates are possible and thus some stability of the mean egg count is established. It has the disadvantage that light infections are not detected as the technique has a lower limit of sensibility of about 200 eggs per gram of stool. It should not be used for diagnostic work and its utility lies in the epidemiological field where egg outputs and hence worm loads in different populations can be compared. It is useful for roughly estimating the degree of reduction of egg output in patients not parasitologically cured after treatment.

Techniques of coproculture are rightly assuming much greater signifi-

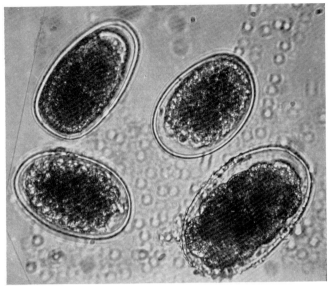

FIG. 22. *N. americanus* ova.

[Courtesy of *Annals of Tropical Medicine and Parasitology*, School of Tropical Medicine, Liverpool]

cance in both epidemiological and clinical studies of hookworm and other nematodes, since they possess sensitivity unequalled by any egg recovery method and, moreover, are species specific. Although laboratory culture methods for recovery of hookworm larvae from faecal samples or soil have long been known to parasitologists, it was not until the concept of filter paper culture in test tubes was introduced that their utility became widely appreciated. Improvements in the original technique such as the adoption of polyethylene tubes for culture and the use of the ancyloscope or the stereomicroscope have made this method indispensable for the study of hookworm.

MANAGEMENT AND TREATMENT

Treatment consists of the correction of the anaemia—usually microcytic but sometimes dimorphic—and the administration of anthelmintics. The responses of *A. duodenale* and *N. americanus* to drugs differ.

*Anthelmintics*
The recommended anthelmintics are relatively non-toxic and in most instances can be given straight away even to debilitated patients. When the anaemia is very severe (less than 5 g per cent) some practitioners prefer to raise the haemoglobin level to about 7–8 g per cent before dealing with the worm

infection specifically. Patients with severe hypoalbuminaemia should be adequately and quickly wormed.

*Tetrachlorethylene* which is still very widely used is given by mouth in a single dose of 0.1 ml per kg body weight with a maximum dose of 5 ml. The drug is given in the morning on an empty stomach. No purgation is necessary either before or after treatment. In heavy infections tetrachlorethylene may have to be given on more than one occasion; if so, it should not be given more frequently than on alternate days. Side-effects are generally mild.

*Bephenium hydroxynaphthoate* (Alcopar) has also been used with good results and minimal side-effects. It is much more effective against *A. duodenale* than *N. americanus* and the dosage varies according to the species being treated. No preparation or purgation is required, but food should be withheld for 2 hours after ingestion of the drug. The dose is 5 g containing 2.5 g base, as a single dose for *A. duodenale*; for *N. americanus* infections, 5 g daily on 3 consecutive days is usually given. In heavy infections, this course may have to be repeated; 15 days should be allowed to elapse in order to properly assess the full effect of the initial treatment.

In the tropics mixed infections of hookworm and ascaris are very common. If tetrachlorethylene is used, *prior treatment* of the ascaris infection must always be carried out with one of the piperazine compounds. Tetrachlorethylene activates ascaris worms in the intestines and in heavy infections a bolus of worms is formed which can lead to intestinal obstruction.

*Mebendazole* (Vermox) 100 mg twice daily for 3 days is also very effective against both types of hookworm.

*Bitoscanate* (Jonit Phenylene-diisothyocyanate 1,4). This anthelmintic is equally effective against both *A. duodenale* and *N. americanus*. The drug is considerably absorbed from the intestine and its mode of action is thought to be twofold; (a) it enters the hookworm when ingestion of the host's blood occurs; (b) it acts directly on the external surface of worms in the lumen of the intestine.

Bitoscanate is administered orally at 12-hourly intervals and only after substantial meals. The adult dose is 100 mg after breakfast, 100 mg after supper on the first day, and 100 mg after breakfast on the second day—i.e. 3 × 100 mg (3 × 2 capsules every 12 hours).

Side-effects are mild and transitory, they include nausea, vomiting, diarrhoea, dizziness, headaches, abdominal pain, and very occasionally fainting. Sometimes an increase of eosinophils following the intake of Jonit can be observed. The safety of the drug in pregnancy has not been finally evaluated and therefore Jonit should not be used in these patients. It has been noted that patients suffering from alcoholism may exhibit an intolerance to the drug. The ingestion of Jonit in combination with coffee may lead to an increase in side-effects and should therefore be avoided. The capsules should not be opened nor chewed as contact dermatitis may be produced.

*Thiabendazole* (Mintezol); *levamizole* (Ketrax); and *pyrantel pamoate*

(Combantrin) are useful broad-spectrum anthelmintics which are also effective against moderate to light hookworm infection.

*Treatment of anaemia*
The response to iron therapy is usually rapid. A cheap and very effective treatment is ferrous sulphate, 200 mg t.d.s. given by mouth and continued for 3 months after the haemoglobin concentration has risen to 12 g per cent. Even without worming, this regime will rectify the anaemia and a rise in haemoglobin of 1 g per cent per week occurs; unless the worms have been removed, however, the haemoglobin will drop as soon as iron therapy is discontinued and anthelmintics are therefore mandatory in heavy infections.

Parenteral iron therapy and blood transfusions are rarely necessary. When indicated, for example if regular oral administration cannot be guaranteed, intramuscular or intravenous total dose iron preparations are very successful. *Ferastral* (a complex of iron and sorbitol gluconic acid) has been successfully used in many tropical countries. A dose of 500 mg for 3–5 injections given as a deep intramuscular injection daily or on alternate days quickly restores the haemoglobin level and replenishes the depleted iron reserves. If concomitant folic-acid deficiency exists, this is treated in the conventional manner.

*Treatment of ground itch and creeping eruption*
Local treatment of ground itch requires the application of antiseptics with the object of reducing the risk of secondary infection. The itching is difficult to relieve but may respond to antihistamine drugs.

*Prophylaxis*
The control of hookworm disease depends on sanitation and mass treatment. Where the latter is effective and faeces are not allowed to remain in surroundings suitable for the development of infective larvae, there will be no infection. In districts in which sanitation has been recently enforced, an attempt should be made at mass treatment with the object of removing the infection from the community. Individual prophylaxis in infected areas includes the avoidance of infection by the protection of parts of the skin; for example, by wearing shoes.

# 12

# LEISHMANIASIS

Leishmaniasis is the result of infection with one or other of a number of species and strains of protozoa belonging to the genus *Leishmania*. Man appears to be the sole mammalian host of some species in some areas; in others, there are additional mammalian hosts or the infection is a zoonosis and man is only a casual host. All the parasites, in nature, are conveyed by sandflies belonging to the genus *Phlebotomus*; in these they undergo a multiplicative cycle of development. It is convenient on clinical grounds to subdivide the leishmaniases into three types: the visceral, the mucocutaneous and the cutaneous.

The organisms recovered from the various types of human infection with *Leishmania* show differences in response to drugs, in susceptibility of animals to infection and in antigenic constitution and immune responses of the host.

The parasites causing the clinical forms of leishmaniasis are:

Visceral: *Leishmania donovani*.
Mucocutaneous: *L. braziliensis*.
Cutaneous: Old World: *L. tropica major*.
      *L. tropica minor*.
  New World: *L. braziliensis*.
      *L. mexicana*.

The biological and antigenic relationships between the species of parasites are not yet fully worked out.

All species of *Leishmania* have specific and group antigens. Complete immunity to the homologous species and strain is established after infection.

Cross-immunity may sometimes develop. An attack of kala-azar confers permanent immunity to *L. donovani* from any geographical area. *L. tropica major* infection provides homologous immunity and usually cross-immunity with *L. tropica minor*; the reverse cross-reaction does not occur. *L. braziliensis* produces permanent homologous immunity and may confer some cross-immunity to *L. mexicana* but not vice versa.

Vaccines have been prepared from cultures of *L. tropica major*, in the form of suspensions of living leptomonads. The suspension is injected intradermally and gives rise to a nodule which seldom ulcerates but may take 6 months to clear. Immunity is developed to *L. tropica major* and *L. tropica minor,* and the leishmanin test becomes positive. A suspension of living leptomonads of *L. mexicana* may also be used as a vaccine. It confers immunity to *L. mexicana* and so protects forest workers from the deforming lesions caused by infection. It does not protect against *L. braziliensis* infections. At present there is no vaccine against espundia.

## VISCERAL LEISHMANIASIS

### DEFINITION

Visceral leishmaniasis, or kala-azar, is a condition due to infection of reticulo-endothelial cells throughout the body with *L. donovani.* The infection is conveyed from man to man by the bites of certain sandflies (*Phlebotomus* spp.). The resultant disease is characterized by a lengthy incubation period, an insidious onset and a chronic course attended by irregular fever, increasing enlargement of the spleen and of the liver, leucopenia, anaemia, and progressive wasting. The mortality is high; death occurs in untreated cases in 2 months to 2 years.

### GEOGRAPHICAL DISTRIBUTION AND EPIDEMIOLOGY

Visceral leishmaniasis is very widespread. It occurs in four main epidemiological forms depending on the geographical area concerned. The clinical features of these forms are essentially similar.

### Indian kala-azar
This form of the disease was practically eliminated by the insecticides used in the widespread malaria eradication campaigns in Bengal, Assam, Madras, South-east India and Burma. In these areas the infection was highly endemic and sometimes occurred in epidemics. The disease has now returned and many thousands of cases have been observed. This recurrence of the disease is due to the local failure of the malaria eradication programmes, based on spraying with residual insecticides, which has led to the reappearance of the vector sandfly.

### Phlebotomus argentipes
Man is the only reservoir of the infection. The disease occurs most commonly in older children.

### Mediterranean kala-azar
This form of the disease classically occurs sporadically in the countries of the Mediterranean littoral. It is also found in Iraq, Iran, parts of the Arabian

peninsula, southern Russia, and in northern China (from where it is now practically eradicated by insecticides and the extermination of the local domestic dog reservoir).

The reservoir of the infection in towns and villages is usually the domestic dog; in rural areas it may be the jackal. The vectors are *P. perniciosus* and *P. chinensis*. The disease is usually seen in infants. It occurs sporadically, not in epidemics.

### African kala-azar

Kala-azar occurs over a wide area of semi-arid country across Africa south of the Sahara, stretching from Senegal to Nigeria in the west, through the Sudan and Chad, to Somalia and Kenya in the east.

The infection is a zoonosis; the reservoirs are usually small rodents. The vectors are *P. orientalis* and *P. martini*. The disease is seen sporadically, occasionally in small epidemics and mostly in adolescents and young adults.

### South and Central American kala-azar

Kala-azar is endemic in northeast Brazil and Paraguay and occurs sporadically in Mexico, Guatemala and contiguous countries, and in Colombia and Venezuela.

The usual reservoir is the domestic dog, sometimes the fox. The vectors vary with the locality; they belong to the subgenus *Lutzomyia*.

The parasite in man lives in the form of morphologically characteristic, inert, oval bodies (leishmania or Leishman–Donovan bodies) in reticulo-endothelial cells throughout the body. These multiply by fission, are liberated by rupture of their containing cells and are taken up by further similar cells in which they again multiply and the cycle is repeated. They appear in small numbers of macrophages in the blood; in this vehicle they are distributed to all parts of the body.

Only female sandflies are blood feeders. After the infective blood meal members of *L. donovani* are liberated in the midgut and rapidly become flagellate leptomonads which migrate forwards to the pharynx and the buccal cavity of the fly. They multiply rapidly and vigorously by simple division and, under suitable conditions, a massive growth of leptomonads blocks the oesophagus and pharynx. On the fly's attempting to take another blood meal some of these flagellates escape from the proboscis into the bite wound, and so the infection is transmitted to a fresh host. The injected flagellates in this host rapidly assume the leishmania form, are taken up by macrophage cells and disseminated as described.

### PATHOLOGY

*L. donovani* parasitizes reticulo-endothelial cells and is found in greatest numbers in those organs which are particularly rich in these cells. Its presence leads to great proliferation of macrophage-type cells. As a result, the liver and especially the spleen enlarge and the red bone marrow extends beyond its normal limits. Reticulo-endothelial tissues in the lymphatic glands, in the lungs, in the intestinal wall, and in the skin, are sometimes heavily parasitized; the degree to which these are affected varies with the strain of parasite and from one case to another. There are almost no tissues from which *Leishmania* have not at some time been recovered on post-mortem of cases of kala-azar and, for this reason, almost every secretion or discharge from the body at some time has been reported to yield parasites.

Histologically the outstanding feature of parasitized tissue is the enormous proliferation of cells of the macrophage type; their presence overshadows the normal structure of the organ and many of the macrophages in the tissue will be seen to contain *Leishmania*. The spleen becomes much engorged and expands until it may largely fill the abdomen; there is little fibrous tissue formation. In the liver the Kupffer cells, which usually are heavily parasitized, proliferate freely. That fibrous tissue formation is not a feature of the histological picture in kala-azar is shown by the return to normal size of an enormously enlarged spleen and liver and the restoration to normal histological structure after effective treatment. The so-called leishmanial fibrosis of the liver is believed to result from fibrosis from other causes, including malnutrition, and not directly from the infection.

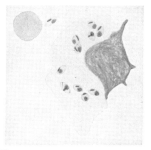

FIG. 23. Kala-azar. Leishman–Donovan bodies in spleen puncture material. [From E.Noble Chamberlain, *A Textbook of Medicine,* John Wright & Sons Ltd., Bristol, 1951]

In the peripheral blood there is an absolute leucopenia (2000–4000 per mm$^3$), due to marked diminution in the number of the granulocytes, as well as mononucleosis. The neutropenia in the later stages of the disease may become a total agranulocytosis, a development commonly followed by the often fatal complication, *cancrum oris*. There is a slowly progressive anaemia, the red cells falling in number to between 2 and 3 million per mm$^3$; the red cells tend to be hyperchromic and macrocytic but nucleated cells are unusual. Red cell fragility is increased; the sedimentation rate is always high; and the platelet count is reduced. The serum bilirubin concentration is usually raised. The total plasma protein is low and there is an inversion of the albumin:globulin ratio, the serum albumin being much reduced as a result of liver dysfunction and the gamma globulin increased partly from increased antibody production. This reversal in the balance of serum protein provides the basis for the formol-gel and other serum tests employed in the diagnosis of kala-azar. In old-standing cases the hypersplenism may influence the blood picture.

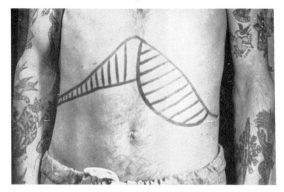

Fig. 24. Kala-azar. Showing enlargement of liver and spleen at time of diagnosis, about 6 months after infection.

[From E.Noble Chamberlain, *A Textbook of Medicine*, John Wright & Sons Ltd., Bristol, 1951]

### CLINICAL PICTURE

The time elapsing between the infecting sandfly bite and the development of clinically demonstrable kala-azar varies greatly. The incubation period ranges from 2 weeks to 18 months or longer. In view of its usually insidious development, and the characteristic absence of prostration even during periods of high fever in this disease, many patients present themselves for diagnosis weeks or months after the onset, commonly because of abdominal swelling caused by enlargement of the spleen and the liver. In cases of this type the patient usually seeks advice between 3 and 6 months after infection, sometimes longer. He may appear looking desperately ill but not feeling it. Though the onset commonly is insidious, in some cases it is acute and simulates the start of an attack of some enteric infection or malaria.

In its early stages kala-azar is not easy to diagnose on clinical grounds when its presence is unsuspected. There is indefinite ill-health and lassitude but there are no constant physical signs. There are irregular fever, a low blood pressure, and a high pulse rate; the changes in the blood picture soon become evident and these, particularly the leucopenia, suggest the diagnosis.

The outstanding physical signs are progressive enlargement of the spleen and, to a lesser extent, of the liver. In the early stages the spleen usually enlarges downwards about 3 cm during each month of the disease; ultimately it may largely fill most of the abdomen and extend into the pelvis. The liver enlarges more slowly, but commonly reaches more than half way to the umbilicus. From time to time patients may be encountered in whom the spleen enlarges but the liver does not or there may be gross enlargement of the liver unassociated with enlargement of the spleen. The enlarged spleen and the enlarged liver are neither painful nor tender. Sometimes there is jaundice, especially late in the disease; it is held to be of bad prognostic significance. In cases of kala-azar from China and the Sudan general enlargement of the lymphatic glands has been reported, but this is not a feature of the disease elsewhere. Though the appetite is usually good, and indeed may be voracious, there is steady bodily wasting. In time the patient becomes emaciated, with a protuberant abdomen due to the gross swelling of the spleen and of the liver.

The fever, which is intermittent, remittent, or continuous, recurs irregularly at intervals of days or weeks. The temperature at some time during the course of a febrile attack may show a double, or a treble, diurnal rise to high peaks. The patient is rarely prostrated and does not usually suffer from the subjective symptoms of fever. Delirium, even in the last stages of the disease, is unusual. Sometimes there is no fever.

The skin is dry and rough; in darkskinned races the natural pigmentation of the skin over the malar bones and temples, and around the mouth, is deepened; it is from this that the disease derives its name (Black Sickness). The hair becomes dry and brittle and tends to fall out; even children may become almost bald, but the hair grows again after specific treatment of the infection.

Oedema of the extremities is not uncommon, particularly in the undernourished and debilitated.

The lungs are invariably involved to some degree; an irritant cough is usual, though physical signs of pulmonary lesions adequate to account for it are absent. Bronchopneumonia and similar complications, due to superadded infections, are common; these are probably attributable to a diminished resistance to infection associated with the leucopenia. Diarrhoea and even dysentery are common, probably arising from superadded infections.

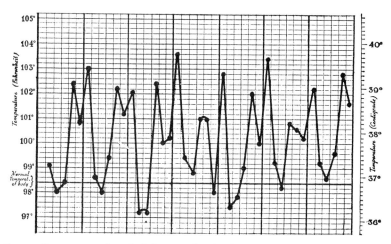

FIG. 25. Temperature chart in kala-azar, showing intermittent or remittent fever with double diurnal rise.

[From E.Noble Chamberlain, *A Textbook of Medicine*, John Wright & Sons Ltd., Bristol, 1951]

Comparatively mild and self-terminating cases of kala-azar may occur. The mortality from the untreated disease is very high; death usually follows within 2 years of the onset.

### POST-KALA-AZAR DERMAL LEISHMANIASIS

An important and not uncommon sequel of visceral leishmaniasis in India, and less frequently in China and the Sudan, is the development of a peculiar dermal localization of the parasite. A year or so after an attack of kala-azar has apparently been cured by specific treatment, lesions of the skin which contain *L. donovani* make their appearance. Their development is not associated with marked ill-health. These dermal lesions vary considerably in appearance; some are erythematous, on the face these commonly assume a butterfly distribution over the nose and cheeks; some take the form of multiple hypopigmented macules, distributed extensively over the trunk and extremities; others, which appear later, take the form of nodules which appear on the sites of one of the preceeding types of lesion, both of which may co-exist on the same patient. The nodules in appearance superficially resemble leprosy nodules; they may be very numerous; they rarely ulcerate; and large numbers of *L. donovani* can be recovered from them. A diagnosis of post-kala-azar dermal leishmaniasis is made on the time of its appearance after recovery from kala-azar and the recovery of *L. donovani* from the lesions.

### DIAGNOSIS

As in every other parasitic infection, the diagnosis of visceral leishmaniasis fundamentally rests on the recovery and recognition of the causative parasite. *Leishmania* can be recovered from the spleen, the bone marrow, the liver or the blood. While the numbers present in any of the tissues, especially the blood, may be so small that direct examination does not reveal them, culture* will usually do so.

Needling and aspiration of material from an enlarged spleen, the sternal or some other red marrow cavity, or the liver afford the best means of finding parasites in ordinary stained smears. Commonly, but not invariably, *Leishmania* are present in great numbers in any of these sites when the disease is well advanced. They are recognized in dried smears of material stained by Giemsa's method, by their characteristic morphology and intracellular

---

* Leishmann–Donovan bodies give rise to growths of flagellate leptomonad forms when sown on media enriched with animal (not human) blood; satisfactory media are N.N.N.Noguchi's leptospira medium, the water of condensation of blood agar, and such special media as Adler's, Lourie's and others. The cultures should *not* be incubated at 37° C; the organisms will *not* grow at this temperature; but they grow at laboratory temperatures (about 25° C). Cultures should be watched for at least 3 weeks before being discarded. Bacterial contamination rapidly kills the protozoa.

location; apparently isolated and free parasites are the result of rupture of the large endothelial cells while making the smear.

In addition to a direct examination of stained smears, culture of parasite material aspirated from such sites should be attempted using single drops of venous blood taken during a febrile period; blood must not be sown in excess on the medium.

The characteristic changes in the blood give an early indication of the development of visceral leishmaniasis. Outstanding is a gross leucopenia, due to a neutropenia, which is associated with a relative mononucleosis; there is a progressive fall in the red cell count and haemoglobin concentration.

Various serum tests, depending on a marked increase in the globulin content, are helpful in diagnosis, though they are not specifically diagnostic of this condition. The formol-gel (aldehyde) test is performed by adding two drops of commercial formalin to 2 ml of the patient's serum in a tube; the mixture is shaken and left to stand at room temperature. A positive reaction is indicated by opacity of the serum, which may also become solid and resemble boiled white of egg, within 20 minutes. The formol-gel test becomes positive within a month or two of the development of the disease, and returns to negative within 6 months of successful treatment and restoration to normal of the plasma proteins. The test is negative in other forms of leishmaniasis, but may be positive in other infections in which there is hypergamma-globulinaemia.

The complement fixation test (using an antigen made from acid-fast bacilli) usually becomes positive early and negative after cure. It is negative in all other forms of leishmaniasis. Results of tests are sometimes unreliable. 'Specific' tests, using antigens made from artificially cultured organisms, or from the spleens of infected hamsters, are also available and equally unreliable.

Fluorescent antibody tests are being used for the identification of this and of other forms of leishmanial infection.

Unfortunately both complement fixation and fluorescent reactions may also show 'false' positive results in trypanosomal infections, and are thus of limited value diagnostically and epidemiologically in areas where both infections exist (not unusual).

The ordinary laboratory animals are insusceptible to infection with *L. donovani*, but the hamster is very susceptible and is much used in experimental work on the parasite.

*Leishmanin skin test* (Montenegro test)
This is a delayed hypersensitivity reaction following intradermal injection of 0.2 ml of a suspension of leptomonads in formolized saline. The test is read 48–72 hours after the injection. A positive reaction is a local induration at least 5 mm across; it represents immunity against reinfection with the homologous strain of *Leishmania*. Its use is not a means of diagnosis of the actual disease.

The test is negative in active kala-azar, but it becomes positive within 2 months of successful treatment and remains so for some years thereafter. It thus is of value in surveys for the presence of the disease in an area; a positive leishmanin rate above 5 per cent is indicative of endemic kala-azar.

PROPHYLAXIS

Certain living strains of *L. donovani,* notably that isolated from ground squirrels in Kenya, when introduced intradermally or subcutaneously, result in a local leishmanial infection (leishmanioma) at the site of inoculation, but not a visceral infection. The local infection persists for 3 or more months and the patient subsequently enjoys a slowly fading immunity against infection with visceral leishmanial infections (*L. donovani*), but not against *L. tropica* infections. This suggests a means of prophylaxis in a community subject to epidemic kala-azar.

In East Africa in some populations there is a high incidence of immunity to experimental infection with human strains of *Leishmania,* possibly the result of previous exposure to non-human strains.

TREATMENT

The trivalent antimonial, potassium antimony tartrate (tartar emetic), was the first drug shown to be therapeutically useful in visceral leishmaniasis. No other trivalent antimonial compounds are of value in the therapy of kala-azar.

Pentavalent antimonials are much more effective. These compounds are not so irritant and are less toxic than are the simple trivalent salts. A high proportion of cases of kala-azar in most areas of its endemicity can be cured by treatment with these pentavalent antimonial drugs. In the Sudan and East Africa the disease has shown itself to be unusually refractory to treatment. Inadequate, or unsuccessful, treatment with antimony of any case of kala-azar may subsequently render that particular case of infection less amenable to it; a greater dosage of the metal becomes necessary to obtain response. If subcurative antimony treatment is continued a stage is reached when the infection becomes completely refractory to the maximum tolerated dosage. When a course of treatment with antimony is begun, therefore, it should whenever possible be continued to its completion without interruption. Fortunately, when resistance to antimony is developed the infection remains susceptible to treatment with certain other drugs.

An effective alternative to the antimonials, which is of particular value in cases of visceral leishmaniasis refractory to antimony treatment, is the diamidine series of drugs. The diamidines are synthetic aromatic preparations which contain no heavy metal; they are therapeutically active against several protozoal infections of man and of animals. Pentamidine isethionate and hydroxystilbamidine isethionate do not cause the troublesome neurological toxic side-effects produced by some other diamidines. They are effective in the radical cure of most forms of kala-azar but are not effective in the treatment of post-kala-azar dermal leishmaniasis, which also is more refractory to the antimonials than is the primary visceral infection. In cases proving refractory to repeated treatment with a variety of drugs, and with greatly enlarged spleen and hypersplenism, splenectomy followed by further intensive treatment may lead to cure.

*Antimonials*

*Urea stibamine.* This compound contains antimony in the pentavalent form and it has been widely and successfully used in the treatment of kala-azar in India and elsewhere. It is a mixture of urea and *para*-aminophenyl stibinic acid of inconsistent constitution. The drug is given in solution in water daily, or on alternate days intravenously for 6–10 doses; it is painful on injection into muscle. The initial dose for an adult is 100 mg, the second is 200 mg; the third and subsequent injections contain 250 mg. For Indian kala-azar a single course totalling 2.5 g (adult dose) is usually adequate. For other forms of kala-azar, 2 or 3 courses, separated by intervals of 14 days are needed. Children are given doses in proportion to kg body weight. Urea stibamine must not be boiled in solution and it must not be left exposed to the air, as it becomes toxic under such conditions. It is contra-indicated in jaundice, cirrhosis, and nephritis.

When the injections are given slowly, side-effects are minimal. Nevertheless there may be coughing, nausea, retching, and vomiting, and in some patients joint pains, abdominal pain, and diarrhoea.

*Sodium stibogluconate* injection (BP). *Pentostam* (BW) is very successful given intramuscularly. Dosage (adult) 6.0 ml (= 600 mg total antimony) daily for 6–10 days. More than one course is necessary for Mediterranean, African, and South American kala-azar, given after intervals of 14 days.

During treatment with the pentavalent antimonials a condition resembling anaphylactic shock may occur very rarely, usually after the fifth or the sixth injection. The temperature rises sharply, often with rigor, and there may be an urticarial eruption, oedema, difficulty in breathing, and cyanosis; hyperpyrexia, shock, and sometimes a fatal issue.

Adrenaline injection (BP) 1.0 ml should be given immediately intramuscularly, followed by 0.5 ml. half-hourly on not more than 2 occasions if the blood pressure remains low. The hyperpyrexia is treated as described on p. 148.

Subsequently, treatment of the leishmaniasis should be continued using an alternative drug and beginning with low dosage.

*Diamidines*

*Pentamidine isethionate* is an aromatic diamidine compound issued as a powder in ampoules. It is given intramuscularly dissolved in water. The dosage is ten daily injections of 3–4 mg of the base per kg body weight (maximum single dose 300 mg). This dosage is adequate for Indian kala-azar. For other forms a second course should be given after an interval of 14 days and, if necessary, repeated after a further interval of 14 days.

Side effects are mild. Toxic reactions may include hypoglycaemia which may be countered by intravenous glucose.

*Hydroxystilbamidine isethionate.* This diamidine is given intravenously by slow infusion in 5 per cent dextrose. The daily dose for adults is 150–250 mg. For children of 5–14 years of age, 125 mg; for children of less than 5 years of age, 60 mg. The dosage is continued for 6–10 days in Indian kala-azar. In other forms of the disease the initial course is given for 10 days and repeated after an interval of 14 days; a third course may be needed after a further interval of 14 days.

Phenergan or other antihistamine drugs should be given concurrently to prevent side-effects, which may include hypotension.

The response to specific treatment of kala-azar with antimonials, or diamidines, is often delayed. The early stages of drug administration are commonly associated with an increase in the temperature and an exacerbation of the symptoms and these may persist throughout treatment. The temperature than falls to normal and shortly afterwards the spleen returns in size to normal with remarkable rapidity; the abnormalities in the blood picture, especially the neutropenia, also rapidly disappear.

### Antibiotics

Amphotericin B has been found to be effective in the treatment of some advanced visceral leishmanial infections which are resistant to other drugs.

The initial dose is 0.1 mg per kg body weight on alternate days, given very slowly (over 4–6 hours) as intravenous infusion in 5 per cent glucose, rising by increments to 1 mg per kg after 10 doses, and continued thereafter at this level for 3–8 weeks. The drug is toxic. Reactions include fever, nausea, vomiting, phlebitis, and impaired renal function.

Phenergan or corticosteroids will relieve reactions. Proteinuria or rising blood urea concentration developing during treatment, or present before treatment are contra-indications.

### Assessment of cure

It is unwise to pronounce a patient to be cured of the disease until at least 2 years without clinical or parasitological evidence of relapse have elapsed since the end of the treatment.

### Post-kala-azar dermal leishmaniasis

This condition does not respond to treatment with the diamidine drugs and is more refractory to antimony treatment than the initial kala-azar to which it is a sequel. A full course of antimony treatment should therefore be given and this may require repetition.

## MUCOCUTANEOUS LEISHMANIASIS

### DEFINITION

Mucocutaneous leishmaniasis, or espundia, of South America is a condition due to infection of reticulo-endothelial cells, initially of the skin and subsequently of the mucosae of the mouth and nose, with *L. braziliensis*. The infection is conveyed from man to man by the bite of certain sandflies (*Phlebotomus* spp.). The resultant disease, after a variable incubation period, is characterized by the appearance of a variety of skin lesions; these commonly are papular, become nodular, and then ulcerate; later, metastatic lesions develop in the mucosae and these extensively erode the adjacent tissues. The sepsis and mutilation resulting from the destructive lesions are responsible for much suffering and a considerable mortality. This sequence of development is not invariable; the condition may not progress beyond the initial cutaneous lesions.

### GEOGRAPHICAL DISTRIBUTION

Classical mucocutaneous leishmaniasis, due to *L. braziliensis*, is the commonest form of leishmaniasis from Costa Rica, through Central America, and in South America, mostly east of the Andes along the Amazon basin and as far south as Paraguay. It is limited to the hot, moist, low-lying forest regions in which the vectors are abundant and is a sylvan and not an urban disease; it does not occur even in forest regions cleared for settlement. The majority of cases progress to the metastatic stage.

Espundia-like lesions of the mouth and nares have been recorded in the Sudan and Ethiopia and in other regions where *L. tropica* is the prevalent parasite.

### AETIOLOGY

Though *L. braziliensis* morphologically and culturally resembles *L. donovani* and *L. tropica,* it is antigenically distinct from them. The parasite is introduced into man by infected sandflies. Initially, in most cases, the infection is confined to the skin; its appearance later in mucous membranes remote from the initial lesions suggests metastasis through the blood-stream.

*L. braziliensis* is a natural infection of rodents, and is transmitted by sandflies (subgenus *Lutzomyia*), which feed on them and sometimes on man. The sandflies acquire the infection by ingesting *Leishmania* when feeding near a lesion. In the gut of the insect these become flagellate leptomonads, the escape of which into a wound at the time of biting is the means whereby the infection enters a new host.

### PATHOLOGY

The primary lesion is cutaneous and develops at the site of the bite. A papule forms which develops into a nodular granulomatous tumour which contains large numbers of proliferating and parasitized macrophage cells. With the appearance of the earliest skin lesions there is some enlargement of the lymphatic glands draining the area; in these also are to be found many macrophage cells containing *Leishmania*. The skin tumours, which are commonly multiple, may remain small and in due course spontaneously disappear, or they may progress to a considerable size and ulcerate. Pyogenic bacterial infection of the ulcerated area is followed by inflammatory changes. Metastasis of the parasitic infection of the skin takes place in the nasobucco-pharyngeal mucosal surfaces causing foul ulcerative lesions which involve contiguous tissues causing distressing deformity.

### CLINICAL PICTURE

As a rule the time intervening between infecting sandfly bites and the appearance of skin lesions in the bitten areas is 10 and 25 days. The primary lesions are usually located on exposed parts of the body; they generally range from one to three in number but occasionally may be more numerous. These initial lesions commonly take the form of itchy papules.

The lesions may retrogress and vanish or may remain stationary without apparent development. Alternatively, they become nodular tumours, which may or may not ulcerate.

The ulcerated type of nodular lesion is the most characteristic. The ulcers vary considerably in size, often exceeding 10 cm in diameter. They have sharply defined edges and a much depressed base which lies on the structures beneath the skin; an indurated wall projects above the level of the surrounding skin. From the base of the ulcer there exudes a sero-purulent discharge; the surface of which dries and forms a tough, brown, membranous crust.

The non-ulcerating lesions are classified as being impetiginous or nodular. The latter may be verrucose or framboesiform. The verrucose lesion is a firm, wart-like tumour with an irregular surface covered with an exudate which dries into a hard scab. The framboesiform lesion is commoner and forms a soft, papillomatous tumour resembling a yaw.

Regional lymphangitis and lymphadenitis usually accompany the ulcerating skin lesions. Though the glands do not greatly enlarge, the lymphatics are very much thickened and become cord-like; nodular dilatations in them may break down and ulcerate through the overlying skin, forming new lesions.

The outstanding feature of *L. braziliensis* infection is metastasis of the parasites in the mucosae, commonly those of the upper respiratory tract and the mouth, rarely those of the genitals. Though this metastasis may be sometimes due to autoinoculation it is generally the result of dissemination of the parasites in the blood stream or lymphatics. Mucosal metastasis occurs even in patients whose initial skin lesions have run an apparently abortive course. In about 10 per cent of all cases it makes its appearance early, and concurrently with that of the skin lesions; in the others it appears later, often after some years. Leishmanial infection of the nasal mucosa takes place before clinical evidence of its presence is apparent; thus, curettings of nasal mucous membrane may yield *Leishmania* some time before mucosal changes occur. The mucosa of the anterior part of the cartilaginuous septum is usually the first to be affected. It becomes reddened and thickened, an ulcer forms, spreads, and extends deeply into the surrounding tissues; the cartilages (but not bone) are destroyed. Adjacent and opposing mucosal surfaces become infected and the process extends backwards into the nasal cavity. Ultimately the entire cartilaginous framework of the nose disappears; the ulcerative process destroys the lips; it invades the soft palate, the fauces, and the rhino-pharynx; and in due course it extends to the larynx and the trachea. It causes much suffering, hideous mutilations, and deformities which may lead to death from respiratory involvement or from inability to take or swallow food.

### DIAGNOSIS

Recovery and identification of the parasite puts the diagnosis beyond doubt. Parasites may be found in aspirates of tissue juice from the lesions, lymphatics, lymph glands, biopsy of lesions, and scrapings of the nasal mucosa. Where parasites are so few that they cannot be recognized in smears, similar material taken aseptically and cultured on suitable media will often yield a growth of flagellates.

There are no serological tests of practical value for the diagnosis of espundia as distinct from leishmanial infection as such.

### TREATMENT

All leishmanial skin lesions acquired in the endemic area must be regarded as potentially metastatic and require immediate treatment.

Some cases will respond to pentavalent antimonial drugs in full dosage. Certain authorities hold that repeated courses of sodium antimony tartrate, as for schistosomiasis, may be effective if pentavalent antimonials fail. Of those which do not, some will respond to pyrimethamine (also used in malaria and toxoplasmosis) given orally in doses of 25 mg daily for 2 weeks. After a rest of 7–10 days the dosage schedule should be repeated and repeated again after a further interval of 7–10 days. Folic acid and vitamin B should be given concurrently.

Cases which do not respond to the above treatment or in which metastatic lesions have developed may be given a full course of Amphotericin B (see p. 127).

Local treatment of the lesions includes cauterization with heat and diathermy, infiltration with solutions of emetine, mepacrine, berberine sulphate, phosphorated oil and other preparations.

# CUTANEOUS LEISHMANIASIS

### DEFINITION

Cutaneous leishmaniasis is a condition due to infection of reticulo-endothelial cells of the skin and, in some cases, also of mucosa, with *L. tropica, L. mexicana* and possibly *L. braziliensis.* The infections are conveyed by sandflies (*Phlebotomus* spp.) in the Old World and by the subgenus *Lutzomyia* in the New World. The resultant diseases are characterized by single or multiple indolent skin lesions and, in some cases, mucosal lesions without systemic involvement. The infections may disappear spontaneously, leaving disfiguring scars or persist for very long periods causing mutilation.

### GEOGRAPHICAL DISTRIBUTION

Cutaneous leishmaniasis due to infection with *L. tropica* (called by local names such as Oriental sore, Delhi or Aleppo boil. Baghdad or Biskra boil or button) occurs sporadically in the countries of the Mediterranean littoral, especially southern Europe and North Africa, in Africa south of the Sahara and in the Middle East, southern Russia, northwest India and northern China. It is usually found in arid areas with marked diurnal temperature variations.

Cutaneous leishmaniasis due to *L. mexicana* and *L. braziliensis* occurs in certain areas in Central or South America.

### CUTANEOUS LEISHMANIASIS OF THE OLD WORLD

These lesions result from infection with *L. tropica.* They appear in three major forms: moist (*L. tropica major*), dry (*L. tropica minor*), and lupoid.

### *Moist (or rural) cutaneous leishmaniasis*
Man is infected sporadically from sandflies infected from the wild rodent reservoirs. Epidemics occur occasionally in villages. The infection is largely transmitted out of doors.

The lesion is self-limited. It develops at the site of the bite, enlarges rapidly, and then subsides within about 6 months, leaving a scar the severity of which depends on the state of secondary infection. Infection may also result from extension from an existing lesion by contact, scratching, etc. In this way, a single individual may develop several lesions.

### Urban (dry) cutaneous leishmaniasis
*L. tropica minor* infects man and the domestic dog. Man to man infection via the sandflies *P. sergenti* or *P. papatasii* can occur, usually indoors.

The lesion is strictly cutaneous and is nearly always single. It grows slowly and may ulcerate. Healing is slow but commonly complete with little scarring after a year. The tissue reaction is much less intense than in *L. tropica major* infections; there are no metastases. Multiple lesions occur in some cases.

### Lupoid (relapsing) leishmaniasis
This infection is seen in countries in the Middle East. The lesions closely resemble those of *lupus vulgaris*. The lesion spreads slowly, leaving a healed area in the centre and advancing at the edges. The progress takes years. *Leishmania* are present in small numbers; the leishmanin skin test is positive.

*L. tropica* attacks non-immune persons of all races, any age, and either sex. Among the indigenous populations the lesions are commonly seen in children. Recovery from an infection affords immunity to reinfection. Where the incidence of the disease is high most of the adult population have suffered from it in childhood. Immunity to reinfection has long been appreciated by some peoples who deliberately infect young children from a sore to forestall infection of the face with its disfigurement.

### PATHOLOGY

In *L. tropica* infections the pathological changes are limited to the areas of infected skin. The local reaction to the infection is the multiplication of infected macrophage cells in the area and swelling and proliferation of infected endothelial cells lining small vessels. A small granulomatous nodule forms which increases in size; the damage to and proliferation of the lining cells obstructs the blood vessels, and necrosis of the centre of the tumour follows. An ulcer is formed. The ulcerated surface becomes infected with pyogenic bacteria and chronic mild inflammatory changes develop, with lymphangitis and lymphadenitis. The leishmanial infection gives rise to no remote or constitutional changes.

### CLINICAL PICTURE

The time elapsing between an infecting sandfly bite and the development of the ensuing skin lesion at its site varies from a few weeks to as much as 3 years; usually it is between 3 and 6 months.

The initial moist or rural lesion caused by *L. tropica major* occurs on a part of the body normally unprotected by clothing and available to attack by the flies. The face, the forearms and backs of the hands, and the thighs, legs, and dorsal aspects of the feet are the most common sites in those wearing European-type tropical clothing. The scalp is not involved even when unprotected. Normally the lesion initially takes the form of a small red itching papule; this becomes a small nodule which is surrounded by a zone of erythema. The centre of the granulomatous tumour then breaks down and an ulcer forms. From this, when it is secondarily infected, there exudes a small amount of mucoid pus which dries and forms a crust. The lesion increases in size; it becomes more indurated; and the area of ulceration correspondingly increases. The mucoid pus exuded from the ulcer base forms a leathery scab, in which sand, dirt and other particles become imbedded.

The walls of an Oriental sore stand up above the surrounding skin, and the edges of the ulcer in it are precipitous and sharply defined. On pulling off the scab a granulating base covered with viscid pus containing a varied bacterial flora will be exposed. No *Leishmania* will be found in this exudate, as these parasites do not survive in the presence of gross bacterial contamination. If, however, the base of the lesion can gently be cleansed without causing bleeding some serous fluid exudes from it, and this will usually contain parasites.

Secondary sores may form immediately around the initial sore and these are extensions due to contamination. Other more remote secondary sores may form following transference of the infection by scratching or by contact of a sore with an abrasion on an opposing skin surface.

An ulcer, if neglected, may develop to the size of a thumb nail or larger. It becomes grossly septic and, under such conditions, it at last heals spontaneously with much scarring; if on the face, this may cause a cosmetic deformity.

While single sores are most common in clean and well-cared-for people, multiple sores are usual in the poorer native population of an endemic area. Nevertheless, 200–300 small sores distributed over the face, forearms, and backs of the hands have developed on a European visitor after a short visit to a Middle East endemic area.

In addition to this, the 'normal' form of Oriental sore, non-ulcerative verrucous or fungating types of lesions are seen to a lesser extent in the same areas of endemicity; these appear to be especially prevalent in south-eastern Russia and Turkestan. In the latter areas the lesions assume a fungating papillomatous, or cauliflower-like, form without ulceration.

On occasions an espundia-like condition, with progressing involvement of the mucosae of the mouth and nose, has developed as a sequel to a cutaneous lesion.

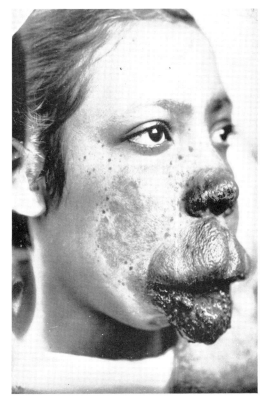

FIG. 26. Leishmaniasis tegumentosa with elephantoid swelling.
[By couresty of Professor C. da Silva Lacaz, Brazil]

### DIAGNOSIS

The diagnosis is established when the causative parasite has been recovered and identified. In moist cutaneous leishmaniasis, before the sore reaches the stage of self-healing, *Leishmania* are present in enormous numbers in the indurated walls and in the tissues underneath the base.

A portion of the unbroken skin in the outer wall of the indurated tumour is cleansed; a fine needle on a syringe, or a capillary glass pipette with a compressed rubber teat, is pushed well into it and a tiny sample of tissue juice is aspirated. The aspirated material is smeared on a slide, which is stained by Giemsa's method. Numerous intracellular *Leishmania* will probably be found. Material obtained in the same way, with strict aseptic precautions, should be sown on a medium suitable for the culture of *Leishmania*. This is kept at room temperature and examined over a period of 3 weeks before discarding. In the absence of bacterial contamination, if *Leishmania* are present there will be a growth of flagellate leptomonads. Methods of diagnosis are similar in other cutaneous leishmaniasis, in which, however, the parasites are fewer.

Treatment of moist and dry cutaneous leishmaniasis is the same. General treatment is needed when lesions are multiple or when there are metastases. Single lesions are self-limiting and need only local treatment and exclusion of autoinfection of other skin areas.

Antimonial drugs may be given parenterally as in kala-azar. They are also infiltrated locally around the edge of the lesion. Mepacrine hydrochloride [200 mg (2 tablets) in 5.0 ml sterile water] may also be used to infiltrate the surrounds. Other local infiltrates that have been used with some success are 5 per cent emetine hydrochloride and 2 per cent berberine sulphate.

Diffuse cutaneous (lupoid) leishmaniasis sometimes responds to infra-red therapy, probably as a result of improved circulation of blood. Chemotherapy as above is also required.

## CUTANEOUS LEISHMANIASIS OF THE NEW WORLD

The infecting agents are (i) *L. braziliensis,* leading to mucocutaneous leishmaniasis (Espundia) which is described separately above, to Uta, the so-called primary cutaneous leishmaniasis of Peru and to Diffuse Cutaneous Leishmaniasis, (ii) *L. mexicana,* which causes Chiclero Ulcer or Bay Sore.

## UTA

This infection is found in valleys in the Western Andes in Peru. It has been eradicated in areas where DDT has been used in malaria eradication. The reservoir is the domestic dog and the vector the house-dwelling *P. peruensis.* The lesions are small, single, and dry, and usually confined to the skin, though they may occur occasionally on exposed mucous membranes. There are no metastases.

Treatment is the same as for *L. tropica* infections.

## DIFFUSE CUTANEOUS LEISHMANIASIS

(Leproid or cheloid leishmaniasis: Leishmaniasis tegumentosa diffusa)

This form of leishmaniasis was first described in Venezuela. A very similar picture has since been described in Ethiopia. Both resemble lepromatous

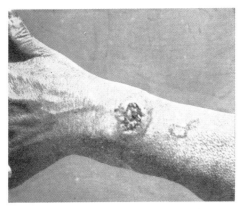

FIG. 27. Cutaneous leishmaniasis Oriental sore.
[From E. Noble Chamberlain, *A Textbook of Medicine,* John Wright & Sons Ltd, Bristol, 1951]

leprosy and are often mistaken for it. The primary lesion forms in the skin and spreads locally. Eventual lesions are pleomorphic and include erythematous macules, papules, and nodules, which may reach considerable size. Diffuse infiltration of large areas may also occur, with roughness and dryness of the affected skin. Lesions are commonest on the face, nose, ears, arms, fingers, hands, elbows, legs, toes, and knees. The lesions develop slowly and persist; they seldom ulcerate.

The disease is very resistant to treatment. Amphotericin B used as in kala-azar is regarded as the best therapy in the South American form. Repeated parenteral courses of Pentamidine have been used with modest success in the Ethiopian form.

The South American form is due to infection with *L. braziliensis*; the Ethiopian variety results from infection with *L. tropica*. It is not known whether the lesions develop because of special host sensitivity to the infecting agent or whether the *Leishmania* represent special variants of the parent species.

## CHICLERO ULCER (FOREST YAWS, BAY SORE)

This syndrome is found in the lowland rain forests of Central America, especially Guatemala, and in parts of Mexico. It occurs in similar areas in all other Central American states, including Panama. In some areas it co-exists with Espundia.

It is caused by *L. mexicana* which is an enzootic of small forest rodents. It is transmitted by sandflies (*Luzomyia* spp.) which seldom bite man unless disturbed. There is evidence that the culpable sandfly rests in the fallen leaves of the forest trees and is disturbed in the early morning by the workers. The

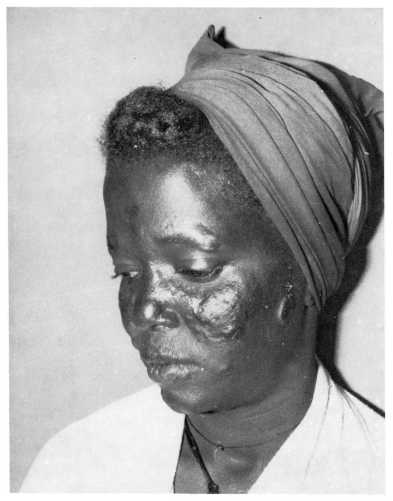

FIG. 28. Diffuse leishmaniasis: Ethiopia.
[By courtesy of Professor W. Peters]

disease is most commonly seen in gum collectors (Chicleros) and other forest workers.

The lesions are single and self-limited. They do not metastasise but when they develop in some anatomical regions they may cause extensive, slow, and irregular local necrosis. The lesions are particularly common on the pinna of the ear and other parts of the face; they also occur in the neck and limbs, at the site of the sandfly bites.

Lesions are normally self-limited and will heal without treatment. Some scarring results, the degree depending on the secondary infection. Bay sores on the ears need treatment. Cycloguanil pamoate (also used as a depot suppressive in malaria) in a dose of 6 mg (base) per kg body weight in an oil matrix, injected intramuscularly, has been found successful. One injection of this depot substance is sometimes sufficient. It may be repeated in cases which relapse.

# 13

## LEPROSY

### (Contributed by S.G.Browne)

DEFINITION

Leprosy is a complex clinical condition resulting from infection with a specific micro-organism, *Mycobacterium leprae* (called Hansen's bacillus, after the Norwegian doctor who first described it in 1874). The disease is characterized by a long and variable latent (incubation) period, a protracted course, and lesions in the skin, the upper respiratory mucosa, and the peripheral nerves. Its course, clinical manifestations, and prognosis demonstrate an extreme range of host–parasite response, from a banal self-healing and localized cutaneous infection to a relentlessly progressive and generalized mycobacteriosis of the tissues affected.

GEOGRAPHICAL DISTRIBUTION

The oldest indubitable written records of leprosy are from India, dated about 600 B.C., but they may embody earlier oral traditions. The disease was apparently unknown in the Western world until the return to Europe from the Indian campaign of Alexander's troops in 327–326 B.C., though Nubian slaves may have meanwhile brought it into Egypt. Thereafter, it was spread around the Mediterranean littoral and to the countries of northwestern Europe by traders, soldiers and pilgrims. Today, leprosy is a problem of serious dimensions mainly in the populous lands of the tropics and subtropics, though very few countries are completely free from the disease. The greatest concentration is to be found in India and the highest prevalence rates in tropical Africa. All the countries in South-east Asia are affected, most of South America, and the Pacific Islands. Leprosy is present among the Australian aboriginals, in the Papua New Guinea Highlands, in the cold uplands of Central Asia, and the equatorial forests of Africa. The total number of sufferers may reach the figure of fifteen millions. Endemic leprosy still occurs in Europe—in Iceland, and more particularly in the southern countries bordering the Mediterranean, and in southern U.S.S.R. The conditions said to favour its maintenance and spread are intimate human contacts in overcrowded and unhygienic conditions; the influence of such environmental factors as temperature, humidity, and elevation is indirect.

AETIOLOGY

The causative organism, *M. leprae*, is an acid- and alcohol-fast organism that in appearance closely resembles *M. tuberculosis*. Despite many claims, it has not yet been successfully and reproducibly cultured in artificial media, nor until recently has it been successfully transmitted to laboratory animals. Recent claims of successful culture of the causative organism have been based on modifications of Eagle's or Hanks' media, on semi-solid agar, and on the addition of various possible adjuvant factors or mycobactins. Hyaluronic acid is claimed to facilitate growth. Much effort is being devoted to this aspect of leprosy research, and interesting findings of diverse aberrant bacterial forms (coccoid, spore-like, and mycoplasma-like bodies, diphtheroid forms, elongated, club- and L-forms) obtained from patients suffering from multibacillary forms of leprosy, have been published. The long generation time (of 12–14 days), and the strict criteria for multiplication based on complicated laboratory techniques, have eliminated many rapidly growing mycobacterial contaminants, and the need for experimental demonstration of neurotropism has excluded other claimants. The production of a bacillary and tissue extract, similar to lepromin, giving a similar range and intensity of reactions as classical lepromin, furnishes another criterion for identifying a mycobacterium as *M. leprae*. Limited local multiplication in the mouse footpad has, however, been achieved, and systemic multiplication accompanied by widely disseminated bacilliferous granulomata in the extremities has been obtained in mice rendered immunologically incompetent by thymectomy and whole-body irradiation. This elegant model has already proved of great usefulness in the identification of *M. leprae*, the demonstration of its viability, the screening of drugs, the proof of drug-resistance, the effect of BCG vaccination in enhancing potential resistance to mycobacterial challenge, the elucidation of cell-mediated immunity to infection, etc. These experimental findings confirm the repeated observation that *M. leprae* are consistently present, though in widely varying concentrations, in lesions clinically diagnosable as leprosy. Koch's postulates are in the process of being fulfilled. More recently, the nine-banded armadillo, found wild in the southern States of U.S.A., Central and South America, has been shown to be susceptible to experimental inoculation of living *M. leprae*, 40 per cent of inoculated animals succumbing to a generalized infection resembling lepromatous leprosy. The armadillo has a long life span, a low body temperature, and an immunological capacity resembling in many respects that of humans; it produces identical quadruplets (but does not reproduce in captivity). Considerable quantities of *M. leprae* are now available for study of the biochemical constitution and immunological properties of the many distinct antigens present within the organism and in its cell walls. Recently, a leprosy-like disease has been reported in wild armadillos in Louisiana.

## EPIDEMIOLOGY

*Source of infection*
Bacilli are shed in enormous numbers from the nasal mucosa and from

ulcerating skin lesions of patients with bacilliferous forms of leprosy. Although they are present in the dermis of such patients, the subepidermal zone and the epidermis itself are usually free from bacilli. They may, however, emerge to the surface from the cells lining the hair follicles, the sweat glands and the galactophorous ducts. Since leprosy bacilli may remain viable for possibly longer than 9 days after being shed from the nose, contaminated fomites may constitute a source of infection. Biting insects may also mechanically introduce viable organisms into the dermis: they have been demonstrated in the mouth-parts of biting insects that have fed on patients suffering from lepromatous leprosy and such insects have experimentally infected laboratory animals. The discharge from neuropathic ulcers only very rarely contains viable bacilli. On standard methods of examination, the lesions of tuberculoid leprosy contain extremely few non-viable bacilli, but patients with such lesions are apparently the source of secondary contact cases with far greater frequency than the scanty infection would suggest. The urine, faeces, and semen may rarely contain leprosy bacilli.

*Infection*

The mode of acquisition of leprosy is not known for certain. Prolonged and intimate contact of a susceptible subject with an index case shedding viable bacilli is generally held to be necessary, but many exceptions to this rule are well authenticated. By far the most prolific source of viable bacilli is the mucoid nasal secretion of persons suffering from lepromatous leprosy. Droplet infection is thus probably more important than the transcutaneous implantation of bacilli through a breach in the skin surface. Ingestion or swallowing of contaminated particles cannot be excluded. The site of inoculation is not necessarily the site of the initial lesion. Infection is generally acquired in childhood or adolescence but this apparent age-susceptibility may be related to opportunity for exposure rather than to innate lack of resistance. No age is exempt. The actual succumbing to leprosy infection, and the development of one or other of the determinate varieties of leprosy, appear to depend predominantly on an inherited ability of the individual to lyse, or not to lyse, *M. leprae*. Nothing is known with certainty about healthy carriers or convalescent carriers of leprosy bacilli, but recent findings suggest that healthy carriers, as well as apparently healthy contacts in the pre-clinical phase of infection, may harbour viable bacilli. Subclinical infection is apparently very common; most persons who have been exposed to leprosy in a closed community for more than a few months show evidence in their lymphocytes of such exposure.

*Development*

The fate of the leprosy bacilli that successfully arrive in the dermis depends on the immunological capacity of the individual to mount a cell-mediated immunity. Either, on the one hand, the bacilli fail to multiply, and the degenerating forms provoke a diffuse non-specific, round-cell reaction or a more vigorous tuberculoid response; or, on the other hand, there is no significant cellular reaction, and the organisms multiply unrestrictedly and disseminate both in the local tissues and systemically. The vigorous cellular reaction may localize the organisms and destroy them, thus averting a more general infection. In patients in whom the defence mechanism is less effective, the organisms pass beyond the papillary layer of the skin and apparently are phagocytosed by the Schwann cells of the smaller ramifying nerve fibres. Some are taken up by wandering reticulo-endothelial cells in the dermis; in them, they appear to multiply freely, causing no recognizable damage to the host cell. Eventually such cells may become replete with fifty or more organisms (*globi*). Organisms are found at certain sites of election in the dermis, as follows: in the vicinity of nerve tissue, in the arrectores pilorum muscles, and in the endothelial cells and media of the small blood vessels. In addition to haematogenous spread when a heavily laden endothelial cell ruptures and discharges its contents into the blood-stream, organisms also travel in the skin lymphatics to distant areas, sometimes bypassing lymphatic nodes and sometimes multiplying freely in such nodes.

Although *M. leprae* are present in greatest concentration in the dermis, the upper respiratory mucosa and the peripheral nerve trunks, organisms will be found if looked for in a variety of deep tissues, i.e. liver, bone marrow, spleen, kidney glomeruli, lungs, lymphatic nodes, all the superficial structures of the eye, posterior root ganglia, etc.; the central nervous system (including the optic and olfactory nerves), however, seems to be almost completely spared, although organisms have been found in the brain of experimentally infected animals.

While the development of multibacillary disease in the individual may reasonably be related to the dissemination of *M. leprae* in tissues that offer both the essential biological micro-environment and an absence of inimical factors, the mode of the spread of other forms of leprosy to different parts of the body is by no means clear. It may be that a few scanty organisms, alive or dead, or their breakdown products, are transported by the blood stream to sites previously sensitized, and there provoke the typical cellular response to their presence.

*Immunity*
Recent work suggests that the basic difference in individuals that determines response to infection is their innate (perhaps in part genetically determined, and inherited) way of dealing with *M. leprae* once it enters the tissues. If the individual reacts by lysing the organisms, which in him evoke a cell-mediated immunity—a tuberculoid response—then he will show the signs of tuberculoid leprosy. If, on the other hand, he belongs to the 1 per cent who are unable to do this, he will suffer from lepromatous leprosy. Not so easy to explain, on this basis, is the great range of intermediate types of leprosy, in which the degree of immunity not only varies within wide limits, but may apparently display wide variations in the individual from time to time.

*The lepromin test*

While the lack of a skin screening test comparable to the Heaf or Mantoux in tuberculosis continues to hamper epidemiological investigations and population surveys for leprosy, the lepromin test does provide a valuable indication of the potential reactivity of the body when the individual is challenged by a mixture of antigens derived from lepromatous tissue. ('Lepromin' consists essentially of leprosy bacilli, intact and fragmented, tissue elements (cellular and acellular), and tissue fluid, prepared in various ways from lepromatous nodules, etc. It is sterilized, purified, and biologically standardized. An amount of 0.1 ml is introduced intradermally in the hairless, anterior forearm skin.) The early (Fernandez) reaction, read after 48–72 hours, consists of an area of erythema and oedema, and is roughly comparable with the Mantoux reaction in tuberculosis, representing sensitivity to injected protein. The late (Mitsuda) reaction, usually attaining its maximum in 3–4 weeks, indicates the degree of sensitivity to the mixture of antigens injected. It is this latter reaction that is important in leprosy.

In patients with lepromatous leprosy, the late (Mitsuda) reaction is completely negative. In patients with tuberculoid leprosy, it is variably positive, the degree of positivity being correlated with the vigour of tissue response, i.e. the diameter of the erythematous papule and its ulceration will be parallel with the cellular response in the skin and peripheral nerves. In the intermediate forms of leprosy, the reaction is weakly and variably positive.

The reaction (read at 48–72 hours, and about the twenty-first day) is expressed in millimetres (of diameter of the papule), with or without ulceration.

Only very rarely of use in diagnosis, the lepromin reaction provides valuable confirmatory evidence for classification and for prognosis. The positivity of the reaction tends to increase with age, with urban residence, with exposure to tuberculosis and to anonymous mycobacteria. It may become transiently negative in an acute inflammatory phase of tuberculoid leprosy. Its negativity in lepromatous leprosy (despite the presence of circulating $\gamma$-globulin antibodies and the tendency to develop signs of erythema nodosum leprosum), is a paradox that awaits elucidation and explanation.

### IMMUNOLOGY

The study of the immunology of leprosy, employing modern investigative techniques, is shedding welcome light on the fundamental processes of cell-mediated immunity in resistance to infection and in determining the outcome of an established infection. The lymphocyte transformation test indicates that over a quarter of subjects living in an area in which leprosy is endemic give a positive response to *M. leprae*. Patients with lepromatous leprosy fail to inhibit *M. leprae*-induced leucocyte migration.

The serum proteins are usually raised in multibacillary leprosy and the albumin:globulin ratio is reversed. The increase in γ-globulins has been shown (by immuno-electrophoresis) to be due to increase in both IgG and IgM. Further evidence of serological disturbance is shown by the following changes: The Rubino test (rapid sedimentation of formalized sheep cells) is frequently positive; false reactions for syphilis may occur; during reactional episodes, C-reactive protein may show a high titre and the erythrocyte sedimentation rate may be raised; cryoproteins, euglobulins, thyroglobulin antibodies, antinuclear factor, rheumatoid factor, and LE cells have been demonstrated. These changes are generally registered in patients with lepromatous or near-lepromatous leprosy, especially when passing through a reactional episode, but they also occur to a much less degree in the serum of patients suffering from tuberculoid leprosy.

The specific immunological defect in leprosy has not yet been identified, but the importance of thymus-dependent lymphocytes (T cells) in determining the outcome of leprosy challenge is now generally accepted. The factors concerned in the capacity of macrophages to facilitate the intracellular multiplication of ingested organisms, are being investigated.

Specific- and group-antibodies present in quantity in the serum of patients suffering from leprosy—especially multibacillary forms, and such forms during episodes of acute exacerbation—exert apparently no restraining effect upon the multiplication and dissemination of leprosy bacilli, and may by themselves be responsible for tissue damage.

Many of the phenomena associated with the acute inflammation experienced by patients suffering from lepromatous leprosy are seen to be manifestations of tissue sensitivity and resulting from antigen–antibody confrontation and complement, and the deposit of immune complexes. When such phenomena occur in target organs (such as dermis, the uveal tract, peripheral nerves, kidney glomeruli, etc.), the clinical results may be disastrous.

### PATHOLOGY

The contradictions and discrepancies apparent in much of the older literature dealing with the pathology of leprosy, and associated with imprecise nomenclature and ill-based generalizations, are now giving place to a more rational (and understandable) picture that takes cognizance of the extremely wide range of the host–parasite relation in leprosy. Recent advances in the microbiology and immunology of leprosy are providing the essential background for understanding the pathology and histology of this fascinating disease.

### TYPES OF DISEASE

It is now generally agreed that there are two extreme or 'polar' types of leprosy and that in between these two polar types is a whole range of intermediate types variously referred to as borderline or dimorphous.

The first polar type is 'lepromatous' leprosy, which is characterized by apparently unfettered multiplication of the causative organisms and their ready dissemination in the body without provoking any specific cellular reaction to their presence. The second type is 'tuberculoid', in which the multiplication and dissemination of the organisms are restricted by an active defence mechanism of the tissues locally, a cell-mediated immunity. (The term 'tuberculoid' refers to the histological 'tubercle', a non-specific response induced by a wide range of particulate foreign bodies, biological or chemical in origin, in individuals apparently pre-determined to react in this fashion.) Patients with lepromatous leprosy show no evidence of tissue sensitization to *M. leprae*, and are completely negative to the lepromin test; whereas the variably positive lepromin test of patients with established tuberculoid leprosy indicates some degree of tissue sensitization to *M. leprae* or its breakdown products. The histological features characteristic of these extreme clinical types of leprosy differ within wide limits, and the various intermediate types may partake to a greater or less degree of the features of the extreme types, depending on their nearness to the lepromatous or to the tuberculoid pole.

In the early stage of leprosy infection, before the disease has clinically or immunologically shown a definite orientation towards one or other pole, the lesions are described as 'indeterminate'. The infection is definitely ascribed to *M. leprae* (which are, however, extremely scanty), but there is insufficient evidence to indicate towards which of the 'determinate' or determined types of leprosy (lepromatous, tuberculoid, or intermediate) the infection will eventually orientate itself, or whether this phase will prove to have been transient and self-limiting.

The histology of these types of disease will now be considered.

### 1. *Indeterminate leprosy*

The only departure from the normal is the presence of scattered collections of round cells in the dermis, with no apparent localization. There is nothing to indicate any specific disease, and certainly nothing to indicate leprosy. Prolonged examination of serial sections, however, of lesions confidently called 'indeterminate' by an experienced leprologist, will reveal certain valuable pointers to the true aetiology, namely scattered clumps of histiocytes and epithelioid cells in the dermis, a few lymphoid cells surrounding a single nerve fibre and perhaps infiltrating the fibre itself and eventually destroying it and making it unrecognizable; a little collection of acid-fast debris in the form of a bacillus in nerve tissue or in a little group of epithelioid cells. A series of sections taken from a developing lesion over the course of months will suffice to establish its nature. It is leprosy; it is early leprosy; but the specific histological evidence is hidden and scanty.

### 2. *Lepromatous leprosy*

In the earliest (or pre-lepromatous) lesion, *M. leprae* are already visible in sections stained by modified Ziehl–Neelsen's method (Fite–Faraco, or TRIFF). They are present in small localized groups of histiocytes or reticulo-endothelial cells in the upper layers of the dermis, within Schwann cells or lying between the fibres of the small dermal nerves in the deeper layers of the dermis, and in the arrectores pilorum muscles. At first discrete and scattered, the bacilli-containing free cells of the dermis tend to aggregate in masses in the neighbourhood of nerve tissue, i.e. near sweat-glands, pilosebaceous follicles, neurovascular bundles, etc. At first, the organisms are scanty and scattered (and hence might be missed by the standard slit-smear examination), but in established lepromatous disease, the whole dermis is occupied by a highly bacilliferous granuloma. The normal architecture of the skin is destroyed; the epidermis is reduced in thickness, the rete pegs diminish in elevation, becoming rounded and flattened before finally disappearing; below a bacillus-free, subepidermal clear zone, the skin appendages are invaded and replaced by an uninterrupted granuloma containing innumerable bacilli in globi enclosed within a glial membrane. The histiocytes, loaded with bacilli, become globular and vacuolated. It is these cells that constitute the foamy (or physaliferous), lipid-laden lepra cells of Virchow, characteristic of lepromatous leprosy. The virtual absence of inflammatory cells, acute and chronic, is noteworthy. The overlying epidermis is apparently unaffected, except by disturbance of the function and appearance of the pigment-forming cells in the basal layer. The subepidermal clear zone is characteristically present in lepromatous leprosy and characteristically absent in tuberculoid. Lepromatous nodules are aggregations of highly bacilliferous tissue.

As the result of treatment, resolution may occur after a prolonged period of granulomatous infiltration, destruction and fibrosis, by no means confined to the areas of visible cutaneous lesions. Deeper tissues, such as cartilage and bone, may be specifically damaged by the bacilliferous granuloma, or secondarily invaded by pyogenic organisms. The intact skin becomes atrophic, dry, hairless, hypopigmented, shiny and parchment-like, and the dermis is replaced by fibrous tissue. The localized nodular masses retract into fibrous scars.

### 3. *Tuberculoid leprosy*

The earliest, or pre-tuberculoid, lesion, arising as it frequently does from an indeterminate lesion, develops the characteristic histological features of high resistance to a localized pauci-bacillary infection. Round cells are the distinguishing element in the picture; arranged initially around nerve fibres and the cutaneous adnexa, they appear as well-defined cords following these structures into the deep dermis. Typically, these tuberculoid follicles contain giant cells and masses of epithelioid cells and histiocytes. The focalization of these lymphocytic infiltrations around the adnexa is suggestive of leprosy, but the involvement of nerve tissue is pathognomonic. It is to the neurovascular bundles, in the inter-rete region and in the dermis, that attention is to be directed, for the lymphocytic infiltration around and within the nerve fibres distinguishes leprosy from all other conditions that evoke the non-specific sarcoid response. The fibres themselves may appear either normal, or so degenerate that they are quite unrecognizable except from their situation. Bacilli are present, but are very scanty. They should be sought in the cellular exudate in the vicinity of nerves and in the nerves themselves. When the lesions are undergoing acute inflammation, however, *M. leprae* may be present in far greater numbers, especially in the raised succulent edges of the lesion, perhaps in clumps of a dozen or more. It is obvious that only in the latter case would bacilli be found by the slit-smear technique. Some workers have successfully used concentration methods to demonstrate bacilli.

As the lesion develops, granulomatous tubercles composed of proliferating round cells and epithelioid cells extend to engulf the superficial nerve plexuses, the non-medullated fibres supplying the arrectores pilorum muscles, the vasa vasorum of the muscular media of the vessels, the hair follicles, and the sebaceous and sweat glands. All varieties of tuberculoid leprosy (termed major and minor, macular, low-resistant, maculo-anaesthetic) consist essentially of the above picture, modified by such factors as cellular concentration, tissue oedema, stage of the disease, and presence or absence of signs of acute inflammation.

As the localized and focalized granuloma develops around the appendages, the cells are gradually replaced by fibrous tissue, impairing their function; the clinical counterpart is diminution or loss of tactile sensitivity, pigmentation, sweating, and hairs.

4. *Intermediate leprosy* (*commonly known as borderline or dimorphous*)
The range and variety of the histological picture may be reminiscent of tuberculoid or lepromatous leprosy, or of almost any combination of both. Present simultaneously may be immunologically incompatible features. Not only may the cellular picture vary from site to site, and according to the depth from the skin surface, but the total picture in the individual may change from time to time, depending on such factors as the natural course of the disease, the effect of treatment, and subtle changes in the immunological state that produce 'down-grading' or reversal responses.

The subepidermal zone is usually clear and both cell- and bacillus-free. The typical cell is epithelioid, but round cells and histiocytes are also found, sometimes in considerable numbers. The typical concentration of the granuloma is periadnexal but focalization may be replaced by a more generalized infiltration. Bacilli may be scanty, or quite numerous. Nerve fibrils may be invaded by round cells or by bacilli, sometimes by both.

With time, the usual course is for the histological picture to become more lepromatous, and for the granuloma to extend widely in the dermis.

## THE NERVE LESIONS

Nerves appear to be the target structures for *M. leprae*. The Schwann cells offer a protective nidus for their multiplication, and the nerves themselves appear to be particularly vulnerable to the low-grade inflammatory response that follows death of the organisms. No apparent damage is sustained by a peripheral nerve trunk harbouring millions of viable *M. leprae* during the invasive stage of lepromatous leprosy. On the other hand, given degeneration of a few organisms in tuberculoid leprosy, or the more rapid destruction of greater numbers in lepromatous and borderline leprosy, a severe and permanent disintegration of nerve tissue becomes apparent. The precise mechanism of this process has yet to be worked out, but interesting parallels may be seen with acute experimental allergic polyneuritis.

In *lepromatous leprosy* enormous numbers of organisms within the nerve trunk provoke no commensurate tissue response. The endoneurium may become swollen and hyaline in appearance, and contain numerous bacilli, but the cellular infiltration is slight and non-specific. During periods of exacerbation, however, the whole trunk and the fibrous sheath may become acutely swollen from oedema and inflammatory engorgement; immune complexes may be demonstrated by appropriate immunofluorescent techniques; the vasa vasorum are compressed and occluded; nerve fibres are subjected to increasing pressure within the unexpansile sheath. The result is local pain, interruption of nerve pathways, and perhaps irreversible damage to the nerve itself.

The ascending invasion by scanty bacilli of the branches and main trunks in *tuberculoid leprosy* is associated with a very vigorous cellular reaction, comparable to that seen in the skin. The nerve thus becomes clinically enlarged and hard and the pressure of the granulomatous mass within an unyielding fibrous sheath, which becomes increasingly harder and thicker, causes secondary neural changes throughout the area of its distribution. This tuberculoid mononeuritis is usually localized to one or a few nerve trunks, develops relatively early in the course of the disease, and in the absence of treatment is frequently progressive.

Pseudo-caseation with tissue autolysis may occur and the softened material may be spontaneously extruded. Evacuation of the sterile pus, or its retention *in situ,* may be followed by a patchy localized calcification or, more rarely, by a tubular calcification involving a considerable length of the nerve trunk. Such features as irregularities and varicosities of the nerve, the abrupt distal delimitation of abnormalities at the level of a fibrous constriction, etc., may be visualized by injection of the perineural lymphatics with radio-opaque micronized lipiodol.

*Intermediate leprosy*
The nature and extent of the histological changes observed in the nerves are

related to the clinical picture. Patients with near-tuberculoid leprosy will show a predominantly round cell and epithelioid type of infiltration, both in the small dermal nerves and the main trunks, while those with near-lepromatous leprosy will have numerous bacilli in the nerves, a relative freedom from cellular exudate, and a tendency to widespread, symmetrical, and late nerve damage. Within a single, small nerve trunk, the two types of response may be seen. The final result is a thin fibrous cord containing no functioning fibres.

### LESIONS OF OTHER TISSUES

*M. leprae* are widely disseminated in the body in lepromatous leprosy; and in tuberculoid leprosy tubercles arise in many organs.

A mycobacterial bacteriaemia may be demonstrated by staining (Ziehl–Neelsen's method) dehaemoglobinized, thick-drop preparations of peripheral blood, in lepromatous leprosy and during acute exacerbation of tuberculoid leprosy. Despite higher temperatures (sometimes held to be inimical to multiplication), *M. leprae* apparently multiply in bone marrow, spleen, liver, lymphatic nodes, testes, etc. The typical histological response to their presence is evoked, similar to the response apparent elsewhere. The Kupffer cells of the liver may harbour innumerable bacilli; tuberculoid follicles are found in Glisson's capsule.

The medullary cavity of the phalanges may be expanded by granulomatous tissue and adjacent cancellous bone may be eroded into cyst-like spaces near the epiphyseal lines, reminiscent of changes observed in sarcoidosis.

The anterior nasal spine and the alveolar process of the maxilla are specifically eroded, and the upper central incisors may be prematurely shed.

In the eye, bacilliferous granulomata may be found in any structure. Quite distinct are the hypersensitivity reactions occurring in the uveal tract during the acute exacerbation of lepromatous leprosy, and the paralytic lagophthalmos that leads to perforating corneal ulceration, hypopyon ulcer and their sequelae.

The testes are commonly affected in lepromatous leprosy; bacilli may be found in the seminal canals; the glandular tissue and the Leydig cells are damaged, and the consequent impairment of function may be a factor in the production of gynaecomastia in longstanding cases.

### ACUTE EXACERBATION

The histological picture presented in acute lepromatous exacerbation is a patchy polymorphonuclear panniculitis, with endarteritis and micro-abscesses.

Using modern techniques of immunofluorescence, workers have demonstrated granular deposits of immune complexes in the dermis, the glomeruli of the kidney and other tissues—findings reminiscent of the Arthus phenomenon. Progressive iridocyclitis and renal failure (related to nephrosis and amyloid deposit) are essentially due to damage resulting from repeated or prolonged immunological insult.

This series of phenomena has been called 'downgrading reaction' on the grounds that the increase in bacillary activity and reduction in specific cellular response constitutes evidence of a decrease in cell-mediated immunity, possibly consistent with a kind of immunological exhaustion due to overwhelming mycobacterial multiplication.

The peripheral nerves bear the brunt of the tissue damage arising during an increase in the degree of cell-mediated immunity that occurs in the course of 'reversal reaction'. This reaction is characteristic of the clinical course of the various immunologically unstable forms of intermediate leprosy (borderline or dimorphous). During treatment—and according to some workers, as the result of treatment—the immunological state of the patient tends to veer towards the tuberculoid pole. The skin lesions begin to repigment and cicatrize, but the clinical results of damage to mixed peripheral nerve trunks may appear for the first time or increase in severity: dropfoot or upper facial paralysis may occur. The nerves themselves may become acutely tender at the sites of predilection, and show changes in size and consistency depending on the underlying pathology.

### CLASSIFICATION

Once the diagnosis of leprosy has been made—by considering the clinical, bacteriological, histological and immunological findings (in that order of importance), the type of leprosy should be established. This is important from all points of view: the patient's, since the length of treatment, the management, and the prognosis depend largely on it; the patient's family, possibly exposed to infection; the community, interested on financial, social, and economic grounds. The stage of the disease should also be assessed, the presence of neurological deficit, orthopaedic impairment and eye trouble, and the need for medical (including surgical) and social rehabilitation. Leprosy is far more than a mycobacterial infection of the skin and peripheral nerves; it has psychological and social overtones that may exceed in importance the purely physical damage.

A practical and clinical classification which can be used by medical auxiliaries working in field conditions is shown in the Table (p. 208).

### CLINICAL PICTURE

*Incubation*
The silent or latent period between the successful transcutaneous or transmucosal implantation of *M. leprae* and the appearance of the first lesions noticed and diagnosed as leprosy, varies within wide limits. Exposure to leprosy

### PRACTICAL AND CLINICAL CLASSIFICTION OF LEPROSY

| Type of leprosy | Lepromin test | Nerve damage |
| --- | --- | --- |
| *Indeterminate* | ? | Nil |
| *Determinate* | | |
| *Tuberculoid* | | |
| Minor | + or + + | Nil or slight |
| Major | + + + | Early; severe; localized at first to one or a few nerve trunks |
| Macular | ± or + or + + | Variable |
| *Borderline* | | |
| | ± or + | Often early; widespread; severe; unpredictable |
| *Lepromatous* | | |
| Pre-lepromatous macular | | |
| Macular | | |
| Nodular | − | Late; symmetrical; generalized; severe |
| Diffuse | | |
| (Lucio) | | |
| *Pure primary polyneuritic* | Correlated with basic type of histology | Variable |

infection is by no means equivalent to contracting the disease; the exact date of infection must generally, in the nature of things, be completely unknown. However, this silent period may be taken to be from 2 to 4 years in the majority of instances; occasionally, it seems to be but a few months (a baby of 5 months has been diagnosed with typical lepromatous leprosy), and exceptionally, it may be prolonged for upwards of 10 years, but longer periods can be accepted only after account has been taken of forgotten or unrecognized skin lesions.

*Onset*

The onset is usually insidious and unnoticed. Sometimes it is heralded by transient or persistent or recurrent paraesthesiae and numbness, confined to a localized area of skin. A short-lived erythematous mottling of the forearms or thighs or pectoral region may be the first abnormality noticed.

Unusual prodromal phenomena, mostly neurological and usually better recognized in retrospect, have been reported, such as upper facial weakness, herpes zoster, causalgia, hypersensitivity, or hyperalgesia in a delimited area of skin, transient generalized paraesthesiae. The symptoms formerly regarded as being indicative of incipient leprosy, like diarrhoea, headache, malaise, etc., are valueless.

*Indeterminate leprosy*

The earliest indubitable sign is some visible change in a delimited area of skin and the commonest of these is, in the pigmented skin, a slightly hypopigmented, ill-defined macule, retaining tactile sensitivity, sweating function, and hair growth—the *indeterminate* macule. This lesion may persist as such, with minimal change, for years, but it more often represents a transient stage in the evolution of a determinate type of leprosy (if it does not regress spontaneously before disappearing completely). Indeterminate leprosy is very common, accounts for up to two-thirds of the cases in Africa (and rather less elsewhere), and is indicative of an endemic affecting the bulk of the population. Most parents recognize it for what it is and do not bring the child for medical examination or treatment unless the macule persists or develops into a determinate type of leprosy. Regular and frequent whole-population surveys will reveal both the frequency and the banality of these lesions, and only careful follow-up and histological examination of individuals in whom the lesions persist or develop, will reveal the cause and the cellular picture.

*Tuberculoid leprosy*

If it persists, the indeterminate lesion becomes better defined and ceases to be truly macular, developing a raised papular edge. It is passing through a

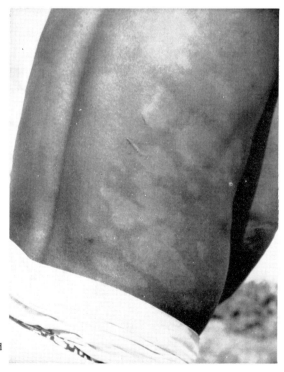

FIG. 29. Borderline-tuberculoid leprosy—macular variety.

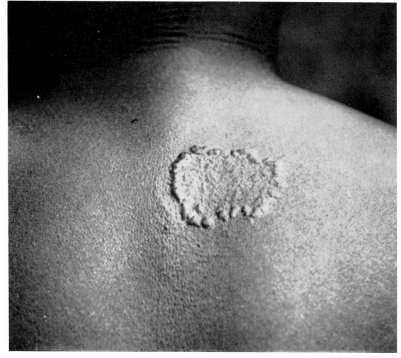

FIG. 30. Tuberculoid leprosy.

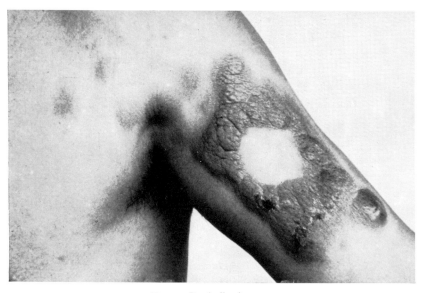

FIG. 31. Borderline leprosy.

pre-tuberculoid, and into a definitely tuberculoid, stage. The surface becomes more markedly hypopigmented; tactile misreference and lack of discrimination are found; hair growth is impaired; sweating is disturbed. This is now a fully developed tuberculoid lesion. Bacilli are rarely found by the slit-smear method in the lesion itself, and never in the nasal mucosa. The histological picture is, however, typical and pathognomonic, and the lepromin test is variably positive.

The clinical presentation covers a wide range, but the essential element is simple; i.e. a well-defined hypopigmented area of skin, characterized (except on the face) by diminished sensation, sweating, and hair growth, and either disappearing spontaneously or else enlarging gradually, new lesions appearing. The skin overlying the lesions may be either smooth and shiny, or rough and dry. The edge is usually raised and may—in the case of major tuberculoid leprosy—become positively hard and craggy, perhaps irritating and ulcerating. Central healing, with dyschromic repigmentation and patchy cicatrization, accompanied by indolent peripheral extension, may occur, producing the most varied clinical picture. Healing with complete resolution and restoration of adnexal functions may occur in patients whose lesion was slight and superficial. Crops of similar lesions may appear, or each successive crop may be less typically tuberculoid than its predecessors. Tuberculoid lesions may occur on any part of the body, but the hairy scalp and the axillae are usually spared.

The descriptive terms applied to this type of leprosy refer in a loose and inconsistent way to the size, elevation, and number of the skin lesions. Thus,

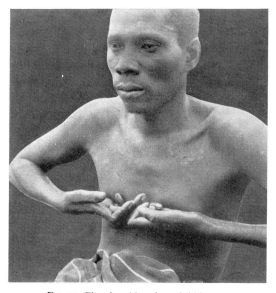

Fig. 32. Claw-hand in tuberculoid leprosy.

'minor' would indicate single, small, and with slightly raised margins; 'major', multiple, large, or with grossly elevated margins; 'macular', completely flat, well-defined, multiple, 'low-resistant'; 'maculo-anaesthetic', well-defined, often single, indolent, micropapulate, or truly macular.

The nerves in relation to a tuberculoid lesion are invariably affected, perhaps only on microscopical examination. Frequently, an unnamed cutaneous nerve passing through or near such a lesion (especially in the scapular region, or near the knee or elbow), is greatly enlarged and easily palpable by the finger nail passed around its borders. The adjacent mixed nerve trunk (if the lesion is on a limb) may be enlarged, hard, and tender, especially at a site of predilection, i.e. where its course is superficial (and hence possibly subject to lower temperatures), passes over a bony prominence, lies near a joint, and is proximal to a constriction. Thus, the ulnar just above the elbow, the posterior tibial below the internal malleolus, the external popiteal winding round the neck of the fibula, and the upper branches of the facial splayed out over the malar bone, are the sites most commonly affected. The median in the antecubital fossa and above the anterior annular ligament of the wrist, and the radial in its humeral groove are next in order of frequency.

Of the superficial sensory nerves, the most commonly affected are the great (posterior) auricular displayed on the surface of the sterno-cleido-mastoid muscle, and the radial cutaneous winding outwards and downwards over the lower end of the radius. Small twigs on the dorsum of the hand, made prominent by flexing fingers and hand, may be palpated with the nail of the index finger. In patients with major long-standing lesions of the pectoral girdle, the branches, trunks, and even roots of the brachial plexus may be hard and tender. The more widespread and long-standing the cutaneous lesions, the greater the possibility of general involvement of the peripheral nerves; unexpectedly widespread and severe nerve damage (often symmetrical) may be present in patients with apparently trivial cutaneous lesions.

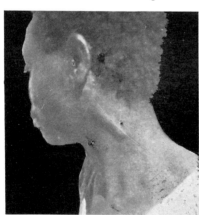

The results of damage to the peripheral nerves constitute the principal reason for the morbidity, the economic cost, and the dread and stigma of leprosy. Sensory and motor modalities are generally affected *pari passu,* but one may be affected in the same patient more than the other; thus, the right hand may be functionally useless by reason of intrinsic paralysis, the sensation being but slightly impaired, while the musculature of the

FIG. 33. Enlargement of great auricular nerve in tuberculoid leprosy.

[From E.Noble Chamberlain, *A Textbook of Medicine,* John Wright & Sons Ltd., Bristol, 1951]

left hand may be surprisingly intact in the presence of severe shortening of the fingers and complete peripheral anaesthesia.

Damage to the motor fibres of the mixed nerve trunks entails the usual succession of paresis, followed by paralysis. Thus, damage to the ulnar nerve leads to weakness and wasting, followed by complete paralysis and atrophy of the ulnar-innervated interossei, lumbricals, hypothenar muscles, and deep thenar muscles, with the characteristic clinical pictures picturesquely termed by the French: *main de prédicateur, main de singe, main en griffe, main de cadavre,* and *main succulente.* The paralysis is accompanied by overaction of the unaffected antagonist, with resultant clawing, fibrous ankylosis, contractures, and hyperextension of the phalanges. Destruction of the fibres subserving sensation is manifested by anaesthesia and analgesia of the skin of the appropriate areas of the hand and forearm.

Changes in the skin, formerly designated 'trophic' and probably multifactorial in origin, are common: the epidermis becomes shiny and thinned, cold and cyanotic; it may be dry and hypoidrotic. The following are also seen: capillary lability; disturbances of pigmentation; wasting of the finger pulp, and disappearance of the ridge-patterns; disturbance of nail-growth, the nail becoming ridged, curved, and subject to infection. The legs and feet suffer changes comparable with those in the forearms and hands. Enlarged external popliteal nerves may be felt, and often seen, as they pass around the neck of the fibula. Collapse of both longitudinal and transverse arches occurs, with inversion (and sometimes, and later, eversion) and dropping of the foot, which becomes flail and useless.

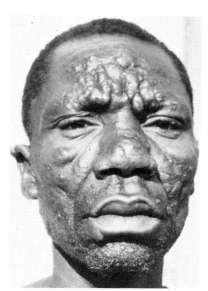

The insensitive tissues are readily injured, and become secondarily infected. Neuropathic (perforating, or 'trophic') ulcers arise over sites of standing pressure or walking shear, for example under the heads of the metatarsals, under the base of the fifth metatarsal, the os calcis, and the toe pulps. The ulcer is preceded by a painless localized subcutaneous haematoma. The phalanges and metatarsals become fragmented from repeated traumata and gradually absorb. Infection of deep tissue

FIG. 34. Lepromatous leprosy.

follows—reaching the bones, and eroding them, with the production of sequestra. All patterns of mid-tarsal bone destruction are observed, recalling Charcot's arthropathy.

Peripheral nerves other than the main mixed nerve trunks of the extremities may be damaged. The great auricular nerve is often palpable and perhaps also visible, when the head is turned in the opposite direction, so tensing the sterno-cleido-mastoid muscle. Paralysis of the facial nerve affects the musculature of the lids, with paresis or paralysis of the orbicularis palpebrarum, loss of the protective lid reflex, corneal ulceration, hypopyon ulcer, and destruction of the globe. The trigeminal nerve may also be damaged—an unusual neurological combination—with resulting corneal hyposensitivity. Tuberculoid leprosy is thus responsible for much blindness. Although, as far as the actual infection is concerned, this form of leprosy is relatively benign, destruction of peripheral nerves (and hence deformity and mutilations), may be early and serious.

*Lepromatous leprosy*

The first sign in most cases is an indeterminate macule, abnormally shiny—the pre-lepromatous macule. It is seen only when a good light falls obliquely on the skin. The macule persists, and is joined by crops of similar lesions—all small, and vague, and slightly erythematous. These are the 'hazy patches' of child, juvenile or adolescent leprosy. There is no demonstrable sensory or thermal loss, or diminished sweating, but slit-smear examination may disclose millions of *M. leprae*.

With greater pigment loss within these flat and ill-defined areas, the lesions are called lepromatous macules. New lesions appear and may become confluent, covering the whole face, trunk and limbs (except the axillae, the inguinal regions and the lumbosacral region) with a confluent hypopigmented rash.

It is on to this type of skin that the infiltrative (or diffuse) or nodular type of lepromatous leprosy is grafted; there is no clear-cut distinction between them. When the infiltration is extensive and generalized, and the skin thickening considerable, the integument of the face becomes corrugated into the 'leonine facies'. The eyebrows (beginning with the outer halves) disappear, and even the lashes and the beard patchily. Except in Japan, leprous alopecia is a rarity.

Nodules, which are localized aggregations of lepromatous tissue, usually sessile, make their appearance especially and initially on the earlobes and face. They are painless and symptomless, varying in number from a few to hundreds, in size from a lentil to a hazelnut, and in site from one ear to the whole of the face and trunk. Sometimes they ulcerate, discharging enormous numbers of leprosy bacilli.

The mucous membranes of the nose and mouth, the naso-pharynx, the pharynx down to and including the larynx, are commonly involved in the lepromatous process, the whole mucosa being replaced by a highly bacilliferous and irregularly thickened granuloma that may ulcerate. Secondary infection of the lesions causes gross destruction of the various structures. The nasal and laryngeal cartilages may be specifically eroded by the granuloma before being invaded by a rapidly progressing secondary infection.

Leprosy bacilli are deposited into any ocular structure by direct extension of peri-orbital lesions, or by the blood-stream; a sensitivity state may be induced during a reaction.

In Mexico and Central America, and elsewhere, a distinct variety of diffuse lepromatous leprosy is found, in which a generalized infiltration of highly bacilliferous tissue appears in the dermis with no accompanying changes in the skin surface and no nodules. The skin is thick and doughy; the fingers tapering; the complexion clear. But wherever the skin is scratched, millions of *M. leprae* are seen. This is Lucio leprosy. A sudden explosion of numerous small superficial polygonal ulcerations is termed the Lucio phenomenon.

### Borderline (*dimorphous*) *leprosy*

In many ways, borderline leprosy is the most difficult type to define, to describe, to diagnose, and to differentiate. Its clinical manifestations range from the near-tuberculoid to the near-lepromatous, the bacterial concentration in the skin lesions may vary from scanty to high, and the lepromin reaction may indicate minimal to moderate tissue sensitivity.

The initial lesion is often an indeterminate macule, which increases slowly in size, becomes slightly infiltrated, and produces 'daughter' lesions; a succession of rashes ensues, each containing elements more succulent and erythematous than the last. The individual lesions tend to be more raised in the centre than around the edge. The centre then becomes depressed to the level of the surrounding skin, and flattened; pigment returns almost completely, so that at this stage a central flat 'immune area' is surrounded by a succulent reddish ring. Tactile sensitivity is slightly impaired, as are sweating and hair growth.

It is in the peripheral nerves that borderline leprosy shows its serious nature: these are often, and at an early stage, enlarged and tender at the sites of election. Nerve damage, perhaps widespread, may even occur before any cutaneous abnormality has become apparent.

### Primary (*persistent*) *polyneuritic leprosy*

While neuritis arising in a patient with skin lesions characteristic of leprosy is the rule rather than the exception, and while it is true that skin lesions may disappear and nerve damage persist, there are nevertheless patients (not infrequently encountered in India, very rarely in Africa) in whom nerve changes typical of leprosy are found with no evidence, past or present, of skin lesions. Nor do skin lesions subsequently develop. After exclusion of the causes of neuropathy common in these countries, recourse may be had to histological examination of an enlarged superficial sensory nerve. Evidence of tuberculoid or borderline leprosy may be obtained, or (much less frequently) scattered groups of *M. leprae* may be seen in Schwann cells.

*Acute inflammation.* One or several or all the tuberculoid skin lesions may, for no apparent reason (or after injudicious therapy, or the exhibition of iodides), become red and swollen, especially around the edges. As a rule, systemic symptoms are absent: the local tissue response, if the lesions are few and small and minor, is of good omen. The marginal papulation is succeeded by fibrosis and repigmentation of the whole lesion. In the case of multiple or large or major lesions, however, while the local tissue response may herald cicatricial resolution, the accompanying acute inflammation in the peripheral nerves is anything but favourable: the sudden inflammatory oedema may result in temporary interruption of motor and sensory pathways, and be followed by irreversible paresis, paralysis and anaesthesia of the structures supplied. Thus, sudden dropfoot, facial palsy, and paralysis of the intrinsic ulnar-innervated hand muscles may result from a mononeuritis or as part of the picture of acute mononeuritis multiplex. Furthermore, succeeding episodes of acute inflammation usually indicate a reduction in clinical resistance, i.e. the near-tuberculoid becomés more and more borderline. The lepromin test may be transiently negative during such a phsase, and may thereafter become progressively less positive with each inflammatory episode.

In borderline leprosy, reaction is more serious and more persistent, entailing progressive pathological changes in peripheral nerves. All or most of the lesions become red and raised and increase in size, new lesions appear, and the whole picture tends to become lepromatous. Other manifestations are: lenticular papules on earlobes and face; polymorphic skin lesions, nodules, papules, plaques; large serpentine erythematous bands; hypopigmented haloes surrounding wine-coloured lesions (sometimes mistaken for sarcoid). With each inflammatory episode, the lesions tend to become more bacilliferous, the intervening skin and the nasal mucosa to become infected, peripheral neuropathy to increase in intensity and range, and the lepromin test to become less positive.

In lepromatous leprosy, acute exacerbation is ushered in by systemic manifestations and febrile disturbance. It may be precipitated by any febrile illness, by mental stress, smallpox vaccination, pregnancy, or parturition. The onset is frequently marked by an attack of erythema nodosum leprosum, the lesions appearing in crops in superficial or deep tissues, on the forearms, thighs, face, and trunk. Polyadenitis, polyarthritis (perhaps with effusion), and orchitis may occur, but the commonest and most serious manifestations are polyneuritis and acute iridocyclitis. New skin lesions appear and old lesions become oedematous and erythematous and may break down and ulcerate. These signs may be slight and transient, or extremely severe and persistent. They may merge imperceptibly into the sorry state known as progressive lepra reaction, in which generalized malaise is accompanied by the development of a thick dark leathery skin having a tendency to multiple ulcerations, the discharge from the ulcers containing innumerable bacilli. The immunological basis for these phenomena has been indicated.

## DIAGNOSIS

The diagnosis of leprosy may be made in the great majority of cases on the history and the pathognomonic signs of the different types of the disease. This is confirmed either by the recovery of *M. leprae* from the lesions in lepromatous or borderline leprosy, or by the demonstration of the typical histology, including damage to the nerve tissue in tuberculoid leprosy. The lepromin test is almost valueless as a diagnostic aid.

### Lepromatous and borderline leprosy

Microscopical examination of material obtained from the dermis and the septal mucosa of the nose, suitably stained for acid-fast organisms, provides confirmatory evidence of leprosy infection: the nearer borderline leprosy is to lepromatous, the greater the chances of the nasal mucosa being positive.

*Technique* of the slit-smear examination: The skin of the most active edge of a typical lesion having been cleansed with a liquid antiseptic, a fold is pinched between thumb and forefinger. An incision 5–10 mm long, piercing the epidermis and entering the superficial layer of the dermis, is made with a sharp, sterile scalpel. The scalpel, turned through a right angle, is then drawn firmly down the length of the incision, scraping as it does so a small amount of tissue fluid from its gaping edges. This material is transferred to a clean, dry, fat-free microscope slide (preferably unused) and spread as for a thick-drop blood preparation. It is then fixed by passing through a spirit-lamp flame, and stained in the cold by Ziehl–Neelsen's method.

Under the oil-immersion lens, the concentration of recognizable *M. leprae* is determined for the average field, and expressed according to a standard notation (the Bacterial Index), the best-known being a geometrical (Ridley) scale, in which the average concentration per field is expressed on a scale ranging from 1 (= 1 organism per 100 fields) to 6 (over 1000 organisms per field).

The average percentage of morphologically normal organisms ('solid rods'), known as the Morphological Index, may be determined from the same preparation.

Both the Bacterial and the Morphological Indexes may be expressed as average figures of the results of the examination of material obtained from several body sites. For ordinary purposes, smears from the edges of the lesions and from one or both earlobes provide sufficient information for diagnosis and control of treatment.

The mucoid discharge from the nasal mucosa furnishes evidence of the presence of leprosy bacilli, i.e. of the actual (not merely potential) infectivity of the patient. In India, the mucus may precociously contain leprosy bacilli before skin lesions appear. Examination of the nasal mucus is simple: a drop is allowed to fall on a microscope slide. It is spread with a platinum loop, allowed to dry, fixed, and stained.

The mucosa of the nasal septum and of the inferior turbinates furnishes information that is usually confirmatory, and may be supplementary. Thus, the nasal mucosa may on occasion continue to be bacilliferous when the skin smears are no longer so; on relapse, it may become positive earlier than the skin; and viable bacilli ('solid rods') may persist in the nasal mucosa, singly and in globi, longer than in the skin. Although isolated acid-fast organisms present in the nasal mucus may occasionally cause confusion, organisms in globi can be none other than *M. leprae,* and there is no mistaking them.

The technique of obtaining material from the mucosa of the septum is as follows: under direct vision, the nares being dilated with a Thudicum's speculum, remove mucus from the lower part of the septum with a dry swab

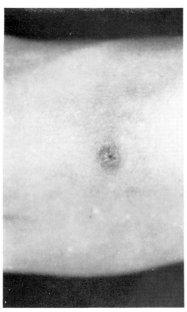

FIG. 35. Positive Mitsuda.

held on angled forceps. (The actual examination should, when conducted gently and deliberately, be merely uncomfortable, but not painful.) Then, with a small angled spud (a splayed-out bicycle spoke is excellent), scrape the mucosa at a site where it is hyperaemic or nodular, removing a small portion of the mucosa. This is spread on a microscope slide, fixed and stained in the usual way.

*Removal of material for histological examination.* Small elliptical portions of skin, about $10 \times 3$–4 mm and thick enough to include the deep dermis, may be removed under local anaesthesia from the active edge of a lesion, fixed in Ridley's solution, and stained by a modified Ziehl–Neelsen technique (Fite–Faraco or TRIFF). The typical histology of the various determinate types of leprosy may be thus made available for immediate or deferred study, together with the visual demonstration of the number, concentration, morphology, and disposition of *M. leprae*.

### Tuberculoid leprosy

Any non-irritating, persisting, skin lesion, in which tactile or thermal sensitivity is reduced, and especially when accompanied by enlargement of a related nerve trunk, in a person who has lived in a country where leprosy is endemic, should be regarded as being due to leprosy till proved otherwise. Skin smears never yield bacilli, except when the lesion is undergoing acute exacerbation, nor does the nasal mucosa.

Histological examination of a portion of skin removed from a suspected lesion, however, provides conclusive evidence. The focalization of the non-specific, round-cell, tuberculoid granuloma in the vicinity of the cutaneous adnexa is suggestive of leprosy (and many other conditions), but invasion and destruction of nerve tissue occurs only in leprosy. Very rarely, removal of a small sensory nerve (e.g. from the wrist or the dorsum of the hand) or a sliver of such a nerve, may be indicated and justifiable. A characteristic histological picture may clinch the diagnosis.

*Borderline leprosy*
The diagnosis is made on the clinical examination, confirmed by bacteriology and histology. The lepromin test may help in classification.

A diagnosis of leprosy should never be made lightly or hastily, nor should treatment be given on suspicion. The psychological and social consequences of a diagnosis of leprosy are sufficiently serious to warrant the utmost prudence. The practitioner may reasonably temporize while awaiting conclusive proof, reassured by the knowledge that if he is in doubt the patient cannot be suffering from a rapidly developing and serious and contagious form of the disease. For all practical purposes, patients suffering from tuberculoid or indeterminate leprosy may be regarded as non-contagious and as administratively 'closed', while those suffering from lepromatous or borderline types of leprosy are rendered non-contagious after a few months of standard treatment. Although they may be for a time potentially contagious, they do not constitute a public health danger provided they take precautions against intimate contact with others, especially children.

DRUG TREATMENT

In the past, for lack of any rational screening technique (*in vitro* culture, or susceptible animal model), drugs that were effective in experimental tuberculosis, or other mycobacterial infections (such as rodent leprosy, caused by *M. lepraemurium*) were selected for trial in human volunteers suffering from leprosy. Although this haphazard procedure indicated some series of drugs useful in leprosy, it became evident that the susceptibility to drugs of *M. leprae* was different in many respects from that of *M. tuberculosis*. More recently, with the perfecting of the elegant mouse footpad inoculation technique for the screening of drugs, the determination of the minimal inhibitory concentration, and the estimation of dietary and serological concentrations of active principle, the experimental evaluation of drugs for use in leprosy has taken on a new sophistication and precision.

Dapsone (diaminodiphenylsulphone, or DDS) is still the sheet-anchor of leprosy treatment. It is bacteriostatic to *M. leprae*, probably by reason of its activity as a partial antimetabolite. It is active in all types of leprosy; it is generally well tolerated; it can be given by the mouth or parenterally for long periods without serious side-effects; and it is very cheap. Its action is, however, slow; it may appear actually to make worse the manifestations of leprosy (by increasing, for example, intraneural fibrosis); its toxic effects, though uncommon, are real; according to some workers it may precipitate polyneuritis, or acute exacerbation; and it may cause anaemia.

In view of the disturbing incidence of sulphone resistance, associated with irregular treatment and also probably with low dosages and slow build-up to the optimal dosage, monotherapy with dapsone alone is no longer to be recommended for patients suffering from multibacillary forms of leprosy, i.e. lepromatous and borderline. To judge from more adequate data derived from experience with tuberculosis, another drug should be given in addition to dapsone, and this for as long as possible, in order to postpone the emergence of dapsone-resistant leprosy bacilli. Problems arising from the increased cost of these other drugs, from the difficulties of ensuring patient compliance, and from the public health and public relations aspects of this change of policy, must be realistically faced by governments and medical staff engaged in the anti-leprosy programmes. Retraining of subordinate auxiliaries, better laboratory cover, and improved supervision of leprosy treatment activities are implied by the more serious attention called for by this new factor of drug resistance.

For patients suffering from tuberculoid or near-tuberculoid forms of leprosy, in whom the bacterial population is relatively small and cell-mediated immunity is well developed, monotherapy with dapsone is still recommended at a standard dose of 50 mg daily for an adult. Indeterminate leprosy is in general to be treated as for tuberculoid leprosy, with the proviso that patients in whom the lepromin reaction remains negative should be treated as for early lepromatous leprosy.

Patients suffering from multibacillary forms of leprosy should be given dapsone at a total weekly dose of 6–10 mg per kg body weight, which works out at 50–100 mg per day. The drug should be given daily, and the maximum daily dose should be administered from the beginning of treatment and continued without interruption. In addition to dapsone, another drug should be given initially. The World Health Organization recommends that this other drug should be either rifampicin, given at a daily dose of 450–600 mg for 3 weeks, or clofazimine (Lamprene, Geigy) given at a dose of 100 mg every other day for 3–6 months. Thereafter, dapsone is continued—in either case—for as long as it would have been had the second drug not been given. In addition to the postponement of the emergence of dapsone-resistant bacilli, each of these regimens has certain advantages: rifampicin rapidly renders the patient non-contagious and clofazimine reduces the risk of acute exacerbation arising.

The thorny question of the introduction of a second drug temporarily for those patients already under treatment for multibacillary leprosy, some of whom may possibly be in the incubation stage of drug-resistant disease, must be left to the discretion of the local authority in charge of the leprosy programme, the ideal advice being in favour of such introduction.

The advocacy of continuation of treatment during reactional episodes is given despite the accumulated evidence of the alleged reactogenicity of anti-leprosy medicaments, and presupposes a control programme in which patients needing special care and treatment during such episodes—however caused—may be assured of speedy help at a central hospital.

The other recently discovered fact complicating leprosy treatment is the presence of 'persister' leprosy bacilli, dormant in bone marrow, lymphatic nodes, superficial muscular tissue, and deep organs, viable and drug-sensitive, but probably non-metabolizing and certainly unaffected by mycobacteriostatic concentrations of anti-leprosy drugs in their immediate vicinity. Such bacilli have been the occasion of relapse, when normally adequate treatment has been stopped; thus, after 12–15 years of dapsone, 5 years of clofazimine, and even 2 years of rifampicin treatment, such bacilli have begun to multiply again, causing clinical and bacteriological relapse.

For this reason, it is now recommended that patients who have had adequate treatment for multibacillary forms of leprosy, and in whom clinical and bacteriological quiescence has been attained, should continue to take dapsone 'for life'. They should no longer figure in the statistics of cases of active leprosy, but should continue to be regularly examined.

*Side effects of dapsone* are seen in the skin (papulo-macular rash, fixed eruption, exfoliative dermatitis, toxic epidermal necrolysis, 'fifth week dapsone dermatitis') and in other organs (hepatitis, nephritis) and systems (acute psychosis, 'drug fever'). There is evidence that dapsone, injudiciously given, may precipitate erythema nodosum leprosum in the predisposed and even in minute doses may cause its return.

Dapsone is also given parenterally as a 20–25 w/v suspension in vegetable oil (arachis usually). The dose of 0.25–2 ml may be given weekly or even fortnightly. A long-acting repository sulphone, acedapsone (DADDS) synthesized primarily for use in chloroquine-resistant malaria, given intramuscularly, releases therapeutic concentrations of sulphone for 75–90 days. Despite the obvious advantages of giving a depot drug at long intervals, the low-serum concentration may favour the emergence of sulphone-resistant bacilli, and sulphone-related exacerbation in the predisposed may prove difficult to control. The World Health Organization recommends that if acedapsone is given, it should be supplemented by oral dapsone in order to bring the serum concentration of active principle up to a more acceptable level. Solapsone (Sulphetrone, B.W. & Co.), a complex di-substituted sulphone, provides a convenient mode of administering a small and graduated dose of soluble sulphone for slow desensitization in patients with dapsone dermatitis.

*The long-acting sulphonamides,* particularly sulfadoxine (sulphormethoxine, sulphorthomidine, Fanasil (Roche)), are much used in certain countries and appear to give results, clinical and bacteriological, comparable with those obtained with dapsone. Their cost, and their tendency to produce untoward side-effects, militate (in the eyes of many) against their widespread use in mass campaigns, and the small margin between the therapeutic and the toxic doses is a distinct disadvantage.

*Antibiotics* have little place in leprosy treatment. Streptomycin may be useful in certain forms of lepromatous leprosy characterized by multiple ulcerations and capreomycin shows some activity experimentally.

*Rifampicin* (Rimactane, Rifadin), a semi-synthetic derivative of *Streptomyces mediterranei*, is a mycobactericidal drug that rapidly sterilizes the nasal mucosa and the dermis, though lurking viable but dormant bacilli may persist for years in bone marrow and elsewhere unaffected by mycobactericidal concentrations of the drug. It is given to patients with widespread lepromatous leprosy, at a dose of 600 mg a day for 2–3 weeks; dapsone at the standard recommended dose regimen is given concurrently and continued.

*Clofazimine* (B663, Lamprene Geigy), a riminophenazine derivative, is an antimycobacterial drug possessing anti-inflammatory properties. It has given good results in severe lepromatous leprosy, long-standing and liable to acute exacerbation, and in patients harbouring dapsone-resistant bacilli. The dose generally advocated is 100 mg daily by mouth, but a lower dose may be equally effective. Bacterial resistance to the drug has so far not been reported.

Much work of potential interest, if not of practical value, has been reported of attempts to create or enhance specific or non-specific immunological resistance to leprosy infection. Thus, injections of whole blood have been given, and of leucocytes, of lymphocytes from healthy donors or from patients with tuberculoid leprosy. Transfer factor has shown promising, if transient, results. Ducton (derived from *Neisseria parva*) and thymosine have also been used, as has levamisole, but no practical line of immunotherapy, from repeated lepromin microvaccination to the introduction of clones of lymphocytes or grafting of thymus glands, has emerged to date.

### Duration of treatment

For tuberculoid and indeterminate leprosy, treatment is advised for at least 2 years, or for at least a year after all signs of clinical activity have ceased; for lepromatous and borderline leprosy, at least 4 years, or at least 2 years after all clinical and bacteriological evidence of activity have disappeared. In this context, and to err on the side of safety and prudence, it is recommended that 'bacteriological activity' should comprise the presence of degenerate *M. leprae* in material obtained by the slit-smear technique. Treatment with dapsone is then continued for life; by these means, any emerging and multiplying organisms arising from 'persisters' will be subject to mycobacteriostatic concentrations of dapsone, and the total bacterial population should not at any time give cause for disquiet regarding the appearance of dapsone-resistant organisms.

*Follow-up.* After discharge from treatment patients should be seen every 3 months for a year, every 6 months for 2 years, and annually thereafter. Skin-smear examination is important in those who have had lepromatous or borderline leprosy.

*Relapse.* If these recommendations are followed, the proportion of patients relapsing will be small. In the case of tuberculoid leprosy, adequately treated, relapse is unlikely, and if it does occur it is generally amenable to treatment.

In the case of lepromatous leprosy, however, relapse may occur from one or other of the following causes: inadequate treatment; multiplication of persister organisms; appearance of dapsone-resistance.

In the past, relapse was most frequently seen in patients in whom the signs of borderline leprosy had rapidly disappeared, giving the misleading impression of rapid and adequate response to the drug and hence inducing premature cessation of treatment.

Nothing is known about acquired reinfection, since it is never possible absolutely to exclude recrudescence of activity from an active focus of facilli that have been dormant for months or years.

Increase in the extent of cutaneous anaesthesia and motor loss, and persistence of localized tenderness over nerve trunks, are not indubitable signs of activity.

*Drug resistance* is to be suspected in patients with multibacillary forms of leprosy who have been taking monotherapy (usually dapsone), usually irregularly and sometimes in inadequate dosage. Skin lesions apparently quiescent may become red and raised; new lesions of similar appearance may arise; small softish papules may be seen anywhere on the body; or a more general maculopapular rash may appear, often on the skin of the forearms.

These lesions contain morphologically normal leprosy bacilli, and so may the apparently normal skin and the nasal mucus, whereas no such bacilli may have been found for months or years at any site examined.

Suspicions of the occurrence of dapsone resistance are confirmed clinically if morphologically normal bacilli persist (or even increase), despite the daily supervised intake of 100 mg of dapsone: usually this clinical confirmation is apparent in 3–6 months. Experimental confirmation is obtainable by injecting a suspension of bacilli from a lesion into the footpads of mice given known amounts of dapsone in the chow. If bacillary multiplication occurs despite the presence of mycobacteriostatic concentrations of drug in the tissues, then drug-resistance is confirmed. Resistance apparently develops in a stepwise fashion, so that bacilli resistant to low concentrations of dapsone may be temporarily susceptible to higher concentrations.

Secondary resistance to dapsone may be expected to occur annually in 1–3 per cent of patients with multibacillary forms of leprosy who have been under treatment with dapsone alone for several years (5–15, commonly). Resistance has also been shown to occur to rifampicin, but not to clofazimine.

Primary resistant leprosy, of whatever form (depending on the potential cell-mediated immunity of the exposed individual), has already been recorded. The gravity of this possibility is emphasized by the difficulty of rapidly recognizing the non-effectiveness of dapsone given as monotherapy to patients suffering from any form of leprosy where infection was contracted from a patient shedding dapsone-resistant bacilli from nose (and perhaps skin).

*Acute exacerbation*

The treatment of the acute inflammatory episodes occurring in the course of leprosy calls for accurate diagnosis and competent medical and nursing care.

In indeterminate and polar tuberculoid leprosy, the acute condition is usually self-limiting and of slight gravity. If, however, a lesion on the cheek suddenly becomes red and oedematous and painful, it must be treated seriously because of the danger of damage to the fibres of the small branches of the underlying facial nerve. The treatment is essentially systemic corticosteroids in appropriate doses to control the inflammation; the conjunctiva should be protected, if exposed, by bland oily drops, and bandaged.

The situation in borderline and lepromatous leprosy is in general potentially serious. In cases showing an increase in cell-mediated immunity (i.e. reversal reaction), the brunt of the threat is borne in the peripheral nerves, and the best treatment apart from rest, splinting in the optimum position, and analgesics and sedatives, is prednisolone. The drug is usually given in fairly high doses—40–60 mg daily for an adult—in order to reduce local swelling, pain, and tenderness in the nerve or nerves. As a rule, the maximum dose is given for a few days only, before being rapidly reduced, so that the patient ceases taking the drug by the end of the fourth week. Cases vary so much in gravity and in response that clinical experience plays a crucial role in their management.

In patients presenting in the throes of classical erythema nodosum leprosum, the general treatment consists of physical and mental rest (usually in bed if symptoms are severe). Slight degrees of reaction, as shown by a few superficial and transient rose spots with no constitutional disturbance, are treated with rest and sedatives.

Patients who are more ill require drugs with some anti-inflammatory activity, such as antimony (potassium antimony tartrate, or a proprietary preparation) or chloroquine (given at a dose of 150 mg base twice daily for a week).

Patients who are more seriously ill from the beginning, or who do not respond to the above measures (continued for two weeks), should be given either prednisolone or clofazimine.

It is this 'hard core' of patients who tax the resources of the medical attendant. He will try to ensure psychological calm for his patient, good nursing care, and a helpful environment, but his reputation stands or falls on his management of the distressing general and local symptoms of this reactional state. Rest is essential. More powerful sedatives (e.g. chlorpromazine) may help. If the patient is still in the unrelieved thores of acute exacerbation, the choice then lies between the corticosteroids and clofazimine (or, if he considers it ethically justifiable to have recourse to a known neurotoxic and teratogenic drug, thalidomide).

The corticosteroids when given in adequate dosage will control severe exacerbation. They may be given in several ways: high doses for a short period, or lower doses for longer, or rapidly increasing doses. The difficulty is to know when to stop, and how to stop without incurring the risk of serious rebound phenomena or habituation—with all its consequences. Sometimes a short course of oral or injectable cortisone (5 ml daily for 5 days, with rapid tapering off) will suffice; or prednisolone given in divided doses totalling 40–50 mg daily for 5 days. The drug must be given in doses just adequate to control the distressing symptoms, and then reduced prudently and as rapidly as possible. With some patients, a single course is sufficient. Others need several courses. Still others seem to require a maintenance dose of 5–10 mg daily, under cover of which dapsone therapy can be cautiously resumed.

Clofazimine appears to prevent the appearance of signs of acute exacerbation in the majority of patients suffering from lepromatous leprosy. In established severe exacerbation, controllable perhaps only with prolonged corticosteroid therapy, clofazimine is a valuable drug. It is given in doses suited for the individual patient and discovered by trial; doses up to 400 mg a day are usually adequate. Under this regime, corticosteroid dependent patients can be weaned, as clofazimine is given in doses sufficient to control the exacerbation and then to exert its anti-mycobacterial action.

The eyes (in acute exacerbation) need especial care. The earliest signs of incipient damage to the uveal tract should be known by every medical auxiliary and treatment (mydriatics) should be given immediately and routinely as soon as eye involvement is suspected. Thereafter, systemic corticosteroids, instillation of hydrocortisone drops or ointments, and perhaps subconjunctival injections of hydrocortisone—may be necessary to control the condition.

Because of the real risk that irregular treatment with dapsone may be a factor in the emergence of dapsone-resistant leprosy bacilli, it is now advised that anti-leprosy treatment be continued without interruption during a reactional episode, and that recourse be had to either prednisolone or clofazimine earlier than was previously recommended.

In the case of patients with lepromatous leprosy undergoing treatment with both dapsone and clofazimine, the incidence of severe reactional episodes is likely to be low. In the cases that do arise, an increase in the dose of clofazimine to 200 mg or even 300 mg daily is advised. The higher dose should not be continued for more than 3 months. If the exacerbation is not controlled by clofazimine at a dose of 200 mg a day, the best course is to give prednisolone in addition at a dose at which no further rose spots appear and nerve pain becomes bearable.

Thalidomide, given under carefully controlled conditions to male in-patients at a dose of up to 400 mg daily, exerts a rapid effect on the manifestations of erythema nodosum leprosum. Despite fears of its neurotoxicity, nerve damage attributable to the drug has not been reported in leprosy, but its use cannot be recommended by the World Health Organization because of its recognized teratogenicity.

### SURGICAL ASPECTS OF LEPROSY

The non-specialist practitioner will find much to interest and to challenge him in the surgical complications of leprosy.

Acute neuritis, particularly of the ulnar nerve above the elbow, will require rest and analgesics. If local pain and tenderness persist, injection of 5 ml of 1 per cent procaine into the nerve sheath may relieve the symptoms for a week or longer; more successful and more lasting may be infiltration of the nerve sheath with the same solution to which 25 mg of hydrocortisone and 1500 units of hyaluronidase have been added per millilitre. If tenderness is exquisite and localized, longitudinal incision of the nerve trunk under local anaesthesia may relieve the pain and save the nerve fibres from compression and destruction.

Dropfoot, treated conservatively, may recover, even after several months. The claw hand may be salvaged by mobilization and physiotherapy, and perhaps made usable by tendon transfer and diverse reconstructive surgical procedures. Persistent dropfoot may be restored by posterior tibialis tendon transfer or relieved by a spring prosthesis. Flail foot and inverted foot require some form of arthrodesis. Chronic plantar ulcers will mostly heal if rested, perhaps in a walking-plaster; recurrence is prevented by protective footwear and education of the patient.

Acute facial palsy is a medical emergency to be treated by corticosteroids in high doses.

Cosmetic surgery calls for special skills and, where indicated for removing stigmatizing afflictions, has great value for the individual patient and for the leprosy campaign. Lagophthalmos is corrected by tarsorrhaphy, nylon sling or temporalis transfer; the saddle-back nose is reformed by cartilage and bone grafts and epithelial inlay; eyebrows are remade from hair-bearing temporal skin; redundant earlobes are refashioned, sagging faces lifted, embarrassing enlargements of the male breast removed, prominent fibrosed nerves excised, and the contours of stigmatizing atrophy of the first interosseous space are restored by injected silicone compound or fibro-fatty insert.

Protective footwear, moulded microcellular rubber, or Plastazote insoles, artificial limbs, protected handles for tools, implements, crockery, cutlery, cooking utensils—all should be provided or adapted.

Patients need educating in the use of their anaesthetic extremities; they need vocational training in farming and saleable skills; and society needs educating about leprosy—its recognition, its treatment.

## LEPROSY CONTROL

The control of leprosy should ideally be viewed in the same way as the control of any other slightly contagious disease. Unfortunately, it is still hampered by ignorance, stigma, and prejudice. Ideally, too, the diagnosis and treatment of leprosy should be integrated into the general public health services, but this is rarely practised.

Leprosy could, in theory, be controlled by sterilizing bacteriologically the reservoir of infection, and minimizing potentially infective contacts. It could also be controlled if an effective preventive measure (e.g. vaccination, or drug prophylaxis) could be universally applied. The ecological factors associated with the decline of the leprosy endemic in northwestern Europe in the past few centuries have not been identified, but it is more than possible that they may yet play a considerable role in leprosy control.

At present, the most effective campaigns are based upon the following: early diagnosis, adequate treatment based on urban or rural dispensaries in charge of polycompetent medical auxiliaries, well-trained and adequately supervised; a central acute leprosy hospital, or a wing in a general hospital catering for those in need of short-term, in-patient care, for example for investigation, and initiation of treatment; for acute exacerbation (especially when eyes and nerves are in danger), drug sensitivity, change of drug, desensitization; for reconstructive surgery (and physiotherapy before and after operation); and for education. Regular whole-population surveys are at present a counsel of perfection, but examination of contacts and of subjects at special risk is invaluable.

Use should be made of existing facilities for reconstructive surgery, rather than expensively reduplicating such services. Scarce funds should not be diverted from prevention of deformity by early treatment to surgical reconstruction of anaesthetic extremities. If the leprosy patient can be treated in his home, from a static or mobile clinic, he will not become socially dislocated, and hence will not require rehabilitation.

The training of trustworthy medical auxiliaries, and the instruction of medical students, doctors, and other medical workers, is a most important part of leprosy control.

The public at large should be educated by all available means—the printed word, radio and television, lectures, seminars, exhibitions, films—the scope is wide and the opportunities limitless. To be avoided at all costs is an insistence on leprosy as a unique disease: this is as unhelpful in the long run as ignorance.

The cooperation of voluntary agencies and international organizations in leprosy control schemes organized by governments brings not only flexibility and initiative, but also continuing expertise and dedicated service. Local participation in such schemes may also be enlisted with advantage.

There is some experimental evidence that BCG vaccination given to mice at a certain moment before or after challenge with *M. leprae* will enhance resistance to infection. The results of field-work are less clear-cut, and the discrepancies between the figures obtained in the well-conducted mass trials of BCG have not yet been explained or resolved. In Uganda, the protection apparently afforded to children exposed to intrafamilial leprosy infection is of the order 80 per cent; in Papua New Guinea, 56 per cent; and in Burma, 0 per cent. Various explanations have been offered. Further work is required, and perhaps the development of a vaccine containing specific antigens, before wholesale BCG vaccination can be advocated solely on the grounds of its protective value against leprosy. However, in view of the positive evidence, it would be wrong to deny BCG to individuals definitely exposed to the risk of infection.

There is also evidence that dapsone given prophylactically at half the therapuetic dose to child contacts of open cases of leprosy may protect about three-quarters of them from developing overt disease. No information is available concerning the period during which dapsone should be taken in relation to the infectivity of the index case, and to the duration of exposure, nor have the questions of cost, distribution, and possible risks of giving a toxic drug to healthy subjects for prolonged periods—been resolved. However, in certain circumstances, drug prophylaxis may have a place.

International cooperative work is being prosecuted vigorously at present, utilizing the relatively huge amounts of *M. leprae* now available from experimentally infected armadillos. It is likely that a specific skin test indicating past or present leprosy infection may soon be forthcoming. Further work is needed for the production of a vaccine that will specifically stimulate cell-mediated immunity in those persons congenitally unable to respond adequately when exposed to infection with *M. leprae*.

# 14

# LEPTOSPIROSIS

## DEFINITION

Weil's disease, spirochaetal jaundice, mud, field or swamp fever, and Japanese seven-day fever are among the names applied to diseases of man due to infection with species of spirochaetes belonging to the genus *Leptospira*. These organisms occur commonly in rats and other small animals and are found in stagnant water. The infection of man is incidental, and often occupational, following contamination of the skin or mucous membranes or the pollution of foodstuffs, usually indirectly, by the urine of infected animals. The clinical picture and mortality vary greatly in severity depending on the infecting species. The severe illness is characterized by fever, toxaemia, jaundice, haemorrhages into the skin and mucous membranes, renal damage, and increasing albuminuria. The mortality in many infections is low.

## GEOGRAPHICAL DISTRIBUTION AND AETIOLOGY

Leptospirosis has a world-wide distribution, irrespective of climate.

Leptospirae are slender, closely wound, actively mobile spirochaetes of varying lengths which commonly have extremities bent in the form of a crook. They stain well with Romanowsky dyes or silver and are easily cultured on simple bacteriological media. They are commonly classified by agglutination reactions and cross-absorption. The type species is *Leptospira icterohaemorrhagiae*, in which there are several subtypes. Many other serotypes have now been identified as causes of human disease.

*L. icterohaemorrhagiae* causes severe illness in man (Weil's disease) but is essentially a zoonosis; the common mammalian host in Europe is *Rattus norvegicus*, but the infection occurs in many parts of the world as an enzootic in other rats and voles, field mice, and small rodents which may harbour the infection for long periods without obvious clinical effects. It sometimes occurs in dogs. The urine of the infected reservoir animal may contain large numbers of organisms which directly or indirectly contaminate food, soil, sewers, paddy rice fields, swamps, and rivers. Man becomes infected usually by ingesting infected water or food; the organisms may also gain entry through cuts and abrasions of skin and mucous membranes.

*L. canicola* is usually found as an enzootic in dogs; it does not occur in rodents. The urine of the infected animal contains leptospirae and the organisms are spread to man via contaminated food or water. The organism causes a mild disease in man, sometimes called 'canicola fever'.

There are many other forms of leptospirosis caused by species which are sometimes widespread, sometimes remarkably localized. Over thirty serotypes (of the 130 in the pathogenic and parasitic strains comprising the complex *L. interrogans*) are known to cause disease in man. These include *L. bataviae* and *L. hebdomadis,* which are found in many parts of South-east Asia including Thailand, Malaysia, and Indonesia and may also occur in the Middle East and in Eastern Europe.

PATHOLOGY

The leptospirae, after gaining entry through the skin and mucous membranes, rapidly multiply and are widely distributed through the body. They tend to localize in certain tissues, especially the kidneys, suprarenals, liver, meninges, and the lungs. They can be cultured from the blood and urine during life and sometimes from the tissues, particularly the kidneys, after death; culture from the kidney tissue of animal reservoirs is sometimes used in epidemiological surveys.

In most severe cases there is usually jaundice and small haemorrhages occur into the skin and mucous membranes. The organs, especially the liver, are bile-stained and often seeded with petechial haemorrhages. The latter are common in the lungs, pleura, pericardium, and in the intestinal and gastric mucosa and may occur in skeletal muscle. Haemorrhages are usually found also in the kidney substance and beneath the capsule.

The liver is usually not enlarged. When death has occurred within the first week of the disease scattered necrotic foci may be found, involving the parenchymal cells; there is centrilobular congestion and parenchymal degeneration and sometimes necrosis. The areas involved are usually infiltrated with polymorphs and lymphocytes. In individuals dying later in the disease the necrotic foci may be partly replaced by regenerating parenchyma. Fatty changes are uncommon.

Bile is present in the intestinal contents and the general consensus is that the jaundice arises from hepatitis resulting from invasion by the spirochaetes, which are present in the tissues in the early stages, and probably also from toxic factors.

In some cases, even where deep jaundice is present, the changes in the liver may be minimal.

The patient may die from hepatic failure but the usual cause of death is renal failure, which is essentially of the same type as that occurring in shock, blackwater fever, and other acute medical states. The kidneys are somewhat enlarged and pale, with haemorrhages under the capsule. The epithelium of the proximal and distal tubules and the ascending loop of Henle show signs of degeneration and necrosis, with shedding of tissue into the lumen, which is irregularly dilated and often contains hyaline, cellular, and blood casts. The glomeruli are little affected. Some are ischaemic, others congested. The medullary vessels are congested. The interstitial tissue is heavily infiltrated, largely with lymphocytes. *Leptospiras* are sometimes present in large numbers, especially when death has occurred in the first fortnight of the infection; thereafter they become scanty. There are often haemorrhages into the mucous membranes of the calyx, ureters and sometimes the bladder. Frank vesicle bleeding may lead to haematuria.

Vasodilatation and congestion and petechial haemorrhages may be found in most organs. Small, localized, or sometimes diffuse, haemorrhages also occur and are found particularly in the spleen and the lungs. There may be subdural and subarachnoid petechiae or frank haemorrhages.

Haemorrhages also occur in the skeletal muscles, especially the gastrocnemius.

The overall picture is one of capillary damage. Clotting time and the platelet count are normal.

Occupational outbreaks or sporadic cases of leptospirosis occur from time to time in men working in rodent-infested surroundings, particularly in sewers, canals, mines and tunnels, swamps and paddy fields, farmyards, and other places liable to contamination with rat urine.

## CLINICAL PICTURE

The classical picture of leptospirosis is seen in *L. icterohaemorrhagiae* infection (Weil's disease).

The incubation period ranges from a few days to 3 weeks.

The onset is usually sudden, with rigors and a sharp rise in temperature, headache, conjunctival congestion, extreme tenderness in the muscles, especially of the legs, and severe muscular pains, and gastrointestinal disturbances with nausea and vomiting. In the early stages the throat is usually sore and deeply congested; local glands are commonly enlarged and tender. There may be a hard dry cough, with small amounts of sticky sputum which is sometimes blood-streaked. The patient becomes increasingly confused and disorientated. Insomnia is common. On the fourth or fifth day, during the febrile period, jaundice appears in many but not all cases. The jaundice steadily deepens for a week or 10 days. When the jaundice is marked the stools become clay-coloured. Skin rashes are often present; there may be petechiae; herpes labialis is usual; and the vesicles may become haemorrhagic. The tendency to bleeding in all tissues is shown by epistaxis, blood-staining of the sputum, and the presence of red cells in the urine. The urine contains much bile pigment; there is always albuminuria; there are usually casts and blood cells; there is oliguria and, in very severe cases, there is anuria and uraemia. Occasionally there are meningitic signs, with raised CSF pressure and up to 100 lymphocytes per mm³ in the fluid. The protein content is moderately raised. *Leptospira* are present in the CSF, sometimes in large numbers.

There is usually some anaemia and there is an early leucopenia followed by a polymorphonuclear leucocytosis, with a total leucocyte count of 10,000–15,000 and in severe cases 25,000 or more. The sedimentation rate is always raised. The platelet count is normal. There are no changes in coagulation patterns.

The remittent fever subsides in the favourable case in 7–10 days. Recovery thereafter is slow, with weakness and persistent malaise. Convalescence begins at the end of the second or at the beginning of the third week; at this stage the organisms are most readily found in the urine. The jaundice, haemorrhages, and albuminuria gradually disappear, and recovery is complete by the fifth or sixth week. In about one-third of the cases, when convalescence is beginning during the third week, the temperature suddenly rises to a high level. This 'after-fever' may persist for 4–20 days; it is not associated with a recrudescence of the classical symptoms and signs of the disease. The constitutional symptoms during it as a rule are less intense than during the initial stages of the disease, and it does not unduly delay full recovery. 'After-fever' is considered not to be a relapse of the Weil's disease, but to be a form of sensitivity reaction.

Attacks of leptospirosis vary greatly in severity. The degree of jaundice is an index of the virulence of the infection. Some are very mild and there is no jaundice; others are of the severity described; others may be fulminating, with severe toxaemia, delirium, meningeal and central nervous symptoms, and cardiovascular failure. Death occurs most frequently during the second week. The mortality varies greatly; in European cases it is usually below 20 per cent, but in South-east Asia it may be 50 per cent. The patient commonly dies of renal failure with anuria, rising blood urea concentration, and uraemia. This syndrome is often accompanied by signs of hepatic failure, with enlarging liver and deepening jaundice (bilirubin 20 mg per cent or higher).

The above pattern appears in varying degrees of intensity after infection with other *Leptospira*. Renal damage, with the organisms in the urine, is seen in most infections. Some cause very severe disease, others very mild or inapparent clinical effects. The clinical picture is decided by the serotype of *Leptospira* responsible and is thus essentially local. Thus *L. canicola* causes a mild disease, *L. bataviae* commonly a severe one.

### DIAGNOSIS

Initially it may be impossible to distinguish leptospirosis from infective hepatitis, yellow fever, or relapsing fever, on clinical examination. Fever, severe conjunctivitis, and intense muscular tenderness and pain, especially in the calves and other leg muscles, are early indications of the infection in an endemic area in particular.

During the first week or 10 days *Leptospira* can be recovered from the blood by the following methods:

## Triple centrifugation

Spin 2 or 3 ml of citrated blood at 1500 rev min$^{-1}$ for 5 minutes; remove the supernatant fluid and again spin the fluid at 1500 rev min$^{-1}$ for 10 minutes; again remove the supernatant fluid, add saponin to the fluid to a concentration of 1 in 1000, and spin at 3000 rev min$^{-1}$ for 30 minutes. Examine the deposit with dark-ground illumination.

## Blood culture

Inoculate some drops of the blood on modified Fletcher medium made by diluting 0.5 ml of Lemco broth, pH 7.4, with 3 ml of distilled water and, after autoclaving, adding 0.25 ml of inactivated rabbit serum passed through a Seitz filter. Incubate at 30° C, and examine in 3 or 4 days.

## Animal inoculation

Guinea pigs inoculated intraperitoneally with infected blood develop fever and jaundice within 2 weeks. If the animal is then killed *Leptospira* will be found in smears or sections of kidneys or liver, or by culture of the blood.

The organisms disappear from the blood after the first week. They then begin to appear in the urine, where they are present in large numbers by the end of the second week.

In epidemiological studies, or at autopsy, ground-up tissues, especially from the liver and kidney, are injected into guinea-pigs which become infected in 2–3 weeks. Organisms can be identified in smears from the animal organs by dark-ground illumination or may be cultured from blood or tissues.

## Immune reactions

For examination for immune bodies, blood can be collected and stored on filter paper and later soaked off for use.

Agglutinins appear in the serum about the sixth day and reach a maximum titre by the third week of the disease. Titres as high as 1 : 10,000–1 : 30,000, when tested against stock cultures, are commonly reached; the agglutinins may persist in the serum for years.

A positive reaction in a dilution of 1 : 100 by the tenth day is diagnostic. Zones of inhibition are prone to occur in this test; it must therefore be set up in a full range of dilutions.

Complement-fixing bodies appear at about the same time. Diagnosis by identifying genus-specific agglutinins or complement-fixing bodies is made easier if serial samples of serum are collected over the period of the illness, from the onset, if possible. Identification of the specific serotype requires the use of specific antigens, which can be determined in a given area, for example Thailand, by some knowledge of the local distribution of the strains.

The *Escherichia coli* adhesion test is also sometimes helpful, using the patient's serum, a suspension of living *Leptospira,* and fresh guinea pig serum. When the test is positive the *E. coli* are seen to be firmly adherent to the *Leptospira.*

### TREATMENT

Penicillin and tetracycline are successful if given in substantial dosage early in the disease. They should be given in the first few days of the overt disease; they have little effect after a week.

Benzyl penicillin, in doses of 600 mg 4-hourly for 24 hours, then 6-hourly for the next 6 days, is commonly used.

Tetracycline, 500 mg 4-hourly, continued for 2 days after the temperature has become normal, is recommended.

Nursing, restoration of water:electrolyte losses, and dealing with renal failure are essential.

# 15

# LYMPHOPATHIA VENEREUM

Lymphogranuloma inguinale, climatic bubo, poradenitis nostras, or Dur-and–Nicolas–Favre disease is a venereal disease due to a virus. It is character-ized by an insignificant primary lesion followed by an associated lymphangitis and lymphadenitis, and usually some minor systemic upset. The affected lymph glands tend to undergo multiple focal suppuration with the formation of sinuses. In women with involvement of the lymph glands within the pelvis great deformity of the pelvic organs may result. The mortality is very low.

### GEOGRAPHICAL DISTRIBUTION

World-wide in distribution, it is most common in the warm climates and more prevalent in the coloured races than the white.

### AETIOLOGY

The causal agent is a virus belonging to the psittacosis–lymphogranuloma–trachoma (PLT) group of atypical viruses; these are intermediate between the typical large viruses, such as those of the pox group, and the rickettsial organisms. They undergo an intracellular cycle of multiplication with large forms approaching the size of bacteria. Unlike the typical large viruses they are susceptible to sulphonamides and to some antibiotics. The members of the PLT group have certain complement-fixing antigens in common. The virus measures from 120 to 180 $\mu$m. It is readily destroyed by environmental changes and by weak antiseptics; it will retain its viability for long periods when kept at $-70°$ C. It can be cultured in living tissue cultures, and on the yolk sac of the developing chick embryo. It can be introduced into monkeys, mice, and guinea pigs, and less readily into other animals, locally by inocula-tion of infective material, but can be maintained for one or two passages only by this means. It cannot be introduced into birds and by this fact can be distinguished from the psittacosis virus. It can be maintained serially in some animals, in particular mice, by intracerebral inoculation. When thus intro-duced the virus causes a characteristic meningo-encephalitis. In nature the virus has been recovered solely from man.

The infection is usually transmitted venereally, and the disease it causes is detected much more frequently in males than in females. This may be due to the fact that in women the primary lesion is often concealed in the vagina and, in such cases, the pelvic lymphatic glands and not the more accessible inguinal glands are affected.

## PATHOLOGY

The small primary lesion, which usually is seen only when it occurs on the external genitalia, is very superficial and consists of an infiltration of the subepithelial layer of the corium with mononuclear cells, lymphocytes, plasma cells and histiocytes, and a few polymorphonuclear leucocytes. The endothelial cells of the small blood vessels of the affected area swell and obstruct them; as a result there is central necrosis in the lesion and a small shallow ulcer forms in it.

The virus passes up the draining lymphatic channels to the associated group of lymph glands. The vessels in the affected glands become congested; there is cellular proliferation, particularly with lymphocytes and mononuclear cells, at the germ centres and in the endothelial lining of the lymph spaces. The normal structure of the gland largely disappears; throughout it appear focal accumulations of proliferating mononuclear cells with some giant cell formation, of plasma cells, and of polymorphonuclear leucocytes. Focal abscesses develop where there is epithelioid transformation of the macrophages, and the resultant tubercule-like nodules undergo necrosis. These slowly developing, irregular, or 'stellate', abscesses in the lymph glands are characteristic of the infection. When near the surface of the gland these abscesses discharge into or through the adjacent tissue, so forming sinuses. Those deeper within the gland may be secluded by proliferating connective tissue, and are eventually replaced by fibrous tissue.

There is an intense connective tissue reaction around the affected glands, which become firmly adherent to the neighbouring structures. The affected glands of the group become matted together and, in the case of the inguinal glands, adherent to the overlying skin and to the underlying connective tissues.

## CLINICAL PICTURE

The incubation period is from a few days to 2 or 3 weeks; usually it is about a week.

The primary lesion is very small and is painless; it rarely lasts for more than a week and as a result it is often overlooked. In males it is usually located on the coronal sulcus, but it may be on the glans, on the prepuce, or within the urethra. At first it is a papule about the size of a pin's head; in the centre of this there soon forms a shallow ulcer which has clear-cut edges. The herpetiform ulcer is surrounded by a reddened zone; it is not indurated and it does not itch.

In females it may be situated anywhere on the external genitalia, but probably most frequently it is within the vagina. In either sex it may be on the perineum; not uncommonly, it is in the rectum. Extragenital sites of primary infection have been recorded occasionally.

In males, and in women who acquire a primary lesion on the external genitalia, there is a feeling of stiffness and an ache usually in one groin 10–30 days after exposure. A single gland becomes enlarged and can be seen and felt at this time; it is slightly tender. Mild lymphangitis extending from the primary lesion to the affected gland may occur but usually escapes notice. The enlarged gland is discrete and at first is freely movable. If the patient is kept at rest it may subside within about a week, and there may then be further development.

Usually the infection spreads to the neighbouring glands of the group and they also enlarge. The affected glands as a result of periadenitis become adherent to one another and to the skin and the underlying tissues. Eventually the group forms a large, lobulated, oval or sausage-shaped mass, over which the adherent skin is shiny and purplish in colour. The lymphadenitis usually is unilateral but it may be bilateral. Resolution may occur even at this stage; but more commonly multiple small stellate abscesses form in the glands. These increase in size and tend to fuse; those which are superficial and can be felt as areas of softening individually open on to the surface of the skin, and form multiple small sinuses. These sinuses are simple; they are not indurated and the skin is not undermined. From each exudes a small amount of thick, glu-

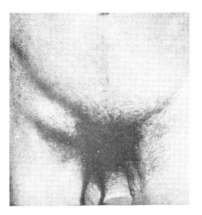

Fig. 36. Lymphopathia venereum with unilateral inguinal adenitis.

[Courtesy J. Brady]

tinous, yellowish-white mucoid pus; this at first is bacteriologically sterile. The discharge from the sinuses continues over many weeks or months but eventually the condition subsides and healing takes place with scarring.

Early in the disease, when the lymph glands are first becoming involved, there may be a febrile constitutional disturbance lasting 1–2 weeks. This is rarely severe, but it may be associated with a sore throat, sometimes with ulceration of the pharynx and tonsils. In some cases there is a generalized slight lymphadenitis during this disturbance; and there may also be painful swelling and redness of joints, and a generalized skin eruption of a non-specific character.

In those cases in which later there is extensive destruction of the lymph glands and surrounding tissues there may be a secondary elephantiasis of the pudenda or of the legs. Rarely, in the case of a purely external genital infection such as is usual in males, the virus infection may travel from the inguinal glands to the iliac glands. In women in whom the primary lesion is intravaginal the virus is conveyed directly in the lymphatics to the pelvic lymph glands. Suppuration and sinus formation in these glands extend into the neighbouring pelvic organs and the virus infection may be further diffused into the other glands within the pelvis. The sinuses cause fistulation of the vagina, rectum, and other viscera; secondary bacterial infection results in chronic inflammatory and fibrotic lesions which involve and damage extensively the contents of the pelvis. There is adhesion and fixation of the pelvic organs; there are commonly elephantiasis of the external genitalia, strictures of the urethra, vagina and rectum, tumour formation, and various ulcerative lesions, recto-vaginal, or urethro-vaginal fistulae, or even the production of a cloaca into which the rectum, vagina, and urethra all open. This progressive, chronic and disabling condition is known as the genito-ano-rectal syndrome, or esthiomène. For obvious reasons it is much more prevalent in women than in men, but it is sometimes encountered in the latter when the primary seat of infection is rectal.

### DIAGNOSIS

Of the various methods devised for diagnosis of the disease the most conclusive is isolation of the virus. This is best done by the inoculation of pus aspirated from a bubo intracerebrally into mice or monkeys; the virus causes a characteristic meningo-encephalitis. Less effectively, the virus can be isolated by inoculation of the material on to the yolk sac of a developing embryo chick.

The Frei skin test is an allergic test of value in the diagnosis of lymphopathia venereum. It is performed by injecting into the patient intradermally an antigen containing heat-killed virus. An antigen may be made from pus aspirated from the unopened stellate abscesses in the inguinal glands of a case of the disease. The antigen most free from impurities is that made from cultures of the virus on the yolk sac of the chick embryo; it is available commercially under the name 'lygranum'. The test is read at 48 hours and 96 hours after the injection of 0.1 ml of the antigen into the skin of the patient, and preferably also into a normal uninfected control. If positive, there is an infiltrated, inflammatory, dome-shaped swelling at least half a centimetre in diameter, which can be both seen and felt. In the centre of the swelling there may be a small area of necrosis surrounded by a red zone. The nodule often persists for 2–3 weeks.

The Frei test becomes positive 1–3 weeks after the development of adenitis. False positive reactions are very rarely encountered; but as the antigen contains a heat-stable component common to other viruses of the PLT group a positive test might be accounted for by infection with one of these. The test remains positive for a very long time, possibly for the remainder of the patient's life. The interpretation of the Frei test therefore must be made in the light of the immediate clinical and other findings.

An effective complement-fixation test, which is also group specific, can be performed using Frei test antigen.

### TREATMENT

Complete rest in bed should be insisted on if the disease is diagnosed in the early stages. Under this measure alone a case of external genital infection may be arrested and may spontaneously resolve at any stage of its development before formation has occurred. If at this time softening can be felt in the affected glands, indicating stellate abscess formation, these should be aspirated under strict aseptic precautions to forestall spontaneous sinus formation.

If an enlarged gland does not begin to subside after a week or so of bed rest but continues to enlarge, complete and clean surgical removal of the affected inguinal gland will terminate the condition. Under no circumstances must the glands be incised, or there will be an indolently discharging granulomatous wound for many months, which finally will only heal with great scarring.

Sulphonamides given early may effect a cure. Sulphadiazine, sulphadimidine, or sulphathiazole may be given in doses of 4–5 g daily in divided doses for 5–10 days. Long-acting sulphonamides, such as sulfadoxine, may also be used.

Tetracyclines are the antibiotics of choice. They exert a rapid specific action on the infection. The dose is 500 mg 6-hourly for 10 days, with complete bed rest. Combined antibiotic and sulphonamide treatment is considered the most effective by some workers.

The treatment of the manifold complications encountered in the genito-ano-rectal syndrome, following pelvic involvement, after initial antibiotic treatment is palliative and surgical.

# 16

# MALARIA

Malaria is a disease caused by sporozoa of the genus *Plasmodium*. It is characterized clinically by fever, which is often periodic; varying degrees of anaemia; splenic enlargement; and various syndromes resulting from the physiological and pathological involvement of certain organs including the brain, the liver and the kidneys.

## GEOGRAPHICAL DISTRIBUTION

Malaria is one of the most widespread of all parasitic diseases. It is found in regions lying roughly between latitudes 60° N and 40° S. The distribution of the plasmodial species is not uniform. Vivax malaria is widespread in the tropics and subtropics and in some temperate regions. It occurs in areas of the Middle East, Iran, Pakistan and Bangladesh, India, Sri Lanka, Burma, Thailand, Malaysia, Indonesia, East and Central Africa, but not in Negroes in West Africa. It is present in Central and South America. Falciparum malaria is found most commonly in warm moist climates. It is the dominant form of malaria in tropical West, Central, and parts of East Africa, in regions of the Middle East, South, Central, and Northern India, in parts of Bangladesh and Pakistan and in Burma, Thailand, Laos, Malaysia, and Indonesia. It occurs in the Philippines, certain Pacific Islands, Haiti in the Caribbean Islands, and in Central and South America. Malariae malaria occurs throughout the tropics, chiefly in Africa, South America, India, Sri Lanka, and Malaysia. It is not as common as either vivax or falciparum malaria. Ovale malaria is uncommon; it occurs in East, West and Central Africa, parts of North-east Africa, and in South America; a few cases have been reported in the Far East.

The distribution and significance of malaria in the world have been modified and in some cases reduced by the global eradication campaign sponsored by the World Health Organization and put into effect by the respective nations. The objective was to end transmission, leading to complete world eradication of the disease. The basic idea was to destroy the vectors in the adult stage by the use of residual insecticides which would kill them days before the parasites could mature to the infective sporozoite forms and also to eliminate the reservoirs of gametocytes in infected human cases.

For many reasons, not least the difficulties of training personnel and costing the operations, the overall eradication scheme has failed. Other factors concerned in this failure have been the growing resistance of the mosquito to the whole range of insecticides and the resistance of some parasites to anti-malarial drugs.

In some areas the eradication scheme worked well and the objective was achieved. For instance, malaria is now regarded as being eradicated from Europe and most of the Caribbean Islands. In many highly endemic areas the eradication programmes greatly reduced the incidence of the disease, but in some of these malaria has re-appeared and the picture is complicated by the loss of immunity in the relevant populations.

The approach has had to be changed and many of the older methods, aimed at control rather than eradication, have had to be introduced. These methods, including larval control and drainage, were successful in some areas at the turn of the century, particularly in islands such as Singapore.

The situation at the moment is fluid. Malaria has returned to many of the countries from which it had been regarded as eradicated or nearly eradicated. In a few it has not reappeared. In Africa, especially sub-Saharan Africa, the distribution of malaria has remained essentially unchanged, as very little eradication was attempted.

## Imported malaria

Travellers and immigrants are taking malaria with them all over the world, to many places where the disease did not formerly exist. Malaria must therefore be regarded as an important possibility in the differential diagnosis of the cause of any febrile illness in anyone who has recently been in an endemic area, or has been living in one. Imported malaria is usually a personal problem for the individual concerned. If *Plasmodium falciparum* is involved it may kill him if not diagnosed and treated. It is of public health importance only in areas in which the vector is present and active, for example in parts of Europe from which the disease has only recently been eliminated.

Malaria may exist where the following conditions for transmission obtain: (i) the presence of suitable anopheline mosquitoes, (ii) a reservoir of malaria infection (usually the local population), (iii) suitable non-immune or partly immune hosts, and (iv) an environmental temperature of between 18 and 29° C with suitable humidity. It does not as a rule occur in regions higher than 2000 m above sea level.

### AETIOLOGY

## The causative organism

Human malaria may be caused by the following plasmodia. Mixed infections occur:

*P. falciparum* (malignant tertian, subtertian or falciparum malaria).

*P. vivax* (benign tertian malaria or vivax malaria).

*P. malariae* (quartan malaria or malariae malaria).

*P. ovale* (ovale tertian malaria or ovale malaria).

Of these infections the commonest and most important are those caused by *P. falciparum* and *P. vivax*.

The nomenclature is confused by the use of descriptive terms, such as 'benign tertian', which change with the language of the country concerned. It is generally agreed that the best way to overcome this internationally is to use the specific name for the infection. Thus malaria caused by *P. vivax* infection becomes 'vivax' malaria, and so on.

A single case of simian malaria (*P. knowlesi*) acquired naturally has been reported. This parasite and other simian malarias (notably *P. cynomolgi, bastianellii*) have been transmitted artificially to man in the laboratory.

*Life cycle*
The life cycle of the parasite is essentially similar in all species of plasmodia.

(a) *The life cycle in the mosquito* (Sporogony)
In the mosquito the plasmodium develops from sexual forms (gametocytes) ingested by the insect during a blood meal. The ingested male gametocyte undergoes rapid development in the fluid of the mosquito's stomach, extruding several motile flagella, one of which fertilizes a female cell or gamete developed from an ingested female gametocyte. The fertilized parasite (the zygote) penetrates the stomach wall and develops beneath the lining membrane, eventually becoming a large cyst within which appear the infective forms of the parasite, called sporozoites. After 7–20 days, depending upon the external conditions, the cysts rupture and the sporozoites migrate, many reaching the salivary glands. The infected mosquito injects sporozoites into the host's tissues during a blood meal.

(b) *The life cycle in man* (Schizogony)
Sporozoites rapidly disappear from the blood stream after infection. During the succeeding 5–7 days the parasite develops further in the polygonal cells of the liver and possibly elsewhere [the so-called *pre-erythrocytic* (*PE*) *phase*]. At the end of this period (called the *pre-patent* period) the products of development in the cells, called *merozoites,* enter the blood and invade erythrocytes, starting the *asexual life cycle* (*Erythrocytic* or *E cycle*) which is repeated at regular intervals. In the erythrocytes the youngest forms appear as unpigmented discs or rings of cytoplasm containing one or more small masses of the nuclear material (chromatin). As the parasite grows it becomes actively amoeboid and granules of brown pigment called haemozoin, formed from haematin and denatured protein, appear in the cytoplasm. Eventually, the parasite divides by schizogony, forming a collection of merozoites, each

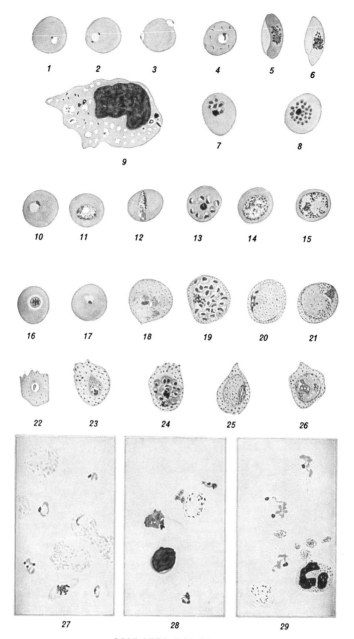

## MALARIA PARASITES

Nos. 1—26. As seen in thin films (Leishman); 27, 28, 29. As seen in thick films (Field).
Nos. 1—4. Malignant tertian rings; 5, 6. Malignant tertian gametocytes; 7, 8. Malignant tertian schizonts (from smear of spleen in fatal case); 9. Macrophage containing ingested malaria pigment.

|  | Quartan (P. malariae) | Tertian (P. vivax) | Ovale tertian (P. ovale) |
|---|---|---|---|
| Rings, trophozoites and schizonts | Nos. 10—13 | 17—19 | 22—24 |
| Gametocytes | Nos. 14—15 | 20—21 | 25—26 |

No. 27. Malignant tertian malaria. Thick film (P. falciparum). Rings and a gemetocyte. Other bodies are masses of platelets.
No. 28. Quartan malaria (P. malariae). Thick film: two trophozoites and a schizont. Also in the film are a lymphocyte and another white cell with unstained nucleus.
No. 29. Benign tertian malaria (P. vivax). Thick film. Three trophozoites, also neutrophil leucocyte and scattered platelets (pink).
No. 16. Platelet superimposed on erythrocyte.

[From E. Noble Chamberlain, *A Textbook of Medicine*, John Wright & Sons Ltd., Bristol, 1951.]

consisting of a small mass of cytoplasm containing a 'nucleus' of chromatin. The erythrocyte ruptures, liberating the new brood of parasites into the plasma and the process is repeated. The ring and growing forms are called *trophozoites*, the dividing forms *schizonts*. The process of rupturing of the infected erythrocytes and consequent escape of merozoites is known as *sporulation*.

Some merozoites enter erythrocytes. Many appear to be destroyed in the plasma before entering an erythrocyte. It is usually assumed that once the latter is penetrated, the parasite proceeds to full development within it. There is, nevertheless, the possibility that in some cases the life cycle is not completed and the parasite may leave the cell. Information on this point is lacking. In the majority of freshly infected erythrocytes the asexual cycle is repeated but in some, the sexual forms, the male and female *gametocytes*, develop. The latter remain within the erythrocytes which continue intact for their full life of up to 120 days. The gametocytes in the blood undergo no further development unless ingested by the mosquito.

In vivax, malariae and ovale infections a liver or *exoerythrocytic (EE)* phase of the parasite occurs, probably originating from the pre-erythrocytic phase. Relapses of these forms of malaria result from the persistence of the exoerythrocytic parasites which from time to time eject infective merozoites into the blood stream and eventually re-establish the erythrocytic (E) cycle. In falciparum malaria such persistent exoerythrocytic forms do not develop and the pre-erythrocytic forms do not persist. Recrudescences thus result from the multiplication of existing blood (E) parasites and relapses arising from persistent liver forms do not occur.

The life cycles of the parasites may be summarized thus:

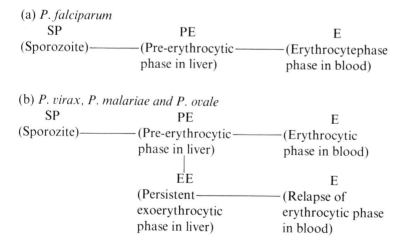

(a) *P. falciparum*

| SP | PE | E |
| --- | --- | --- |
| (Sporozoite)————— | (Pre-erythrocytic phase in liver) ————— | (Erythrocytephase phase in blood) |

(b) *P. virax, P. malariae and P. ovale*

| SP | PE | E |
| --- | --- | --- |
| (Sporozite)————— | (Pre-erythrocytic phase in liver) ————— | (Erythrocytic phase in blood) |
| | EE | E |
| | (Persistent exoerythrocytic phase in liver) ————— | (Relapse of erythrocytic phase in blood) |

*Note.* By the time clinical malaria has developed in *P. falciparum* infection, the only form of the parasite life cycle present is the E phase. In infections with the other species, both the E phase and the liver phase (EE) are present.

As will be seen later, the chemotherapy of malaria is based on these points.

*Endemicity*

Malaria in a community may be either stable or unstable. Stable malaria occurs in regions in which there is constantly repeated infection. The population has a high degree of immunity and epidemics do not occur. Unstable malaria occurs in regions in which transmission is intermittent, for example, where it is seasonal or in populations inadequately protected by drug suppression or entomological control. In such areas the population has a varying degree of immunity and epidemics are liable to occur.

The endemicity in a given area depends on the insect transmission and the host response. Where there is continuous heavy transmission the malaria is called holoendemic. Endemic areas are classified as hyperendemic, mesoendemic and endemic depending on the findings in the population in regard to parasitaemia and spleen rates in relation to age groups.

*Acquired resistance to malaria*

The severity and duration of malaria attacks depend on many factors, including the nutritional status of the host and the virulence of the infecting strain. The most important modifying factor, however, is the development of resistance or immunity in the infected individual.

Certain individuals are naturally more resistant than others to malarial infection. They may live continuously for years in endemic areas without developing a clinical attack, or may fail to become infected after artificial inoculation with parasites. Most subjects, however, are readily susceptible to infection and continuous reinfection or long-continued infection over many years usually leads to the establishment of some degree of acquired resistance, especially to superinfection (i.e. infection with the same strain of parasite). The immunity in malaria, in terms of resistance to reinfection with the homologous parasite, is apparently engendered by the E phase of the parasite. Persistence of resistance thus depends on persistence of the parasite in this form. In artificially induced infections it has been shown that eradication of the erythrocytic infection is followed in a few months by loss of resistance to superinfection. Humoral antibodies, including complement-fixing and fluorescent antibodies, are produced during an infection but do not appear to be directly related to resistance to the parasite.

However, the development of immunity is accompanied by an increase in circulating gamma globulin and the administration of this globulin isolated from semi-immune individuals infected with falciparum malaria will destroy the E forms of the parasite and cure the infection in young children.

Resistance takes time to build up, so that as a rule non-immune individuals suffer most severely from malaria in their early years of exposure.

In the indigenous population of a malarious area the active disease is usually rare in very young infants probably because of a combination of the high proportion of Haemoglobin F in the infant, the passive transfer of immune bodies from the mother and of the inhibitory effect of the milk diet itself on the multiplication of the malaria parasite. It becomes more common and severe in the latter half of the first year of life and in the first few years of childhood, when attacks are often very severe and not infrequently fatal. As the surviving children grow older, however, the attacks get milder and, provided there is continued reinfection by the same strain of parasite, the overt disease eventually becomes very much modified and ameliorated in the older child and the adult.

Where infection is interrupted for even a few months the acquired powers of resistance rapidly decline and the individual becomes open to severe attacks on reinfection or recrudescence. In communities such diminution of resistance may be the forerunner of epidemics.

Genetic factors also modify the effects of infection. In individuals possessing Haemoglobin S, the effects of *P. falciparum* are modified and the severe pathological lesions seldom occur, even in the children. There is evidence also that similar protection against the ravages of the disease is offered by erythrocyte glucose-6-phosphate dehydrogenase deficiency (see Chapter 9).

### PATHOLOGY

The immediate pathological significance of the pre-erythrocytic phase and the EE cycle, beyond the destruction of a few liver cells, is unknown. The E phase of the parasite is the basic pathological agent in clinical malaria.

The powers of invasion of the species of plasmodia differ considerably. *P. vivax* develops most easily in the youngest erythrocytes, so that at any one time not more than 2 per cent of erythrocytes are invaded. *P. malariae* develops chiefly in the older red cells, the infection rate seldom exceeding 1 per cent. *P. falciparum* invades all ages of erythrocytes indiscriminately so that very high infection rates may occur.

With each sporulation, the invaded red cells are destroyed. Furthermore, varying numbers of uninvaded red cells are lysed during the attack, and both parasitized and unparasitized cells are phagocytosed in large numbers by the macrophage cells especially of the spleen and liver. Anaemia develops, the severity of which depends as a rule on the species of invading plasmodia. Anaemia is most pronounced in falciparum infections, where the loss of red cells may be very extensive and rapid.

The anaemia causes some degree of anoxaemia, but this is seldom significant so far as the basic metabolic processes of the host are concerned. Much more important is cellular anoxia arising from cytotoxic factors released during the infection.

It has been shown that the serum of an infected patient contains a factor which inhibits respiration and oxidative phosphorylation in liver cell mito-chondria. This may be one of the basic processes by which the parasite affects the host.

This and other factors initiate and maintain a chain of physiological and patho-physiological responses which create the disease in the host. This expanding chain reaction involves many interlinked and interacting processes which include, amongst others, local and general dynamic vascular distur-bances and their consequences, alterations in hormonal balance, and in membrane permeability, the function of organs such as the liver and kidneys, the release of pharmacologically active substances such as histamine and kinins. The results vary with the individual host; the local and general distur-bances are at first reversible but, with time, may become irreversible and lead to tissue destruction and the death of the host. Many of these processes and the pathological patterns arising from them are basically inflammatory and are not specific to malaria, but occur in other acute medical states.

The pathological patterns developing in the tissues are influenced by changes in the general circulation of the blood in the body and in the local circulation in the organs. Factors which may affect the general circulation are the physiological responses to high fever and the profound effects of medical shock. Local circulatory phenomena include the development of 'inflamma-tory' stasis in vessels usually impermeable to large molecules. In the brain this leads to increased permeability, with local loss of protein and water and, in falciparum malaria, to so-called 'plugging' of the small vessels, many of which are filled with cells containing parasites, usually all in the late stages of schizogony. Local leakage of erythrocytes results in ringing of these vessels with erythrocytes, many of which are free from parasites, or contain parasites in any stage of schizogony. It is possible that a contributing factor may be some deposit of antigen–antibody–complement complexes on the vessel walls, but similar deposits occur in other vessels elsewhere in the body, without similar reactions. The 'blockage' of the vessels has also been blamed on increased rigidity of infected erythrocytes caused by the presence of the parasite, but there is no biological evidence to support this view. The reduc-tion and redistribution of the renal circulation with the development of renal anoxia, and changes in the liver blood flow which lead to centrilobular congestion and cellular degeneration and necrosis illustrate the basic factors.

Some mechanical interference with local circulation may also be caused by other changes in the blood cells, such as the development of 'stickiness' in relation to phagocytes and the vascular endothelium, or the 'sludging' of erythrocytes, and by the swollen phagocytic cells such as the Kupffer cells of the liver.

The role of coagulation and thrombosis of small vessels has not been established. It is probably of little importance. There is some evidence of coagulopathy (which indicates *reduced* capability of clotting) in falciparum malaria but clotting as such is seldom seen at autopsy.

Malaria pigment is derived from haemoglobin. It is particulate, insoluble and not itself toxic. The general pathological pattern is, however, influenced by its appearance in the tissue spaces and in phagocytic cells. The iron contained in the malarial pigment is not available for the reconstitution of haemoglobin except after a very long period.

Details of the lesions are unnecessary here. It is essential for the physician, however, to understand that many of the pathological processes concerned in malaria are reversible and prompt treatment may prevent or modify their development.

As in most other acute/chronic infections, it is now realized that the tissue immune reactions play an important part in the synthesis of the host reaction to malaria infection. The complexity of this reaction has been demonstrated in the Gambia, where the plasma of infected individuals were found to contain soluble malarial antigens and antibodies to them. Malaria infections are followed by changes in the serum immunoglobulins, with increases in both IgG and IgM. Haemolysis, as Gear suggested 30 years ago, may be partly due to antibody–antigen plus complement reaction. Renal damage due to the formation of antibody–antigen complement complexes is demonstrated in *P. malariae* nephrosis. It has been suggested that the widespread intravascular coagulation (which has never really been demonstrated) could reduce the complement levels. Excessive destruction of erythrocytes, infected and uninfected in *P. falciparum* infection, could arise from autoimmune response or opsonization. Splenomegaly may result in part from aberrant immune response to the infection. There is evidence that malaria may affect the immune response to unrelated antigens from infectious agents in particular. This could be related to Burkitt's lymphoma. Immune reactions are dampened down in pregnancy; the placenta is an area in which immune reactions tend to be minimal.

CLINICAL PATHOLOGY

Alterations in erythrocyte counts and plasma haemoglobin concentrations occur in proportion to the degree of erythrocyte destruction and haemozoin formation.

The erythrocyte count is an indication of the degree of anaemia present except in cases complicated by vascular failure, where loss of blood volume may cause haemoconcentration.

In uncomplicated malaria the measurement of haemoglobin concentration is sufficient for estimating the degree of anaemia. In blackwater fever, where there is severe haemolysis and there may be an appreciable concentration of haemoglobin in the plasma, measurement of the circulating erythrocyte mass requires an erythrocyte count.

The thin blood film may show considerable variation in the size of uninfected erythrocytes. There may be poikilocytosis and punctate basophilia. In severely anaemic cases nucleated red cells may be present.

The bone marrow response is essentially normoblastic. During the infection there is often considerable erythroblastic activity without corresponding reticulocytosis in the peripheral blood. Reticulocytosis appears a few days after successful therapy.

The chemical make-up of the blood depends on factors such as the state of the liver and kidney function and the water–electrolyte balance of the body. There are no chemical findings specific to malaria. In some cases there may be raised plasma potassium, especially during severe lysis. Sodium and chloride concentrations are frequently low, especially where there is severe vomiting or diarrhoea. Cases in which hepatic dysfunction is evident show an increase in bilirubin in the plasma and sometimes in the urine. Hepatic function tests usually show some deviation from normal during the acute attack.

Where renal dysfunction or failure has appeared, the blood urea nitrogen rises considerably.

In severe lysis there may be haemoglobin and methaemalbumin in the plasma.

The total plasma protein concentration may be unaltered or low; in acute falciparum infection the albumin concentration falls after the first 7–10 days, due to failure of synthesis and loss from the blood into the tissue spaces. In all infections, in the course of time, usually some weeks, the albumin : globulin ratio may change, due to decrease in the former and increase in the latter, usually in the gamma globulin fraction, indicating production of immune bodies.

The urine should always be examined in malaria. The volume passed is important. The volume of *each* specimen should be recorded as well as the 24-hour total. This ensures the early diagnosis of oliguria or anuria. The chloride concentration is low in any case in which the renal tubules have been damaged. Even when the concentration is low, however, the total output may be normal. Where there is severe loss of electrolytes by vomiting, sweating or diarrhoea, there may be no measurable sodium chloride in the urine. Similarly, urea nitrogen concentration is often low, although the total output may be within normal limits.

The urine has no characteristic reaction in malaria. It is just as often neutral or alkaline as acid. Protein may be present in otherwise uncomplicated cases. Considerable amounts may be passed, particularly if haemoglobin is also present. Hyaline and granular casts are common and may be present in large numbers together with erythrocytes in cases in which acute renal dysfunction develops. Haemoglobin is present in cases in which there is severe lysis (see blackwater fever, p. 261).

## CLINICAL FEATURES

*Incubation period*

The time elapsing between the inoculation of sporozoites in man, i.e. the infective bite, and the appearance of clinical signs (rise of body temperature above normal, with E parasites present in the erythrocytes) is referred to as the *intrinsic incubation period*. The length of this period varies with the plasmodial species involved. It is usually 10–14 days, but may be some weeks or months. There is often some delay in individuals who have been taking antimalarial drugs irregularly.

The time elapsing between the ingestion of infected blood by the mosquito and the appearance of sporozoites in the salivary glands, i.e. the period required before the insect becomes infective to man, is known as the *extrinsic incubation period*.

## Periodicity

The periodic elevations of temperature and associated phenomena, i.e. the *paroxysms*, occurring in the classical malarial attacks are roughly contemporaneous with the sporulation of the parasite. The interval at which they recur is known as the periodicity of the fever. When the cycle of schizogony is so adjusted that sporulation occurs at about the same time in the majority of groups or broods of parasites, the periodicity is determined by the length of the asexual life cycle. In *P. vivax* and in most strains of *P. falciparum* infections, sporulation occurs every 48 hours, so that the paroxysm occurs every third day, and the periodicity is tertian. The periodicity of paroxysms in falciparum malaria sometimes indicates a parasite life cycle of rather less than 48 hours; paroxysms in such infections occur at intervals of less than 48 hours and the fever peaks consequently occur slightly more frequently than every third day, giving rise to the so called subintrant fever (hence the term subtertian malaria). In *P. malariae* infections the erythrocytic cycle takes 72 hours. Fever peaks occur every fourth day, and the basic periodicity is thus quartan. In all infections, sporulation may occur daily, with daily paroxysms (quotidian periodicity).

## The attack

*Primary attack*. The attack immediately succeeding the intrinsic incubation period is known as the primary attack.

*Relapse*. A relapse is a recurrence of the clinical signs and symptoms of malaria and the reappearance of parasites in the peripheral blood following a period of quiescence after the subsidence of the primary attack. *True relapses* arise in vivax, ovale, and malariae infections as the result of fresh infection of erythrocytes by merozoites derived from active persistent liver forms (EE forms) of the parasites. They may occur at intervals and are usually shorter in duration and milder than the primary attack. The periodicity is usually similar to that of the primary attack.

An attack of malaria should be considered as a relapse only when the possibility of reinfection can be excluded.

*Recrudescences*. In *P. falciparum* infections, since there are no persistent EE forms, true relapses do not occur. Recrudescence of the clinical attack results from the continued existence of the original erythrocytic (E) phase in the blood. In patients who have left the endemic area the parasites rarely persist for more than 1 year; probably never more than 3 years. Recrudescence of other forms of malaria may also occur after incomplete treatment.

*Reinfection.* A reinfection is a fresh infection in an individual who has previously had malaria. Reinfections with the same strain follow much the same clinical course as the primary attack except when the host has residual acquired resistance. In the latter case the clinical course is much milder than in the primary attack.

### CLINICAL MANIFESTATIONS OF MALARIA

The most severe clinical form of malaria is that caused by *P. falciparum* infection. When neglected or when complicated this disease is usually fatal in non-immunes.

Malaria caused by the other plasmodia (*P. vivax, P. malariae,* and *P. ovale*) may be severe and unpleasant in non-immunes but is very rarely fatal.

In view of these clinical differences, and the differences in the life cycle in the human host quoted above, falciparum malaria should be considered separately from the others, which in many respects may be grouped together as the relapsing malarias.

Mixed infections occur. In these circumstances the clinical effects of *P. falciparum* infection predominate. *P. ovale* infection is easily suppressed in this way and may appear months after the dominant parasite (usually *P. falciparum*) has been successfully eliminated by therapy.

In dealing with malaria, the physician must determine not only the species of infecting parasite but also assess the degree of resistance to infection offered by the patient; that is, whether he has acquired resistance or not.

The descriptions which follow refer separately to malaria in 'non-immunes' and in 'semi-immunes'.

A 'non-immune' is an individual who has not been exposed previously to the infection.

A 'semi-immune' is an individual who has been exposed and infected at some time. His state of resistance to the infection on exposure will depend on many factors, including the successful eradication—or otherwise—of his previous infection, the length of time spent away from exposure to fresh infection, the strains of past and present parasites to which he had been and is exposed, and the potential genuinely protective antibodies he possesses. It is conceivable that the latter might be absolute; in such a case the individual could be considered 'immune' and not 'semi-immune'. Experience indicates, however, that there is a vast range of protective antibody in previously exposed people. In holoendemic areas, where the attack is greatest, the majority will become re-infected and most will develop parasitaemia and some will exhibit modified clinical signs of the infection. Such individuals cannot be regarded as 'immune'. They are classified here, as in most texts, as 'semi-immunes' and dealt with accordingly.

For convenience of description of phenomena such as the febrile paroxysm, which may not always be present in falciparum malaria, the relapsing infections are considered first.

## THE RELAPSING MALARIAS

### VIVAX MALARIA*

#### INCUBATION PERIOD AND PRODROMAL SYMPTOMS

The intrinsic incubation period is usually 10–15 days. In a few strains it may be some months. The appearance of the primary attack is often considerably delayed in individuals who had been receiving suppressive chemotherapy during exposure. In such individuals, the first clinical attack may not appear until some months after the drug dosage has been stopped.

In the last 2 or 3 days of the incubation period prodromal symptoms are common. The patient frequently complains of headache, limb pains, backache, anorexia, and sometimes nausea and vomiting. There may be mild shivering attacks during which the patient complains of feeling cold. In relapses prodromal symptoms are often absent.

#### THE CLASSICAL ATTACK

*Onset.* In the primary attack the onset may be associated with a rigor but this is unusual. For the first few days the fever is irregularly remittent or intermittent. During this period rigors are uncommon. The pattern of intermittent, regularly recurring, febrile paroxysms is usually established by the end of the first week.

*The paroxysm.* For some reason paroxysms occur as a rule more commonly in the afternoon and evening than in the morning. The fully developed paroxysms may be divided into three clinical stages; the cold, the hot, and the sweating stage.

*The cold stage* is short, lasting from 15 minutes to 1 hour. In a few cases it may be considerably longer. The patient feels chilly, begins to shiver, and finally passes into rigor. The temperature at the start of the shivering is usually below 37.8° C. It rises rapidly, sometimes reaching 40° C or even higher at the height of the rigor. At this point the skin is cold and pale. The pulse is fast and thready, the blood pressure often raised. Nausea and vomiting are common

---

* Ovale malaria is very similar to vivax malaria. The course is usually mild, but febrile paroxysms are sometimes severe. Periodicity is slightly longer than that of vivax malaria. The density of parasitaemia is low, since reticulocytes are preferentially invaded. The spleen enlarges more slowly.

and may be severe enough to suggest food poisoning. Frequency and polyuria are usual.

*The hot stage* succeeds the cold. The rigor ceases; the subjective feeling of cold disappears and the patient complains of being uncomfortably hot. The temperature frequently remains at about the level reached at the end of the cold stage, but occasionally may rise, and in rare circumstances may reach hyperpyrexial levels. The pale skin now flushes and feels hot and dry. The blood pressure may fall moderately; the pulse is full and bounding. Respiration is rapid, nausea and vomiting are common, and the patient frequently complains of severe thirst. At this stage he becomes restless and excitable and may go into delirium. One of the most severe subjective complaints is that of post-orbital headache.

*The sweating stage* follows the hot stage which lasts longer than the cold, frequently 2 hours or more. Sweating first appears at the temples, and rapidly becomes generalized and copious. The temperature falls to normal or subnor-

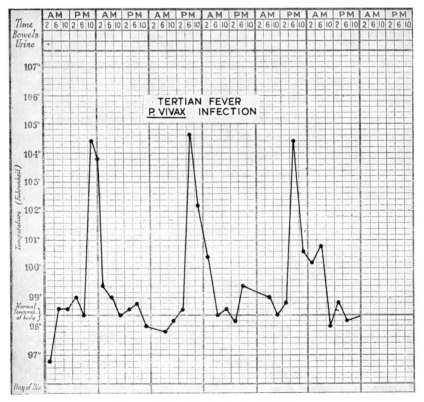

Fig. 37. Tertian fever in *P. vivax* infection.

[From B.G.Maegraith, *Pathological Processes in Malaria and Blackwater Fever*, Blackwell Scientific Publications, Oxford, 1948]

mal in the course of an hour or so. The pulse rate becomes normal and with the subsidence of the temperature the patient usually passes into an exhausted sleep from which he awakes considerably refreshed.

*The interval.* The period between the subsidence of fever and the appearance of the next paroxysm is known as the interval. In the interval the patient feels well and the temperature is within normal limits in the majority of cases, although it may occasionally rise to 37.8 or 38.3° C.

*Erythrocytes.* Parasitized erythrocytes are enlarged; they are destroyed at sporulation and unparasitized cells may also be lysed. Anaemia therefore develops after the disease has been overt from some time. This is not often severe in vivax malaria, although it may occasionally reach serious proportions in children. The bone marrow reaction is normoblastic. There may be a slight increase in reticulocytes during the early stages of the paroxysms, but these cells do not perceptibly increase in numbers as a rule until after administration of specific drug therapy.

*Leucocytes.* There may be a mild leucopenia due to polymorph depression.

*Parasites in the peripheral blood.* Representatives of all forms of the asexual parasite from the early ring to the mature schizont may be recognized in the peripheral blood at any one time, though one particular stage greatly preponderates at certain stages once regular periodicity is established. The number of invaded erythrocytes is seldom over 2 per cent of the total cells. Gametocytes usually appear after the infection has been going on a week or more.

*The spleen and liver.* The spleen is often sufficiently enlarged to be palpable by the end of the second week of the attack. It may sometimes be felt to increase in size during the paroxysm. The liver enlarges and may be palpable in the acute attack.

*Herpes labialis.* This is present in about one third of all cases. It frequently precedes the malarial attack and disappears rapidly after antimalarial treatment has commenced.

Complications are very rare.

## COURSE AND PROGNOSIS

In untreated primary infections paroxysms recur regularly for 6 weeks to 3 months or more, depending upon the strain of parasite, before spontaneous clinical cure occurs. Spontaneous cure is frequently heralded by the lengthening of the intervals between paroxysms, and by reduction in their severity both in regard to the appearance of rigors and the temperature reached.

*Relapse.* Relapses occur after a period of clinical quiescence which may last for some weeks or months. The clinical features of a relapse are similar to those of the first attack, except that the initial period of irregular fever is absent. The onset is accompanied by rigor and paroxysm, and periodicity similar to that of the parent attack is established from the start. The relapse is commonly less severe and of shorter duration than the first attack. It is unusual in vivax malaria for relapse to occur more than 3 years after the patient has left the endemic area.

## MALARIAE MALARIA: QUARTAN MALARIA

### INCUBATION PERIOD AND PRODROMAL SYMPTOMS

The incubation period is frequently longer than that of vivax malaria. It may be as long as 30–40 days and in some cases even several months. Prodromal symptoms similar to those of vivax malaria develop in the last few days of the incubation period. Parasites may be observed in the blood before symptoms develop.

### THE ATTACK

*Onset.* The onset of the disease is often insidious. The clinical picture may be more severe than that of vivax malaria. The primary attack frequently starts with a paroxysm, followed by regular periodicity, which is quartan in type when the majority of broods of the parasite undergo schizogony together. All variations from quartan to quotidian periodicity may occur but quartan is the commonest. In this form of malaria, the periodicity may vary from time to time in the same individual during the same attack.

*The paroxysms and interval.* The three stages of the paroxysms are clearly distinguished. Rigors may occasionally be absent; on the whole they are commonest in attacks in which the periodicity is quartan. Sometimes the cold stage is prolonged. The hot stage frequently lasts several hours. Nausea and vomiting are extremely common during this stage. The sweating stage is often followed by a fall of temperature to well below normal and may end in the partial collapse of the patient.

*Erythrocytes.* The anaemia is usually less pronounced than in vivax malaria, but may occasionally be severe.

*Leucocytes.* There is usually some leucopenia.

*Parasites in the peripheral blood.* Representatives of all stages of the asexual parasites are usually present at any one time, the dominant form depending on the periodicity. As a rule less than 1 per cent of red cells are infected. Gametocytes appear within a few weeks of the onset of clinical signs.

*The spleen and liver.* The spleen is not usually enlarged to the same extent as in the other infections. It is, however, commonly palpable within a fortnight from the onset. The liver enlarges and may be palpable in the acute attack.

*Herpes labialis* is common.

*Oedema,* especially of the ankles, may appear in the acute attack.

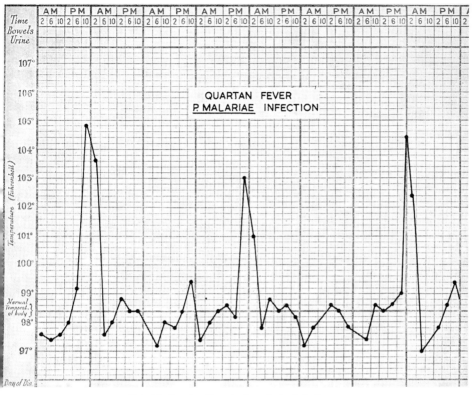

FIG. 38. Quartan fever in *P. malariae* infection.

[From B.G.Maegraith, *Pathological Processes in Malaria and Blackwater Fever*, Blackwell Scientific Publications, Oxford, 1948]

### COURSE AND PROGNOSIS

The acute attack of quartan malaria is self-limited. It may last for several months before spontaneous clinical cure. The disease is rarely fatal and seldom gives rise to complications. Quartan malaria is the most persistent form of human malaria. Relapses are common, and may occur irregularly many years after the primary attack.

An association has been established between *P. malariae* infection and a nephrotic syndrome in children. The peak incidence is around 5 years of age. The child presents with generalized oedema, oliguria, massive proteinuria, and severe hypoproteinaemia. Renal biopsy shows tubular degeneration and glomerular lesions ranging from thickening of the basement membrane to fibrosis. Pathogenesis depends on laying down of soluble antigen–antibody complexes which can be demonstrated in the glomeruli by fluorescent antibody techniques. IgG, IgM, and $B_1$ complement are present and, sometimes, antigen. Tubular damage is minor; there may be hyaline cytoplasmic droplets and protein debris in the lumen. Parasitaemia is usually low and it is considered that the lesions are not directly initiated by the presence of the parasite as such. Treatment is difficult and prognosis is poor.

## FALCIPARUM MALARIA

This is the most serious form of malaria. Attacks may be uncomplicated or associated with serious and often fatal complications.

## THE UNCOMPLICATED ATTACK

### INCUBATION AND PRODROMAL SYMPTOMS

The incubation period varies from 8 to 15 days. Prodromal symptoms, which are often severe, occur during the last few days of the incubation period. The patient is depressed and unwell. He complains of severe headache, bone and muscle pains, especially nagging backache in the lumbar or sacro-iliac region. Shivering feelings, nausea, and vomiting or diarrhoea are frequent.

*Onset.* Parasites may exist in the blood for long periods before the onset of severe symptoms, especially in individuals who have built up some acquired resistance or who are misusing suppressive drugs. In such cases the onset is insidious, with symptoms such as diarrhoea, persistent dyspepsia, malaise and backache, which may not at first suggest malaria.

The onset of the overt attack is, however, usually well defined. Shivering feelings and chills are common, but there is commonly no well-defined rigor.

*The attack.* The patient usually presents with obvious fever, flushed dry skin, and bright eyes. He looks like a case of moderately severe influenza and may not appear very ill. This appearance is deceptive, however, since serious complications may arise at any stage of either a primary attack or a relapse.

The headache, bone and muscle pains and malaise of the prodromal period persist and increase as the attack develops.

Anxiety, mental confusion, and delirium are common. The patient is more asthenic and prostrated than in vivax infections and, in those cases in which periodic fever becomes established, the feeling of well-being which normally accompanies the interval between the paroxysms in vivax malaria is absent.

*Fever.* The fever is usually irregular at first and shows no sign of periodicity. In about one-third of cases periodicity becomes evident after the first few days and is commonly tertian or quotidian. The paroxysms are often not as regular as in vivax infections and the temperature during the intervals may not fall to normal. In many cases, there is no periodicity and the fever becomes remittent, intermittent, or continuous. Even in severe attacks the fever may not be high. It may be absent until towards the end of the attack or until the appearance of complications. Occasionally there may be no fever at any stage, even in the presence of heavy blood infection.

*Sweating.* Where paroxysms are present sweating follows the hot stage, as in vivax malaria. When the fever is persistent or intermittent, but without paroxysms, sweating is common and is often persistent. The pale, moist skin in such cases has a characteristically earthy toxic appearance. In some cases in which the temperature is high, sweating may be absent.

*Erythrocytes.* Because of the rapid and progressive lysis and phagocytosis of both parasitized and unparasitized erythrocytes, severe anaemia is common in falciparum malaria. Erythrocyte counts of fewer than a million cells per $mm^3$ with a corresponding fall in haemoglobin concentration may be recorded. In cases of average severity the red cell count varies from 2.5 to 3.0 million cells per $mm^3$ with corresponding low haemoglobin concentration. In mild cases there may be little or no obvious anaemia. In severe cases the loss of red cells may be so rapid that haemoglobin is liberated into the plasma and passed in the urine, giving rise to the syndrome of blackwater fever, sometimes referred to as 'malarial haemoglobinuria'.

The degree of anaemia is not always an indication of the severity of the attack; fatal complications sometimes occur in cases with apparently little red cell destruction. The red cell count and haemoglobin concentration may be temporarily much increased by the appearance of shock and the associated sudden loss of circulating blood volume.

The anaemia is normocytic. The bone marrow reaction is usually normoblastic, but in very rapid and severe cases this reaction may be depressed.

*Leucocytes.* There is usually a leucopenia with a count of the order of 3000–4000 cells per $mm^3$. Granulocytes are reduced and there is an increase in large mononuclear cells. In severe cases haemozoin pigment may be present in circulating polymorphs and monocytes.

*Parasites in the peripheral blood.* In this infection the later stages of schizogony take place in tissue vessels so that normally only the younger growing forms (rings) of the parasites appear in the peripheral blood. In heavy infections all forms may be present. Very high rates of infection of erythrocytes (e.g. 20 or 30 per cent) may occur. Gametocytes appear within a few days of the onset of the primary clinical attack and persist for up to 3 months after cure.

In the untreated case the parasitaemia increases as the disease progresses, but there may be appreciable daily variations in the parasite density, which may demand repeated examinations of the peripheral blood at intervals of a few hours.

*Cardiovascular system.* The blood pressure may fall from the outset. Systolic pressures of 90–100 mmHg and diastolic pressures of 40–50 mmHg are common, even in the absence of complications. The pulse is usually full and fast but may, in the late stages, become slow in relation to the fever. If shock develops the blood pressures fall dramatically and the pulse rate may exceed 150 per minute and be barely perceptible.

*Abdominal symptoms.* Nausea and vomiting are common from the onset and may be very severe. Epigastric discomfort, anorexia, and dyspepsia are common. Watery diarrhoea is frequent and is particularly notable in infections with certain strains of the parasite, especially those prevalent in West Africa.

*The spleen.* The spleen enlarges rapidly in all cases, and is usually palpable within 10 days of the onset. Its size sometimes increases during paroxysms, decreasing in the interval. The enlarged organ is usually tender and there may be tenderness in the splenic region even when the organ is not palpable. After repeated attacks, especially in children, the spleen may become enormous. In frequently reinfected adults it is sometimes fibrotic and may be smaller than normal.

Sudden splenic infarction and perisplenitis may cause acute tenderness over the splenic area in the left hypochondrium or pain in the left shoulder region. Surgical emergencies may arise from sudden rupture of the spleen or torsion of its pedicle.

*The liver.* Deviations of 'function' tests and enlargement of the liver probably occur in all cases. In some, especially where gastro-intestinal symptoms are evident, the liver may be tender and palpable below the costal margin. Jaundice appears in severe cases and may be rapidly progressive.

*Respiratory symptoms.* The respiration rate is usually increased and in infection with some strains, notably those formerly found in Eastern Europe and those in West Africa, there is often some involvement of the lungs producing signs and symptoms varying from cough associated with a few scattered moist sounds to signs of bronchopneumonia or frank pulmonary oedema. The latter may occur in shocked cases.

*Renal symptoms.* Indication of renal disturbances may occur. There is protein present in the urine and granular and hyaline casts are common. The concentration of urinary chloride is often low, even in the absence of dehydration, indicating some tubular dysfunction.

More severe renal involvement occasionally develops, with oliguria, sometimes proceeding to anuria, and non-specific acute renal failure, with associated uraemia symptoms (see p. 281). A syndrome similar to acute nephritis with oliguria and the passage of urine containing albumin, blood cells, and casts may also occur.

*Herpes labialis* is present in about one-third of cases.

### COURSE AND PROGNOSIS

If the acute attack is adequately treated and no pernicious symptoms develop there is little risk to life. The acute attack is usually of shorter duration than that of either vivax or malariae malaria. Recrudescences are not uncommon in inadequately treated cases. They do not usually appear later than 9–12 months after the initial attack but have been reported as long as 3 years later. Severe anaemia and splenomegaly develop in patients constantly exposed to reinfection or to a series of acute attacks. The frequently infected patient may pass into the state of malarial cachexia, the clinical picture of which is often complicated by malnutrition. The condition in children may be fatal.

As noted on p. 245, the attack may be considerably modified in individuals with Haemoglobin S or with G-6-Pd-deficient erythrocytes.


## THE COMPLICATED ATTACK

Clinical complications (also called pernicious malaria) may develop without warning at any stage in falciparum malaria. Complications appear most commonly in individuals who have suffered repeated attacks, especially when these have been inadequately treated.

Pernicious symptoms may be anticipated if more than 5 per cent of the erythrocytes are infected; if 10 per cent of the infected cells contain more than one parasite, or if many schizonts are present in the peripheral blood. On the other hand, complications may develop when the blood infection is apparently light.

The syndromes of pernicious malaria are usually grouped according to the organs which are principally involved. The major forms are: (1) cerebral malaria, (2) hyperpyrexia, (3) gastro-intestinal malaria, (4) algid malaria, and (5) blackwater fever.

In any of these complications and in apparently uncomplicated falciparum malaria, acute renal failure may develop (see p. 245).


### CEREBRAL MALARIA

This syndrome commonly unfolds over a period of days of uncomplicated febrile illness. It may, however, appear suddenly with rapid development of coma. The patient complains of headache and of drowsiness. If untreated, he passes into coma with the pupils contracted (often unequally) and deep reflexes abolished or exaggerated. All kinds of neurological signs may be present: the Babinski sign may be positive, hemiplegia may develop, there may be stiffness of the neck, or muscular twitching and convulsions resembling those of epilepsy. Acute mental disturbances are common; in endemic areas such disturbances should be considered malarial in origin until proved otherwise. The clinical picture is frequently a mixed one from the point of view of the nervous system, but forms of cerebral malaria are sometimes referred to as epileptiform, cataleptic, meningeal, paretic, and so forth, depending on the prevailing nervous signs. There is usually irregular remittent fever and often severe anaemia. Parasites, including schizonts, are usually present in large numbers in the peripheral blood.

Hyperpyrexia may appear early (usually in a neglected attack) or may develop during the course of an apparently mild attack. It sometimes occurs in association with cerebral malaria. The skin is hot and dry and there may be some cyanosis in the extremities. It is important to note the dryness of the skin, which indicates inhibition of sweating. By the time the patient is seen he is disorientated, in delirium or coma. Incontinence of urine and faeces is common.

The peripheral blood is usually heavily infected; schizonts as well as ring forms and pigmented trophozytes are commonly present.

Malarial hyperpyrexia may be clinically indistinguishable from heat hyperpyrexia (see p. 144). It is thus always essential in a holoendemic area to exclude malaria before a diagnosis of heatstroke can be safely made.

## GASTRO-INTESTINAL SYNDROMES

### Bilious remittent fever
This syndrome arises from severe liver damage. It varies considerably in severity. The patient suffers from acute epigastric discomfort from the onset, and in the severest form rapidly passes into a typhoid state with characteristic remittent fever. He complains of nausea; vomiting comes on early and is persistent, the vomit containing bile and often 'coffee-grounds' or unchanged blood. Diarrhoea develops early; the stool is watery and contains both blood and bile. The liver becomes enlarged and tender from about the second day, and icterus appears on the first or second day, becoming progressively more severe. The urine volume is scanty and the urine contains granular and hyaline casts, albumin, and bilirubin. The picture closely resembles acute infectious hepatitis or yellow fever. Renal failure may supervene with the development of anuria and acute uraemia. Death occurs in severe cases from vascular collapse or acute renal or hepatic failure. Parasites, including schizonts, are present in large numbers in the peripheral blood.

### Dysenteric malaria
This may be clinically indistinguishable from acute bacillary dysentery. It is characterized by the passage at frequent intervals of stools containing blood, mucus, epithelial and other cellular debris, and, in some cases, pus cells. The abdomen is tender and retracted. Nausea and vomiting are common and the temperature is usually high and remittent. There is nearly always heavy parasitaemia.

*Choleraic malaria*

The patient suffers from profuse watery diarrhoea, nausea, and vomiting, muscular cramps in the limbs and abdomen, and progressive dehydration. The stool is mainly fluid, containing particles of faeces and sometimes small quantities of blood and mucus. The salt content of both blood and urine is low. Medical shock or acute renal failure with anuria and rising blood urea concentration may occur, as in cholera. Parasites in all stages of development are usually present in the blood in large numbers.

### ALGID MALARIA

In this condition the patient passes rapidly into medical shock, frequently associated with coma. The facies are drawn and pinched, the eyes sunken. The skin is inelastic, pale, and covered with clammy sweat. Although the skin feels cold the rectal temperature may be raised to 38.5–39° C. The breathing is shallow and sighing. The pulse is thin and fast; both systolic and diastolic blood pressures are low, the diastolic being frequently unmeasurable. There is often acute reduction of circulating blood volume, evidenced by haemoconcentration.

There may be intense epigastric discomfort, persistent vomiting, and sometimes choleraic diarrhoea. Parasites, including schizonts, are commonly present in very large numbers in the peripheral blood. Algid malaria often develops during an apparently mild attack of falciparum malaria. Its onset is independent of the prevailing degree of parasitaemia or anaemia.

The untreated condition is fatal, the patient dying from vascular failure. The clinical picture in some ways resembles that of acute adrenal insufficiency.

### BLACKWATER FEVER

Blackwater fever is a state of acute intravascular haemolysis accompanied by haemoglobinuria occurring as a complication of *Plasmodium falciparum* infection. The syndrome does not complicate the other plasmodial infections.

It may occur in non-immune persons after irregular exposure to infection in highly endemic areas for months or years. Most individuals give a history of irregular chemosuppression and inadequate chemotherapy of attacks or recrudescences of falciparum malaria. It also occurs occasionally in natives of endemic areas, living under conditions of incomplete entomological or drug protection against infection.

*Pathogenesis.* The essential feature of blackwater fever is sudden acute haemolysis, the pathogenesis of which is not fully understood. No abnormally haemolytic strains of *P. falciparum* have ever been identified; there is no evidence of a circulating haemolysin and the saline fragility of the erythrocytes is not increased.

It is now believed that the haemolysis is precipitated by an immunosensitivity reaction. Irregular exposure to the E phase of *P. falciparum* creates an autogenous sensitivity which causes an antibody–antigen haemolytic reaction when the individual is reinfected with the same strain of parasite, usually after a period of freedom from reinfection. It may appear without warning and without an associated attack of malaria.

Blackwater fever was common in caucasian troops exposed to *P. falciparum* infection in West Africa in the Second World War at a time when quinine was the only drug available for treatment and suppression of malaria. When antimalarial measures were tightened up and mepacrine and later paludrine were substituted for quinine, the disease disappeared in the troops. On the other hand, when West African Negro soldiers returned home after a long sojourn in Burma, during which time they were exposed under irregular mepacrine suppression to Burmese *P. falciparum* parasites (to which they were notably resistant), blackwater fever appeared in some of them when they became reinfected with the local African strains of *P. falciparum*. More recently, in American troops infected in Vietnam with chloroquinine-resistant strains of *P. falciparum,* and repatriated to the U.S.A., blackwater fever appeared during recrudescence of the infection some time after suppression by sulphon-amides, or other chemotherapy. In these cases the haemolysis presumably developed in the same way as in the African troops on return from Burma, except that the sensitizing parasitaemia was a recrudescence of an existing infection and not a reinfection with the original strain.

Irregular therapeutic and suppressive dosage with antimalarial drugs is an important factor in many cases. The habit of taking quinine irregularly, particularly at times of 'fever', was a common prelude to blackwater. Before the introduction of modern synthetic drugs, blackwater appeared in cases of falciparum malaria undergoing quinine therapy.

There is evidence indicating that the role of quinine in initiating lysis is occasionally a direct one, but it is now believed that the drug, because of its general inefficiency as a suppressive when taken irregularly, fostered the development of an immunosensitivity state in the individual patient resembling that which initiates acute lysis in the incompletely protected native of an endemic area returning after an interval and becoming re-infected with a trigger dose of local *P. falciparum* (as in Africans returning from the Burmese campaign—see above). Possibly both processes may be involved in some individuals.

*Pathology*. The haemolysis produces a sudden and sometimes catastrophic reduction in the circulating erythrocyte mass.

A few *P. falciparum* parasites are present in the peripheral erythrocytes in about half the cases when first seen, but usually disappear as haemolysis progresses. They may reappear in convalescence.

In some cases there may be clinical cardiac failure, but death results most commonly from renal failure, vascular collapse or hepatic failure. The heart muscle may show some change including granular fatty degeneration, fragmentation, and loss of striation; brown pigment is often found deposited in the cytoplasm near the nuclear poles. The pathological changes in the liver and kidney and their pathogenesis are essentially the same as in falciparum malaria. In cases complicated by vascular collapse, the autopsy findings include those of shock.

During active lysis, haemoglobin is present in the plasma. Another pigment, methaemalbumin, has also been detected (Fairley) and was at one time thought to be derived from albumin and haematin split from the free haemoglobin. The hydrolysis of the latter, with liberation of haematin, is, however, now under considerable doubt.

The blood urea nitrogen concentration is raised slightly in practically all cases, irrespective of the existence of renal insufficiency. When renal failure develops the blood urea nitrogen rises to great heights as in other similar forms of acute uraemia. After recovery from renal failure it rapidly returns to normal.

Plasma protein concentrations are usually low, the reduction being mainly in albumin. There is sometimes an accompanying increase in globulin. Plasma bilirubin is raised, especially in cases with obvious hepatic dysfunction. There may be some acidosis.

## CLINICAL PICTURE

Blackwater fever sometimes occurs in individuals who have never taken antimalarial drugs, but it is common to find that the patient has been taking suppressive therapy irregularly or has been treating himself for malarial attacks with occasional heavy doses of antimalarials.

The appearance of haemoglobinuria is usually sudden. It may appear during a falciparum attack or during apparent health. The onset is proclaimed by a sudden rise in temperature which reaches 39–40° C in the course of a few hours. Rigor is common. The fever is usually remittent and associated with heavy sweating. In a few cases hyperpyrexia develops. Some mild cases and others in shock may be practically afebrile. The onset of shock is followed by a dramatic fall in temperature.

Haemolysis may occur only once or may recur at intervals. Each haemolytic phase may last a few hours to 36 hours or longer. Occasionally the haemolysis is continuous and overwhelming.

During haemolysis the red cell count falls rapidly and may fall to fewer than 1.0 million or fewer cells per mm$^3$ in a few hours.

*The urine.* Haemoglobin appears in the urine shortly after the commencement of haemolysis and persists for some time after haemolysis has stopped. From the clinical point of view, however, haemolysis and haemoglobinuria are considered contemporaneous. During the lytic phase the urine contains a mixture of oxyhaemoglobin (red) and its derivatives, principally methaemoglobin (dark brown). The colour of the specimen depends on which pigment predominates. Oxyhaemoglobin is in excess in alkaline urine. The first specimen of urine passed after haemolysis is often the darkest. As the lysis abates each specimen becomes successively less pigmented until finally clear.

Protein is present in high concentration throughout the lytic period. When the pigment clears, the albumin usually goes with it. The urine of the interlytic phase is thus non-pigmented and practically free from albumin. The urine passed during haemolysis may be acid, neutral, or alkaline.

During haemoglobinuria there is always a massive brown deposit containing hyaline and granular casts, amorphous epithelial debris and haemoglobin pigments.

The urine passed during, and for some days subsequent, to haemolysis is unconcentrated so far as its electrolyte concentration is concerned, although its specific gravity may be high as a result of its protein content.

Renal failure may develop independently or during medical shock. Anuria is seldom absolute; the patient commonly passes during the day 30–40 ml thick, black, tarry urine loaded with albumin. Anuria comes on suddenly and its onset may be missed unless the volume of each specimen of urine passed is measured separately. It may occur during the passage of pigment or in an interlytic phase. It is independent of the reaction of the urine.

The patient proceeds into acute uraemia with rising blood urea nitrogen, oedema, disorientation, and sometimes coma. The syndrome is usually fatal without treatment, but recovery may occur spontaneously, the patient passing rapidly into a period of diuresis passing very dilute urine.

Practically all cases show signs of hepatic dysfunction soon after the onset. The liver edge becomes palpable and tender. The enlargement may proceed rapidly until the edge presents several fingers-breadth below the costal margin. Jaundice is often visible by the end of the first day and deepens fast. Bilirubin appears in the urine, and may be masked by the blood pigments. The faeces are watery and often contain bile. There is sometimes severe watery diarrhoea. Vomiting may be intractable and accompanied by hiccup. Sometimes the liver failure may advance so rapidly as to suggest acute infectious hepatitis.

Medical shock may develop. If the shocked patient survives for some time petechial haemorrhages may appear in the skin and mucous membranes and the vomitus and faeces may both contain altered blood.

The vomiting, watery diarrhoea, and sweating commonly lead to severe dehydration.

The mortality rate varies from 20 to 30 per cent of all cases.

In the uncomplicated case recovery is rapid and convalescence uneventful. Malaria parasites may appear in early convalescence and require treatment.

Complications are frequently fatal. More than half the deaths arise from renal failure, most of the others from vascular failure, hepatic insufficiency, or uncontrollable lysis. Occasionally there may be cardiac failure, sometimes occurring during apparently satisfactory convalescence.

Because of the risks of further attacks of blackwater fever, the individual should be advised to leave the region in which the attack occurred. Some have survived several attacks.

## *Diagnosis*

Blackwater fever is the probable diagnosis in cases of abrupt haemoglobinuria and increasing anaemia in a patient who is exposed to *P. falciparum* infection, particularly if there is a history of irregular chemosuppression or other protection against malaria. It is necessary in suspected cases to measure *both* the erythrocyte count and the blood haemoglobin, since the latter is compounded of both the haemoglobinaemia and the pigment in circulating erythrocytes, so that a completely false impression of what is happening may be obtained by measuring haemoglobin concentration only.

Causes of haemoglobinuria other than blackwater fever must be excluded. The most important of these (which does not concern the Anglo Saxon caucasian who was once so prone to blackwater fever) is the induction of haemolysis in a glucose-6-phosphate-dehydrogenase-deficient carrier challenged by chemical or infective agents (see p. 139). Consuming the Fava bean or its products may precipitate disastrous haemolysis in such patients. The syndrome, which is called favism, occurs commonly in certain geographical areas, notably Sardinia.

Haemoglobinuria can be distinguished from haematuria due to schistosomiasis, etc., by the presence of haemoglobin pigments and not erythrocytes in the urine. Bilirubinuria can be distinguished chemically or spectroscopically. Myoglobinuria in viperine snake bite may be mistaken for haemoglobinuria; it can be distinguished spectroscopically.

The recognition of renal failure is very important in blackwater fever. Every specimen of urine passed should be examined separately and its volume measured and recorded.

The absence of malaria parasites from the peripheral blood in a well developed case of blackwater fever has no diagnostic significance.

*Treatment* (see p. 280).

## MALARIA IN 'SEMI IMMUNES'

In individuals who have acquired some resistance to any local plasmodial strains the clinical effects of malaria resulting from infection with these strains may be greatly modified. Irregularly spaced febrile attacks of short duration occur, which do not usually resemble ordinary malaria. There is malaise, headache, often backache, anorexia, and sweating. The response to treatment is rapid. More severe attacks develop as immunity is weakened or lost, for instance as a result of the irregular or careless use of antimalarial drugs or incomplete entomological protection. Blackwater fever may follow reinfection with *P. falciparum*, as described above.

## MALARIA IN INFANTS AND CHILDREN

In tropical countries malaria is one of the great causes of morbidity and mortality in children. The clinical attack is rare in the first months of life, but thereafter for several years children are prone to pernicious forms of malaria and even vivax and malariae malaria may occasionally be fatal to them. Rupture of an enlarged spleen following external violence is a serious risk in falciparum and vivax infections.

The clinical picture of malaria in children depends on whether they are suffering from acute recent infection, or from the effects of frequent reinfection, or long-continued infection, or both.

The acute form is often totally different from the adult disease. It is seen most commonly in children who have not had the full benefit of protective measures, or who live in areas where malaria is seasonal.

The infected child is dull, restless and miserable with no appetite. It resents feeding and food is often vomited back. Bile may be present in the vomit. There is frequently severe abdominal colicky pain, considerable wind and diarrhoea, the stool sometimes containing bile. The abdomen is distended and tender, especially in the hepatic and splenic areas. The spleen is usually palpable and commonly the liver also. As the result of the prevailing anaemia the mucous membranes are pale and in Europeans the skin has an earthy tinge. There may be some flush and where fever is present the skin is often dry; it may, however, be cool and clammy with sweat. The temperature usually ranges from 38.0–40.6° C and the fever may be continuous, remittent or intermittent. Rigors are uncommon. Convulsions are common; there may be meningismus.

If the condition is allowed to continue for long, the anaemia becomes more severe, the abdomen more distended, the spleen (and often the liver) larger, and there is often rapid loss of weight and wasting of the limbs, sometimes associated with puffiness of the face.

If the malaria remains untreated the child may become rapidly worse and die, or it may temporarily recover with the abatement of most or all of the signs and symptoms and gradually slip into the progressive ill-health and recurrent fever of so-called 'chronic' malaria.

This form of malaria is commonest in falciparum areas and is seen in children of all ages up to adolescence. The normal growth and development of the child is retarded. The patient is listless, wasted, with thin skinny flaccid limbs and a huge, protuberant abdomen. There is chronic dyspepsia and flatulence. Anorexia may be extreme and complicating factors arising from deficiencies of essential food substances and minerals are usually accompanied by purpura and epistaxis. Mucous membranes are pale; the skin is sometimes tinged with jaundice. Fever is common, not invariable, and may never be prominent. It is usually remittent, occasionally intermittent, but not periodic.

Anaemia is often severe with haemoglobin concentrations of 5 g per 100 ml or lower. By this time, as a rule, the parasitaemia is low, but it may rise considerably—even to 10 per cent or higher—in exacerbations or fresh infections. Normally, only ring forms and gametocytes are seen in the peripheral blood, but in severe cases pigmented trophozoites and schizonts are present.

The spleen is very large and tender and may present into the pelvis. The liver is frequently enlarged and tender. Rupture of the enlarged spleen may follow external violence or the organ may twist on its pedicle, causing an acute abdominal crisis.

The condition, if untreated, becomes progressively worse and passes into the state of malarial cachexia, which ends fatally.

### CONTROL OF MALARIA IN INFANTS AND YOUNG CHILDREN

In endemic areas the malaria parasite is suppressed during the first 2–3 months of life in breast-fed infants not receiving dietary supplements. Infection occurs, but severe attacks and high degrees of parasitaemia are rare. This may in part be due to the Haemoglobin F present in the infant erythrocytes and to some extent to immune bodies transmitted through the placenta and the mother's milk. However, a milk diet (breast, bottled or dried) will equally well suppress the parasite in experimentally induced infections in non-endemic areas. Milk is deficient in *p*-aminobenzoic acid (PABA) which the parasite needs for synthesis of folic acid. Unlike the infant, the parasite is unable to use the preformed folic acid present in the milk.

In most countries, by the end of the third month the infant on the breast is also receiving food additives, which contain PABA. The parasite is no longer inhibited and the infants begin to suffer the consequences of the infection, with high mortality.

In mesoendemic areas, no suppressive drug regimens may be needed and each attack of malaria is fully treated and followed for a short time by a period of chemosuppression. This helps build up protective immunity. In holoendemic areas, the consensus is that the indigenous child up to the age of 5 years should undergo incomplete suppression of the parasite, by being given antimalarial drugs at longer intervals than would be needed to produce full suppression (as in the expatriate child, who will not eventually be exposed to further infection). In this way, some protective immunity will develop, so that the child can deal better with infection after the drug is withdrawn. This technique, of course, must be combined with full therapy of any attacks of malaria which may develop.

A common regimen is as follows:

Rely on unsupplemented breast feeding for the first 2 to 3 months, treating any attacks which may occur. Then give suppressive antimalarial drugs. Of these, pyrimethamine is recommended in a single dose of 12.5 mg up to the age of 3 years, thereafter 25 mg. The drug should be given once every 3 or 4 weeks, or, if possible, every 2 weeks. The interval depends largely on whether the mother is consistent in bringing the baby regularly to the dispensary.

If there is resistance to pyrimethamine, combinations of long-acting sulphonamides and pyrimethamine may be substituted, or the appropriate dose of chloroquine may be given, provided the parasites are sensitive to the drug. All overt attacks *must* be treated.

(For prophylaxis and suppression of malaria in general, see pp. 784–788.)

## MALARIA IN PREGNANCY

Malaria is a common cause of premature labour and abortion, especially in the last months of gestation. The mother may die from malaria following childbirth if the disease is untreated. Women exposed to frequent reinfection in an endemic area appear to lose some of their acquired resistance during pregnancy and may consequently develop severe malarial attacks. Clinically severe attacks also often appear in the puerperium.

In hyperendemic areas pregnant women not infrequently come to term with severe anaemia, enlarged spleens sometimes presenting into the pelvis, and enlarged livers. In such women, mechanical factors may lead to elevation of the diaphragm and difficult delivery. The anaemia will respond to antimalarial therapy.

A malarial attack in a pregnant woman, particularly in a primipara, must be regarded as a possible cause of abortion. Full drug therapy is required for overt malaria during pregnancy; it will not increase the risk of abortion. Antimalarial suppression is advised in highly endemic areas in the third trimester and also in SS homozygotes. Post-partum rises of temperature are often caused by malaria. Malaria may be transmitted occasionally from mother to child across the placenta. It is not decided whether this occurs as the result of some intra-uterine placental accident. Congenital malaria is more frequent in infants born of non-immune subjects.

## THE DIAGNOSIS OF MALARIA

### PARASITOLOGICAL DIAGNOSIS

*The certain diagnosis of active malaria depends upon the identification of the Erythrocytic (E) parasites in the peripheral blood or elsewhere* (e.g. the sternal marrow). Where the parasites are difficult to find in the blood, examination of the marrow is unlikely to help the diagnosis.

The presence in the blood of trophozoites or later growing forms, indicating the progress of an active asexual cycle, must be established.

*The discovery of gametocytes only is not suffient to confirm the diagnosis of active malaria.* Gametocytes are not usually formed until schizogony has been proceeding for some days. They may be found in the peripheral blood weeks and even months after the overt attack has subsided or been cured.

*Blood-films.* For the diagnosis of the presence of parasites the examination of stained thick blood-films is sufficient. The species of plasmodium present can usually be indicated in the thick film but must be confirmed by examination of a thin film, prepared in the ordinary way and stained by Giemsa's method.

*The thick film.* Clean the tip of a finger or lobe of an ear with alcohol and allow to dry. Prick with a cutting needle and squeeze gently until a large globule of blood exudes. Pick up the blood with the undersurface of a clean glass slide. Spread it evenly over a circular area about 2 cm across with the needle or corner of another slide.

Allow the film to dry thoroughly before staining.

Field's stain or dilute Giemsa are recommended for general use.*

Lysis of the erythrocytes with loss of haemoglobin occurs during staining. In the final preparation the parasites are stained (cytoplasm blue, chromatin reddish). White cell nuclei and platelets stain deep blue and pinkish respectively.

All stages of the asexual parasite are to be found in the peripheral blood in vivax, malariae, and ovale malaria. Only ring forms are as a rule found in the peripheral blood in falciparum malaria unless the rate of infection of red cells is very high, when pigmented growing forms and schizonts appear.

In all infections, gametocytes may be present after the first few days of illness, and may remain after treatment.

The blood should be examined frequently during an attack. This is particularly necessary in falciparum malaria in which the numbers of parasites present may vary considerably during the day. Failure to find parasites in one specimen is not significant. Repeated examination of films made morning and evening over periods of days may be necessary, particularly if the patient has been taking suppressive antimalarial drugs. In the latter case the patient should, unless there are good clinical grounds otherwise, be taken off drugs until the diagnosis is confirmed or unless it has already been confirmed.

Differentiation of species depends on factors outlined below.

* Field's stain is supplied in two sets of tablets, A and B. These are each dissolved in water and kept in wide, open-mouthed jars. The thoroughly dried thick film is immersed in solution A for a few seconds, washed in water, and dipped in solution B for a few seconds. After washing, the slides are dried in the vertical position. Giemsa stain is diluted 1:30 with buffered water (pH 7.0–7.2). The slide is immersed film downwards for 20 minutes or longer. The stain is washed away rapidly and the film dried at an angle.

*Plasmodium falciparum*

*Thin film.* Parasites numerous; may be 10 per cent or more erythrocytes infected. Multiple infection of erythrocytes common. Usually ring forms only, with one or two chromatin dots. Pigmented late trophozoites and schizonts present only in heavy infections; pigment is coarse, dark brown or black, conglomerated into a single mass in schizonts which contain up to thirty-six merozoites. Infected erythrocytes are not enlarged; may be coarsely stippled (Maurer's dots). Gametocytes crescentic.

*Thick film.* Many non-pigmented ring forms with one or more chromatin dots; cytoplasm usually delicate but may be dense. Other forms seen only in heavy infections. In infections which have continued for a week or more or in recurrent infections, crescentic gametocytes may be present.

*Plasmodium vivax*

*Thin film.* Parasites few; not more than 2 per cent erythrocytes infected. Multiple infections rare. All stages of E phase may be present. Rings are large. Trophozoites large, irregular, and pigmented. Usually only one chromatin dot. Pigment granules are fine and yellow-brown. Large pigmented schizonts (containing about twelve merozoites) are common. Infected erythrocytes are enlarged and finely stippled (Schüffner's dots). Gametocytes are round and fill cells.

*Thick film.* Rings large but few. One chromatin dot. Coarse cytoplasm. Pigmented trophozoites and schizonts present. Gametocytes rounded. Although outlines of infected erythrocytes are not visible, the Schüffner's dots may often be seen.

*Plasmodium malariae*

*Thin film.* Parasites few. Ring forms, pigmented trophozoites, schizonts, and gametocytes may be present. Multiple infections rare. Rings are small and sturdy, with one chromatin dot. Trophozoites occur in band forms running across the erythrocyte. Pigment granules are coarse and dark brown. In schizonts, which fill the cells, there may be a central clump of pigment around which the merozoites group to form a rosette. Infected cells are not enlarged; some may show fine stippling. Gametocytes are rounded, compact, with abundant peripheral granules of pigment and single central chromatin mass.

*Thick film.* Few parasites. Rings usually small with compact cytoplasm. Band-form, solid-looking trophozoites are usually present. Single chromatin dot. Pigmented trophozoites and schizonts (sometimes with central pigment mass and rosette of merozoites). Gametocytes are rounded, compact, with central chromatin mass and peripheral granular pigmentation.

*Plasmodium ovale*

*Thin film.* Few parasites. All forms may be present. Parasites resemble *P. vivax*. Granules of pigment are coarser than in *P. vivax* and dark brown.

Schizonts may have a central pigment mass and from six to twelve merozoites. Gametocytes round and fill cell. Infected erythrocytes are enlarged and pale, peppered with Schüffner's dots; they appear oval and may be fimbriated at one or both extremities (probably artifacts derived from making the film).

*Thick film.* Rings large but few. Parasites resemble *P. vivax.* Schüffner's dots easily visible. (Examination of the thin film necessary for confirmation.)

### CLINICAL DIAGNOSIS

Until proved otherwise, malaria must be suspected in all cases of fever in endemic areas or in individuals recently exposed in an endemic area. Diagnosis can be made only by finding the E phase of the parasite in the erythrocytes. Clinically, the regular succession of paroxysms and fever-free intervals should make the physician suspect the presence of malaria. The combination of fever, anaemia, and enlarged spleen is highly suspicious in an endemic area. Falciparum malaria may often clinically resemble other diseases. For instance, it may evoke a set of symptoms very similar to those of acute surgical abdominal conditions, such as appendicitis or peritonitis, or may simulate pneumonia or pleurisy, especially in cases where spontaneous splenic infarcts or subcapsular haematomata have occurred. Examination of the blood should never be neglected. Watching the response of the fever to the administration of antimalarial drugs is no substitute for searching for the parasites. The fever will subside in any case if the patient is suffering from a short-term arbovirus infection. On the other hand, failure to control the fever with, say, chloroquine may be due to the presence of a resistant parasite, or to some other infection. The presence of quinine, mepacrine, or proguanil can be chemically checked in the urine.

If facilities for blood examination are not available and malaria is suspected, a full antimalarial therapeutic course should be given.

## THE TREATMENT OF MALARIA

### THE BASIS OF CHEMOTHERAPY

The treatment of malaria aims at eradication or control of the parasite and dealing with clinical complications.

The clinical effects of malaria result from the presence of the E phase of the parasite in the erythrocyte. Control of the attack depends on the removal of these parasites from the blood and on the anti-inflammatory activity of the drugs used.

Drugs which destroy the E forms are called *Schizonticides.* The classical compounds are the 4-amino-quinolines, quinine, mepacrine, proguanil, pyrimethamine. The first three are strongly anti-inflammatory.

Proguanil and pyrimethamine destroy the initial liver infection (PE or first

EE phase) in *Plasmodium falciparum* infection. In the other three infections the destruction of the persistent liver infection (exoerythrocytic or EE phase) is achieved by only one group of drugs, the 8-amino-quinolines, for example Primaquine.

### AVAILABLE DRUGS

The following compounds all have their uses in the treatment of malaria:

(a) *Chloroquine* (Aralen, Resochin), *Nivaquine*, and other 4-amino-quinolines, including *Amodiaquin* are bitter colourless drugs. *Chloroquine* and *Nivaquine* tablets contain 150 mg of the active base, chloroquine; *Chloroquine* is the phosphate, *Nivaquine* the sulphate of this base. *Amodiaquine* tablets contain 200 mg or 150 mg of drug base.

Ampoules containing solutions of various salts are prepared for parenteral use, for example, *Nivaquine soluble*, provided in ampoules of 5 ml containing 200 mg (base).

*Action*: These drugs act against the erythrocytic or E cycle of all parasites, i.e. they are schizonticides. They destroy the gametocytes of *P. vivax*, *P. malariae*, and *P. ovale* but not those of *P. falciparum*.

*Toxicity:* Side effects are few when given orally. Occasional gastro-intestinal discomfort, sometimes transient pruritus. There may be temporary blurring of vision and sometimes scotomata. On high dosage over long periods serious effects on vision, leading to blindness, have been reported. Given intravenously they may cause shock. In suppressive dosage over long periods, side effects may occur. See page 286.

*Parasite resistance* to 4-amino-quinolines, with cross-resistance to mepacrine, has been demonstrated in South-east Asia and south America but not in Africa. (see p. 288)

(b) *Quinine:* a bitter crystalline alkaloid prepared as bihydrochloride, hydrochloride, or bisulphate. Of these, the first is the most soluble.

The drug is prepared as:

(i) *Tablets,* containing 260–325 mg of the alkaloid as one of the above salts. The sulphate is the least soluble and is best given in acid solution. The bihydrochloride is most commonly used. (ii) *Powder,* in ampoules for solution in water. Usually the hydrochloride in doses ranging from 500–650 mg of the alkaloid. (iii) *Solutions,* in ampoules, otherwise similar to (ii). (iv) Various less bitter compounds such as quinine ethylcarbonate (euquinine), are prepared for administration to children.

*Action:* Quinine is a very effective schizonticide acting on the early schizonts of the asexual parasite in all infections. It destroys the gametocytes of *P. vivax*, *P. malariae*, and *P. ovale*, but *not* those of *P. falciparum*.

*Toxicity:* Some tinnitus, deafness, and dizziness may be expected and sometimes nausea, occasionally vomiting. ·

Erythematous rashes (sensitivity) may occur; quinine may rarely give rise to haemoglobinuria even in the absence of malaria.

In large doses it may promote abortion; this is unlikely in therapeutic doses. Very large doses may cause blindness. In suppressive doses, see page 286.

*Parasite resistance* in *P. falciparum* infections only has been reported very occasionally at RI levels in South-east Asia.

(c) *Proguanil* (Paludrine; Chloroguanide): a colourless bitter synthetic biguanide.

The drug is prepared as *Tablets,* containing 100 mg hydrochloride.

*Action:* Proguanil is a schizonticide acting a little later in the life cycle and a little more slowly than quinine or chloroquine. It is now seldom used therapeutically. It is a causal prophylactic for falciparum malaria *only*, destroying the initial lower PE phase and so preventing the blood infection. It produces radical cure in cases in which the E phase of the parasite has been established and inhibits the development of the sexual cycle in the mosquito. It is a very good suppressant for all forms of malaria. It has little action on gametocytes in the blood.

*Toxicity;* There may be slight gastro-intestinal disturbances, including vomiting, and occasional haematuria, with high dosage, but with normal therapy and when used as a suppressive the drug is non-toxic.

*Parasite resistance* is widespread but localized and erratic in its distribution and degree. Cross-resistance to pyrimethamine usually occurs.

(d) *Pyrimethamine* (Daraprim): A colourless relatively tasteless drug, prepared as tablets containing 25 mg of the base. Widely used as a suppressant, it produces radical cure in established *P. falciparum* infection but not in other infections. Also used as an adjuvant to sulphonamides in treatment and control of chloroquine resistant parasites.

*Action:* Same as Proguanil. It also destroys the primary lower PE forms and inhibits the sexual cycle in the mosquito.

*Toxicity:* Very low. Seldom used therapeutically. In suppressive dosage: see page 286

*Parasite resistance* is widespread. Cross-resistance to Proguanil occurs.

(e) *Mepacrine* (Atebrin, Atabrine, Quinacrine): a bitter yellow acridine compound prepared as the hydrochloride or methane sulphonate now seldom used.

The drug is prepared as: *Tablets,* containing the equivalent of 100 mg of the base as hydrochloride. It is now seldom used orally or parenterally (only intramuscularly, *not* intravenously).

*Action:* Mepacrine is a schizonticide acting on the asexual E cycle of all parasites. It has an action on gametocytes similar to that of chloroquine.

*Toxicity:* Therapeutic doses given orally are not toxic in the majority of patients. Occasionally severe psychotic symptoms may develop, disappearing rapidly after cessation of the drug. Toxicity in suppressive doses: see page 286.

*Parasite resistance* to mepacrine has been reported. Parasites resistant to 4-amino-quinolines usually show cross-resistance to mepacrine.

(f) *Primaquine* and *Pamaquine* (Plasmoquin, Plasmochine): bitter colourless synthetic 8-amino-quinolines.

Primaquine is much the most widely used. It is prepared as tablets containing 7.5 mg or 15.0 mg of the active base respectively.

Pamaquine is prepared as tablets containing the equivalent of 8–10 mg of the base.

*Action:* The 8-amino-quinolines are relatively weak schizonticides but have considerable activity on all tissue phases of *P. vivax, P. malariae* and *P. ovale.* They are active against the P.E. phase of *P. falciparum* but only in toxic doses. In combination with active schizonticides such as quinine, they produce radical cure of vivax, malariae and ovale malaria. They actively destroy gametocytes of all species.

*Toxicity:* There is little margin between therapeutic and toxic doses. Cyanosis due to the presence of methaemoglobin, and colicky abdominal pains are signs of toxicity; their appearance rarely indicates the stopping of the drug. Acute self-limited haemolysis with haemoglobinuria may develop in individuals whose erythrocytes are glucose-6-phosphate dehydrogenase deficient.

(g) *Drugs in treatment of drug-resistant parasites:* see page 289.

### OTHER DRUGS

Certain sulphonamides and sulphones act as schizonticides in *P. falciparum* infections especially in the semi-immune host. Both groups of compounds show some activity against 4-amino-quinoline-insensitive strains of *P. falciparum.*

*Sulfadoxine,* a long-acting sulphamide, has considerable schizonticidal activity and is given (usually in combination with pyrimethamine) for chemotherapy and chemosuppression of chloroquine-resistant and proguanil/pyrimethamine-resistant *P. falciparum* strains.

*Diaphenylsulphone* (Dapsone, DDS), widely used in leprosy, has schizonticidal activity against *P. falciparum* in semi-immunes and is also being tried against chloroquine-resistant strains. It is usually given in combination with pyrimethamine which potentiates its activity. It may induce haemolysis in G-6-Pd-deficient subjects. It is active against Proguanil resistant strains of *P. falciparum* and has been used successfully as an adjuvant with Proguanil in areas, as in Vietnam, when seasonal high incidence of infection is accompanied by correspondingly high incidence of resistant strains.

Repository or depot compounds intended to provide anti-parasitic activity over a long period after administration are being tested for mass control of infection especially in *P. falciparum* endemic areas. The most widely used drug is Cycloguanil embonate, a derivative of the dehydro-triazine metabolite of Proguanil. Protection against *P. falciparum*, *P. vivax*, and *P. malariae* infections exists for several months after intramuscular injection of 6 mg per kg body weight (adults) or 5–15 mg per kg body weight (children). It is sometimes given in combination with Sulphadiamine, DADDS in infections with chloroquine and Proguanil-insensitive *P. falciparum*, and Proguanil-insensitive *P. vivax*.

New drugs are under constant examination (see later).

### THE CHOICE OF ANTIMALARIAL DRUGS

In a given case, the choice of drug to be used and the dosage to be given will depend on its speed of action and the point in the parasitic life cycle at which it exerts its maximum effect.

The choice also depends on (i) the species of infecting parasite or parasites, (ii) the state of acquired resistance to infection which has been achieved by the patient—i.e. whether he may be regarded as immune, semi-immune, or non-immune, and (iii) the sensitivity or otherwise of the infecting parasite to individual antimalarial drugs.

Antimalarial drugs should be given orally if possible unless parenteral administration is indicated. Once the disease has been controlled by paren-teral dosage, oral administration should be resumed.

Eradication of the E phase of parasites which leads to the cure of the basic clinical patterns of malaria is achieved by the use of schizonticides.

Of these, only the 4-amino-quinolines and quinine are commonly used. Mepacrine is equally effective but is now seldom given. Proguanil and pyri-methamine are less effective and are not used for this purpose except in special circumstances. They are only weakly anti-inflammatory.

In *P. falciparum* infections the eradication of the E phase with a schizonti-cide is the only objective.

In the relapsing malarias (*P. vivax*, *P. malariae*, *P. ovale*) eradication of infection is achieved by removal of the E phase with a schizonticide and of the EE phase with an 8-amino-quinoline.

Chemotherapy in the individual case may be modified by two factors: the immune status of the patient and the existence of drug-resistance in the parasites.

*Immune status.* In the infected non-immune the objective of chemotherapy is complete eradication of all forms of parasites.

In the semi-immune, eradication of all forms is needed only if the patient is unlikely to be re-exposed to infection.

In an endemic area or in individuals about to return to an endemic area, it usually suffices to suppress rather than eradicate the infection since complete eradication of the E forms would lead to rapid loss of protective immunity, and in any case reinfection is likely.

The treatment of non-immunes and semi-immunes is considered separately below.

*Drug resistance:* In some areas of the world parasites have developed resistance to the 4-amino-quinolines and mepacrine (*P. falciparum* only) or to Proguanil and pyrimethamine (all parasites); in some places they have become resistant to all four synthetic drugs (*P. falciparum* only). So far, strong resistance to quinine or to the 8-amino-quinolines has not been encountered.

Where the parasite is resistant to a specific drug, the compound cannot be used successfully and an alternative is needed.

The problems of drug resistance are discussed separately below (p. 288).

## ADMINISTRATION OF DRUGS

Drugs are given orally except where complications exist, in which case they are given parenterally.

Parenteral therapy is required when oral administration is impossible or when the blood infection is heavy and rapid control of parasites is essential. The indications are the same for all drugs, and include intractable vomiting; vascular collapse (shock); coma or delirium; hyperpyrexia; hyperparasitaemia; other forms of pernicious malaria.

## THE TREATMENT OF MALARIA IN NON-IMMUNES

### THE ACUTE UNCOMPLICATED ATTACK

ADULTS

1. *Falciparum malaria.* Any of the following courses of treatment will bring about clinical cure and will in most cases produce radical cure. A good drink of water or other bland fluid should be taken with each dose of the drug. A watch must be kept on vomit in case the tablets are returned. If they are, the course must be repeated. Treatment must be followed in an endemic area by suppressive therapy.

(a) The drug of choice (in the absence of parasite drug resistance) is a 4-amino-quinoline, usually chloroquine (diphosphate of chloroquine base) or nivaquine (sulphate or chloroquine base).

| *Chloroquine or Nivaquine* | 4 tablets (600 mg base) on admission<br>2 tablets (300 mg base) 6 hours later<br>2 tablets (300 mg base) once daily for<br>2–3 days |

(b) *Quinine*　　　　　　　　650 mg b.i.d. or t.d.s. for 10 days

(c) *Mepacrine* is effective, but seldom used because of side-effects.

300 mg t.d.s. for 1 day; 200 mg t.d.s. for 1–2 days; 100 mg t.d.s. for 5 days

2. *Vivax malaria:** Any of the above courses of treatment will be effective for clinical cure. Combined therapy is needed for radical cure. In such treatment, any schizonticide except mepacrine (which potentiates the toxic effects of the 8-amino-quinolines) may be used to deal with the E form of the parasite, and an 8-amino-quinoline such as primaquine is needed to eradicate the EE phase and so exclude the possibility of relapse. Resistance to chloroquine has not been reported.

Examples of combined therapy:

(a) *Chloroquine*　　　　　Day 1: 4 tablets (600 mg base) followed in 6 hours by 2 tablets (300 mg base)
Days 2, 3, 4: 2 tablets (300 mg base) once daily

*Primaquine*　　　　　7.5 mg twice daily or 15 mg once daily for 10–14 days

*Note:* The 8-amino-quinoline can be started at the same time as the chloroquine or follow it. There is some evidence that potentiation of drug activity occurs when the compounds are given simultaneously.

(b) *Quinine*　　　　　　　650 mg twice daily for 10 days

*Primaquine*　　　　　7.5 mg twice daily or 15 mg once daily for 10 days, beginning on day 1.

*Note:* Because of possible toxic effects of the 8-amino-quinolines patients must be kept quiet and, if possible, in bed during treatment and persuaded to drink fluid freely. Individuals with G-6-Pd deficient erythrocytes may suffer haemolysis when taking these drugs. This is self-limited, but if there is severe haemolysis with haemoglobinuria the drug is usually withdrawn.

CHILDREN

All drugs are well tolerated by children. Chloroquine is probably the most

* Applies also to malariae and ovale malaria.

satisfactory. The basis of treatment is the same as in adults for all forms of malaria.

*Chloroquine or Nivaquine*

| Age | | Dose |
|-----|-----|------|
| Up to 1 year: | Day 1: | ½ tablet followed by ½ tablet in 6–8 hours |
| | Days 2–5: | ½ tablet once daily |
| 1–3 years: | Day 1: | 1 tablet followed by ¾ tablet in 6–8 hours |
| | Days 2–5: | ½ tablet once daily |
| 3–6 years: | Day 1: | 2 tablets followed by 1 tablet in 6–8 hours |
| | Days 2–5: | ½ tablet once daily |
| 6–12 years: | Day 1: | 2 tablets followed by 1 tablet in 6–8 hours |
| | Days 2–5: | 1 tablet once daily |
| 12–15 years: | Day 1: | 3–4 tablets followed by 1–2 tablets in 6–8 hours |
| | Days 2–4: | 1–2 tablets once daily |

*Note:* 1 tablet of chloroquine or nivaquine contains 150 mg base.

*Quinine.* Children tolerate quinine very well, but ordinary salts are often too bitter and *quinine ethylcarbonate* (*euquinine*) is easier to administer.
Birth to 1 year, give one-tenth adult dose

$$\text{Subsequently give } \frac{\text{age}}{20} \times \text{adult dose}$$

(Example: at age of 5, dose is one-quarter of the adult dose. At 10, one-half of the adult dose.)

*Primaquine.* Doses for combined therapy, given with a schizonticide over 10 days:

Aged 4–8 years: 5.0–7.5 mg (base) once daily or in two divided doses.
Aged 8–15 years: 11.25–15 mg once daily or in two divided doses.

*Note.* Younger children are not usually given the drug.

### SEVERE AND COMPLICATED ATTACKS (*P. falciparum*)

Drug treatment is, of course, essential in dealing with complicated or pernicious malaria and no delay should be tolerated. At the same time, *it is imperative to see that the complication itself is treated at once.* In some instances, for example in cases of shock or hyperpyrexia, this may be necessary even before chemotherapy can be commenced.

For details of the treatment of complications, see below.

### PARENTERAL CHEMOTHERAPY

Parenteral injection of drugs is required.

The choice lies between intravenous or intramuscular quinine and a 4-amino-quinoline, for example chloroquine.

Intravenous injections are the most immediately effective.

There is some risk in intravenous administration of quinine and chloroquine in the shocked patient, since both drugs may lower the blood pressure. If shock occurs during treatment it is dealt with as below.

Because of the existence of chloroquine-resistant strains of *Plasmodium falciparum* in South-east Asia, South Asia, and South America and the suspicion that some strains in Africa, while not showing full resistance, may respond slowly to chloroquine, it is at present the custom to *use quinine in all serious cases, wherever they come from.*

### DOSAGE IN ADULTS

(a) *Quinine.* Not more than three doses should be given in 24 hours. *Oral administration of some other antimalarial should be commenced as soon as possible.*

   (i) *Intravenous injection of quinine.* Quinine (bihydrochloride) 500–650 mg depending on body weight.

   The first injection is normally given by syringe. The drug is dissolved in 10–15 ml sterile water or saline and taken up into a wide-bore syringe. *The injection is made slowly through a fine needle,* taking 10–15 minutes. The second injection should not be given until 8 hours after the first; this and subsequent doses may be added to a saline drip.

   (ii) *Intramuscular injection of quinine (hydrochloride).* The same dose is taken up into solution in 5–10 ml sterile water and injected with aseptic precautions deep into the gluteal muscles. The injection is painful and may occasionally lead to abscess formation, usually only if the bihydrochloride has been used. Again, the second dose can be given, if desirable, after 8 hours and not more than 3 doses should be given in 24 hours.

(b) *Chloroquine (4-amino-quinoline).* Intravenous and intramuscular dosage is 200–300 mg of the base. Not more than three doses should be given in 24 hours. Some authors advocate 200 mg (base) for the first dose, followed by 200 mg after 8 hours and then again after 8 hours if required. Technique of administration is as for quinine.

A common preparation is wide use is *Nivaquine soluble,* a solution of chloroquine sulphate made up in ampoules of 5 ml, containing 200 mg of the base. The contents of the ampoule are diluted to 15–20 ml with pyrogen-free water and administered intravenously as for quinine. Thereafter the drug may be given with a saline drip.

(c) *Mepacrine: intramuscular injection only.* Mepacrine should be used *only* when other drugs are not available and should be avoided in children. Musonate, 350 mg; hydrochloride, 300 mg.

The powder is dissolved in about 10 ml sterile water and the injection is made with aseptic precautions into the gluteal muscles. It may occasionally cause abscess.

The dose may be repeated 8-hourly, until oral administration is possible. *Mepacrine should never be given intravenously.*

CHILDREN

Parenteral therapy should be given to children with great care. Dosages of chloroquine and quinine are calculated in terms of body weight working back from the adult dose. Solutions should be dilute and are preferably given in divided doses over some hours. The dose of chloroquine should not exceed 5 mg per kg body weight. Intravenous injections should be avoided in very young children. In general for children, but not for adults, the intramuscular route is to be preferred.

*Complications of parenteral therapy.* Quinine and chloroquine are both hypotensive compounds and rapid administration or excessive dosage may produce shock. In patients already in or verging on shock, extreme caution is needed and the drugs are better given by intravenous drip or intramuscularly. Shock is treated simultaneously.

## TREATMENT OF COMPLICATIONS

*It is essential to treat the complications and the malaria concurrently.* Treatment of the one without treatment of the other will be ineffective.

### Acute haemolysis and anaemia
Transfusion of blood is necessary when the numbers of erythrocytes are so low as to affect seriously the oxygen-carrying powers of the blood, i.e. when the count has fallen to 2 million or fewer cells per $mm^3$ or the haemoglobin concentration is below 6 g per cent. Citrated blood can be safely given. The amount required must be judged from the red cell count and the patient's general condition. When transfusion is given solely for the purposes of

restoring the circulating erythrocyte numbers, 1 litre given over 24 hours is usually sufficient. Where lysis is proceeding vigorously it may be necessary to repeat the transfusion. The amount of blood given must be carefully measured and should be included in the input–output fluid balance chart.

Choosing the donor is a particularly important procedure in malaria, where the agglutinin pattern of the patient's blood is often temporarily disturbed. Blood which is apparently of the right group may prove to be incompatible and *it is therefore essential to cross-match the patient's cells and plasma with the plasma and cells of the donor before transfusion.*

Corticosteroids are recommended, as in the other lytic anaemias. Prednisolone phosphate, intramuscularly, may be given in doses of 40–60 mg daily over the period of the haemolysis or until the haemoglobin concentration is maintained at over 7 gm per 100 ml.

### Blackwater fever

Treat haemolysis as above.

Treat dehydration and shock as described below.

In the rare event of many parasites being present in the peripheral blood, a full course of schizonticide is needed. In the absence of resistance, chloroquine is indicated. If the parasites are chloroquine-resistant Proguanil or the combination of sulfadoxine and pyrimethamine may be tried. *Quinine should be avoided.*

Suppressive drug dosage should be continued in convalescence using proguanil or pyrimethamine. Where there is a clear history of previous attacks of falciparum malaria, a therapeutic course of suitable schizonticide may be given before suppression is re-established.

Vomiting or hiccup may be relieved by sucking ice, or by giving morphine. The latter may be used for the restless patient. Chlorpromazine, in doses of 50–100 mg given intramuscularly, is also useful in anxious and restless patients. Valium orally in doses of 10 mg twice daily is equally effective.

The patient should be given light foods if he will take them. Glucose should be added to all drinks and, if necessary, to infusions.

### Haemolysis and G-6-Pd deficiency

Treatment of haemolysis arising in G-6-Pd-deficient patients challenged with drugs or with the Fava bean (Favism) consists primarily in removing the activating agent and dealing with the haemolysis and its complications as described above. In deficient subjects challenged with 8-amino-quinolines, the haemolysis is usually self-limited.

### Shock

Patients in whom shock has appeared, including those with algid malaria, require immediate infusion of fluid to restore the blood volume. The first administration should be one litre of plasma or saline containing dextran, given rapidly, i.e. in about one-half to one hour. This should be followed by a more slowly administered litre of isotonic saline or isotonic glucose. If further fluid is required because of dehydration or salt deficiency, proceed as for replacement of fluid (see Cholera, p. 60).

Corticosteroids may be helpful, for example hydrocortisone sodium succinate, 100 mg, may be given intravenously or intramuscularly 8-hourly during the crisis. Thereafter the dose is reduced rapidly.

*Acute dehydration*

In patients in whom there has been severe loss of fluid from vomiting or from choleraic diarrhoea, replacement of water and salt is essential, even in the absence of vascular failure. Intravenous injection of isotonic saline or isotonic saline glucose solutions should be given as required (see p. 60). More than 3–5 litres of fluid is seldom needed in 24 hours.

In all cases a fluid input–output balance chart must be kept: infusions must be included in the total input of fluid for the 24 hours.

*Treatment of renal failure*

The renal failure in malaria and blackwater fever is an illustration of the renal anoxia syndrome, first described in blackwater fever, in which the operative cause is failure of the intrarenal blood flow with reduction or even cessation of glomerular filtration and the secretion of urine. When renal failure is established oliguria becomes anuria, a state in which very small volumes of urine are passed or none at all; the blood urea nitrogen rises rapidly, usually at a rate of up to 60 mg per 100 ml serum daily. There is a rise of plasma potassium, acidosis, and sometimes clinical evidence of pulmonary, cerebral, and peripheral oedema often exaggerated in the unfortunately common event of overhydration from excessive administration of parenteral fluid.

Rising blood urea and increasing signs of uraemia call for dialysis. In the tropics the facilities for haemodialysis are seldom available, but peritoneal dialysis is a good substitute provided the cost of the dialysis fluids can be met. Dialysis is usually needed daily for 10–14 days.

Many cases of renal failure in the tropics will have to be treated conservatively. An attempt is made to lower the rate of protein catabolism by providing the maximum number of calories of non-protein origin which can be carried by the limited fluid intake demanded, carbohydrate being used in preference to fat. The carbohydrate is given as lactose rather than glucose by nasopharyngeal tube, with intramuscular chlorpromazine to reduce the vomiting. If the patient is unable to accept the sugar in this way it must be given parenterally, with the accompanying risk of thrombosis following intravenous administration of hyper solutions.

The diet otherwise should contain up to 20 g protein and should be restricted in sodium chloride.

Anabolic steroids should not be used.

Estimated losses in sweat, diarrhoea, and vomiting should be replaced quantitatively but overhydration must be avoided at all costs.

Overhydration may be relieved by diarrhoea induced by oral administration of 50 ml of 70 per cent solution of sorbitol 2-hourly.

The heart should be monitored by regular ECG examinations if possible in order to watch for evidence of potassium intoxication, indicated by widening of the QRS complex and heightened T waves. When biochemical estimations can be made, the serum potassium should be kept below 7 mEq per litre. Temporary reduction in serum potassium by increasing the intracellular concentration can be achieved by giving soluble insulin (20 units) and glucose (50 g) simultaneously. More continuous control can be obtained by the use of ion-exchange resins which increase the loss of potassium in the faeces. Calcium-zeocarb resin is recommended for this purpose. Intravenous dosage of calcium gluconate 10–20 ml of 10 per cent solution may be given to protect the heart from the effects of current hyperkalaemia.

Recovery from renal failure is followed by a period of diuresis during which large amounts of low-concentration urine may be passed for a week or more. The extent of the diuresis depends partly on the existence or otherwise of previous overhydration. Where excessive amounts of urine are lost, electrolytes, particularly potassium, have to be replaced orally. Loss of potassium may be balanced by giving up to 10 g potassium chloride in the course of the day; this is safe so long as more than 1 litre of urine per day is secreted. In some cases excessive loss of potassium causes the clinical effects of hypokalaemia and potassium may have to be replaced by intravenous infusion of 500 ml of dextrose (5 per cent) saline containing 25 mEq potassium.

If infection is a hazard, as in peritoneal dialysis, penicillin is the antibiotic of choice. Tetracycline should be avoided because of its stimulating effect on protein catabolism.

*Treatment of other pernicious complications*

(i) *Cerebral malaria.* The neurological and psychological syndromes are treated on general lines. Prompt treatment of the underlying malaria will bring rapid relief in most cases, provided the condition is diagnosed early. Corticosteroids should be given in comatose patients. Dexamethasone is recommended.

Refractory headache following recovery from the acute attack may be very difficult to manage, but relief may sometimes be obtained by the use of nicotinic acid.

Mental sequelae require expert psychiatric treatment.

(ii) *Hyperpyrexia.* The basic factor here is the same as in heat hyperpyrexia, i.e. the inhibition of the sweating mechanism and consequent failure of heat loss.

Sweating must be re-established and this is best done by reducing the temperature by evaporation of water from the body surface. The patient should be covered with a wet sheet and fanned vigorously.

In the first instance the cooling should be stopped when the rectal temperature reaches about 39° C. From this point the temperature usually continues to fall and natural sweating may appear. The temperature may rise again and fever may persist until the malaria infection is controlled, but return of hyperpyrexia is rare. If high fever reappears it must be treated as above.

(iii) *Bilious remittent fever*. Treatment is that of liver insufficiency. Early treatment of the malaria is the only real hope of success.

In the severe case transfusion or infusion of plasma or saline may be necessary, depending on the degree of anaemia, the presence or absence of shock, or the loss of fluid and salt.

(iv) *Malarial dysentery*. The ordinary general treatment of acute dysentery is required, including parenteral replacement of water and salt.

(v) *Choleraic diarrhoea*. Replacement of fluid is essential. If shock has supervened one half litre of plasma given fast is indicated, followed by saline as required (see Shock, p. 60). In cases suffering from dehydration or salt deficiency without shock, one half litre of saline should be given rapidly followed by further infusion as required. The concentration of urinary chlorides should be watched during treatment.

### TREATMENT SUBSEQUENT TO RECOVERY FROM THE ACUTE ATTACK

*Prophylaxis and suppression*

Non-immune patients living in endemic areas must continue prophylactic or suppressive therapy after treatment of an acute attack.

This is unnecessary in non-malarious areas except for special purposes, for example the suppression of vivax malaria. Efficient treatment of falciparum malaria leads to radical cure.

There is usually no need to remove the patient from the endemic area, except after severe, complicated, or frequently repeated attacks.

*Anaemia*

Recovery of the erythrocyte content of the blood is usually rapid after treatment of malaria.

Patients in whom severe anaemia persists into convalescence may benefit by blood transfusion. A litre of citrated blood given slowly is usually adequate.

Iron salts in the ferrous state should be given orally in anaemic cases, in a dose of 600–1000 mg ferrous sulphate daily in divided doses three times during the day. If the patient finds this salt causes gastro-intestinal disturbances, the gluconate may be substituted.

## THE TREATMENT OF MALARIA IN SEMI-IMMUNES

In such individuals all forms of malaria are usually mild and respond readily to treatment.

Single doses of proguanil, 300–500 mg; pyrimethamine, 50 mg; chloroquine or some other 4-amino-quinoline, 600 mg (base); or quinine bihydrochloride 1.3 g for 2 successive days will usually be effective. Children receive doses in proportion to body weight.

More serious cases need treatment similar to that of non-immunes.

Parasite resistance to drugs must be taken into consideration in deciding which compound to give.

## PROPHYLAXIS AND SUPPRESSION

For suppression in infants and very young children see p. 267.

Drug control of malaria in individuals exposed to infection could be achieved in two ways:

(a) by *prophylaxis,* which implies the prevention of infection after the bite of an infective mosquito and,

(b) by *suppression,* which means the suppression of the erythrocyte infection to subclinical levels.

In the subject who has not been exposed to infection previously, the ideal is prophylaxis. Since no known drug is capable of destroying the sporozoite, true prophylaxis is not at present possible in any form of malaria. Proguanil and pyrimethamine, however, have been shown to destroy the PE forms of *Plasmodium falciparum* and, if given over the pre-patent period, may thus prevent the initiation of the E cycle in the erythrocyte. This action is regarded by some as a form of prophylaxis which has been named *causal prophylaxis.* Since the end effect is the same as that of the suppression plus radical cure, which is achieved in this infection by any active schizonticide, the use of this term is not universally acceptable. Causal prophylaxis cannot at present be achieved in vivax, malariae, or ovale infections but the 8-amino-quinolines which kill the EE forms of these parasites will also destroy the PE form of falciparum malaria, thus acting as a 'causal' prophylactic for this infection only. Unfortunately high dosage is required for this effect.

Suppression of all forms of malaria may be achieved by the use of paludrine, chloroquine and, somewhat less efficiently, quinine. In using a particular drug due consideration must be given to the likelihood of parasite drug resistance. Mepacrine is now very seldom used.

In falciparum malaria the proper use of proguanil, pyrimethamine, or chloroquine in suppressive doses leads to radical cure. This is not so in other forms of malaria, which tend to relapse after the cessation of suppressive therapy.

Individuals under exposure and known to be already infected with falciparum malaria must be given a full therapeutic course of chloroquine (or an alternative if there is chloroquine resistance) before prophylaxis or suppression is attempted.

In frequently reinfected individuals in whom some immunity has developed, suppression is usually the only reasonable and easily attainable objective. Prophylaxis under such conditions is to be obtained by entomological and other control measures rather than by chemotherapeutic methods.

Prophylactic or suppressive therapy with all drugs except mepacrine should be commenced immediately before entry into an endemic area and continued for some time after leaving. Mepacrine must be given in the proper daily dosage (100 mg) for at least 14 days before entry, since it takes this time to establish an active concentration of the drug in the blood.

*In order to obtain the full effect of any drug, regular dosage during exposure is essential. Dosage must be continued for 28 days after leaving the endemic area.*

The drugs should be taken with ample fluid; there is no contra-indication for alcoholic drinks. Drugs are best taken during or shortly before the evening meal.

### CHOICE OF DRUG

For most areas, chloroquine (or some other 4-amino-quinoline), proguanil or pyrimethamine, or quinine should all be successful if taken regularly in adequate doses. Proguanil-resistant strains of parasites exist in some regions. They will be equally resistant to pyrimethamine, but will be susceptible to the other schizonticides. Chloroquine-resistant parasites are usually also insusceptible to mepacrine but not to quinine. They may appear in areas in which proguanil and pyrimethamine resistance has already developed. In areas where resistance does not exist, proguanil and pyrimethamine have the advantage of inhibiting the development of the sexual cycle in the mosquito, thus reducing the infectivity of local vectors.

Attempts are being made to synthesise suppository drugs which will act for long periods after a single dose and so help to break the cycle of man–mosquito–man in the community. One such drug, cycloguanil or camolar, has already been found to protect against certain strains of *P. falciparum* and *P. vivax* for many months.

Unfortunately, this compound is a derivative of dehydrotriazine, the active metabolite of proguanil, and is consequently inactive against proguanil- and pyrimethamine-resistant parasites.

Despite a common belief to the contrary, in the doses recommended the drugs have no efect on sexual potency or pregnancy.

DOSAGE

**Non-immune** (*visitors and foreign residents in endemic areas*)
  (i) *Proguanil*
    Adult: One tablet of 100 mg daily.
    Child: Birth to 1 year: 25–50 mg daily; 2–5 years: 50–100 mg daily.
    Begin at the time of entering endemic area. Continue for 28 days after leaving area.
  *Side-effects.* None.

  (ii) *Pyrimethamine*
    Adult: One (25 mg) or two (50 mg) tablets once weekly.
    Child: Birth to 3 years: $\frac{1}{2}$ tablet (12.5 mg) once weekly.
        Thereafter to 12 years, 25 mg, then 25–50 mg weekly.
    Begin at the time of entering endemic area. Continue for 28 days after leaving area.
  *Side-effects.* None.

  (iii) *Chloroquine (or other 4-amino-quinolines)*
    Adult: 2 tablets (300 mg base) given once weekly.
    Child: Age 0–1 year, $\frac{1}{4}$–$\frac{1}{3}$ tablet; 1–3 years, $\frac{1}{2}$–$\frac{2}{3}$ tablet; 4–6 years, $\frac{2}{3}$–1 tablet; 6–10 years, 1 tablet; over 10 years, adult dose.
  *Side-effects.* There may be some gastro-intestinal discomfort, occasionally vomiting, but this seldom appears after the first few doses. After long continued use slight skin changes have been reported. The vast majority of patients suffer no side-effects.
  *Parasite resistance.* In view of the increasing evidence of parasite resistance to chloroquine, it has been proposed by some authorities that, in order to limit the spread of resistance and to preserve the drug for therapeutic purposes, it would be better in future not to use it on a wide scale alone or in combination with other drugs as a suppressive. If this suggestion were to be adopted, proguanil, pyrimethamine or quinine or, in some areas, sulfadoxine plus pyrimethamine are the alternatives.

  (iv) *Quinine*
    Adult: 1 tablet of 260 or 325 mg daily.
    Child: In proportion.
  *Note.* Quinine is efficient but is used for suppression *only* where other drugs are not available.
  *Side-effects.* Dizziness; tinnitus with some degree of accompanying deafness; nausea, sometimes vomiting, skin sensitivity rashes.

  (v) *Mepacrine* (now seldom used)
    Adult: One tablet of 100 mg daily.
    Child: Mepacrine is not advised for children.
    *If it is to be used, begin 14 days before entering endemic area.* Continue for 28 days after leaving area.

*Side-effects.* There may be some slight gastro-intestinal discomfort after the first few doses. This drug will stain the skin yellow and is excreted in the hair. The colour is sometimes mistaken for jaundice, but can be differentiated from the latter by the absence of coloration of the conjuctivae.

Late effects are rare but include the development of browny-blue pigmentation of the finger nails and thickening and blue coloration of the skin and mucous membranes. Skin eruptions similar to those due to *lichen planus* may also occur.

The psychotic effects of mepacrine have not been observed on suppressive dosage.

## Semi-immunes
   (i) *Proguanil:* 300–500 mg once weekly.
  (ii) *Chloroquine:* 300 mg (base) once weekly.
 (iii) *Quinine:* 650 mg once weekly.

These dosage regimes will secure a high level of suppression. They are economically feasible in large groups, such as labour personnel, in which it is desirable not to interfere too much with existing immunity.

### OTHER TECHNIQUES OF SUPPRESSION

*Chloroquine and primaquine*
This combination was used by Americans in Vietnam as a suppressive regime against *P. vivax* and chloroquine sensitive *P. falciparum* infections.

Dosage, once weekly: Chloroquine    300 mg (base)
                         Primaquine     45 mg (base)

*Chloroquine and pyrimethamine*
This combination (given once) has been used in malaria eradication campaigns for presumptive treatment and also for suppression (at 3-weekly intervals).

Dosage: Chloroquine     600 mg (base)
              Pyrimethamine   50 mg (base)

*Pyrimethamine and primaquine*
Because of its schizonticidal, gametocytocidal, and sporontocidal potentials, this combination has been tried at 2-weekly intervals in eradication campaigns.

Dosage: Pyrimethamine   50 mg (base)
              Primaquine     40 mg (base)

*Sulfadoxine and pyrimethamine*
This combination (Sulfadoxine 1·0 g plus pyrimethamine 50 mg) is given once every 2 weeks. The one drug potentiates the effect of the other, once they both act in the early stages of nucleic acid synthesis.

It is very successful in suppression of *P. falciparum* infections (including chloroquine-resistant strains) and *P. vivax* infections.

Resistance has been defined as the ability of a parasite to survive and/or multiply in a concentration of a drug equal to or higher than that attained by normally recommended dosage and within the limits of the tolerance of the subject.

Resistance develops more easily against the schizonticides proguanil and pyrimethamine, which block the folic acid:folinic acid cycle of the parasite than the 4-amino-quinolines and mepacrine, which block both the nucleic acid and the glycolytic cycles. Resistance to quinine is so far minimal.

Drug resistance is found most commonly in areas of unstable malaria, or where the drug has been or is being misused; it has developed in areas in which the antimalarial drug has been added to table salt for control purposes. It also occurs in areas in which there is no evidence of misuse (or even the use) of the relevant drug. It can be produced experimentally in rodent and simian malaria by repeated drug challenge.

### Resistance to proguanil and pyrimethamine

Parasite resistance to these drugs in *P. falciparum* and *P. vivax* infections was first detected in South-east Asia. Resistance in all parasite species is now widespread in Malaysia, Indonesia, East, Central, and West Africa, and South America. Parasites resistant to proguanil are usually resistant to pyrimethamine (which is derived from a metabolite of proguanil) and *vice versa*. There is cross-resistance to the related compound cycloguanil embonate but not to quinine, chloroquine or mepacrine.

### Resistance of P. falciparum to the 4-amino-quinolines

Resistance to chloroquine of *P. falciparum*, but *not* of other species of parasite, was first noted in Brazil and Venezuela and shortly afterwards in Thailand. It is now common in most South-east Asian countries, as far East as Papua New Guinea, and in northern and central South America. So far, it has not been demonstrated in Africa. However, RI resistant parasites have been detected in two individuals (in the U.S.A. and Scandinavia respectively), after recent visits to Kenya and Tanzania.

Grades of resistance to therapeutic drug dosage are classified as follows (based on grading of resistance of strains of *P. falciparum* to chloroquine):

*Sensitivity*  (S) Clearance of asexual (E) parasites within 7 days of beginning of treatment. No recrudescences.

*Resistance*

   (RI)  Clearance of asexual (E) parasites as in sensitivity, followed by recrudescence within 28 days.

   (RII)  Marked reduction in numbers of asexual (E) parasites, without clearance, followed by recrudescence.

   (RIII)  No reduction of asexual parasitaemia.

It should be noted that resistance is graded in terms of the effect of the drug on the parasites in the peripheral blood, not on the effect on clinical signs. In the non-immune these aspects run in parallel. In the semi-immune clinical relief may be produced without great reduction in parasitaemia.

### Resistance to primaquine
*P. vivax* is not at present known to be resistant to the 8-amino-quinolines, but there are strains in the Solomon Islands and in Sumatra in which double the dose is needed (30 mg daily) for radical cure.

## TREATMENT AND SUPPRESSION OF DRUG-RESISTANT PARASITES

### Treatment of chloroquine-resistant *P. falciparum*

*Quinine*
So far practically all strains have been found sensitive to quinine but, in some, the dosage of quinine has had to be high and continued for longer than normal. Grade RI resistance to quinine has been reported in some South-east Asian strains.

Quinine may be given alone, although a long course has unpleasant side-effects for the average patient.

Dosage recommended: 1.3 g in two divided doses (0.65 g) daily for 14 days. Where resistance is pronounced, the daily dose may be increased to three doses but this may be beyond the endurance level of the patient. Parasitic and clinical response is usually rapid.

Quinine therapy is now usually limited to 3 days at 650 mg 12-hourly. On the fourth day sulfadoxine 1500 mg plus pyrimethamine 75 mg is given as a single dose. A single dose of the new drug mefloquine 1.5 g has been successfully substituted for the sulphonamide and pyrimethamine.

Where parenteral therapy is needed in a case of chloroquine resistant malaria, quinine 650 mg is given intravenously twice on the first day, the second dose 12 hours after the first. Oral quinine is continued as above for the next 2 days. On the fourth day sulfadoxine and pyrimethamine are given, as above.

### Combination of sulphonamides or sulphones with pyrimethamine
For the treatment of chloroquine-resistant *P. falciparum,* or where RI resis-

tance to quinine is suspected, the following is recommended orally: sulfadox-ine 1.5 g or 15 mg per kg body weight plus pyrimethamine 50–75 mg. The pyrimethamine may be repeated on the following day. This combination, given once only, is effective in most cases both in non-immunes and semi-immunes. The clinical response is slow, but may be speeded up by anti-inflam-matory drugs. Sulfalene (2 g) may be substituted for the sulfadoxine; dapsone 200 mg may be used instead of the sulphonamides.

In the event of recrudescence dosage may be repeated.

### Tetracycline
Tetracycline hydrochloride 500 mg four times daily for 5 days will provide radical cure of falciparum malaria. The infection is slow to respond, however, and a more rapidly acting schizonticide such as quinine, which is also an anti-inflammation drug, should be given at the beginning of the course.

### Suppression of chloroquine-resistant *P. falciparum*
Various compounded tablets are now recommended for successful suppression of chloroquine-resistant *P. falciparum*. Maloprim (12.5 mg pyrimethamine plus 100 mg DDS), one tablet weekly: Fansidar (25 mg pyrimethamine plus 500 mg sulfadoxine), one tablet weekly.

Proguanil and pyrimethamine in the usual doses will suppress the infec-tions so long as they are not resistant to these drugs. The chloroquine-resistant strains are usually resistant to mepacrine but are sensitive to quinine.

In some areas parasites are resistant to all forms of major synthetic drugs. These will usually respond to quinine.

Diaphenylsulphone (dapsone, DDS) has been used experimentally to supplement proguanil suppression in areas where there is seasonal increase in transmission of parasites with proguanil:pyrimethamine resistance, as in the highlands of Vietnam.

A combination of cycloguanil embonate and sulphadiamine (DADDS), called CI564, used as a depot, has been given successfully where chloroquine resistance exists.

### Treatment and suppression of other drug-resistant infections
Proguanil- and pyrimethamine-resistant parasites (*P. falciparum, P. vivax, P. malariae,* and probably *P. ovale*) respond to the 4-amino-quinolines, mepa-crine, or quinine.

Proguanil–pyrimethamine-resistant strains of *P. falciparum* in some areas respond to the combination of sulfadoxine and pyrimethamine, or to the CI 564 (Cycloguanil embonate and DADDS). Proguanil-resistant strains do not respond to the latter.

### New drugs
The search for better drugs continues. Over 200,000 compounds have been tested in the last decade.

Interest has centred recently on derivatives of 4-quinolinemethanol. The compound, 142490 WR (a trifluoromethyl 4-methanol derivative) now called 'Mefloquine' has been found very efficient in clearing chloroquine-resistant *P. falciparum* infections and is also a good suppressive against normal and resistant strains. As noted above, it also acts as an adjuvant to quinine in place of sulfadoxine and pyrimethamine in the treatment of chloroquine-resistant strains of *P. falciparum*. Dosage: 1000–1500 mg, once.

# 17

## MISCELLANEOUS DISORDERS

### AINHUM

Ainhum is a fissured constriction, of unknown aetiology, which affects usually the fifth or fourth toes, and less commonly other digits of the feet or occasionally of the hands. The progress of the lesion is very slow and ultimately it causes sequestration of the distal part of the affected digit.

Ainhum occurs widely throughout the tropics and subtropics in the dark-skinned races. It is predominantly a disease of Negroes but also occurs in India and in Polynesia; it does not occur in the white-skinned races. It may develop in Negroes who have been resident in temperate climates for many years. Adult males are far more commonly affected than are adolescents or females. It is not found in those habitually shod and is unusual in children.

The cause is unknown, but the tendency to ready keloid formation in Negroes may be a contributory factor; the fissuring with hyperkeratosis may sometimes be due to yaws.

Ainhum starts as a fissure, usually on the plantar and outer surface of the fifth toe. There is marked hyperkeratinization around the lesion which, in due course, extends round the affected digit. A constricting fibrous band finally encircles the digit at the level of an interphalangeal joint. The tendons are involved and movement becomes impossible. The distal part of the digit becomes bulbous, misshapen, and everted; though painless it causes mechanical inconvenience and is prone to be injured. In time, often after many years, the distal part spontaneously sequestrates without bleeding. One toe only is usually involved. The condition may be bilateral; several toes and, very occasionally, a finger may be affected.

There is no specific treatment. Amputation of the digit is the only satisfactory way of ending the inconvenience.

### THE CHIGOE FLEA

*Tunga penetrans,* the chigoe or jigger, is a flea, both sexes of which feed on warm-blooded animals. The pregnant female buries her head, thorax, and abdomen in the skin where she stays until she oviposits. Commonly she infests the feet, causing discomfort and lameness and often, as a result of her presence, secondary sepsis.

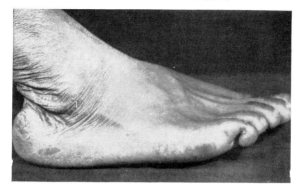

FIG. 39. Ainhum of the fifth digit of the foot of an African.

Originating in South America, the chigoe has now established itself in many parts of the tropics. It occurs extensively over tropical Africa; but although it must repeatedly have been introduced into India and the Far East it has not spread there.

The adults of both sexes of *T. penetrans* live in dust or sand in the floors of huts and houses. They take blood meals from any warm-blooded animal. After fertilization the female bores, head first, into the soft epidermis of man and other animals, especially the pig, until her head lies in the dermis and the posterior end of her abdomen is just beneath the skin surface. For over a week her abdomen steadily hypertrophies until it is about the size of a small pea; this is largely a physiological development but, in part, it is due to distension with blood and the developing ovaries and eggs. The eggs are then extruded through the posterior abdominal aperture to the exterior; 150–200 escape at intervals over 7–10 days; the flea after this shrinks and dies *in situ*. A larva emerges from each egg 3 or 4 days after deposition; this lives in dust, undergoes two moults, and pupates; an imago then emerges. The developmental cycle occupies about 17 days.

The sites most frequently attacked are the spaces between the toes, under and around the toe nails, and the soles of the feet, especially the instep; occasionally other parts of the body are infested. In children, especially native children, there may be dozens of chigoes in the feet, the thighs, the perineum and external genitalia. In adults, especially Europeans, the numbers usually are fewer, commonly only in the feet.

The first symptom is itching; later there is inflammation and swelling; later still ulceration, sometimes followed by gross sepsis.

The pregnant female should be eased out with a sterile needle and the wound cleaned and dressed. If this is done early, and the flea is not ruptured in the process, the lesion soon heals. Secondary sepsis is the main source of trouble; the aim is to avoid this. The bare skin should not be allowed to come into contact with the floor. Shoes should always be worn. Cleanliness in the home is of obvious importance. Insecticidal treatment of the floor may help.

## GRANULOMA VENEREUM

Granuloma venereum, or ulcerative granuloma is a veneral disease due to infection with the organism *Donovania granulomatis* (also called *Calymmato-bacterium granulomatis*), a short, bacillus-like organism, found in large numbers within endothelial and large mononuclear cells in the lesions of skin and mucous membranes. It is characterized by chronic, progressively extending, superficial, granulomatous ulceration of the genito-inguino-crural regions.

It is widely distributed in India, South-east Asia, Papua New Guinea, Northern Australia, the Pacific Islands, Brazil, Guyana, and the Caribbean Islands. It occurs also in West and East Africa, the southern United States and southern China. A few cases have occurred in Europe. It does not occur in temperate and cold regions.

The disease is transmitted venereally. It is much more common among the coloured races than the white and is said to be more common in women than men. The greatest incidence of the disease is in the period of greatest sexual activity.

Sections of the spreading edge of the skin lesion show an infiltration of the superficial portions of the corium and of the papillae by lymphocytes. The lesions are superficial and affect only skin and mucous membranes. Local lymph glands are not involved unless there is secondary infection. The dermis is highly vascularized. Large mononuclear and endothelial cells packed with *Donovania* (formerly called 'Donovan bodies') are present in the granulomatous areas. In older portions of the lesion there is fibrosis, with the production of scars which break down easily.

The initial lesion consists of a papule or vesicle and in the great majority of cases is found somewhere on the external genitalia, usually the penis or labia minora, within about a week of sexual contact. The lesion remains superficial and spreads centrifugally, and by autoinfection, to opposing surfaces. It exhibits a predilection for moist warm surfaces, particularly the glans penis and scrotum in the male, the labia, fourchette and vagina in the female, and the inguinal folds, the perineal and perianal regions. In some cases the skin of the face and the mucous membrane of the mouth may be affected.

The disease extends so slowly that years may elapse before a large area of skin is involved, but in mucous membranes the spread is more rapid.

Three clinical types of lesions have been described: (1) a nodular dry type characterized by a painless, granulomatous area raised above the surrounding skin and studded with nodular or sometimes papillomatous, dry granulations; this is the commonest type; (2) an *ulcus molle* type, in which the ulcer is large and spreading with a depressed base, thin edges, and a glazed, moist, pale-red surface almost devoid of granulations; there is an offensive discharge and the condition is painful; (3) a sclerotic type characterized by much hard fibrous tissue. Islands of active disease become surrounded by the rapid formation of fibrous tissue and consequently breaking down of the scar is frequent.

Owing to cicatrization, pseudoelephantiasis of the female genitalia, stenosis of the vagina and of the urethral and anal orifices, and recto-vaginal fistulae may occur. Lesions limited in distribution to the vulva or to the cervix are readily mistaken for malignancies. The lymphatic glands are not primarily or conspicuously involved and the general health is, as a rule, unaffected unless there are anatomical complications or severe secondary infection.

Diagnosis depends upon the great chronicity of the superficial granulomatous condition occurring in the genito-inguino-crural region and upon the absence of enlarged lymphatic glands. *Donovania* can be found in mononuclear cells on biopsy of the lesions or on examination of the exudate from them.

The lesions should be cleaned. Chloramphenicol (2 g orally, daily for 1 week, then 1 g daily for 2 weeks, with the usual watch on the white blood cell count), tetracycline (in similar dosage), and streptomycin (4 g intramuscularly, daily in divided doses of 1 g each for 7–10 days) are effective in checking the local spread of the lesions and promoting healing.

Owing to the chronicity of the condition, and the tendency of the lesions to break down after apparent healing, treatment may have to be repeated. In these cases, after cleansing of the ulcers by suitable dressings, physical applications such as diathermy or X-rays may aid resolution. Where fistulae, strictures, and other deformities have developed, surgical interference may be necessary after the primary infection has been dealt with.

## KURU

Kuru is a fatal disease due to degeneration in the central nervous system, particularly the cerebellum and its connections.

It is confined to the Fore people in the Eastern Highlands of New Guinea; to a limited extent it may be encountered in a few tribes who have intermarried with these some generations ago. It has certain features similar to 'scrapie' in sheep.

Kuru was first recognized as an entity in 1951, though there was a history of its occurrence for some 50 years. From 1 to 5 per cent of the susceptible clan population may be affected. It is found only above 4 years of age, and chiefly in adults; in youth both sexes may be affected, but in later life females predominate.

During the last decade the incidence has declined, and there have been changes in age and sex distribution. There are now few cases in children under 12 years of age, and a third of those affected have been adult males. Recent surveys show the case incidence to have been episodic; after several cases have developed and died in an area it remains free from further cases.

Chimpanzees inoculated intracerebrally with Kuru brain tissue have developed a condition indistinguishable from Kuru 3–4 years later This, together with the picture of cerebellar derangement and terminal spill-over into other central nervous systems, and the epidemiological evidence, suggests that Kuru may be due to a slow virus infection in a susceptible population.

It is believed that the virus may have been transmitted as a result of the cannibalistic rite of eating the brains of enemies, which was confined to the women and children of the tribe and is now becoming old-fashioned.

But for a variable degree of shrinkage of the cerebellum there is no macroscopic change to be seen on autopsy. Histological studies reveal widespread neuronal vacuolar degeneration, but no inflammatory cellular response, predominantly in the cerebellum and its connecting tracts, the basal nuclei, extra-pyramidal tracts, and the frontal cortex.

### CLINICAL PICTURE

This is characteristic and constant. Initially there is an ataxic gait; this progresses over 3–6 months to a stumbling, weaving walk and fine and coarse tremors. Choreiform and exaggerated athetotic movements develop when the patient stands upright, but he relaxes at rest and during sleep. Later, walking becomes impossible; gross dysphagia and dysarthria develop; and, finally, aphagia and aphonia. Extreme depression, punctuated by episodes of euphoria and melancholy, characterize the progress of the disease; and there may be terminal dementia. Death occurs in decubitus with incontinence, in 6–18 months after onset, commonly as a result of bronchopneumonia and other secondary infections and starvation.

The outstanding physical sign is muscle incoordination, with disorder of the finger–nose and heel–knee tests, rhombergism, and an irregular nystagmus. There are no sensory, or fundal, changes; the cranial nerves are not involved, apart from malfunctions of speech and swallowing and a terminal convergent squint. Reflexes and muscle tone remain normal until hypotonia or spasticity terminally appear.

The disease is fatal. There is no specific treatment.

## LYMPHOBLASTIC LYMPHOMA ('BURKITT TUMOUR')

This malignant, undifferentiated, lymphoblastic lymphoma has a distinctive anatomical location and is virtually confined to children. It has been known for many years in moist warm areas of tropical Africa but occurs also in Papua New Guinea and in South America. It is reported occasionally in the eastern U.S.A., Western Australia, India, Vietnam and South Africa.

In the areas concerned, it is the commonest malignant condition in children between 2 and 14 years of age, irrespective of sex or race, and in tropical Africa is more prevalent than the total of other forms of malignant disease. It is most frequent in the age group 5–9 years. Its incidence and distribution suggest that it may be virus caused and possibly vector-borne.

The tumours, of reticulo-endothelial lymphomatous type, involve structures otherwise rarely the seat of malignancy in children, such as the ovaries and the testes, the thyroid and salivary glands, the extradural space in the spine and more especially the orbit, excluding the eye, and the jaws. There is often multiple distribution in these sites; but the associated lymph glands are rarely involved even terminally. It looks as though dissemination takes place through the circulation. Tumour deposits are found at any one time not only in widely separated sites, but as multiple lesions within a single organ before they coalesce into a tumour mass. The progress of the condition is rapid. The tumours consist of a poorly differentiated, lymphocyte (lymphoblastic) lymphoma with a variable admixture of non-malignant histocytes.

One side of a jaw, either upper or lower, characteristically is first involved. A soft swelling forms on either side of an alveolus and rapidly develops with displacement and then shedding of the teeth; the tumour does not ulcerate through the skin or mucosa. Often two or more quadrants of the jaws are concurrently involved, usually the maxilla and mandible on the same side; only exceptionally are the cervical lymph glands involved. Multifocal jaw tumours in a child or the combination of a jaw tumour with tumours in the thyroid, kidneys, or ovaries, are virtually diagnostic of the condition. Alternatively, a tumour invading the orbit and displacing the eye, and probably originating in the upper part of the maxilla, may be the first sign; the eye itself is not involved until a late stage. In other cases tumours may develop in the abdomen, commonly either in one or both loins indicating renal involvement, or as enlargements of the liver or in the epigastrium, or as bilateral ovarian tumours; these last are characteristic and diagnostic. Extradural space invasion in the spinal canal may lead to paraplegia and is the most common cause of the latter in children in parts of Africa. Increasing enlargements of the thyroid or salivary glands herald tumour formation in these; unilateral testicular tumours are not unusual; the breast or subcutaneous tissues are occasionally the initial site. Spontaneous remission, even temporary, does not occur. The rate of growth of the tumours is very rapid. Diagnosis is confirmed by biopsy.

Radical surgical removal should not be attempted in view of the dissemination of the lesions. 'Bulk reduction surgery' may be permissible as the response to chemotherapy appears to be related to the size of the tumours. Success has attended vigorous chemotherapy in some cases, but it is not constant.

The nitrogen mustard drugs give the best results: nitrogen mustard (mustine hydrochloride, mustagen) is a severely toxic drug. It is given in a dose of 0.1–0.3 mg per kg, for 5 days; it is best given intra-arterially. Leakage into tissues causes necrosis. Administration by aortic catheterization, with the intention of infusing the entire body, has led to recession of original tumour but occasional redistribution of tumour masses. Cyclophosphamide (endoxan) can be given orally or intravenously. Given by the latter route the dose is 20–40 mg per kg body weight as a single injection, repeated in 14 days if local tumour regression is incomplete. A follow-up of oral dosage (5 mg per kg body weight) is sometimes used. The dose may be repeated when the bone marrow has recovered from the usual depressant effects of the drug.

Methotrexate, in doses of 5 mg orally for 7 days, is successful but slower in action. Toxic effects may be severe, especially in patients with low folic acid levels. The drug is usually regarded as a second line drug in cases resistant to the mustard compounds.

Other compounds have been tried, including Chlorambucil (leukeran) and Cytosine arabinoside with some success. Recurrences occur in the original tumour site. Pyrimethamine, as a folic acid antagonist, produces limited, local tumour response and subsequent poor survival rate.

After treatment with these compounds there have been good recoveries with apparent disappearance of the lesions and survival for some years. The results, however, are unpredictable. In isolated cases tumours may regress spontaneously, suggesting the development of an immunological factor. Host defence mechanisms are involved, but these may be depressed temporarily by the cytotoxic drugs, especially when used over long periods. This may explain the better results obtained in Africa than in more sophisticated areas in Europe and North America.

## MELIOIDOSIS

Melioidosis is due to infection with *Pseudomonas pseudomallei* a bacterial organism of the glanders group, which normally infects rodents. The disease in man is rare, and usually takes the form of a pyaemia, with multiple caseous nodules and abscesses in various organs and tissues. The mortality is extremely high, and the diagnosis is often made at post mortem.

Most cases of melioidosis have been recorded in South-east Asia; others have been reported in Burma, the U.S.A., Africa, Europe, and Australia.

*Ps. pseudomallei* is a Gram-negative aerobe which closely resembles *Pf. mallei,* the organism causing glanders.

The method by which man acquires the infection has not been established, but it is generally thought that ingestion of foodstuffs contaminated by the urine and faeces of infected rats is the usual route. Infection may also result from inhalation of infected material. There is no evidence that the disease spreads from man to man, and all human cases are apparently the result of sporadic infection from the natural animal reservoirs. In infected rats the disease is a subacute or chronic one; the rats continue to discharge the organisms over a considerable time in their faeces and urine.

Lesions much resembling those of glanders occur in almost any of the tissues in the body. They consist of caseous nodules which form around embolically conveyed foci of *Ps. pseudomallei*. As the nodules enlarge, their centres become necrotic. Extensive multiple caseous abscess formations are found in the lungs, liver, and spleen at post mortem; similar abscesses may occur anywhere in the body. *Ps. pseudomallei* can readily be recovered in pure culture from all the lesions. Lymph gland involvement is not usual.

In view of the varied location, number, and size of the abscesses characteristic of melioidosis the detailed clinical picture is extremely variable. Broadly, the disease can be divided into two clinical types; the septicaemic, which is rapidly fatal; and the pyaemic which progresses more slowly, and from which a small percentage of patients may recover if their lesions are restricted in number and superficial in location.

The septicaemic type of the disease resembles any other severe septicaemia. There is delirium and severe toxaemia, continued fever, and signs of pulmonary involvement. The liver and the spleen enlarge. There is usually a dysenteric diarrhoea. Patients with fulminating infections may die within a few days; those with a less severe septicaemia may survive for periods up to 3 weeks.

The pyaemic type of the disease is more common than the septicaemic. Necrotic lesions and abscesses appear one after another in a number of internal organs. The lungs are affected early in the condition; the liver is nearly always involved; the genito-urinary tract is commonly the seat of lesions. The central nervous system, in common with every other structure of the body, may contain abscesses. Pyaemic melioidosis may simulate many grave infective diseases. It usually ends fatally within 2 months, but at times may continue over several months or even for a year or more. In rare cases of pyaemic melioidosis the lesions occur superficially in the skin, the subcutaneous tissues, and the immediately underlying muscles, bones, and joints. These cases may ultimately recover spontaneously if assisted by suitable local treatment.

Isolation and identification of the causative organism from the tissues or from pus, blood, urine, cerebrospinal fluid, or sputum establishes the diagnosis.

The isolated organism should be tested for sensitivity to a wide range of antibiotics and sulphonamides. Chloramphenicol and the tetracyclines have proved valuable in certain cases when given over long periods orally or parenterally. A close watch must be kept on the white cell count, which falls sharply, especially when chloramphenicol is used. Other antibiotics have also been of use in some cases. The sulphonamides, particularly sulphadiazine, are successful on occasions in large doses. Aspiration and drainage of superficial abscesses should be carried out when possible; antibiotics can be introduced into the cavities when drained.

## TROPICAL MYOSITIS

Localized inflammation and abscess formation in the muscles of the limbs and trunk is found in many parts of the tropics, particularly in Africa, areas of South America, and Japan. It has not been decided whether there is any one common causative agent.

The pus from the abscess is bacteriologically sterile in about 10 per cent of cases; in most it contains *Staphylococcus aureus* or streptococci. Some cases may result from secondary infection of filarial abscesses or the lesions of tropical phlebitis or sickle cell anaemia. Secondary infection of extravasated blood following haemorrhage from injury or scurvy is sometimes thought to be responsible.

The syndrome occurs mainly in the indigenous population or those of mixed blood and only very rarely in Europeans.

It may appear at any age but is most common in the second or third decade. Men, especially agricultural workers, are more often affected than women.

The commonest site of the lesions is in the lower limb (thighs, calves, and buttocks). The arms, chest wall, and abdominal wall may be affected in that order. There is usually only one abscess. Sometimes, especially in staphylococcal infections, there may be several.

The lesion usually develops for a week or more before the symptoms become severe enough for the patient to seek advice. There may be a history of local trauma or an episode of local lymphangitis. In some cases the history is much longer, the lesion developing slowly over some weeks.

The patient complains of severe local pain which immobilizes the part affected. He is often apprehensive and resents examination.

The general condition is usually good but he may be suffering from some fever and general constitutional symptoms. When pus is forming quickly the temperature may become high and swinging, and there may be a high leucocyte count or general toxaemia.

In the area affected there is a hard diffuse circumscribed swelling, usually extremely tender, sometimes hot, tense, and sometimes fluctuant. There may be some more generalized local pitting oedema.

In the majority of cases the lesion resolves without pointing or requiring surgical treatment. In some untreated cases pus may be discharged and indolent sinuses left after healing. Death may occur in rare instances from the toxaemic effects of infection.

The causative factors concerned being largely unknown, the immediate diagnosis is simply that of a muscle abscess. The aetiological factors involved, for example phlebitis, haematoma in scurvy, and filarial abscesses, require general investigation. Confusion may arise with osteomyelitis and arthritis.

The patient should be nursed in bed. The affected part, if it is a limb, should be rested, if necessary in splints. Analgesics may be administered for pain. Local treatment includes fomentation and either aspiration or open incision, drainage, and packing, if the general condition (for example high swinging fever and leucocytosis) demands interference. As much as a pint of pus may be removed from a large abscess. Some authorities claim that aspiration is preferable to open incision. Sulphathiazole or sulphadiazine 1.5 g three times a day for 1 week are successful in some cases.

Antibiotics may be given with effect in some, especially where the infective agent is staphylococcus. Tetracycline is likely to be more effective than penicillin.

## TROPICAL PHLEBITIS

A primary thrombophlebitis occurring in Africa.

Tropical phlebitis was first described in East Africa but is now known to have a widespread distribution throughout Africa.

It occurs most often in otherwise healthy young male adults. There is no obvious occupational incidence. It is predominantly a disease of Africans, but has been reported in a few Europeans working in Africa.

There is no seasonal incidence, but outbreaks, resembling small 'epidemics', occur from time to time.

It is believed, on the grounds of the pathology and clinical appearance, that the causative agent may be a virus; it has been suggested that in some cases it may be syringe-transmitted.

There is gross interruption of the vessel wall in all its divisions by granulation tissue containing multitudes of newly formed blood vessels, fibroblasts, endothelioid cells, giant cells, and macrophages, some of which contain so-called cytoplasmic inclusion bodies. The lesion is especially prominent in the media and extends into the connective tissue surrounding the vessel. The vasa vasorum are not cuffed. In the immediate vicinity of the lesion there is a thrombus firmly adherent to the vessel wall with distal secondary thrombosis. Considerable organization and recanalization of the clots occurs as the condition progresses.

There are two main clinical forms, differing only in severity, namely, *phlebitis major* and *phlebitis minor*. In the former, large veins are involved and the general reaction is severe. In the latter small veins are involved and the general reaction is mild or negligible.

*Phlebitis major:* This condition is acute and usually non-recurrent. It may affect both superficial and deep vessels. The syndrome commences suddenly with intense pain in the affected area. There is acute tenderness along the course of the affected vessel and some protective spasm of regional muscles. Within a few hours local swelling occurs and the tenderness and pain increase and make examination difficult. The distal veins become engorged and oedema may develop, especially if a limb vein is involved. Fever and constitutional signs develop. In some cases the fever is high, especially when very large vessels are involved. In the normal course of events the temperature returns to normal and the local signs subside in a few days. Occasionally in severe cases, especially when there is secondary thrombosis, the temperature may remain elevated for 2–3 weeks.

Palpation of the inflamed vessel is usually possible only after the subsidence of the acute local signs. It discloses a smooth, thick, hard cord, which may remain tender for weeks. The swelling is not attached to the skin and can usually be felt clearly along the path of the vein which, because of the extensive local connective tissue reaction, is often thickened considerably more than would be expected if the lesion were confined entirely to the vessel wall. There may be one or more swellings on the vein, measuring several centimetres in length. More than one vessel may be involved.

Healing is slow, but in uncomplicated cases the swelling eventually disappears and circulation is ultimately restored. Suppuration does not usually occur, but it is possible that phlebitis may explain occasional cases of tropical myositis.

The local picture is complicated by the vascular effects of obstruction to circulation. These effects depend on the vessel affected. In the leg the femoral vein is often involved. The leg becomes oedematous, the oedema subsiding slowly. The distal vessels become congested early and some form of collateral circulation may eventually be established.

Any large vein may be affected, including the superior or inferior vena cava. In the former case both arms and the neck and face become oedematous and congested. In the latter, oedema of both legs, the pelvis and lower abdomen may develop. Thrombosis may also occur in the venous sinuses of the skull, or in the mesenteric veins. In the latter case there develops an acute abdominal crisis with severe epigastric pain, vomiting, and shock; blood may be passed per rectum.

It is believed that the splenic vein is involved occasionally, leading to multiple or total infarction; this may be a cause of primary splenic abscess. It has been suggested that tropical phlebitis may be responsible for some cases of gangrene in the extremities. Secondary embolus is very rare. Oedema may be the only presenting sign after deep thrombosis.

The prognosis depends mainly on the vessels affected. Thrombosis of the vena cava, or visceral veins, may be fatal.

*Phlebitis minor.* Mild cases may exhibit sudden local pain, tenderness, and oedema without fever or other constitutional signs. The patient may notice painful lumps in the extremities. These are found to be related to veins. There may be several along the line of a single vessel and a number of veins may be involved. The swellings are firm, tender, up to 5 cm in diameter. They usually subside completely in a few weeks. There may or may not be accompanying distal congestion and oedema.

Outbreaks of acute cervical phlebitis accompanied by constitutional symptoms have been described. The patients may develop stiff neck and slight fever, sometimes with no obvious signs suggesting local thrombosis. They may go on to recovery, relapse, or subsequently develop thrombophlebitis elsewhere. During these so-called 'epidemics' some subjects develop fever only.

The clinical condition in a case in which a superficial vessel is involved is usually easy to diagnose. When the vessels are deep the diagnosis has to be considered along with many other conditions and may be very difficult. Associated arteries may occasionally be involved, but the very acute local changes accompanied by fever and constitutional signs will usually distinguish the condition from other forms of thrombophlebitis such as Buerger's disease. Tropical myositis may be difficult to distinguish when the phlebitis occurs in the deeper small veins, especially those of the neck. Local lymph gland enlargement must be excluded.

There is no specific treatment. Local treatment consists of rest and elevation where possible. Sulphonamides or antibiotics do not seem to affect the clinical course except where secondary infection has occurred. Anticoagulants such as heparin may be indicated but there is no record of their use.

# 18

# NUTRITIONAL DISORDERS

INTRODUCTION

Nutritional requirements in the tropics are basically the same as in temperate regions. The diet of populations indigenous to the tropics is, however, largely governed by custom and supply and tends to be based on some staple carbohydrate foodstuff, such as rice, maize, or cassava, to which other substances are added fortuitously. Such a diet tends to be badly balanced and lacking in total protein, especially animal protein, and deficient in many essential substances, including minerals and vitamins. Community-wide poverty and disease, climatic extremes such as droughts and floods, and inefficient agricultural methods combine, moreover, to make food supplies inadequate. It is not surprising, therefore, that nutritional disturbances in which any dietary element may be involved are common in the tropics and represent a constant background against which other disease processes develop.

Most nutritional disturbances are directly related to the diet and arise from such factors as inadequate intake, imbalance of the various constituents of the diet, and deficiencies of essential substances. Some, however, may be independent of the diet and originate from faulty intestinal absorption, as in sprue, or from interference with the intake, absorption, or utilization of nutrients, arising from parasitic or bacterial infection. However they develop, primary quantitative or qualitative deficiencies are potentially injurious to health and may themselves influence the pathological effects of other disease states, especially parasitic infections.

Finally, several endogenous food poisons are known or believed to cause clinical disorders such as epidemic dropsy, lathyrism, vomiting sickness of Jamaica, and hepatic veno-occlusive disease.

## VITAMIN DEFICIENCY SYNDROMES

### (Contributed by H.Alistair Reid)

Vitamins are accessory food factors essential for normal body metabolism and for maintenance of health. Some vitamins may be synthesised within the human body but the amounts are insufficient for normal requirements and primary dietetic deficiency states are common in the tropics. Secondary deficiency is also common and is usually due to disorders of the alimentary tract.

Vitamins may be subdivided into the fat-soluble group (A, D, E, and K) and the water-soluble group (B complex and C). The most important clinical syndrome of vitamin deficiency in the tropics is xerophthalmia (vitamin A deficiency). Beriberi (thiamine deficiency) can be lethal. Xerophthalmia is a common cause of blindness and is dangerous to life when complicated by keratomalacia and secondary infection. Rickets and osteomalacia due to lack of vitamin D are rare in the tropics but may be found in towns if conditions preclude exposure to sun or sky-shine. Mucocutaneous lesions are common and are sometimes ascribed to riboflavine deficiency, although response to this single vitamin is often disappointing. Pellagra due to lack of nicotinamide is unusual but is sometimes found amongst maize eaters or alcoholics. Deficiencies of vitamin $B_{12}$ (cobalamin) and folic acid (pteroylglutamic acid) are considered in the chapter on anaemias. Diseases due to lack of vitamin E, vitamin K, pyridoxine, pantothenic acid, biotin, and ascorbic acid are very uncommon in the tropics.

Although clinical syndromes are diagnosed according to the predominant nutrient thought to be deficient—for example, beriberi, xerophthalmia, and so on—it should be realized that multiple deficiency states are much more common than disease due to a single deficiency. Deficiencies of protein and calories are often co-existent, as are bacterial or viral infections and infestation with parasites. It is therefore essential to treat the patient rather than the diagnosis and, in most parts of the tropics, this will involve giving extra calories, protein, vitamin A, and vitamin B complex, as a routine, in addition to dealing with parasites and infections which are so commonly present. The latter may include infective diarrhoea, thrush, measles, and respiratory infections.

## XEROPHTHALMIA

Xerophthalmia (vitamin A deficiency) is a common cause of blindness among pre-school children throughout the tropics, specially in Asia. Xerophthalmia is more common in towns than in rural areas. It is often associated with protein energy malnutrition and it is therefore important always to examine the eyes of infants and toddlers with malnutrition.

*Physiology and pathology*
Retinol is a fat-soluble alcohol found only in animal foods. It is formed in the wall of the small intestine from a precursor, carotene. Carotene is abundant in green vegetables, red palm oil and yellow fruit but carotene is not as readily absorbed as preformed retinol. Retinol is readily available in fish-liver oils, milk, butter, liver, and egg-yolk. There is negligible retinol in skimmed or

condensed milk and no carotene in rice (or most cereals except maize). Retinol is stored in the liver and it is metabolized and excreted very slowly so that a normal liver stores retinol sufficient for about a year.

The term 'vitamin A' covers all compounds with vitamin A activity. About 1000 international units of vitamin A, equivalent to 300 μg retinol, are needed each day up to the age of 5. Thereafter requirements rise to 2500 (750 μg retinol) daily and 4000 units (1200 μg retinol) for lactating women. Infants obtain vitamin A from milk, in which the concentration of vitamin A is kept high at the expense of the mother, hence the need for extra vitamin A during lactation.

Vitamin A is important for retinal adaptation for vision in dim light and is essential for the integrity of epithelial cells. It may also function in the synthesis of glucocorticoids. The aldehyde formed from retinol is an essential component of visual purple and bleaching of visual purple in the rods of the retina enables the human eye to see in dim light. Victims of vitamin A deficiency are often troubled with 'night blindness' although it is not practicable to detect this in young patients. Deficiency also causes a morphological change in epithelial cells which undergo squamous (scaly) change (or metaplasia), becoming flattened, dried, and heaped up one upon another. This change in the conjunctiva is called *xerosis conjunctivae* and in the cornea, *xerosis corneae*. If the deficiency of vitamin A continues and is severe, necrosis of the cornea or keratomalacia develops, resulting in permanent damage. Rupture of the eyeball can cause rapid blindness; and subsequent heavy scarring of the cornea can also cause blindness if it is over the pupil area. Experimentally, vitamin A deficiency can result in blocking of the sebaceous glands of the skin and this causes a roughness of the skin or follicular keratosis. However, follicular keratosis is not specific to vitamin A deficiency; it has been observed in West Africans on a high intake of vitamin A.

### Clinical features
Xerophthalmia affects mainly pre-school children aged 1–4 years. The causal factors are very similar to those resulting in protein–energy malnutrition, namely weaning on to an inadequate diet, and infections, especially infective diarrhoea and measles. Therapeutic starvation instituted as treatment for infections often contributes to a vicious circle.

### Conjunctival changes
In xerosis conjunctivae or dryness of the bulbar conjunctiva the eye loses its lustre and shine, and this is best appreciated by holding the eye open. The dryness is bilateral and usually generalized throughout the exposed part of the bulbar conjunctiva or it may be localized to a small part. Later there is thickening, stiffness, and wrinkling with small vertical folds. A fine diffuse greyish pigmentation may develop (but a patchy coarse pigmentation can occur normally in healthy subjects).

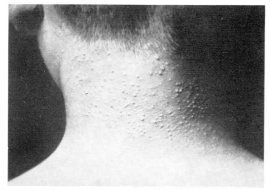

FIG. 40. Retinol (vitamin A) deficiency. The skin of the neck is dry and is generally thickened: the hyperkeratotic papules are well marked. These changes are common in Vitamin A deficiency, but not specific.

[Courtesy Roche Products Ltd.]

Bitot's spots are silver-grey foamy spots, usually external to the cornea and often bilateral. Round, oval, or triangular, they are superficial and look rather like a piece of paper put on the conjunctiva. They can be removed by wiping with lid movement, leaving a rough xerotic surface. Bitot's spots are very easy to see and are thus a valuable sign suggesting xerophthalmia. But they are not specific as they can occur in subjects not deficient in vitamin A (and then the spots do not respond to vitamin A therapy).

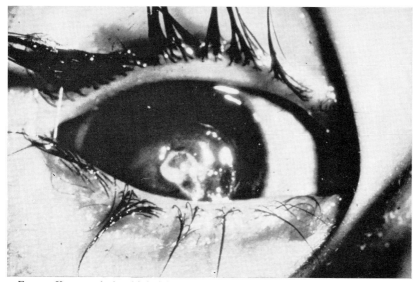

FIG. 41. Keratomalacia with bulging of the centre of the cornea. Perforation leading to rapid blindness is imminent. Even if perforation is averted, later scarring of the cornea, if it occurs over the pupil area, can cause blindness.

[Courtesy Professor D.S.McLaren]

*Corneal changes*

Xerosis corneae follows on conjunctival xerosis and affects both corneas but to widely varying degrees. The dryness gives the cornea a dull, hazy appearance best demonstrated by holding the lids apart for 15 seconds. These changes are reversible and, unless secondary infection complicates the picture, there is a striking absence of inflammatory features such as pain, photophobia, and congestion.

Keratomalacia results in irreversible changes and constitutes a grave emergency. Softening or colliquative necrosis involves the whole thickness of the lower part, or more often all the cornea which melts into a cloudy white or yellowish gelatinous mass (Fig. 41). The process is rapid, particularly in very young children. Perforation of the cornea, prolapse of the iris, extrusion of the lens, and infection of the eyeball can follow and often lead to destruction and shrinking of the eyeball (phthisis bulbi). Later, heavy scarring over the pupil area can also lead to total blindness.

*Night blindness and other features*

Poor vision in dim light is a characteristic feature of experimental vitamin A deficiency produced in adult volunteers. But techniques to demonstrate 'night blindness' are expensive and not applicable to pre-school children. In older children night blindness may suggest the possibility of vitamin A deficiency but in the tropics there are many other possible causes. Follicular keratosis, a roughness of the skin on the front of the thighs and back of the arms (well described as 'permanent goose-flesh'), may be present but it is not specific for vitamin A deficiency. Clinical evidence of kwashiorkor or marasmus almost invariably accompanies xerophthalmia.

DIAGNOSIS

The diagnosis of xerophthalmia is clinical. Early conjunctival xerosis can be made more obvious by instilling a small drop of 1 per cent Rose Bengal. Within a few minutes a triangular pink area appears on one or both sides of the cornea. The colouring disappears within 10–30 minutes. Serum retinol levels (normal 15–90 $\mu$g per 100 ml) may be low but are of no diagnostic help in individual patients because they merely reflect recent intake. Thus the level may be normal in florid xerophthalmia because of recent high intake, or low despite adequate liver stores. Usually conjunctival xerosis precedes the sinister corneal changes but sometimes, especially in younger toddlers, keratomalacia may develop too quickly for conjunctival changes to be observed.

Unless there is secondary local infection, xerophthalmia shows a striking absence of inflammatory changes. Trachoma is also common in the preschool age group. Trachoma can be distinguished as it shows these inflammatory changes which have a characteristic distribution affecting the conjunctiva lining the upper lid and the upper margin of the cornea which is invaded by pannus. As already mentioned, xerophthalmia is almost always accompanied by other features of subnutrition, especially kwashiorkor or marasmus; and there are often signs of general infection, especially alimentary or respiratory.

Supportive therapy for the general malnutrition is of the greatest importance in xerophthalmia. This will include treatment of electrolyte upsets, general infections, and coincidental local eye infection if present.

Halibut-liver oil contains 600–700 units of vitamin A (about 200 μg retinol) per drop. One teaspoonful of cod- and shark-liver oil contains 2000 units (600 μg retinol) and 1000 units (300 μg retinol) respectively. In mild cases of xerophthalmia with night blindness and xerosis conjunctivae but no corneal involvement, oral supplements suffice. The daily dose should be 25,000 units (7500 μg retinol) supplied by 30 ml of cod-liver oil. Standardized capsules of 100,000 and 200,000 units of vitamin A are available from UNICEF. If the cornea is involved, water-dispersible vitamin A palmitate should be given by stomach tube if necessary, 10,000 units (3000 μg retinol) per kg body weight daily. A similar amount should also be given by intramuscular injection, using a water-miscible preparation since the usual form in oil may not be adequately absorbed from intramuscular injections. These high doses should be continued for at least 5 days according to the response of the eye lesions and the general condition. Alternatively, a single massive dose of 300,000 units may be given orally and intramuscularly. Cod-liver oil should be continued during convalescence to obtain liver storage and prevent relapse. Night blindness disappears within a few hours or days. Small children behave normally again in a dark room. Older children can count fingers again at a distance of 1 metre. Xerosis usually resolves completely in 2–3 weeks; the response to treatment of keratomalacia depends on the extent of the damage present before treatment is started. Mortality in xerophthalmia is often high. This is mainly due to the accompanying protein–energy malnutrition.

# RICKETS

Rickets is a disease of calcium and phosphorus metabolism occurring in infants and children who receive insufficient vitamin D (cholecalciferol), and often insufficient calcium. Since vitamin D can be manufactured in the skin when exposed to ultraviolet light, rickets is rare in the tropics except in towns.

Vitamin $D_2$ or ergocalciferol is a synthetic substance made by irradiating ergosterol found in fungi and yeasts. Vitamin $D_3$ or cholecalciferol is the natural form of vitamin D; it is produced by ultraviolet irradiation of 7-dehydrocholesterol which is widely found in animal fats such as the oily secretions of skin. Skin pigment reduces the formation of vitamin D and therefore heavily pigmented children are probably more susceptible to rickets. Milk contains negligible vitamin D. Vitamin D is stored in the liver and fatty tissues though to a lesser degree than vitamin A. A daily intake of 10 $\mu$g (400 international units) will prevent rickets in childhood.

Vitamin D is concerned in the absorption and proper use of calcium and phosphate. In rickets there is irregular growth of bone with widening of the zone between diaphysis and epiphysis and poor calcification.

### CLINICAL FEATURES

The earliest lesion which may appear from 2 months onward is craniotabes, a softening of the back of the skull on which the infant lies. The skull may indent like a piece of paper. The anterior fontanelle remains open and its edges soft (normally it is closed by 18 months). Bossing of the frontal and parietal eminences, and rounded swellings over the costochondral junctions near the sternum ('rickety rosary') and at the wrists and ankles appear. Bones soften and bend, resulting in bowlegs or knock-knees, Harrison's sulcus (where the diaphragm is attached), and so on. If rickets continues beyond the second or third year the child will be underweight and underheight, and dentition will be delayed (normally at 1 year old there are two or more teeth).

### DIAGNOSIS

Radiological examination of the wrist shows a characteristic widening of the lower ends of the radius and ulna, with concave cupping and a frayed, hazy appearance. The serum calcium is usually normal, alkaline phosphatase increased, and the phosphate decreased; but the latter two can show normal levels in florid rickets. Skull bossing can occur in any anaemia, especially in haemoglobinopathies, but does not develop as early as in rickets.

### TREATMENT

Milk is of primary importance for general nutrition and at least 1 pint should be drunk daily. Oral administration of 100 $\mu$g (4000 international units) of vitamin D is adequate, given in the form of ergocalciferol or cholecalciferol (as cod-, halibut-, or shark-liver oil). Treatment should be continued until clinical, biochemical, and radiological evidence indicates control and thereafter the dose of vitamin D should be gradually reduced to the prophylactic dose of 10 $\mu$g daily. An early radiological sign of response is an opaque transverse line ('Müller's line') of calcification appearing within 3 weeks at the growing end of long bones.

If rickets is secondary to disease such as renal disease, much larger doses of vitamin D are required and may have to be given parenterally. But it is important to remember that hypercalcaemia from hypervitaminosis D can be a far more serious disorder than rickets.

# BERIBERI

Beriberi is a disease with generalized oedema and peripheral neuropathy and, sometimes, heart failure, associated with thiamine deficiency. The word 'beri' means weak and comes from Sri Lanka, although the disease was probably first described in Japan. Beriberi is usually associated with a polished rice diet and is thus most commonly found in Asia. In recent years, beriberi has become a rare disease. But it has also been found in groups eating highly milled wheat, especially when alcohol consumption is high.

## PHYSIOLOGY AND PATHOLOGY

Thiamine is concerned in the intermediary metabolism of carbohydrate; peripheral nerves and cardiovascular tissues are presumably sensitive to the resulting impairment of oxidation of $\alpha$-keto acids. The richest sources of thiamine are yeast, whole cereals, liver, peas, beans, and fresh green vegetables. Rice contains adequate amounts of thiamine but this is largely lost when rice is polished. Little thiamine is stored in the body. Requirements are related to the metabolic rate and to the carbohydrate intake. For an average adult the total daily requirement is about 1 mg, and for a nursing mother 1.4 mg.

In beriberi the oedema is generalized and mainly due to increased permeability of peripheral blood vessels. If the heart is involved, it is usually greatly dilated but there are no pathological changes specific to beriberi. In cerebral beriberi, haemorrhages are found in the mid-brain, the hypothalamus, and the walls of the third ventricle.

## CLINICAL FEATURES

The three clinical syndromes ascribed to thiamine deficiency are acute infantile beriberi, chronic beriberi, and cerebral beriberi (Wernicke's encephalopathy).

### Acute infantile beriberi
This is acute heart failure occurring in breast-fed babies aged 2–5 months when the mother is deficient in thiamine. The mother may or may not show signs of beriberi. She may have noticed restlessness, vomiting, undue crying, and some puffiness of face and feet in her infant but breathlessness with or

without convulsions may be the first sign and death can follow within 24–48 hours. On examination, the infant is cyanosed, the pulse and respiration rate rapid, the liver enlarged, and sometimes abnormal neck vein distension is observed. There is variable but generalized oedema. The apex beat is displaced outwards; the blood pressure may be normal or raised, but in advanced cases may be unrecordable. If the infant survives the first 1–2 days, head retraction, twitchings, and an aphonic cry may suggest meningitis but lumbar puncture yields normal cerebrospinal fluid.

### Chronic beriberi

Chronic beriberi is a disease mainly of adults. It may be precipitated by pregnancy, infections, and a diet change, for example to polished rice, or even an increased carbohydrate intake without a corresponding increase in the intake of thiamine. On rare occasions adult beriberi may present in acute form somewhat similar to the infantile type. A rapidly spreading limb paresis is associated with acute heart failure which may be fatal in a few days; or the subject may pass into the chronic form.

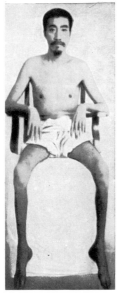

Fig. 42. Thiamine deficiency. 'Dry' beriberi showing wrist drop and marked wasting of the lower extremities. Similar effects may result from viral infections.

[Courtesy Professor B.Platt]

Chronic beriberi consists mainly of peripheral neuropathy and peripheral oedema. Sometimes, though not usually, the heart is also involved. Over some weeks, increasing heaviness, then weakness, affects the lower limbs, the first symptom usually being difficulty in rising from the squatting position adopted for defaecation. Individuals may also complain of cold or burning feet, tingling of the toes, or cramping pains in the calves. Swelling of the face and the feet may be noticed before, at the same time, or after the neuropathic symptoms start. At any stage increasing breathlessness and weakness on exertion due to heart failure may supervene.

Oedema is generalized, being present over face and feet; sometimes it is initially confined to the scrotum. It may mask moderate or gross wasting (though quite often the subjects are obese). Ascites is usually absent or minimal. The most useful neurological signs are inability to rise from the squatting position unaided and marked tenderness of the calves (which are often swollen) to pressure. Cerebration, pupil reaction, and fundi are normal. On rare occasions a central scotoma and nerve deafness are present. The upper limbs are usually normal in mild or early cases apart from absent tendon reflexes. The degree of paresis in the lower limbs varies from mild weakness, best shown by the squat test, to complete paralysis with footdrop and symmetrical wasting. The knee-jerks and ankle-jerks are absent and the plantar responses normal though sometimes absent. All sensation is depressed over the lower limbs, particularly vibration, and position sense.

The heart is usually normal but, if it is involved, there are signs of congestive heart failure with abnormal neck vein distension, enlargement of the liver, and warm extremities. Despite these signs of gross congestive failure, the patient is often able to lie flat on his bed without aggravating the dyspnoea. The apex beat is displaced outwards but is often difficult to feel owing to obesity or oedema, or both. The blood pressure and the heart sounds are usually normal; but the blood pressure can be either low or high. Radiology shows gross enlargement of the heart shadow and the electrocardiogram shows non-specific changes, most commonly symmetrical T-wave inversion in the right chest leads.

### Cerebral beriberi. Wernicke's encephalopathy

Most recorded cases of cerebral beriberi have been in alcoholics; two of Wernicke's original three patients in 1881 were alcoholics. But a series of 52 non-alcoholic cases in a Singapore prisoner-of-war hospital have been very well described; four-fifths of them had classical beriberi in addition. Nevertheless, the comparative rarity of cerebral beriberi among indigenous peoples of Asia where beriberi is common is puzzling, particularly as the clinical picture is very striking (and therefore unlikely to be overlooked). It consists of mental signs, eye signs, and peripheral neuropathy. The mental features include confusion, emotional upset, and loss of memory for recent events resulting in confabulation (a glib form of lying owing to memory gaps). Nystagmus is invariably present; it is usually horizontal but may also be vertical and rotatory. External rectus palsy is present in about one-quarter of the patients and, on rare occasions, papilloedema. The peripheral neuropathy is similar to that described above but ataxia may predominate over motor weakness.

### DIAGNOSIS

The diagnosis of beriberi is clinical. The plasma pyruvate may be raised but this is not specific and of no real help in the diagnosis of individual patients. The transketolase of red blood cell haemolysate is low, usually under 20 units (normal range 30–90 units). Infantile beriberi has to be distinguished from other types of acute heart failure but, provided one thinks of the diagnosis, it is quickly clinched by the dramatic response to specific treatment.

In adults the clinical criteria for diagnosis are: (1) objective signs of peripheral neuropathy; (2) generalized oedema with, or more usually without, heart failure; (3) absence of causes other than beriberi to account for (1) and (2); (4) a dramatic response of (2) to thiamine. Not infrequently, so-called 'dry beriberi' is diagnosed but this is almost invariably a synonym for peripheral neuropathy of uncertain origin. Unless there is a clear history indicating that peripheral oedema has been present at some stage of the illness, the term 'dry beriberi' should be avoided. Whether peripheral neuropathy is in fact due to beriberi or of uncertain origin, the response to thiamine is poor, even in early cases. Absence of proteinuria will usually exclude renal oedema. Protein deficiency leading to oedema in adults is usually associated with low plasma albumin whereas in 'pure' beriberi the plasma proteins are normal. Oedema due to cirrhosis of the liver is usually accompanied by other signs such as ascites, enlarged spleen, and so on. Other causes of peripheral neuropathy in the tropics are legion; even with exhaustive investigations the cause usually remains uncertain. Cardiac beriberi has to be differentiated from other types of high output failure, especially hypertension, severe anaemia, and thyrotoxicosis. The ability to lie flat in bed is suggestive and the dramatic response to thiamine confirms the diagnosis.

### TREATMENT

In acute infantile beriberi, an intravenous injection of 10 mg thiamine results in a dramatic improvement within hours. Often the infant is in a shocked, moribund condition and then the injection should be intracardiac. A depot intramuscular injection of 25 mg thiamine should be given both to the infant and to the mother, both of whom can usually be discharged from hospital the following day. The mother should be advised to eat green vegetables which are usually the cheapest adequate source of thiamine. In adult beriberi, the oedema and (if present) heart failure respond rapidly to oral administration of 10 mg thiamine hydrochloride twice or thrice daily but if heart failure is severe, 10 mg thiamine should be given by intramuscular injection for the first dose. Intravenous injection is best avoided since on rare occasions it has precipitated hypertension and thus aggravated heart failure. The most accurate guide to progress is given by the patient's weight which should be charted daily. Neurological defects respond slowly and may not recover completely. However, a follow-up study of subjects who had cardiac beriberi as prisoners-of-war showed no evidence of heart disease some 10 years later. General malnutrition, other vitamin deficiencies, and secondary factors of infection, liver disease, and so on are often present and require concomitant treatment.

It is preferable to treat cerebral beriberi with large doses of vitamin B complex given by intramuscular or intravenous injection. Parentrovite is a suitable preparation. Ocular signs respond within 24–48 hours but the mental disturbance may take weeks and the ataxia months to resolve.

## BURNING FEET SYNDROME

This distinctive and troublesome complaint is associated with malnutrition, especially involving deficiency of protein and the B group of vitamins. Burning, throbbing pain in the soles of the feet occurs intermittently but especially at night so that sleep is disturbed. Stabbing, shooting pains may spread up the leg as far as the knee. There are usually no objective signs of neuropathy. The treatment is similar to that for mucocutaneous lesions which may also be present.

## MUCOCUTANEOUS LESIONS

Angular stomatitis, cheilosis, dyssebacia, glossitis, facial eczema, and corneal vascularization are common in the tropics. They have been produced experimentally by low riboflavine intake but in clinical practice the lesions rarely respond to riboflavine alone. Angular stomatotis is the most common lesion

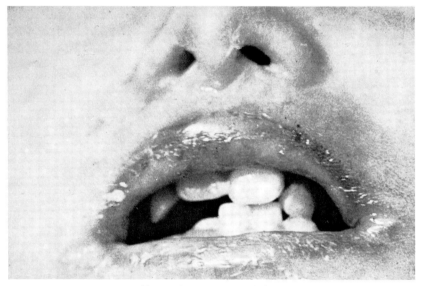

FIG. 43. Mucocutaneous lesions.

and consists of grey-white fissures at both angles of the mouth (Fig. 43).Cheilosis is a sore, cracked condition of the lips. Dyssebacia is a term used for large follicles, plugged with sebaceous material, around the sides of the nose. The tongue may be sore and hyper-red; later, it may be unduly smooth, due to atrophy of the papillae. A scaly, greasy, skin eruption may occur at the angles of the nose, behind the ears, and occasionally around the genitalia (and then the condition is sometimes called the oro-genital syndrome). In treatment, it is preferable to administer the whole vitamin B group as yeast tablets.

## PELLAGRA

Pellagra is a chronic, relapsing disease associated with eating maize and characterized by changes in the skin, alimentary and nervous systems. Formerly common throughout many parts of the world, pellagra is now rare but remains endemic in some areas of India, South Africa, and North Africa. Although deficiency of nicotinic acid is regarded as the chief causal factor, pellagra is a result of multiple deficiencies including protein, riboflavine, and probably other group B vitamins.

### PHYSIOLOGY AND PATHOLOGY

Nicotinic acid is a pyridine derivative which is converted in the body to nicotinamide, the physiologically active form. Tryptophan, an essential amino acid, is a precursor of nicotinic acid and in the presence of other factors in the vitamin B complex, it can be converted to nicotinamide. Another essential amino acid, leucine, may antagonize the function of nicotinamide. Sources of nicotinic acid must therefore be considered for their content of tryptophan and leucine in addition to that of nicotinic acid. Meat, whole grains, and yeast are rich sources; milk is poor in nicotinic acid but rich in tryptophan. Maize contains nicotinic acid in a bound form unavailable to the consumer. There are no distinctive pathological changes in pellagra.

### CLINICAL FEATURES

Pellagra is usually a chronic, relapsing disease chiefly of adults and it can last for years. It may occasionally be acute. The most characteristic feature is the skin change. Skin lesions are strikingly symmetrical, very sharply demarcated, and occur over parts of the body exposed to sun. Thus, lesions occur over the face, especially the forehead and nose, the neck, the back of the arms and hands, and the front of the legs and feet (see Fig. 44). The early change is a sunburn-like erythema which slowly becomes thickened, pigmented at the margins, and after weeks or months may peel in the centre, leaving a red-brown scaly area. Secondary infection is quite common. Mucocutaneous changes as described above, abdominal discomfort, and diarrhoea are common. All levels of the nervous system may be involved in pellagra resulting in a great diversity of neurological features. Mental disturbances including depression, irritability, and poor memory may lead to the mistaken diagnosis of mental illness. These symptoms are later followed by restlessness, tremors, rigidity, and convulsions. There may be evidence of retrobulbar neuritis, nerve deafness, sensory spinal ataxia, spastic paraplegia, and peripheral neuropathy which can be mainly motor or mainly sensory.

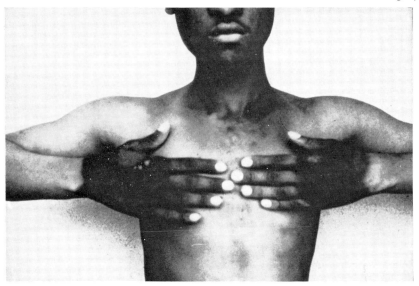

FIG. 44. Pellagra, showing the diagnostic triad of symmetrical skin lesions, sharp demarcation, and distribution in parts exposed to the sun.

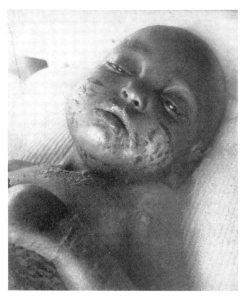

FIG. 45. Multiple deficiency of the B group of vitamins. Nicotinic acid deficiency is shown by the skin changes on the cheeks, thorax, and upper limbs. There is also cheilosis and angular stomatitis, indicative of a riboflavine lack.

[Courtesy Dr D.B.Jelliffe]

## DIAGNOSIS

The skin lesions are the main lead to diagnosis—the symmetry, sharp demarcation, and distribution in exposed parts. Neuropathies involving the spinal cord and peripheral nerves are very common in the tropics. Of the myelopathy syndromes, sensory ataxia is more common than spastic paraplegia. These neuropathies may or may not be accompanied by clinical or epidemiological evidence of nutritional upset, including vitamin and protein deficiencies, and the effects of food toxicants. In many cases, the cause remains obscure despite exhaustive investigations.

## TREATMENT

Although the principal deficiency is nicotinic acid there are always other nutritional deficiencies associated. A well-balanced diet with adequate protein and calories is therefore important. Sedation may be needed if mental symptoms are marked. If the dermatosis is associated with crusting and infection, washing with a dilute disinfectant solution should be followed by application of a cream containing 3 per cent iodochlorhydroxyquinoline (Vioform) and 1 per cent hydrocortisone. If diarrhoea is severe, electrolyte replacement may be necessary and preliminary treatment with tincture of opium should be given until nicotinamide takes effect. The whole vitamin B complex should be administered as yeast tablets. Nicotinamide is also given by oral doses of 500 mg daily. Nicotinic acid is better avoided because of its vasodilator effect. Nicotinamide is absorbed very rapidly from the stomach and small intestine, despite severe digestive disorders; parenteral therapy is therefore unnecessary. The skin and tongue changes respond to treatment dramatically, within hours. Mental features often improve within days but other neurological effects improve only gradually.

# SCURVY

### VITAMIN C: ASCORBIC ACID

Scurvy is a deficiency syndrome primarily due to lack of ascorbic acid in the diet. The vitamin occurs plentifully in fresh oranges, lemons, limes, tomatoes, and raw vegetables. It is quickly destroyed by heat and drying and is absent from most 'tinned' fruit and vegetables.

Experimental pure deficiency of ascorbic acid in animals does not reproduce the syndrome; it is possible that some of the haemorrhagic features derive from concomitant deficiency of citrin (vitamin P).

Daily requirements for adults are about 10 mg. Children need more, weight for weight.

Ascorbic acid is necessary for the formation and maintenance of intercellular mesenchymal 'cement' substance. In deficiency, collagen, matrices of bone, and the intercellular cement between endothelial cells break down, with resultant haemorrhages. The vitamin is also concerned in endochondrial bone formation and the production of the matrix osteoid.

### CLINICAL PICTURE

*Adults*

Scurvy is rare in adults. It is still found in isolated communities and occasionally in elderly people in the 'developed' world who look after themselves, and subsist mostly on tinned food, not bothering to eat fresh fruit. Scurvy also appears in conditions of deprivations, such as obtained in war-time concentration camps.

The early symptoms are fatigue, listlessness, and anorexia. Onset is gradual. The first physical sign is hyperkeratosis of the hair follicles, with plugging of ducts, normally on the thighs and buttocks, but gradually spreading to the trunk and arms. Haemorrhages now develop, often first seen as perifollicular. They occur deep in the muscles, especially of the calf, thigh, and forearm and in the joints, especially the knees. There may be severe subcutaneous haemorrhages following trauma, epistaxis, haematuria, and melaena. Old healed wounds may break down. Characteristic changes occur in the mouth. The gums become proliferative, spongy, and bleed readily. Teeth loosen and fall out. Gum infection leads to foul breath.

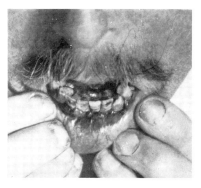

FIG. 46. Ascorbic acid deficiency. Scurvy showing severe gingivitis and loosening of the teeth.

[Courtesy Roche Products Ltd.]

Secondary infection is common.

The majority of the morphological changes are obvious. In children there is deficient dentine and bone formation. The latter may be seen radiographically and there is a wide zone of calcified but non-ossified material just beneath the actively growing epiphyseal cartilages—the scorbutic lattice. Fractures may occur in this area.

*Course*

Unless ascorbic acid is given, scurvy is a progressive disease. It may terminate suddenly in a cardiac crisis or form a massive haemorrhage, but death usually occurs from cachexia and intercurrent infection. Such severe scurvy is rare.

## DIAGNOSIS

Well-developed scurvy is easily diagnosed on the basis of skin and mouth changes. Anaemia is not necessarily present. The saturation test, i.e. giving a large dose of ascorbic acid and measuring the proportion excreted, is not very helpful. Of the earlier signs the appearance of perifollicular haemorrhages is the most important and is almost pathognomonic. The normal clotting and bleeding times, erythrocyte, leucocyte, and platelet counts, exclude many of the haemorrhagic blood diseases. Administration of ascorbic acid as a thera-peutic test is advisable in doubtful cases.

## TREATMENT

Mild scurvy is not a dangerous condition, but all patients should be treated rigorously and immediately and kept at rest until the acute condition has subsided. Although improvement may be expected on only 10 mg ascorbic acid daily, it is advisable to give 100 mg or more orally, either as a single dose, or, preferably, in divided doses, and to supplement the diet with fresh fruit juices, green vegetables, and salads. When these are not available, sprouting legumes can be substituted. Associated deficiencies should receive appropriate treatment, preferably by dietetic means. Improvement is rapid.

A maintenance dose of 10 mg daily is needed where recovery is slow or fresh food is difficult to obtain.

## INFANTILE SCURVY

### (Barlow's Disease)

This form of scurvy may occur in infants in disadvantaged circumstances who are given artificial or overcooked foods. It is rare before the sixth month, as the newborn have adequate stores of ascorbic acid. It is common in the second 6 months and in the second year of life, when growth is at a maximum. The onset is gradual, with the child being fretful and refusing its food. The infant resents handling as the limbs become very tender, due to painful epiphyses and sub-periosteal haemorrhages. The latter show as hot, red, tender swellings near a joint. When these haemorrhages occur near the femoral necks, rigidity and pseudoparesis of the affected limbs may develop. This gives rise to the common attitude adopted by the child, sometimes called the 'pithed frog' position.

The gums bleed easily and haemorrhages occur around erupting teeth. Petechial and larger haemorrhages are also common in the skin, mucous membranes, and soft tissues, especially behind and around the eyeballs. Blood may be vomited; there may be melaena and haematuria.

As bleeding continues, severe anaemia develops.

Diagnosis is made on history, clinical grounds, and X-ray findings. Changes in the bones appear at sites of most active growth, especially in the long bones—the sternal ends of the ribs (noted clinically as costochondral beading, a very common finding), the distal end of the femur, the tibia and fibula, the proximal ends of the humerus, and distal ends of the radius and ulna. There is cortical atrophy, sharp outlining of the epiphysial ends, and atrophy of the trabecular structure, leading to a 'ground glass' appearance. X-rays also reveal a dense epiphyseal line and subperiosteal haemorrhages.

Treatment consists of 100–200 mg ascorbic acid daily by mouth, until recovery (usually a few days). Fruit juices should be added to the diet.

## MEGALOBLASTIC ANAEMIAS

For discussion of folic acid and cyanocobalamin deficiencies, see page 29.

## PROTEIN–ENERGY MALNUTRITION

In most of the disadvantaged world, including the tropics, it is the lot of the majority of infants and children to subsist on an overall deficient diet which is short of calories and qualitatively and sometimes quantitatively lacking in protein. To the hazards of these diets are added specific deficiencies of essential substances and minerals. The syndromes which result collectively make up the spectrum of protein–calorie malnutrition. The clinical picture that develops depends on the age of the victim, the severity of the overall and specific deficiencies, and the relative deficiencies in terms of protein and calories. Modifying factors of great significance are infections and the anorexia and upsets in intestinal absorption and other functions that may accompany them.

The major clinical patterns are kwashiorkor and marasmus. Kwashiorkor results from subsistence on a diet very low in protein, and which also may be low or sometimes adequate in calorie content. The characteristics thus derive primarily from severe protein deficiency; opinion is divided about the significance of the usual excess of carbohydrate. Marasmus is the result of overall starvation; the diet may be balanced, but the primary factor is severe limitation of calories. All kinds of syndrome lie between these two extremes.

## KWASHIORKOR

Kwashiorkor means roughly 'the deposed one'. The syndrome occurs in most parts of the world in children between the ages of 6 months and 4 years, especially in those recently weaned, or in process of being weaned and being placed on a diet consisting of staples which are largely carbohydrate, with little protein content, such as cassava, supplemented with little or no protein, or with protein of poor biological value.

Kwashiorkor is characteristically a disease of artificially fed or early weaned children. It usually first appears weeks or months after weaning, and so may develop in different age groups depending to some extent on local custom. It also appears in infants who are weaned too early and taken from the breast on to some diet which may satisfy hunger but is desperately short of protein and often of requisite calories. The disease occurs in some of the larger towns of Thailand in infants who have been transferred to a diet consisting mainly of condensed milk and water because their mothers have to go out and work. It commonly appears in the second and third year of life in Africa and elsewhere in the tropics where supplemented breast feeding goes on into the second year or longer. The child who develops kwashiorkor has usually been living on an inadequate diet for some time and is already underweight and malnourished. On leaving the breast it is often kept semi-satisfied by ingesting bulky carbohydrate staples like cassava which are practically devoid of protein and which cannot physically be taken in sufficient quantities to provide the calories. In these circumstances the child may have been heading for marasmus due to overall calorie deficit on breast milk, but is pushed into kwashiorkor by the sudden intense reduction of protein intake. The transition phase is sometimes distinguished as a separate entity, called 'marasmic kwashiorkor', which in some respects amounts to marasmus plus oedema.

Kwashiorkor sometimes appears in infants still on the breast. In these cases supplementation with essentially carbohydrate staple foods is already usually considerable and the child is forced by the filling effect of the supplement to take less milk and so reduce its protein intake. Kwashiorkor often appears rapidly in the semi-starved infant, precipitated by dietary changes of this sort or by acute infectious diseases. Of the latter, measles and gastro-intestinal infections are very important.

The organs most affected at necropsy are those with the highest protein turnover—the liver and the pancreas. Pathological changes occur in the skin, the extent varying considerably from one patient to another, ranging from patchy changes in pigmentation to extensive damage resulting from specific vitamin deficiencies; the hair is normally involved, with loss of curl and pigment, as described below.

In the well-advanced case there is marked atrophy of the mucosa of the villi of the small intestine, especially the jejunum, resembling that seen in malabsorption syndromes.

In some geographical areas, as in East Africa, it has been noted that the free amino acid concentration is low in kwashiorkor, the essential acids being largely affected so that their ratio to non-essential amino acids is changed. This has not been observed in other areas, for example the Far East, possibly because of the differing amino acid components of the local staples.

There is always low serum protein content, mainly due to gross reduction in albumin arising from decreased synthesis, but this is not usually considered to be the only or necessarily the major cause of the oedema. In terms of total body water per kg body weight, the child is overhydrated and the osmolarity of the intravascular, extracellular, and intracellular fluid compartments is reduced. Renal function is disturbed and there is usually a notable deficiency in intracellular potassium and commonly of magnesium. Various changes in glucose absorption and utilization have been reported and hypoglycaemia may recur. Intolerance to certain sugars, especially lactose, is common— largely due to relative absence of the appropriate enzymes from the gut lumen.

There is marked reduction in intestinal absorption of fats especially those contained in milk; this can be slowly reversed by treatment.

The liver in early cases shows peripheral lobular fatty degeneration of the parenchymal cells and infiltration. This regresses with treatment and regeneration is complete, without fibrosis. There is often atrophy of the acinar cells in the pancreas, with loss of zymogen granules. Periacinar, perilobular, and even periductal fibrosis is present in some cases. In severely affected cases there is a corresponding reduction in duodenal enzyme content, involving especially lactase, lipase, and trypsin. Other acinar glands may be affected; for instance, the salivary glands. Hyaline lesions of the glomeruli of the kidneys and pericapsular fibrosis have been reported.

The clinical picture is variable. It includes retardation of growth, changes in pigmentation in the skin and hair, alterations in the texture of the hair, oedema of the limbs and body, apathy, irritability, and pathological changes in certain organs, especially the liver and pancreas. Dermatoses derived from nutritional deficiencies are usually present.

The child is retarded in stature and weight for its age. The muscles are wasted but this may be masked by the considerable oedema, which often makes the child relatively heavy; the true state of affairs may be revealed only after the disappearance of the oedema.

The patient is peevish, grizzling, and apathetic. The oedema involves the legs and may extend to the thighs, genitals, and buttocks and at times even the anterior abdominal wall. Ascites is rare. Oedema is very common in the forearms and hands and the face is usually involved, especially around the eyes and malar regions. The common picture is that of a miserable, pot-bellied child sitting upright with legs extended and remaining stationary rather than wandering about like a normal infant. The liver is usually palpable and firm; the edge is about an inch below the costal margin. The spleen may also be palpable in infants with malaria.

Changes in the hair and skin are notable. The hair becomes depigmented, turning grey or white or, especially in Africans, somewhat light-reddish. The natural curl is lost, a feature particularly obvious in Africans, in whom the thick, rich, black curl is replaced by a fine, grey, wavy wisp.

Well-advanced dermatosis is not an essential part of the clinical pattern, but slight changes in pigmentation and texture of the skin probably occur in all cases and, as a rule, by the time the child is seen, extensive dermatoses have developed. These appear mainly in areas of the body exposed to irritation and trauma, for instance the buttocks and 'napkin' area, the back, the thighs, and legs. The lesions are physically not unlike those seen in pellagra, but as a rule the areas affected in pellagra, such as the face, hands, and feet, escape in kwashiorkor. Trowell has described the early hyperpigmented lesions as 'black varnished patches' which rapidly enlarge, crack, and tend to peel off in 'enamel-paint' plaques up to an inch across, leaving depigmented, thinly epithelialized, or ulcerated areas beneath, which may become extensively infected leading to bullous changes and severe ulceration. These changes are particularly common over the buttocks and lower trunk. On the legs the scaling is often less obvious, the general appearance being that of 'crackled' or 'crazy pavement' skin. Many children exhibit in addition dry, slightly scaling, skin changes over the greater part of the body surface. Changes in the eyes, lips, and tongue resulting from multiple specific deficiencies such as varying degrees of xerophthalmia, Bitot's spots, etc., angular stomatitis, cheilosis, and glossitis, occur at all stages of kwashiorkor. Photophobia is common.

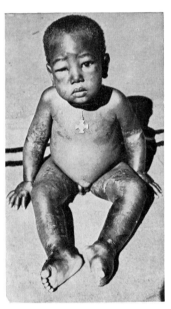

FIG. 47. Kwashiorkor. Note expression, hair, oedema and skin changes. [By courtesy Dr Michael Gelfand]

The child commonly suffers severely from gastro-intestinal upsets. Diarrhoea is usual, with liquid or porridgy yellow or bile-stained stools containing undigested food; offensive steatorrhoea may occur. Vomiting is common and sometimes persistent. Varying degrees of dehydration may result, even in 'oedematous' cases, from loss of fluid and electrolytes from the diarrhoea and vomiting. In very severe cases the dehydration may become extreme, especially where there is secondary gastrointestinal infection. Most cases present with mild, orthochromic, normocytic anaemia. Occasionally there may be macrocytosis, associated with increase in number of reticulocytes. The blood picture to a large extent is decided by the parasitological state of the child; malaria and hookworm may greatly complicate the situation. The bone marrow response is normoblastic.

The untreated case steadily goes downhill. There is a very high mortality. Fortunately, the response to treatment is extremely good and all but the worst cases have a good chance of survival. The difficulty is that, on discharge from a hospital, the baby goes back to a social environment in which the return of the syndrome becomes almost inevitable.

Diagnosis of kwashiorkor is largely clinical. The age and dietary history of the infant are the essential points. Retarded growth, oedema, pot-belly, changes in the hair and skin establish the diagnosis. Biopsy of the liver may reveal the fatty changes, usually in the peripheral regions of the lobules.

Kwashiorkor must be distinguished from other causes of oedema, enlargement of the liver, and skin changes. A very careful examination for evidence of parasitological infections is essential. These may be present in any case.

Kwashiorkor must also be clearly distinguished from *marasmus* arising from overall malnutrition from deficient intake, often associated with infective states (see below).

It may at times be necessary to differentiate kwashiorkor from abdominal tuberculosis in which ascites is common although very rare in kwashiorkor, and from certain stages of *hepatic veno-occlusive disease* (p. 334) and, in India, *infantile (biliary) cirrhosis*. The latter condition affects infants and young children, often of vegetarian families in good economic circumstances, and is characterized by enlargement of the liver and usually of the spleen, protuberant abdomen with prominent superficial veins, sometimes ascites and oedema, and varying degrees of light or severe jaundice. In the late stages there is periportal and diffuse disorganizing hepatic fibrosis with signs of portal hypertension. There are no skin changes. The cause is unknown; a virus hepatitis is suspected.

### TREATMENT

The object is to adjust the diet as quickly as possible and provide a high content of biologically suitable protein, sufficient calories and adequate accessory substances and minerals. The speed of adjustment will depend on the individual child. Too rapid feeding may exacerbate the diarrhoea and worsen existing water:electrolyte imbalance, or intensify the anorexia. Once the latter has been overcome, the child usually becomes eager for food and the adjustment presents few difficulties.

In very sick children attention must first be given to life-saving procedures, chief amongst which is often adjustment of water:electrolyte dehydration. Where diarrhoea has been prominent and continues, severe dehydration develops even in the presence of the accumulated oedema fluid. There is relative sodium loss, hypokalaemia, and depletion of cell potassium, commonly some acidosis except when vomiting is severe, when there may be alkalosis. In addition, there is usually some renal dysfunction in regard to water excretion and the cardiac reserve is low and unable to deal with too rapid replacement of the deficient intravascular fluid compartment.

It is important, therefore, to rehydrate orally if possible, by giving frequent small amounts of diluted dextrose saline, to which 1 g potassium chloride should be added per litre. The child should receive 120–200 ml per kg body weight per day.

When gastro-intestinal disturbances are gross and diarrhoea is severe and continuous, replacement of fluid parenterally is essential. The infusion should be given intravenously where possible, otherwise intraperitoneally or subcutaneously (without sugars). Suitable hypotonic fluids are Ringer's lactate (1 part sodium lactate one-sixth M; 2 parts Ringer's solution; 3 parts 5 per cent glucose solution) with dextrose or Darrow's solution (sodium chloride, 3.0 g; potassium chloride, 2.7 g; sodium bicarbonate, 4.4 g in each litre).

If vomiting is severe, the lactate or the bicarbonate should be omitted from the solutions and chlorpromazine, 0.5 mg per kg body weight, given intramuscularly.

The initial volume of fluid provided should be 40–50 ml per kg body weight (calculated as theoretic weight for age) per day. The infusion should be given quickly in the first instance at 40–50 drops per minute, gradually slowing over the day. As soon as rehydration is established, and the urinary flow improves, the child should continue on oral fluid.

Diuretics must never be used in attempting to reduce oedema or resolve oliguria.

Anaemia is seldom severe enough to need transfusion. If blood is given it must be administered very slowly to avoid embarrassment of the circulation.

Infection must be dealt with as quickly as possible. It is usually impossible to ascertain whether the diarrhoea is due to bacillary dysentery or other organisms, but there is little doubt that some sick children develop, and die from, bacterial bronchopneumonia. Severe cases of kwashiorkor are therefore usually given penicillin over the first week. Some workers advise penicillin and streptomycin, others have used tetracycline with or without streptomycin and some have given chloramphenicol. The broad spectrum antibiotics have their own troublesome complications so that common usage is to provide penicillin as daily procaine penicillin, with or without streptomycin in the usual dosages.

In addition to dehydration and infection, a common serious complication which may be fatal is *hypothermia*. The child is cold and cyanotic, the rectal temperature well below normal. Despite the tropical environment the child needs to be kept warm and given shelter and protection from cold and draught.

Once the life-saving procedures are in hand, the adjustment of the diet should begin. The principle is to offer a high-protein, easily assimilable and calorie-adequate diet, usually based on cow's milk to which must be added the necessary essential substances and minerals. The patient is often unable to take milk or other animal fats so that vegetable fats are substituted. Because of the damage to the pancreas and intestinal wall, it is also unable to deal with certain sugars, particularly lactose, excess of which greatly exacerbates the diarrhoea. Lactose should not therefore be used in the diet; sucrose or fructose are usually the most satisfactory additional sources of carbohydrate.

In many parts of the world easily made mixtures are prepared for use in treatment of kwashiorkor. These are often stored dry in dispensaries, etc., and water is added as required before use.

In Ghana, Sai recommends a mixture made up of equal weights of skimmed milk, casein, vegetable fat, and sucrose. (It is possible that fructose might be better than sucrose, but it is too expensive for ordinary use; banana, which contains fructose, may be substituted.)

For the first few days the child is given food gradually on the basis of 30–60 calories and 1.0–1.5 g protein per kg body weight per day. This may be given either in the form of the mixture or as milk diluted with an equal volume of 5 per cent glucose solution. Using the mixture the diet is increased as fast as the child can manage to 100–200 calories and 3–5 g protein per kg body weight per day (based on theoretical weight for age).

Nursing is essential in the early stages. As the child improves, the mother or relatives should gradually take over.

Vitamins may be given as multivite preparations or in local foods. Where there are signs of xerophthalmia, vitamin A should be given intramuscularly as this condition may develop very quickly and cause permanent damage to the cornea leading to blindness. The usual folic acid deficiency can be adjusted by small oral maintenance dosage and iron is given as the ferrous salt if the anaemia is severe. After rehydration, in severe cases magnesium should be given in the form of a 50 per cent solution of the sulphate intramuscularly in daily doses of 0.5 ml for a child of 5–7 kg body weight rising to 2.0 ml at 15 kg. When the diet is being adjusted, magnesium lactate may be added, but supplements of groundnuts will probably provide adequate quantities of the mineral.

Recovery takes place in two phases. Initial recovery is indicated by the rapid disappearance of oedema fluid, usually with a substantial concurrent temporary fall in weight; the diarrhoea subsides, there is improvement in appetite and mental reactions; the skin lesions begin to heal and the patient becomes less apathetic. This takes 2–3 weeks and is followed by a long consolidation period which may last several months, during which the diet has to be adjusted to switch from the more expensive and exotic hospital foods to one which can be provided locally.

The protein should theoretically be best supplied from animal sources but this is usually impossible for economic and social reasons and some form of balanced vegetable protein mixture, derived from local resources, must be provided, for example, from groundnut extract and soya bean. At this stage it is essential to teach the parents to provide and prepare the diet, otherwise relapse is more than likely.

The relapse may be quite as severe as the original episode, the same syndrome is produced, including the depigmentation of the hair, the colour and texture of which is restored during treatment and recovery; in this way the growing hair may exhibit alternating bands of normal black pigmentation and grey or reddish depigmentation—the so-called 'flag sign'.

Parasitic and bacterial infections must be treated. Malaria and acute bacterial infections should be dealt with immediately. Most helminth infections such as hookworm, unless obviously causing severe anaemia, can be left until convalescence. Lipotropic factors such as methionine and choline are useless.

*Assessment of progress*

The usual way of determining the severity and progress of a given case of protein–calorie malnutrition is by clinical assessment. Some confusion has arisen, however, as a result of giving a single label to two very distinct metabolic situations. Attempts to find a biochemical yardstick have been made without a great deal of success. In kwashiorkor serum albumin levels are low or very low; in marasmus the levels may be a little lower than normal, but are not greatly changed. Little correlation has been found between the clinical state and the balance of essential to non-essential amino acids and the hydroxyproline index, which is basically a measure of growth, is low in both. Recent work in Nigeria has suggested that serum-transferrin levels correlate well with the current nutritional state of the patient. These are very low in kwashiorkor and normal in marasmus. They may be useful in assessing improvement under treatment. The method of estimation can be adopted as a field test.

## MARASMUS

Underfeeding, even when the balance of the diet is maintained, leads to undernutrition which in its advanced form becomes *nutritional marasmus*. The fully developed syndrome is often caused by a mixture of the effects of extreme undernutrition and of infection, especially ascariasis and hookworm infection, and gastro-intestinal disturbances associated with diarrhoea.

The child with marasmus is grossly underweight. There is marked loss of subcutaneous fat. The skin is cold and flaccid. The features are sharpened, the eyes wide and sunken. The typical facies resemble those caused by dehydration, which may also be present. Where there is no dehydration the lips, tongue, and mouth are moist; when the child is dehydrated, which is usually the case when diarrhoea is present, the mouth is dry.

The whole body appears shrunken. The ribs and bony eminences are prominent, the muscles are wasted, and the limbs stick-like. There is usually no oedema. There are no hair changes and often no dermatosis. The abdomen is usually distended, occasionally scaphoid.

The picture is rare in the first few months of life while the child is on the breast. The maximum age incidence is under 18 months.

The child is miserable, whines continuously, and is given to frantic finger-sucking. It usually reaches the clinic only when severely ill and then may survive for months. The appetite is good, maybe ravenous in the early stages; later the child is apathetic and the appetite is completely lost.

Diagnosis depends on appearance and history. The situation of chronic undernutrition may be exacerbated by febrile illness or by heavy gastro-intestinal worm loads.

Total plasma proteins are only slightly reduced, but there is a fall of albumin and nearly always a rise in gamma globulin. The duodenal enzymes, blood sugar, and blood urea are normal. Because of the acute loss of body fat, the proportion of water in the body is high and the plasma volume per kg body weight is correspondingly high.

There are no characteristic autopsy changes, beyond the loss of fat.

Marasmus is difficult to treat and in severe cases the mortality is high. The advanced syndrome requires treatment similar to that for kwashiorkor (see p. 325).

## ENDOGENOUS FOOD POISONING

### EPIDEMIC DROPSY

A condition caused by ingestion of the seeds of the Mexican poppy (*Argemone mexicana*) or their products, particularly in contaminated mustard oil, characterized in severe cases by oedema, vascular dilatation, and cardiac insufficiency.

Epidemic dropsy is seen most commonly in India, particularly in Bengal, where most cases occur in Calcutta, and also in Bihar, Orissa, and Central and United Provinces. It has appeared in Mauritius, Fiji, and South Africa.

The toxic agent is contained in the seeds of *A. mexicana* which grows as a weed amongst edible crops. The seeds are very similar to those of the mustard plant and may be mixed with the latter by accident or deliberately as an adulterant in the manufacture of mustard oil. In the outbreak in South Africa the seeds were found as a contaminant of cheap badly sieved wheat.

In India epidemic dropsy appears amongst rice eaters who use mustard oil for cooking. It is commoner in the middle class than in poor people who cannot always afford mustard oil and have to use substitutes. The incidence varies considerably from year to year. It is highest during the rains or soon after, the maximum occurring in July or August, the minimum in April. The maximum incidence corresponds roughly with the issue of the fresh season's oil.

Breast-fed infants, having no access to mustard oil, are not affected, children under the age of 4 rarely. All other age groups are involved. The sexes are affected equally.

The apparent racial distribution of the condition arises from dietetic habits. Wherever mustard oil can be contaminated, epidemic dropsy may appear.

The syndrome usually appears in groups of individuals on the same diet. Only a few families in scattered districts may be affected, but at irregular intervals there may be serious outbreaks involving large numbers of people.

Various extracts of argemone seeds have been found to have physiological effects resembling some of the features of the syndrome. The toxic factor is an alkaloid called sanguinarine, which interferes with the end stages of carbohydrate metabolism. In this way, sanguinarine poisoning somewhat resembles thiamine deficiency, and epidemic dropsy and wet beriberi are similar enough in clinical features to have been confused in the past. Unfortunately vitamin $B_1$ has no therapeutic activity.

The basic physiological change is a generalized severe vasodilatation affecting capillaries and small vessels, particularly in the skin, heart muscle, and the uveal tract. The early oedema has been explained by increase in capillary permeability; the late oedema results from heart failure.

Irregular formation of new blood vessels is common in many tissues, particularly beneath the skin. In some cases and in some epidemics, but not others, subcutaneous haemangiomata (so-called 'sarcoids') develop which may become pedunculated and bleed freely. Haemorrhage may occasionally occur from mucous membranes. Varying degrees of secondary anaemia may develop, often complicated by the effects of concurrent deficiencies.

Vascular dilatation involving the iris and ciliary body not uncommonly leads to raised intraocular pressure. Optic atrophy develops in untreated severe cases.

At autopsy vascular congestion and dilatation of the skin, the liver, and other organs is notable. In the heart muscle there may be oedema, intense congestion, and considerable new capillary formation. In cases complicated by myocardial insufficiency the characteristic enlarged 'congested' liver develops.

Moderate anaemia develops in severe cases. The cells are normocytic and usually orthochromic.

The volume of urine is often increased. Albumin may be present. The electrolyte concentration is low.

The clinical picture varies widely. It is probable that in many cases the signs are so mild as to be overlooked. In patients in the same feeding group, for instance members of the same family, the syndrome also appears in varying intensity. Some outbreaks are notable for severity; others for mildness. These variations depend to a considerable extent on the dose of toxic agent absorbed.

In most cases the onset is insidious. In severe cases it may be sudden. The patient may give a history of a few days of anorexia, nausea, and looseness or diarrhoea before the onset of oedema. Severe cases begin acutely and may end fatally in a matter of days.

Oedema occurs in all. Other signs vary in incidence and intensity from case to case and from outbreak to outbreak.

The usual moderately severe case complains of weakness, breathlessness on exertion and swelling of the feet and legs. There is often mild fever. Nausea is common and there may be some vomiting. In some patients diarrhoea is a prominent and difficult feature; in others it is absent.

The oedema is soft and easily pitted. It is usually confined to the lower extremities and appears rapidly. In ambulatory patients it becomes worse at the end of the day. Very rarely there may be general anasarca. In severe cases there may be effusions into the pleural cavities and pericardium. Lung oedema may appear in the terminal stages.

The patient's chief concern is usually dyspnoea at rest and this is worsened by exertion. The pulse is fast and thready; the diastolic pressure may be very low. In severe cases the heart is dilated and systolic apical murmurs are common. The electrocardiogram shows signs of myocardial involvement. There may be frequent extrasystoles or sinus tachycardia. In fatal cases signs of acute heart failure develop. The pulse may become irregular and fibrillating. The liver enlarges and becomes tender. Heart failure may develop progressively over a few days, or appear suddenly and lead to a fatal issue.

Peripheral vascular changes are common. Irregular bluish mottling of the skin with dilated vessels may occur. These changes develop a few days after the appearance of the oedema but may be evident from the beginning in acute severe cases.

Subcutaneous telangiectases and haemangiomata appear in some cases. The haemangiomata (the so-called 'sarcoids') develop after the original skin vascular dilatation has subsided and progress steadily to become small tumours up to half an inch across, raised above the surrounding skin and sometimes sessile, which may bleed freely after injury. They gradually reduce in size during convalescence and finally disappear.

In some patients in the acute phase there may be tenderness of the calf muscles, increased or absent knee jerks, and widespread tingling, burning feelings in the skin. Pareses are uncommon, except in the presence of vitamin deficiencies.

One of the most serious complications is the development of glaucoma, which may result in blindness. Evidence of pathologically raised intraocular pressure includes dimness of vision, contraction of visual fields, and subjective rainbow haloes. There is surprisingly little ocular pain.

Abortion or stillbirth is common.

The signs and symptoms in the case of average severity subside on rest in bed. The patient may be little affected so long as he remains at rest, but may suffer exacerbation of the cardiac condition on exertion. Convalescence is slow.

Some cases are very severe from the beginning and fail to respond to treatment, dying in cardiac failure in a few days.

The death rate varies from outbreak to outbreak. It is usually about 5 per cent but may be much higher.

Prognosis largely depends on the cardiac state. It is bad when decompensation has appeared. In some cases severe and even fatal cardiac symptoms may develop during treatment. Prognosis must therefore be guarded in all cases.

The diagnosis is easy in a recognized outbreak. The dietetic history of the patient should give the necessary clue.

The appearance of acute oedema in several members of a family or similar groups known to be using mustard oil is highly suggestive. Cases which begin with diarrhoea may be missed and there may be some confusion with wet beriberi or famine oedema, both of which usually develop more slowly. In beriberi nervous lesions may be prominent and the response to thiamine therapy is usually dramatic. Beriberi may occur concurrently.

The patient is put to rest in bed and given a diet from which the suspected oil or seeds are absent.

A high protein diet with moderate content of fat and carbohydrate is essential.

An initial saline purge is indicated in diarrhoeic cases. Sodium sulphate, 15 mg, is given immediately; 7 mg is given subsequently, as required.

Heart failure may or may not respond to digitalis. In any case this drug should be tried. It is best given in the form of Lanoxin, 250 $\mu$g daily. If unsuccessful a combination of mersalyl and ammonium chloride may be beneficial.

Obvious dietary deficiencies should be corrected. Vitamins B and C are often required to adjust the diet but no immediate response to the former is to be expected. It is probably simpler and equally effective to add yeast or vegetable extracts, cod-liver oil, and citrus fruit. Unlike beriberi, the condition does not respond to parenteral vitamin $B_1$ administration.

In view of the evidence of salt retention the salt intake should be limited during the acute stages.

Haemangiomata do not require treatment unless they bleed, when pressure is usually effective.

Glaucoma may need surgical interference. Pilocarpine is not effective. A careful watch for increased ocular tension should be kept in all patients as the eye changes may appear in apparently mild as well as obviously severe cases.

Public health measures should prevent the use of contaminated oil or wheat and should aim at the extermination of *A. mexicana* and the avoidance of contamination before the mustard oil is processed.

### LATHYRISM

An acute spastic paralysis of sudden onset, associated with weakness, muscular pains, and sometimes incontinence of urine, is a syndrome which has been reported from many countries, and particularly India, Iran, Africa, and the Mediterranean littoral. It occurs among poor people who eat lathyrus peas, and has its highest incidence late in the season when the crop has been stored for some time and also during droughts and famines when malnutrition is rife and the lathyrus crop, a particularly hardy crop, is eaten by more people than usual. It is believed that clinical effects result from the ingestion of a toxin contained in the seeds of the Akta weed, a common contaminant of a lathyrus crop. Treatment is unsatisfactory, but some functional relief may follow administration of vitamins, particularly vitamin A.

### VOMITING SICKNESS OF JAMAICA

This condition occurs only in Jamaica amongst peasants who eat the unripe fruit of the Ackee plant (*Blighia sapida*). The basic pathogenic effect is precipitate hypoglycaemia, apparently arising from a block of gluconeo-genesis, thought to be due to peptides contained in the fruit which have hypoglycaemic effects in animals.

The clinical picture is characteristically seen in children aged 1–10 years, not in breast-fed infants. Attacks may occur in several members of a family at the same time, after eating the fruit, developing some hours afterwards. There are all grades of attack, but two forms of the severe syndrome are recognized: (i) *fulminating*, in which the child collapses, becomes drowsy, does not vomit but goes into convulsions, passes into coma, and dies, and (ii) *acute abrupt*, starting with vomiting without nausea, pain, fever, or diarrhoea, becoming somewhat drowsy and prostrated, then recovering for an hour or so, passing once more into vomiting, convulsions, coma, and death, unless treated.

The child becomes very hypoglycaemic. At autopsy the liver cells are almost completely denuded of glycogen.

Mild cases recover on their own in 48–72 hours; they occur usually in older children and adults. Severe attacks in young children are fatal unless treated; the prognosis depends on the speed of diagnosis and treatment.

The hypoglycaemia responds to sugar replacement. In mild cases where there is no vomiting 50 per cent glucose solution can be given orally. Most cases require intravenous infusion of 50 per cent glucose on the basis of an initial dose of 1 g glucose per kg body weight. Cortisone has been used as an adjuvant by some workers.

The Ackee fruit, which is an important source of food in Jamaica, is not eaten on other Caribbean Islands and is harmless except when unripe. Prevention thus depends entirely on health education.

A somewhat similar clinical syndrome is caused in the U.S.A. by eating the White Snake Root.

### HEPATIC VENO-OCCLUSIVE DISEASE

This occurs in Jamaica and has been reported from Israel and India. In Jamaica, children 1–3 years of age and of poor families are most commonly affected. Older children, and occasionally adults, may also be involved.

The acute stage is characterized by sudden abdominal distension, with slight tenderness over the smooth firm edge of the enlarged liver, which may be palpable anywhere to the level of the umbilicus. Acute ascites is common and there is often some ankle oedema. At this stage the children do not feel very ill and many recover spontaneously or with treatment. Occasionally the syndrome rapidly progresses to fatal hepatic failure. The usual cause of death is haematemesis from varices arising from portal hypertension.

Relapse is common, with moderate liver enlargement associated with recurrent or sometimes persistent ascites; there may be dilated abdominal veins and moderate enlargement of the spleen.

Diagnosis from cirrhosis may be difficult clinically although a history of intermittent subacute attacks is suggestive in the geographical areas concerned. Examination of liver biopsy is usually necessary. The histological picture is one of blocked centrilobular and sublobular veins, with congestion, followed eventually by centrilobular non-portal fibrosis.

Certain herbs which are species of *Senicio* or *Crotolaria* used for beverages or medicines are believed to be responsible for the disease in man and can reproduce the pathological pattern in cattle and rats.

There is no specific treatment. The child should be given a normal diet with normal fluid intake and no added salt. Paracentesis is needed if there is severe ascites and may be repeated when necessary. Diuretics may help to restrict the ascites. Intercurrent infections require treatment. Recovery is usually rapid unless there is already heavy hepatic fibrosis, with varices. In the latter case, a porto-caval shunt may be successful.

# 19

# PLAGUE

DEFINITION

A formerly widespread bacterial disease caused by *Pasteurella pestis*, a primary rodent infection, which is spread to man either by the bite of an infected rodent flea in the case of bubonic plague, or by droplet infection in the case of pneumonic plague.

Plague is a quarantinable disease within the International Health Regulations. In the past it occurred sporadically or in epidemic proportions in congested urban areas as a result of transmission of infection by the fleas of domestic rats. It also occurs in sparsely populated districts amongst those who come into contact with wild rodents which harbour the infection. These infections are commonly called wild plague. The clinical aspects of infection are basically the same whatever the epidemiology.

The clinical course is rapid and the mortality in untreated cases is high.

DISTRIBUTION

Plague is at present widespread in the Socialist Republic of Vietnam as a result of the recent war. It appears sporadically in other tropical and subtropical countries. It is found in small foci in India, Burma, Indonesia, and the Democratic Republic of Kampuchea. Cases have been reported during the last 4 years in Nepal and the Yemen. Plague is reported regularly from Brazil and Peru and has occurred recently in Bolivia and Ecuador. A few cases of wild plague are reported annually from the U.S.A. In Africa it is found in small numbers in Madagascar, Libya, Zaïre, Tanzania and Lesotho. In 1972 cases were reported in Libya and Tanzania. It exists as an enzootic in many countries, including Kenya, Ethiopia, Iran, Nepal, and the U.S.A.

Wild plague occurs, sometimes with associated pneumonic outbreaks, in South-east Russia, Mongolia, North-east China, parts of South Africa including the Transvaal and the Orange Free State, Brazil, Argentina, Peru, Ecuador, and parts of the western U.S.A.

AETIOLOGY

*Causative organism*
Plague is caused by invasion of the tissues by *P. pestis*, a small Gram-negative,

bipolar staining, pleomorphic, non-motile, ovoid, aerobic rod which in the tissues is capsulated. *P. pestis* is very sensitive to heat and direct sunlight. It does not normally survive long outside the body although it will persist for a few days in sputum or dust under cool moist conditions and sometimes for weeks in flea faeces. It survives freezing for longer periods.

Permanent immunity is usually conferred by an attack of plague. Second attacks have occasionally been reported.

*P. pestis* produces a powerful toxin which is believed to be concerned with some of the more serious general effects, especially the central nervous system syndromes. It has been noted in Vietnam that in occasional cases which have apparently not responded to antibiotic therapy although the organisms have been eliminated, suggesting that death may have resulted from toxaemia and possibly Herxheimer reaction.

### Transmission

Plague is naturally an enzootic in a wide group of rodents. It is normally transmitted from rodent to rodent by fleas.

Man may be infected in two ways: (i) through the infected flea (or occasionally the louse or the bed bug) and (ii) through droplet infection spreading from cases of pneumonic plague.

### (i) *Transmission by the flea*

*The common vectors.* Human plague depends for transmission principally upon rat fleas, of which *Xenopsylla cheopis* is the most efficient vector and *X. braziliensis* and *X. astia* much less efficient. The human flea *Pulex irritans* is difficult to infect with *P. pestis* but may occasionally be concerned in transmission. The fleas of cats and dogs and of the rodent reservoirs of sylvatic plague do not readily bite man, but may become infected and transmit plague if they do.

*The mechanism of infection through the flea.* Plague bacilli may be passed in the flea faeces and rubbed into the tissues through skin abrasions or the flea bite. They may also be carried directly on the mouth parts of the flea after previous biting of an infective source. By far the commonest mode of spread, however, depends on the blocking of the proventriculus of the infected flea by rapidly multiplying bacteria. The blocking makes ingestion of blood impossible and the flea becomes hungry and tries repeatedly to feed. Its efforts are rewarded only by regurgitation of blood and bacteria. In this way a single flea, although it lives for only a day or two after blocking, may bite many times and disseminate plague organisms much more widely than a normal flea.

The uninfected rat flea lives as long as 1–2 years in suitable conditions. Survival is longest in a relatively cool moist environment. Hot dry conditions are rapidly fatal.

Unblocked infected fleas do not usually survive for longer than a fortnight.

Under suitable circumstances (e.g. in rat nests), they may remain alive for months and so carry the infection over from one season to another.

(ii) *Droplet infection*
It is probable that the origin of an outbreak of pneumonic plague is a patient infected in the ordinary way by the flea and in whom pulmonary complications have developed. Once established, pneumonic plague spreads from subject to subject by droplet infection. Cold or freezing conditions with relatively high humidity favour droplet spread. Further spread is facilitated by congestion of population and intimate contact between healthy and infected subjects.

EPIDEMIOLOGICAL FORMS

Plague exists in two main epidemiological forms, *urban* and *wild*. The mechanisms of transmission differ somewhat in these two forms but the basic factors are essentially the same.

*The spread of urban plague*
Plague existing as an enzootic in wild rodents is accidentally transmitted to commensal rodents, which largely depend on man for their food supplies and are consequently found in villages, towns, and cities. The rat most commonly involved is the semi-domesticated brown rat *Rattus norvegicus*. The latter dies and infected fleas leave it and migrate to and infect the domestic rat, *R. rattus*. When this in turn dies (in the course of a few days) the infected fleas feed on man and plague appears. The mouse *Mus musculus* may occasionally be similarly involved.

Sporadic cases occur from time to time in this manner so long as the disease remains as an enzootic in the reservoir animals. When it becomes an epizootic, and other conditions are suitable, the disease eventually appears in man in epidemic proportions. The epizootic precedes (usually by some weeks) the epidemic and is commonly indicated by a high rodent mortality. When the rat population has been suitably reduced, the epidemic spread stops. The pattern of an epidemic of plague which is not medically controlled is thus a slow beginning, a rapid rise (as the epizootic develops), and an abrupt fall after some months.

Dispersion from district to district may occur as the result of extension of an existing enzootic or epizootic. Enforced spread of this nature as a result of warfare is regarded as the principal explanation of the recent tremendous upsurge of plague in Vietnam.

Sporadic cases may result in some districts from migration of infected rats, particularly in ships, without the involvement of the local rodent population. Plague has sometimes been spread by the carriage of infected fleas in merchandise and clothing.

Ambulatory cases may carry the disease to new areas and lead to infection of local rodents. This has occurred in Vietnam.

*The spread of wild plague*

Plague persists in certain sparsely populated or rural districts as an enzootic in wild rodents. In these districts it appears sporadically in man, especially amongst people whose work brings them into contact with the reservoir animals. Occasionally it appears in epidemic proportions.

The enzootic is kept going by flea transmission from rodent to rodent. Man may acquire the infection by dissecting or skinning infected wild animals and becoming directly infected through cuts and scratches on the skin or being bitten by their fleas.

Epidemics occasionally arise as in urban plague when semi-domestic rats become infected after contact with wild rodents and convey the infection via fleas to domestic rats. This usually happens during an epizootic amongst the reservoir animals but epizootics probably often occur without epidemic spread.

Unlike the domestic rat, wild rodents may migrate considerable distances and carry plague with them, infecting fresh rodents in new localities. In this way the disease may appear sporadically over very wide areas.

*Factors influencing the spread of plague*

Once the domestic rat has become infected, plague will spread rapidly wherever the human population is excessive and living in insanitary conditions in which rats abound and have easy access to food.

The flea population is very sensitive to climatic conditions and since only relatively few fleas on any given rat become capable of transmitting the infection, factors which limit the number of fleas are often important in determining the spread of the infection in man.

In temperate climates the disease is commoner in summer and autumn when the fleas are most numerous. In the tropics it appears mostly in the cooler weather or during periods of high humidity.

Plague has appeared in regions as high as 2135 m above sea level.

All ages and either sex may be affected. There is no racial immunity.

The incidence of plague varies greatly from year to year in a given area. When conditions have remained unfavourable for the flea for several seasons the incidence in the following year is likely to be low.

Spread to man depends very largely on the closeness of the association of semi-domesticated and domesticated rats once the former are infected. In areas in which the domesticated rat has been largely ousted by the less domesticated brown rat, the spread of plague is considerably reduced, and may practically cease.

## PATHOLOGY

The pathology of plague is non-specific. There is a vigorous but usually unsuccessful inflammatory reaction to the organism, which is accompanied by varying degrees of toxic tissue damage, especially to the endothelial lining of the lymphatics and blood vessels.

In bubonic plague there may be a local lesion at the site of infection, appearing first as a vesicle, later becoming a focus of necrotic inflammation. this is usually inconspicuous.

The bubo forms in the lymph glands draining the point of infection. These glands enlarge rapidly and become matted together in oedematous haemorrhagic connective tissue and may ultimately suppurate. The changes in the glands are essentially inflammatory. The blood vessels are intensely congested; there may be haemorrhages into the substance; there is a massive cellular inflammatory infiltration. Small necrotic foci form and may coalesce to become abscesses eventually discharging to the surface. The affected glands contain enormous numbers of bacilli. In most cases the infection reaches the blood-stream and all organs may become involved. There is generalized vasodilatation, notably in the liver and spleen, both of which enlarge, become congested, and may contain scattered areas of focal necrosis and haemorrhage.

The heart muscle is frequently involved, the tissue becoming oedematous, haemorrhagic, and infiltrated with inflammatory cells. A haemorrhagic pericardial effusion commonly develops.

The lungs may be seriously involved. There may be acute oedema, congestion and haemorrhage into alveoli and small bronchioles, and patches of haemorrhagic consolidation which may coalesce to involve most of a lobe. The affected pulmonary tissue is swarming with bacilli, which are found in the watery, blood-stained or frankly haemorrhagic fluid which partly fills the bronchi and even the trachea. In primary pneumonic plague similar pulmonary lesions develop as the result of inhalation of infective droplets. A bacterial bronchiolitis and alveolitis is set up and extends to become bronchopneumonia and finally lobular consolidation. The bacilli multiply locally in enormous numbers leading to early and severe toxaemia and bacteraemia. The pulmonary lymph glands and contiguous tissues become involved within a few hours; the lesions resemble those of the characteristic bubo but are less intense. Lesions in other organs may appear, similar to those seen in bubonic plague, but death may occur so quickly that these may not develop.

Early prostration, stupor and delirium indicate involvement of the central nervous system, but necropsy does not always reveal concomitant physical damage to the brain which is, however, usually congested and often spotted with petechial haemorrhages. The cerebrospinal fluid may be turbid, containing many neutrophils. Occasionally, there may be a frank pasteurella meningitis, which rarely occurs as a primary lesion.

## CLINICAL PICTURE

The clinical pattern of plague varies. There is serological evidence that asymptomatic infections occur in endemic areas and during outbreaks. A few cases may be so mild as to pass practically unnoticed. There may be merely a small vesicle and light inflammatory reaction at the site of the infected bite, with no constitutional disturbance at all; there may be some local adenitis which persists without general symptoms for a few days or weeks before resolving. Such mild cases are usually called *Pestis minor* or ambulatory plague. Most cases are seriously ill and without treatment the mortality is very high. Plague is commonly classified as bubonic, septicaemic, or pneumonic depending respectively upon whether (i) the processes are limited to the glands draining the flea-bite, (ii) the dominant feature is active bacteraemia, with or without localizing signs, or (iii) the infection is primarily in the lungs following introduction of the organisms via the respiratory tract. The modern tendency is to distinguish only two forms, the bubonic and primary pneumonic. There is evidence that in practically all cases bacteraemia without multiplication of the organisms occurs as a transitory phenomenon, reappearing later in appropriate context as a true septicaemia, with massive multiplication of the organisms. So-called 'primary septicaemia' cases are probably examples of this secondary bacteraemia in which deep-seated buboes have been overlooked or in which the gland reaction has been inconspicuous. There may be some inflammation about the original flea bite, where a small pustule occasionally develops. Such local reactions are seldom severe and are in any case inconspicuous in comparison with the reaction in the glands draining the area.

*Bubonic plague*
The majority of cases develop a bubo in the regional lymph glands draining the area infected. There is commonly only one bubo, but there may occasionally be more.

The incubation period ranges from 2 to 10 days; the commonest period is 3–6 days. Prodromal symptoms consist of headache, backache, malaise, and apathy.

The onset is sudden, with a moderately severe rigor or a series of shivering attacks. There may be convulsions in children. In the course of the first day the temperature rises to 39.4–40° C or higher. The temperature remains elevated and remittent for the next 2–5 days and then falls slowly or suddenly, the fall of temperature usually corresponding to the full development of the bubo. Suppuration and secondary infection of the latter causes a later return of fever.

The general appearance of the patient is characteristic. In the early stages he is dull, apathetic, and confused. He may become extremely apprehensive and complain of backache, headache, muscle pains, vertigo, and increasing prostration; the gait is unsteady. From then onwards, the overall appearance is one of advancing stupor and prostration. The speech may be slurred, there may be muscular tremor and twitching.

The skin is hot and dry. There is general blotchy vasodilatation, especially notable in the face. The conjunctivae are congested. There may be petechial haemorrhages in the skin. Large or small subcutaneous haemorrhages may be prominent in some outbreaks, especially on the trunk. Occasionally patches of skin may become necrotic, suppurate, and form abscesses; purpura sometimes develops and may be associated with local dry gangrene, usually of the extremities.

The tongue is dry and sometimes swollen. The surface may become covered with a dark grey or black coating. Sordes is common.

The pulse in the febrile stage is fast. It may become almost uncountable in the late stages.

In severe cases the heart dilates and death may result from cardiac failure. The blood pressures are often low and vascular failure may supervene terminally, in which case the diastolic pressure may be unmeasurable. The respiratory rate is fast at the onset and may increase as the disease develops. There may be some epigastric pain, nausea, and sometimes vomiting.

The spleen is moderately enlarged and tender. There is usually some polymorphonuclear leucocytosis.

As the condition progresses the mental dullness often gives way to anxiety and restlessness and the patient may become highly excited and even maniacal. On the other hand, the lethargy may deepen and coma eventually develop.

*The bubo.* Extreme local pain and tenderness at the site of the developing bubo are commonly present from the onset, even before the swelling appears. In most cases the bubo appears on the first or second day after the onset of fever. In some it may be the first sign of illness. It takes 2–5 days to reach full size. The affected gland or glands are at first hard and painful and swell rapidly. Their position depends on the site of infection. In over 70 per cent of cases the bite is on the leg and the groin glands are involved; the axillary glands are affected in about 20 per cent. The bubo is very painful and tender. The skin over it is erythematous and hot; the surrounding subcutaneous tissues are infiltrated, oedematous, and sometimes haemorrhagic. Because of the pain the patient adopts a characteristic attitude in an attempt at relief. When the bubo is in the groin he lies on the other side, with the knee flexed and the thigh drawn up; when it is in the axilla the arm is abducted and extended.

The affected glands are not discrete but are matted together. After reaching full development they either recede or suppurate. Suppuration usually occurs early in the second week. It leads to pointing and discharge of *P. pestis* infected pus. Secondary infection is almost inevitable and chronic indolent ulcers or sinuses are often left after otherwise complete recovery. Occasionally large vessels may be eroded and lead to severe haemorrhage. After recovery from plague the patient may die from the results of the local sepsis.

*Course and prognosis*

The course of bubonic plague is short. Without treatment from 30 to 90 per cent of cases die in an average outbreak. Most deaths occur before the fifth day. The outcome depends to a large extent on the degree of secondary septicaemia. Progressive severe septicaemia is indicated by a general worsening of the condition and often by a generalized moderate lymphadenitis. Occasionally plague 'carbuncles' (secondary buboes) may develop as a result of metastatic spread. A sudden fall of temperature about the time the bubo matures is regarded as a bad prognostic sign. In many patients there appear to be irregular bursts of septicaemia but once the local lymphatic barrier has been passed serious lesions may develop particularly in the liver and heart.

*Septicaemic fulminant cases*

As noted above, a primary septicaemia is always present in bubonic plague, followed later by increasing blood infection in the more serious cases. It is sometimes regarded as a primary syndrome, particularly if infection enters through the respiratory system. In such cases death occurs within 1–3 days, before bubonic or pneumonic evidence of infection can fully develop. The onset is sudden with rigor and high fever and severe headache. The patient is prostrated. Restless and anxious at first, he becomes delirious and soon stuporose or comatose. Signs of heart involvement develop quickly and the pulse becomes very fast. There may be severe haemorrhage into the gastrointestinal tract, or from visible mucous membranes.

*Pneumonic plague*

In the terminal stages of bubonic plague, pulmonary complications may appear which are similar to those described below. The term 'pneumonic plague', however, is usually reserved for those cases in which the pneumonic involvement originates from the inhalation of infective material and in which the lung is the primary site of invasion.

The onset occurs abruptly 2 or 3 days after exposure. Prodromata are rare. Rigor is usually absent but there may be early chilly feelings and some shivering. The patient complains at first of headache, backache, and anorexia. The temperature rises to 39.4 or 40° C or higher in the first 24 hours, after which clinical signs of pulmonary involvement appear. A frequent and initially painless and non-productive cough develops and the patient becomes increasingly dyspnoeic. The sputum is at first mucoid or watery; it rapidly becomes tinged with blood and finally bright red or brown, frothy, and loaded with plague bacilli. Pain in the chest becomes severe and breathing more and more rapid and difficult, the patient gasping for breath as the pneumonic process develops. Towards the end there is often considerable cyanosis. The physical signs in the chest are equivocal; there may be fine râles at the bases, some dullness on percussion. X-ray shows rapidly progressive infiltration eventually involving the whole lung fields. Signs of heart involvement are always early and severe. The heart dilates, the dullness extending to the right. The blood pressures fall, the pulse rate quickens and may be almost uncountable. Death occurs usually in 1–3 days, rarely longer.

Bacilli are present in the blood from the beginning, sometimes in relatively large numbers. There is always a considerable polymorphonuclear leucocytosis with a white count of 40,000 cells or more per mm$^3$.

Vascular damage is usually evident. Haemorrhages from the mucous membranes, epistaxis, haemoptysis, haematuria, and widely scattered petechiae or larger haemorrhages into the skin may occur.

Without specific treatment pneumonic plague is almost invariably fatal. Modern chemotherapeutic methods have greatly changed the outlook.

### COMPLICATIONS

Abortion is to be expected in untreated pregnant women.

In septicaemic cases meningismus is common and sometimes frank infection of the cerebrospinal spaces occurs leading to meningitis clinically indistinguishable from other acute forms. There are pus cells and *P. pestis* in the fluid, which is under pressure.

Death from cardiac failure may occur in early convalescence.

### DIAGNOSIS

The clinical diagnosis of bubonic plague is of great importance. It should be easy during a known outbreak and plague should always be regarded as a possibility in cases of adenitis in an endemic area. In any case a geographical history is essential since exposed individuals may be carried by jet far away from the area of exposure during the incubation period. The sudden onset with high fever, prostration, and toxaemia, especially affecting the central nervous system and heart are suggestive. Before establishment of the bubo, or in primary septicaemic cases, diagnosis may be very difficult and confusion may arise especially with typhus.

In mild cases the bubo may be mistaken for lymphogranuloma or other forms of adenitis. Bacteriological examination of the gland juice should settle the diagnosis.

Rapid, if tentative, diagnosis may be possible by identification of characteristic pleomorphic bipolar organisms in smears (stained with Giemsa or Gram) of juice taken by syringe aspiration from the bubo in its early stages. In septicaemic cases the bacilli may sometimes be numerous enough to show in a blood film. Pus from more advanced buboes may not show *P. pestis* clearly.

In primary pneumonic plague the diagnosis should be confirmed by examination of the sputum which swarms with *P. pestis.*

Laboratory aids to diagnosis may be a great help in so far as the community is concerned but, because of the time necessary to carry them out, may be of little value to the individual case.

The examination of dead or trapped rats is nevertheless most important in the control of plague. The animal to be examined should first be immersed in disinfectant solution in order to destroy its ectoparasites. The post-mortem changes of plague are characteristic. There is diffuse intense subcutaneous congestion and ecchymosis. Lymphatic glands, particularly those in the neck and groin, are usually enlarged and necrotic. The serous cavities may contain blood-stained fluid. The liver is large, pale, and peppered with small greyish necrotic areas. The spleen is large, deeply congested, and may show scattered small necrotic foci. The lungs are congested, oedematous, and may contain similar foci.

Material from the infected source—the bubo, blood, sputum—is spread on blood agar and on desoxycholate agar for bacteriological examination.

All organs are teeming with bacilli which are easily seen in smears stained by Grams's method.

Bacteriological confirmation of the nature of the organism is necessary to distinguish it from *P. pseudo-tuberculosis*. This can be had in a few days by bacteriological culture using blood or material aspirated from a bubo. A volume of 5 ml blood should be injected into 25 ml nutrient broth which should then be incubated for 48–72 hours at 37° C. Material obtained by syringe from an enlarged gland into which an equivalent volume (0.5 ml) of sterile saline has been injected may be added to broth and should be examined by direct smears stained with Giemsa. Pus should be treated the same way.

Alternatively, suspected material may be rubbed on to the shaved belly of a guinea-pig. Subcutaneous inoculation of a suspension of ground-up fleas from a suspected rat may also infect the guinea-pig. The animal will die in 3–5 days if plague is present. Blood, bubo aspirates and other clinical material may be sent from remote areas to a laboratory in a so-called holding medium for bacteriological examination, culture and animal inoculation. The autopsy picture is similar to that seen in rats dead of plague.

Bacteriological investigation should be undertaken only under insect-proof laboratory conditions.

Antibodies to the capsule of the plague bacillus (Fraction 1 antigen) can be detected in the serum of patients late in the infection and in convalescence by complement fixation and passive haemagglutination tests. Serological diagnosis is of no immediate value, but is useful retrospectively and in special circumstances for epidemiological surveys including detection of animal reservoirs.

### TREATMENT

The patient should be nursed in bed. Good nursing is a very important part of treatment, especially if the heart is involved. Exertion should be avoided as far as possible until well into convalescence since myocardial inefficiency often persists for some time after the acute illness. The skin requires particular attention where petechial or subcutaneous haemorrhages are present.

Symptomatic treatment may include morphine for restlessness or local pain at the site of the bubo. Fomentation may considerably ease such pain and assist the pointing of an abscess. Incision and drainage of the bubo is not advisable until pointing has occurred; such interference may initiate septicaemia.

Chemotherapy is now very effective and has greatly reduced the mortality, especially in bubonic and pneumonic plague. In Vietnam the mortality rate for untreated bubonic plague ranges from 40–70 per cent, and for pneumonic plague is practically 100 per cent. With prompt specific treatment the fatility rate has fallen to about 5 per cent in bubonic plague and to about the same figure in pneumonic, provided the case is treated within the first 24 hours (for instance, in contacts under observation). Cases seen later in pneumonic plague are usually moribund and cannot be saved by therapy.

The most effective drugs are streptomycin and the tetracyclines. Certain of the sulphonamides, including sulphadiazine and sulphadimidine, are successful in the treatment of contacts of bubonic or pneumonic plague and are useful substitutes for antibiotics when these are not available. Where streptomycin-resistant strains of *Pasteurella* have been reported, tetracycline is effective. Antiplague serum has no place as an adjuvant to chemotherapy.

Specific therapy should be instituted immediately the diagnosis is suspected and must not wait on bacteriological confirmation.

*Streptomycin.* 1 g should be given intramuscularly twice, thrice, or four times daily, depending on the clinical severity of the case, up to a total of 20 g.

*Tetracycline.* The total dose for the adult should be 40 g. The dosage regime should vary according to the clinical condition of the patient. A common dosage schedule in a case of average severity is 500 mg orally 4-hourly until the fever subsides, then 6-hourly. In very severe cases dosages of up to 6 g daily have been given.

Chloramphenicol is active but is seldom used.

*Streptomycin* in doses as above has been combined successfully with *sulphadimidine* in doses of 3 g immediately, followed by 1 g 4-hourly for up to 7 days.

Insensitivity to streptomycin has been suspected in some cases but not fully confirmed. No insensitivity to tetracyclines or to sulphonamides has been detected.

Secondary infections usually react to the tetracyclines, but may require other antibiotics, such as penicillin (inactive against plague).

## Control

*The case.* As far as possible sporadic cases of flea-borne plague should be isolated in hospital. When cases are numerous, they may be successfully treated in their own homes provided immediate measures against fleas and rats are instituted.

Bodies of patients and rats should be handled with care by suitably clothed attendants (gowns, boots, gloves, masks, and caps) and either burned or buried in quick-lime.

Pneumonic cases must be isolated. They should be attended by a minimal nursing and medical staff who must wear protective clothing and face masks.

Overalls, gloves, masks, and caps are advisable during the treatment of all plague cases. DDT-impregnated clothing reduces the risk of flea bite, since fleas cease to be active within 10 minutes of exposure to the insecticide.

*Contacts.* The other occupants of a dwelling in which flea-borne plague has occurred should be regarded as contacts exposed to infective flea bite. They should be given chemoprophylactic treatment as below, and watched for clinical signs.

All those who have been exposed to a case of pneumonic plague are regarded as contacts in considerable risk to themselves and their associates. It has been the practice to isolate them separately if possible or otherwise in groups, and watch them for at least a week, removing for further strict isolation and treatment any who show signs of illness.

Recent successful prophylaxis of contacts with tetracycline or sulphonamides indicates that such antisocial measures are not necessary and that chemoprophylaxis alone may be sufficient.

All those exposed to any form of plague should be given tetracycline, 500 mg 6-hourly for a week, or sulphadimidine, 6 g daily for 3–7 days after intimate contact or 3 g daily for a week for others.

Contacts with pneumonic plague are treated similarly and must be watched, taking the oral temperature 4-hourly, and given a full course of therapy if any signs develop.

*Vaccination.* A considerable degree of personal protection may be obtained with dead or attenuated living vaccines of *P. pestis.* Vaccination is recommended for individuals at risk to infection. Currently, dead vaccines are preferred because of difficulties in handling and transporting the attenuated vaccines. Severe local and sometimes general reactions often follow vaccination. Single dose mass vaccination during epidemics probably lowers the attack rate. Vaccinated individuals appear to respond better to chemotherapy than unvaccinated. "Booster" doses are given every 6 months, so long as exposure continues.

*Control of rats and vectors.* Flea control by all available methods including dusting infested areas with DDT, etc., should be carried out immediately plague has appeared. Resistance to DDT is unfortunately common, but fleas are sensitive to most other insecticides. This will check the spread of plague but not eradicate it.

Rat control is essential and must be carried on continuously by poisoning, trapping, protection of food, and improvement of sanitation. Routine examination of rats for evidence of plague should be instituted in every likely endemic area.

In urban areas such control is manageable with trained personnel. It is difficult in rural areas, for which mobile teams are sometimes prepared.

# 20

# RABIES

### DEFINITION

Rabies, or hydrophobia, is a condition due to infection with the rabies virus. The disease affects a wide variety of warm-blooded animals and birds, but is primarily one of carnivores; infection in man nowadays is usually acquired from the domestic dog. Rabies in man is characterized by a variable, but usually long, incubation period and by an extremely short course which ends fatally once symptoms develop.

### GEOGRAPHICAL DISTRIBUTION

Rabies occurs in many areas in Africa, the Middle East, the East and South-east Asia, Central and South America. It is also present in many countries of Europe, especially West Germany and France, and appears occasionally in western country districts of the U.S.A. and Canada. It does not exist in Australia, the Pacific Islands, the Atlantic Islands, or the United Kingdom, where a system of rigid quarantine for 6 months for all rabies-susceptible animals is enforced. Dogs, cats, and other pets which have been given a course of prophylactic vaccination are all subject to quarantine.

The usual reservoir, so far as transmission to man is concerned, is the domestic dog, less commonly the cat. In parts of Central and South America and the Caribbean, the reservoir is sometimes the vampire bat. In rural areas of Europe the reservoir and sometimes the transmitters are wild animals, especially the fox and the wolf. In India mongooses and jackals and, in Africa, hyenas, are important carriers.

### AETIOLOGY

*The virus*

The causal agent is a neurotropic virus which can be grown only in nerve tissue. The virus particles are large, measuring 120–300 μm in length and up to 80 μm in diameter. The nucleoprotein is RNA. Rabies virus can be cultured in living tissue culture media containing mouse or chick brain, and in the developing chick embryo chorio-allantoic membrane. It is readily destroyed by antiseptics, by heat, by sunlight, and by ultraviolet irradiation; it withstands desiccation, especially when in the frozen state. It survives for weeks at 4° C, and for months at temperatures below freezing; when dried and stored *in*

347

*vacuo* it survives for years. In neutral glycerol at room temperatures it remains viable for weeks, and at 4° C for months.

Agglutinin absorption tests, and a study of antigenic structure, suggest that all strains of the virus are of common origin. It is probable that the virus undergoes changes in virulence and infectivity with changes in the mammalian host and the speed of its transference. Rapid passage increases the speed of multiplication of the virus in the brain but usually diminishes its tendency to invade the salivary glands. Abnormally virulent strains of virus commonly cause a paralytic form of the disease with a diminished tendency of the infected animal to bite; this reduces the opportunity for their transmission. Many named strains of rabies virus showing individual peculiarities have been maintained and investigated in laboratories throughout the world. Though there are antigenic variations between them, these variations appear to be quantitative rather than qualitative.

### Reservoirs

In highly developed and urbanized countries the domestic dog is the usual reservoir of rabies infection; in the less developed and more primitive regions rabies is primarily a disease of wild animals. All common mammals may become infected, including the fox, jackal, and hyena, and dogs may play a minor role in its maintenance and spread. In the spreading enzootics of Europe, in which man is occasionally involved, the fox has been the principal reservoir, and has been responsible for introducing the infection from northern Baltic countries across to France and, particularly, West Germany. So far, the infection has not been implanted into Britain, but this could be a matter of time and failure to control the smuggling of infected pets, especially dogs, into the country. With the travels of man and his dogs rabies has comparatively recently been introduced to many previously uninfected parts of the world. For example, it has become established by this means in the continents of North and of South America. Here at first enzootic in the domestic dog, it has spread to the wild animal populations which now form the main reservoirs of the infection in these regions; the same applies to South Africa. It has been established that in hibernating animals infected with rabies the progress of the disease is suspended. This is a further means of 'reservoiring' the infection.

In Mexico, Central, and South America a paralytic disease in the form of an ascending myelitis, now known to be rabies, has long been extant in cattle and other domestic livestock. Its incidence has not been affected by control of the dog population; there is no epidemiological relationship between it and the usual canine rabies. The infection is conveyed by the blood-sucking vampire bats peculiar to these regions. The bat, *Desmodus rotundus*, feeds nocturnally by incising the skin of recumbent and sleeping animals, including man, and lapping blood which escapes from the wound. This paralytic form of rabies appeared in Trinidad some years ago and human beings were infected. The numerous uncontrolled pariah dogs in the island were free from infection. The outbreak was blamed on the migration of infected bats from the mainland or from unidentified animals, such as introduced Indian Mongooses, which in Puerto Rico and Grenada, were found to be infected.

A feature of the rabies infection in bats was that a proportion of them could transmit the infection in their salivary secretion for months as symptomless carriers; some of them subsequently even became infectious without manifesting signs of illness. Others, however, when infected showed abnormalities in behaviour, such as flying by day and fighting, and subsequently died of the disease.

It has been found that rabies infection occurs also in other bats—fruit eating and insectivorous—in association with infected vampire bats. Presumably it was transmitted to them by the rabic vampires; but these other bats also have attacked mammals as a result of their disease and infected them. Lately, many species of insectivorous bats in Florida have been shown to be rabid; some cases of rabidity in mammals have resulted from attack by them. Infected bats of various species have also been found in Louisana, Texas, California, and others of the southern U.S.A. Still more recently, insectivorous and fructivorous bats elsewhere, notably in Yugoslavia, have been found to harbour rabies.

What is disconcerting is the report on the deaths of two men from rabies after a stay in bat-infested caves in Texas without evidence of their being attacked or bitten by bats or by arthropods. In subsequent experiments various animals in these caves confined in cages proofed against arthropods and bats developed rabies, presumably by air-borne infection.

### Infectivity

Though the saliva of an animal suffering from rabies may be infective it does not follow that all bitten by the animal contract the disease. In a recorded instance, many persons were bitten in rapid succession by a single rabid dog, and only a few contracted the disease. Statistics show that of some thousands of persons bitten by subsequently proven rabid animals, and unprotected by vaccine treatment, only 5–15 per cent contracted rabies.

## PATHOLOGY

### Infection and spread

The virus as a rule is introduced into a wound or abrasion of the skin contaminated by the saliva of an animal suffering from the disease. It enters the small nerves in the immediate vicinity and, by diffusion or multiplication, spreads along the nerves and up the appropriate nerve trunks. The infection ascends the peripheral nerve trunk to the spinal cord and brain, where it diffuses in the central nervous system and spreads centrifugally down the nerves to nerve terminals and ganglia in various organs. If those organs are secretory the secretions may be infective when infected ganglion cells are shed into them; this would explain the infectivity of saliva.

*Morbid pathology*

Post-mortem examination of cadavers of men and dogs dying of rabies shows no gross characteristic changes. There is a diffuse meningo-encephalitis, with oedema and hyperaemia, and there may be small haemorrhages throughout the central nervous system. On histological examination there is some perivascular infiltration and there are collections of proliferating neuroglia cells and of lymphocytes and plasma cells around ganglion cells in the central nervous system and in the sympathetic ganglia. The ganglion cells are swollen and vacuolated, their nuclei are eccentric, and the affected cells disintegrate. The extent of these changes varies greatly; in cases of short duration they may be very slight.

*Negri bodies*

These are inclusions found in the cytoplasm of nerve cells of animals dying of rabies. In man they are most numerous in Ammon's horn, the cerebrum, bulb, and cord; they may also be seen in endoneurocytes in the sensory fibres of the trigeminal and the sympathetic nerves of the face. In dogs the hippocampus is the classical site in which to seek them, but they occur elsewhere in the brain and in the ganglionic nerve cells of the body.

Negri bodies are seen best in smears of brain rather than in histological sections. They are rounded oxyphil bodies which stain readily with eosin, fuchsin, Giemsa's stain, iron–alum–haematoxylin, and various special stains. they range in size from 2 to 25 $\mu$m; the longer the duration of the disease before death the larger they are. The larger bodies contain basophilic nucleus-like granules. Negri bodies are found in the brains of nearly all dogs allowed to die naturally of a street virus infection; they are usually seen in humans dying of rabies; they are only exceptionally found in animals dying of a fixed virus infection. The brains of rabid dogs killed prematurely may not contain them but may nevertheless contain the virus.

### CLINICAL PICTURE

*Incubation*

The incubation period varies greatly; usually symptoms appear between the fifth and eighth week. It is the amount of virus and the tissue into which it is introduced which govern the length of the incubation period. In the experimental disease the incubation period varies inversely with the amount of active virus inoculated and bears no direct relation to the site of the inoculation. The short incubation period following bites on the head and face, or hands, is probably due to severe laceration occurring in well-innervated regions; thus a large amount of virus enters the wound and gets into nerve tissues.

*Furious rabies*

The onset of rabies is sudden; there may be a prodromal period lasting 2–3 days with malaise, nausea, vomiting, a sore throat, and slight fever. The patient then complains of headache and insomnia and, very often, of pain at the site of the infecting bite; this latter is the first symptom of diagnostic significance. He soon becomes uneasy, restless, and a prey to anxiety; the breathing is rapid, with sighing respirations. He is well orientated and while his attention is fixed the speech is normal; then anxiety overcomes him and his speech comes in rushes; he recovers with a sigh and there is a period of calm. The attacks quickly become more frequent, intense, and spasmodic; the pharynx, larynx, and eventually the whole respiratory apparatus, become involved in them; extremely painful spasms are precipitated by attempts to eat or drink, and the patient becomes afraid to swallow. As the spasms intensify even the thought of drinking induces them, as do external stimuli such as sudden movement, a draught of air, a sound, or even a smell. A thick ropy mucus collects in the mouth and throat, and drips from the mouth between attempts to expectorate it. The voice is hoarse and raucous.

As the spasms become generalized convulsive seizures occur; during them the body is arched and rigid and the breath is held. There may be maniacal or 'furious' periods, particularly in manual workers of low intelligence, in which the patient throws himself about and destroys things within reach. During the intervals between the spasms the mind is clear. The reflexes are increased; palsies of groups of muscles may cause lack of expression, a squint, and inability to close the mouth or eyes; there is usually a rapid resting pulse rate, but sometimes bradycardia; Cheyne–Stokes breathing is usual.

Death commonly takes place during a severe general spasm; but if the patient survives the stage of excitement the muscle spasms cease, he becomes quiet, falling into a state of apathy, stupor, and coma. This is soon followed by progressive paralysis, until death occurs. The duration of the illness rarely exceeds 10 days in those infected from dogs, and commonly is no more than 4–5 days.

*Paralytic rabies*
Rarely, the stage of excitement and spasm does not appear or is slight and ephemeral, and depression and progressive paralysis are the predominant manifestations. In such cases the onset usually appears as sudden weakness in an extremity; the usual difficulty in swallowing occurs only terminally. In the human cases of rabies following infection from bats in Trinidad, most primary infections were in the toes. There was an ascending paralysis associated with nerve root pains. An unusual feature of this outbreak was the survival of some of the patients for over 2 weeks, and in one case for 30 days, after the onset of the paralysis.

*Rabies in the dog*
Human rabies in practice is so closely connected with rabies in the domestic dog, that it is important for the physician to recognize rabidity in the dog.

There is evidence that apparently healthy dogs may have rabies virus in saliva which can cause virulent rabies in man, but as a rule rabies in the dog assumes one of two forms: dumb or furious. These occur in about equal numbers. With dumb rabies the dog suffers difficulty in swallowing ('chicken bone in the throat'); it rarely bites; it is lethargic and hides; it dies within 3 or 4 days from a rapidly progressing paralysis. Dumb rabies is not of great significance in the further spread of the infection.

In the early stages of furious rabies a dog may behave normally for some hours at a time. The signs are restlessness, anorexia, and a tendency to hide; an altered appetite, shown by swallowing pieces of wood, straw, stone, and other indigestible objects; and a tendency to bite living and inanimate objects with a deliberate noiseless snapping. Spasms occur which are of the jaw type, manifested by seizing in the mouth anything within reach during the spasm; and of the stomach type, with a spasm of the abdominal muscles often induced by attempts to eat or drink. These spasms end with a violent respiratory effort and the expulsion of greenish or bloody frothy mucus from the mouth, a curious barking sound, and profuse salivation. There is continuous or intermittent panting, with a lolling, dry, brick-red or brown tongue; suffusion of the eyes, which are staring and may squint; and a pawing action at the mouth as if to dislodge a foreign body from the teeth. Finally the limbs and the jaw become paralysed, there is a fall in the respiration rate, and the animal dies, usually within 10 days of the onset of illness. The tendency to bite persists right up to death. Not all of these symptoms are evident at any one time, but most of them will be noted if the animal is closely watched over some days. The saliva of the dog may be infective for a few days before clinical signs appear and remains infective until and after death. In some dogs with furious rabies the virus does not appear in the saliva, which therefore is not infective.

At autopsy the gross findings are not distinctive. There may be haemorrhages and small erosions of the gums; there are usually dried scabs of mucus obstructing the nasal orifices; the peritoneal and mucous coats of the stomach are often congested, and there may be a variety of foreign bodies in the stomach. The head of the dog should be removed, packed in ice, and sent to a laboratory; alternatively, the skull may be split and the whole head sent immersed in formalin solution. The pathological changes in the brain, meninges, and cord resemble those already described in man.

When appropriate laboratory facilities are available a firm diagnosis of rabies can be made in 80 per cent of dogs by the recognition of Negri bodies; in 95 per cent of them by recovery of virus from the brain; and in 80 per cent of them by recovery of virus from the saliva. The most rapid recognition, taking only a few hours, is achieved in specimens of fresh brain by the use of labelled fluorescent antibody for the determination of the presence of the virus.

*The suspect dog*
If the dog has already been destroyed, as is sometimes the case, the body

should be procured for laboratory examination. *After a biting incident the dog, if living, should be segregated and watched for signs of the disease. If the animal survives for more than 10 days it is not rabid; if it dies within that period the brain should be searched for Negri bodies.* Late evidence that the dog is not rabid warrants the stoppage of preventive treatment of the potential patient.

TREATMENT

There is no specific treatment for the disease once symptoms develop. Distress may be lessened by keeping the patient quiet by heavy sedation (120 mg sodium phenobarbitone intravenously) and antispasmodic drugs such as chlorpromazine. Curarization with positive pressure endotracheal ventilation in conjunction with intensive treatment with immune serum and anti-rabies vaccine has suggested a hope of survival of some patients. Patients with rabies are potentially infective to their attendants and suitable precautions must accordingly be taken.

Two forms of preventive treatment are available during the incubation period. These are (1) vaccine treatment and (2) treatment with immune serum. Either or both should be started immediately when careful assessment of the facts of the case indicates a probable infection. *Under no circumstances must the death of the dog with post-mortem proof of rabies infection be awaited before preventive treatment is begun.*

MANAGEMENT OF TH E BITTEN PERSON

As noted above, once the disease has been established there is no specific treatment and the case almost certainly will end fatally, although in the last 3 years two cases have been reported to have recovered.

The objective in dealing with a person bitten by a suspected rabid animal is therefore to prevent the development of infection and the appearance of the disease. The measures which can be undertaken are local treatment of the bite wounds, the induction of passive immunity by giving hyperimmune serum, or the development of active immunity by giving rabies vaccine.

*Local treatment of bite*

Local treatment of the wound is of great value and should be carried out as early as possible. Saliva must be wiped carefully from the surrounding skin, without further contaminating the wound. Bleeding should be encouraged, where possible by the application of a ligature. The wound should be thoroughly cleansed, with a syringe, with soap or detergent solution; every crevice and every tooth puncture must be thoroughly flushed. Caustic or necrotizing applications have been advocated for this purpose, such as the cautery, dilute or pure hydrochloric or nitric acid, caustic soda, or permanganate crystals; they are all very painful and cause subsequent disfigurement;

none is superior to a simple soap solution if the wound is properly flushed with it soon after its infliction. Cleansing of the wound by one of the methods mentioned above affords a high proportion of sterilization of the infection if throughly and efficiently done within a few hours of the injury. Primary suture of the wounds should be avoided.

Excision of the wound may be considered; if efficiently done this may be effective.

VACCINES

The vaccine treatment of rabies was discovered by Pasteur towards the end of the last century. He injected subcutaneously, saline emulsions of the spinal cords of rabbits infected with fixed virus. An active immunity was developed by the patient to rabies virus during the incubation period of the naturally acquired infection.

Modern rabies vaccines may broadly be divided into two types; those containing living and those containing killed virus. Brain substance, which contains a greater concentration of virus than does spinal cord, has now almost entirely supplanted the latter as a natural source of the virus. Killed virus vaccines have become popular as they have proved to be just as effective as those containing living viruses. The agents used to kill the virus in brain tissue have been numerous. Heat-treated vaccines and vaccines treated with phenol, formalin, chloroform or ether, yatren, ultraviolet light, and many other chemical or physical applications have been developed.

Vaccines most commonly used are:

1. Suspensions of infected animal (usually rabbit) brain inactivated by phenol (the Semple type vaccine).
2. Suspensions of duck embryo on which the virus has been grown, inactivated by $\beta$-propiolactone (DEV vaccine).

The duck embryo vaccine is most often used as neurological complications do not occur after its administration.

The standardization and comparison of the antigenic powers of rabies vaccine has for some time been difficult. The Habel potency mouse test has been devised to solve the difficulty. A series of mice is injected intraperitoneally with the vaccine under test and their immunity is subsequently challenged by injecting intracerebrally graduated dilutions of a standard fixed strain of virus. By this means the protective potency of the vaccine is determined.

*Complications of vaccination*

Though most patients treated with the vaccines suffer no ill-effects, in some cases complications have occurred. About a week after the first dose of vaccine there may be erythema, oedema, pruritus, and pain at the site of the inoculation; these subside within a few days, though they may recur in about 10 days if the treatment is continued. The reaction appears usually towards the end of the course of infections. It is commonest in those who have been previously treated and have become sensitized to the vaccine. Sometimes it is severe and is accompanied by fever, glandular swellings, and a general systemic upset; if treatment is not stopped at once there may be graver manifestations in the form of encephalitis and paralyses. Peripheral neuritis, and an ascending myelitis with paralysis, may appear and sometimes end fatally. Complications are not due to the virus content of the vaccine, but to sensitization to the animal tissue from which it is prepared. When they appear vaccination is usually stopped, but if risk of rabies is great DEV vaccine may be substituted for other vaccines which may be being used and vaccination continued under a cortisone cover.

### IMMUNE SERUM

Immune sera are obtained by actively immunizing large animals such as sheep and horses; taking serum and concentrating the specific antibody. The injection of this serum into a patient confers a temporary, strong, passive immunity. Serum followed by a vaccine offers the most effective means of preventing rabies after severe exposure to infection. Serum may also be given in cases of severe bite during the 10-day observation period covering the suspected dog.

### PROPHYLACTIC TREATMENT

*Administration of vaccine*
Semple vaccines are given subcutaneously in daily doses, into alternate sides of the abdominal wall, for periods of 14–21 days, depending on the severity of the bite. Most vaccines are given in volumes of 3–4 ml daily.

The DEV vaccine has the advantage of requiring smaller injection volumes. It is supplied lyophilized and the dose is made up in 1 ml sterile water for each injection. A dose is given daily for 14 days.

Even if serum has been administered, vaccine administration should not be delayed beyond 24 hours despite the risk of neutralization by the antibody.

The doses of vaccine given at each injection and the times of their administration for intensive or for less intensive courses of treatment are laid down by the laboratory issuing the vaccine. Doses are given by deep subcutaneous injection, taking care to use a separate site for each injection. To ensure high levels of antibodies, booster doses of vaccine are usually given at 10 days and again at 20 days after the last dose of the vaccine course. This is useful also to overcome interference with passive immunization where serum has been used.

*Administration of serum*

The serum is given intramuscularly in a single dose of 40 IU per kg body weight. Sensitivity should be checked before administration.

Serum sensitivity (usually to horse serum) should be tested by instilling 0.1 ml of a 1 in 10 dilution in saline of the serum into the conjunctiva. Local vascular dilatation, itching, and heavy lachrymation within 15 minutes indicate a high degree of sensitivity.

Desensitization is then attempted by subcutaneous injection of 0.1 ml of a 1 : 100 dilution of the serum, repeating the injection and doubling the dose every 15 minutes until 1.0 ml has been given. If no reaction occurs, the serum is given intramuscularly at 15-minute intervals, doubling the dose each time. If increasing the dose produces a reaction, the dose should be halved for the next injection. If signs of anaphylaxis appear, 1 ml of 1 in 1000 adrenalin is injected subcutaneously. Reactions are less severe and less common if purified hyperimmune globulin is used.

Serum sickness may appear after 7–10 days. The risk is reduced by antihistamine drugs given at the time of injection and subsequently for 1 week.

Immune serum made from rabbits can be given without risk of sensitivity reactions; human hyperimmune globulin has also been used and avoids the risks of anaphylaxis.

The question of retreatment of a patient not uncommonly arises following a further biting episode or other contact with a rabid animal. If the time since the previous treatment does not exceed 3 months further treatment is unnecessary unless the second exposure to infection is very severe. If the interval does not exceed 6 months two reinforcing doses of vaccine, at an interval of a week, suffice. If it exceeds 6 months a full course of treatment should be repeated. When allergy to the vaccine is manifested by a patient, the vaccine should be changed to one prepared from the brain of another species of animal or an avianized strain may be used.

SUMMARY

A. *Local treatment of bite wound*

(a) Cleanse the wound thoroughly with a soap or detergent emulsion, flushing every crevice and puncture.

(b) Deep wounds, inaccessible for washing, may be cauterized by nitric acid, this being then neutralized with sodium bicarbonate.

(c) Avoid surgical interference or primary suture of the wounds.

B. *Preventive treatment*

(a) If the bites are severe a single dose of hyperimmune antiserum or globulin is given intramuscularly as soon as possible.

(b) This is followed after 24 hours by a course of vaccine in the case of severe bites.

(c) If the bite is not severe vaccine treatment may be given without initial antiserum.

There must be rigid enforcement of quarantine regulations and control of the domestic dog population. The prophylactic immunization of dogs by vaccination is practicable and effective. By this means rabies, which was periodically epizootic and endemic in Japan, has been reduced to negligible proportions. High egg passage vaccine (HEP) has been used successfully for prophylaxis in humans exposed to special risk, for example veterinarians. Booster doses are required every 3 years and recommended after any exposure. The admission of vaccinated animals is not permitted in the U.K. where they must still undergo the full 6 months' quarantine. Animals susceptible to rabies are not admitted into Australia.

# 21

# THE RAT-BITE FEVERS

## DEFINITION

The rat-bite fevers are due to infection with one or other of two distinct organisms, *Spirillum minus* and *Actinobacillus muris*. Both organisms normally occur in rats and in a variety of other small animals. They gain entry to man not uncommonly as the result of a bite by a rat and less frequently by that of another animal; the human cases of infection are incidental and sporadic. The clinical syndromes following infection with either organism are somewhat similar. They are characterized by a febrile illness of long duration, often with recurring inflammation of the bite-wound and local adenitis, and with an evanescent eruption, severe muscular pains, and sometimes arthritis. The mortality is low.

Cases of rat-bite fever due to either organism have been recorded from many parts of the world. Climate plays no direct part in their occurrence.

## AETIOLOGY

For a great many years it has been known that a febrile illness may follow the bite of a rat, and of other small rodents and mammals. Early in the century Japanese workers reported the recovery of a spirillar organism from cases of rat-bite fever (sodoku) in Japan. This organism was named *Sp. minus* and was accepted as the cause of rat-bite fever in man. However, it was not found in all cases. Later it was shown that a streptothrix-like organism now called *Act. muris* (*Streptobacillus moniliformis*) could also cause the syndrome.

Strains of *Sp. minus* have been artificially maintained by serial subinoculation in animals and in man for the treatment of general paralysis; in each case they caused the expected disease syndrome. From human cases of *Act. muris* infection the organisms can consistently be recovered by culture of the blood on suitable media. Either of these two infections in man may result from the bite of a rat, but *Act. muris* infection alternatively may be acquired by swallowing material containing the organism, as occurred in an epidemic at Haverill (Haverill Fever) in the U.S.A. following consumption of infected cow's milk.

*Sp. minus* differs from the true spirochaetes in that its body is rigid; although it is motile, its motility is due to terminal flagella. It varies in length from 2 to 5 $\mu$m; the spirals, which are broad, number two to four or more. The organism stains well with the Romanowsky stains or silver impregnation method. It is readily inoculable into laboratory animals but cannot be cultured *in vitro*. The spirilla can be found widely in the organs of naturally infected rats but not in the saliva. It has been suggested that the infection following a rat bite is due to escape of the organisms into the mouth from abrasions of the gums and of the tongue, in the latter of which they are present in large numbers.

*Act. muris* also has been recovered from sundry organs of naturally infected rats, but appears primarily to be an inhabitant of the nasopharynx. It has been found in this site in a high percentage of a group of apparently normal laboratory rats. In wild rats it has been recovered from the lungs, in which it was held to be responsible for inflammatory and caseating lesions. This organism may cause epizootics in mice, with involvement of the eyes, swelling of the lymphatic glands and of the joints, and paresis of the hind limbs.

### PATHOLOGY

The information available on the distinctive pathology of the rat-bite fevers in man is meagre and somewhat confused. In both diseases there appears to be a septicaemic type of infection. There is generalized hyperaemia of the internal organs; the liver and spleen may be enlarged; there is often a slight general lymphadenitis; and there may be arthritis with effusion, especially in cases of *Act. muris* infection. In fatal cases the liver and kidneys show marked parenchymatous changes.

### CLINICAL PICTURE

The clinical manifestations due to the two types of rat-bite fever are somewhat similar, and purely on clinical grounds it may be difficult to differentiate them. The incubation period of the disease due to *Sp. minus* ranges from 5 to 30 days, the usual being about 2 weeks; that of the disease due to *Act. muris* ranges from 2 to 10 days, the usual being about 5 days. The bite causing the infection in either case appears to be healing, or to have healed, at the time of the onset of symptoms. In the case of the *Sp. minus* infection the lesion becomes inflamed once more and may develop a chancre-like ulceration with marked local lymphangitis and lymphadenitis. The onset of symptoms in either case is usually abrupt with a sharp rise of temperature, often of a remittent or septic type, and sometimes in association with shivering attacks. In *Sp. minus* infections the fever lasts from 2 to 4 days; it then subsides and recurs after an interval of 3–7 days for a similar period; relapses recur fairly regularly on six to eight occasions. In *Act. muris* infections the fever is intermittent and there are no regularly recurring relapses. In either infection an eruption commonly appears; in *Sp. minus* infections this may be an evanescent bluish-red, or purplish, mottled erythema confined to the uppermost part of the trunk; or maculopapular and extend all over the trunk and limbs. In *Act. muris* infections the eruption is macular and petechial. In *Sp. minus* infections arthritis is unusual; but in *Act. muris* infections there is very commonly a polyarthritis with effusions into the joints; this is a constant complication in infected animals. The joint fluid contains many cells, and the causal organisms can be recovered from it by culture; spontaneous suppuration of the affected joints does not occur.

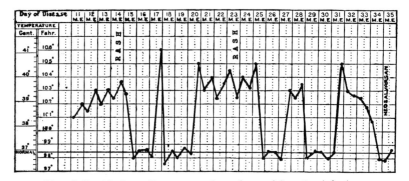

FIG. 48. Rat-bite fever. Temperature chart of case of *Sp. minus* infection.
[By courtesy of E.Noble Chamberlain, *A Textbook of Medicine,* John Wright & Sons Ltd., Bristol, 1951]

The spleen and the lymph glands usually do not enlarge in *Sp. minus* infections but do so commonly in *Act. muris* infections. Although both conditions are debilitating and may cause marked prostration, the mortality from either is low.

DIAGNOSIS

A recurrent, febrile illness occurring after a rodent bite should be suspected of being caused by *Sp. minus* infection. Non-relapsing fever should be regarded as due to possible *Act. muris* infection.

*Sp. minus* infections
The organisms are not present in great numbers in the blood, even at the height of the fever, and it is rarely possible to find them in blood films. They can be seen more readily in oedema fluid aspirated from the inflamed site of the infecting bite. This fluid should be searched with dark ground illumination, or stained with Leishman or Giemsa, or by a silver impregnation method. The most effective way of recovering and identifying the organisms is inoculation of the blood, oedema fluid, or lymph gland puncture material, taken during a febrile period, into susceptible animals such as mice. Some time

may elapse before the infection becomes apparent in the animals, but the organisms can then be recovered from the blood, lymph gland juice, or peritoneal fluid. *Sp. minus* cannot be grown artificially in culture media.

### *Act. muris* infections

Laboratory animals, including mice, are refractory to infection with this organism, but it can readily be cultured from blood taken during fever and inoculated into beef infusion broth enriched with rabbit serum. Agglutination tests may be performed with the patient's serum and a stock laboratory culture of the organism and the organism isolated from the patient can be tested against a known agglutinating serum.

### TREATMENT

### *Sp. minus* infections

Penicillin in the form of Penicillin V (potassium) in doses of 250 mg 4-hourly for 3–4 days is rapidly active in eradicating the infection.

Streptomycin, 1 g daily for 10 days, also effectively eradicates the infection.

The organism is very susceptible to arsenic. Three intravenous injections each of 0.4–0.6 g of neoarsphenamine at 3-day intervals usually suffice to effect a cure.

### *Act. muris* infections

Penicillin compounds, as above, are specific, but there have been some reports of the occurrence of penicillin resistant strains of the organism. Tetracycline is active in *Act. muris* infection, in a dosage of 500 mg 6-hourly for 10 days.

# 22

# THE RELAPSING FEVERS

### INTRODUCTION

These fevers are due to infection with strains of spirochaetes all of which morphologically are indistinguishable. The infections are transmitted by lice or by ticks; the louse-borne and the tick-borne relapsing fevers consistently manifest epidemiological and clinical features which distinguish them.

The organism conveyed by lice is *Borrelia recurrentis*, which infects no mammals other than man. It is transmitted by the human body louse, *Pediculus humanus*. Louse-borne relapsing fever is commonly epidemic and found preponderantly in cold and temperate climates.

The organism conveyed by ticks is *B. duttoni*, which normally infects rodents and occurs only incidentally in man. In central Africa, however, man may be the principal host. Ticks can also act as reservoirs as they have a long life and may transmit the *Borrelia* transovarially. In nature the tick-borne infection is not known to spread from man to man by means of the louse, although *P. humanus* has been infected experimentally, and lice from patients suffering from natural *B. duttoni* infections have been shown to harbour the organism. The regions in which the louse-borne disease and the tick-borne diseases normally occur are entirely distinct geographically; epidemic, louse-borne relapsing fever has never been known to appear spontaneously in tick-borne relapsing fever areas or distribution without its introduction from an outside source.

The starvation, overcrowding, and squalor associated with famines, wars, and other great human catastrophes have favoured major outbreaks of both these diseases.

## LOUSE-BORNE RELAPSING FEVER

### DEFINITION

Epidemic or louse-borne relapsing fever is due to infection with *B. recurrentis*. The organism is conveyed from man to man by the human body louse, *P. humanus*. The clinically severe disease is characterized by periods of fever with toxaemia, body pains, enlargement of the spleen and of the liver, bronchitis, and jaundice. The febrile periods recur usually on one or two occasions. The mortality rate is considerable in epidemics; individual cases respond well to chemotherapy.

The only major endemic area at present is Ethiopia. Foci exist in China, Peru, and eastern Europe. Small outbreaks occur in and spread from itinerant workers, in the Sudan and Ethiopia.

Though primarily a disease of cold and temperate climates, where lice abound, outbreaks have occurred in parts of equatorial Africa, in India, and in South America, where it is a disease in the cold seasons. Serious epidemics have occurred coincidentally with, or have closely followed, outbreaks of epidemic louse-borne typhus.

## AETIOLOGY

Many strains of *B. recurrentis* have been isolated from patients in various parts of the world during outbreaks of epidemic, louse-borne relapsing fever. Despite antigenic variations, however, these are all regarded as belonging to the same species.

*B. recurrentis* can readily be found in films of peripheral blood taken during the febrile periods. In wet preparations they are actively motile; in dried films they stain readily with the usual dyes. Their average length is about 15$\mu$m, and their diameter 0.2–0.3 $\mu$m. They are made up of spiral turns each occupying 2–3 $\mu$m, so that a spirochaete of average length consists of about six to eight spirals. In wet preparations, when not subjected to pressure, the axis is straight; but in dried films the spirochaetes are much distorted and bent. *B. recurrentis* can be cultured on suitable fluid media *in vitro* and in the growing chick embryo. The ordinary laboratory animals are refractory to infection with this organism directly on its recovery from man. It can be introduced into, and maintained in, the usual experimental animals only after passage through monkeys.

The blood of a patient suffering from relapsing fever contains spirochaetes only during the febrile periods. Lice feeding on the blood at this time become infected. Immediately after the blood meal the spirochaetes disappear from the gut of the louse; they are believed to assume some developmental form, such as granules, and after 5–15 days appear in considerable numbers throughout the body. The louse is now infective and remains so for the remainder of its life. The infection is not transmitted transovarially; individual lice must be infected by a blood meal before they can transmit the infection.

Infection of man rarely, if ever, results from the bite of the louse. Lice damaged and ruptured by scratching liberate the contained spirochaetes which are rubbed into abrasions caused by scratching of the louse bite.

Persons of both sexes and of all ages are susceptible to infection, but the incidence of the disease in males is greater than that in females; it is least prevalent in young children. An attack of louse-borne relapsing fever affords complete immunity to reinfection for a time but this wanes and a second infection may occur within a year of the first. The disease in the endemic regions tends to recur epidemically at 2- or 3-year intervals, probably on this account.

There are usually petechial haemorrhages in the skin, the mucous membranes of the mouth, stomach, and intestines. Haemorrhages also occur in the tissues of the kidneys and other organs, and under the endothelial lining of the serous cavities and under the meninges; these haemorrhages may be confluent. The liver is much enlarged and hyperaemic. The spleen is much enlarged, soft, and congested and there may be local necrosis. There may be multiple infarctions and miliary aggregations of mononuclear cells on the periphery of which are large numbers of spirochaetes. Fatty degeneration of the heart, the liver, and the kidneys is common. Intracranial haemorrhage, acute meningitis, hepatitis, or rupture of the spleen are among the immediate causes of death; a secondary bacteraemia may result in death from pulmonary infection. Spirochaetes may be found lying in the intercellular spaces and within endothelial cells throughout the body, particularly in the spleen, the Kupffer cells of the liver, and the endothelial cells of the lymph glands and bone marrow. If the examination is deferred for many hours after death few may be found.

CLINICAL PICTURE

The incubation period ranges from 2 to 12 days; usually it is from 4 to 8 days. After a prodromal period lasting a day or two the onset is sudden. There is shivering, with severe headache, confusion, bodily pains, nausea and vomiting, and profound prostration. The temperature rises to between 39.4 and 40° C. The fever is usually continuous, though it may be remittent. There is great thirst; the face is flushed; the eyes are injected; and commonly there is epistaxis. In severe attacks the spleen and the liver both enlarge and are tender. Jaundice is usual. There is an increased respiration rate, with a cough, and evidence of bronchitis. Sometimes there is a macular eruption on the trunk and limbs, which may be erythematous or haemorrhagic. Petechial haemorrhages and ecchymoses may occur in the skin and visible mucous membranes.

The symptoms and signs continue for 4–9 days. The temperature then suddenly falls to normal or subnormal, often with collapse of the patient. The symptoms and signs rapidly abate, the liver and spleen shrink in size, and the patient's condition improves. There follows an afebrile period which lasts from 4 to 17 days, usually about a week. This is succeeded by a relapse. The first relapse is similar to the primary attack but usually is of slightly shorter duration and lesser severity. Rarely it may be more severe and jaundice may make its first appearance during it. There is then another afebrile period and this may be followed by a second relapse. The second relapse is less severe and of shorter duration than the first. The second relapse is usually followed by convalescence. Rarely there is a third, mild, relapse before the disease finally ends. In about half the cases there are two relapses; and in only 1 or 2 per cent are there three relapses.

The death rate from louse-borne relapsing fever is influenced by the age and the condition of the patient. In those who are ill-nourished and who live under bad conditions the mortalty commonly is over 30 per cent in the absence of efficient care and treatment.

## DIAGNOSIS

The disease is readily diagnosed, when suspected, by recovery of the spirochaetes from the blood in which they are numerous during the periods of fever; they are absent from the blood during the afebrile intermissions of the disease. The parasites can be found in wet preparations by the Indian ink and similar methods, or by examination with a dark-ground condenser. They can readily be seen in thick or in thin blood films stained with Leishman or with Giemsa stain. They may be recovered by culture or by the inoculation of monkeys where facilities are available, then passage via other animals.

## TREATMENT

Prompt steps comparable to those employed in epidemic typhus must be taken to free the patient and all contacts from louse infestation.

*Antibiotics*

*Tetracycline* is the drug of choice. The spirochaetes disappear rapidly from the blood in severe cases after a single intravenous dose of 250 mg. The usual dosage regimen is 250 mg or 500 mg on the first day, followed by 500 mg on the second day. Reactions to treatment may be severe and because of this some authors recommend intramuscular procaine penicillin, 300,000 units initially, followed next day by tetracycline, 500 mg orally as a single dose. As a precaution against relapse, larger doses of tetracycline have been given, such as 500 mg 6-hourly on the first day, followed by 250 mg 6-hourly for a week, the latter course repeated after 10 days. Recent Ethiopian experience has indicated that both for immediate clinical relief and for control of relapse, these long dosage regimens are probably unnecessary.

*Penicillin* will terminate the attack but will not invariably prevent subsequent relapse. The *Borrelia* disappear in about 36 hours. Reactions to treatment are mild. Allergy to penicillin is a risk. Dosage varies considerably. A successful regimen is 300,000 units of procain penicillin on the first day, followed by 800,000 units daily for 3 days.

*Arsenicals* were widely used before the antibiotics but have now been abandoned. Given during the febrile period, neoarsphenamine in a single dose of 400–600 mg given intravenously slowly and well diluted was effective; this was repeated in the event of a relapse. Reactions were severe.

*Reactions to treatment.* These may be severe but are not contra-indications to treatment, since the disease itself may be fatal.

The reaction begins about an hour after any treatment. The patient goes into rigor with a rise of temperature and increase in pulse and respiration rates. The rigor is followed by a febrile period in which the temperature may reach 41 °C. There is a fall in blood pressure and a sharp decline in blood leucocyte count. Spirochaetes disappear from the blood. The patient gradually recovers and the fever subsides over a period of 8–10 hours. Cortisone has no alleviating effect.

*General.* Vitamin K, 20 mg parenterally is useful in cases in which there is evidence of severe tissue bleeding. Dehydration should be dealt with in the usual way, by parenteral glucose saline if necessary. Care should be taken not to overload the circulation. High fever needs sponging with cool water and fanning.

## TICK-BORNE RELAPSING FEVER

### DEFINITION

Non-epidemic relapsing fever is due to infection with *Borrelia duttoni*. The organism normally infects rodents and is conveyed by ticks; under such conditions it occurs only incidentally in man. In central Africa, however, man is probably the only mammalian host; the infection is there conveyed by ticks and is endemic. The clinical features of tick-borne broadly resemble those of louse-borne relapsing fever but the attacks are more severe, of shorter duration, and relapses are more numerous.

### GEOGRAPHICAL DISTRIBUTION

Human infections occur sporadically in Mediterranean countries, especially North Africa, and eastward to Russian Central Asia and northern India, in tropical and subtropical America, and in many parts of the U.S.A. where *B. duttoni* occurs enzootically in small rodents, and in other animals.

In Central, East, and South Africa tick-borne relapsing fever occurs endemically.

### AETIOLOGY

In those areas where the organism is primarily one of the rodent and animal populations the infection is transmitted to man by ticks infected from animals. Some of the animals serving as reservoirs of the infection inhabit holes and caves where the ticks rarely feed on man. Humans entering the caves, however, are attacked. Other animals serving as reservoirs live in bush or scrub country and trappers, travellers, campers, and others passing through the area are liable to become infested by infected ticks which normally feed on the animal population.

In Central Africa ticks infesting human habitations become infected from a human being. Throughout these regions the infection, though widely distributed, tends to be a patchy one. Persons spending the night in a rest house or on an old village site may acquire the disease from the infected ticks. A neighbouring village site may be free from the infection. The African disease differs from other forms of tick-borne fever in that so far as is known no mammal other than man, and, of course, the ticks, maintain the infection.

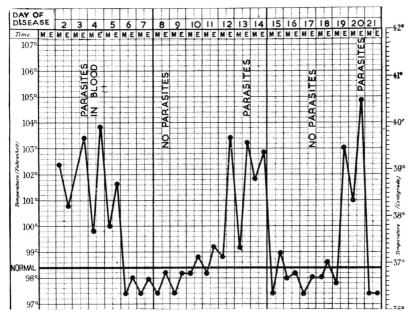

FIG. 49. Temperature chart of case of tick-borne relapsing fever. Primary attack and first two relapses.

*B. duttoni* is morphologically identical with *B. recurrentis*, but differs from it in some biological characters. It is readily inoculable into laboratory animals without preliminary passage through monkeys. In nature it is conveyed from one host to another by a number of ticks, of which the African *Ornithodorus moubata* is one of the most important. The offspring of infected female ticks are infected transovarially; thus the infection may persist through several generations of ticks. It follows that only rare contact with a source of infection is necessary for the maintenance of the infection in a colony of ticks and that members of the colony may be infective over very lengthy periods of time after the last contact with infected hosts.

When *O. moubata* takes a blood meal containing *B. duttoni* the organisms rapidly disappear from the gut; after a time they reappear in large numbers in the body cavity. In the female ticks spirochaetes can be found in the ovaries, as well as in other solid organs; in this respect infection of the tick differs from that of the louse, where the spirochaetes are found only in the fluid media. In ticks the invasion extends to the Malpighian tubes, the salivary glands and the saliva, and the coxal fluid. In feeding, a tick pierces the skin and excretes saliva; it evacuates its bowel towards the end of a meal and discharges coxal fluid. By all these channels spirochaetes may be discharged on to the skin. They enter the wound made in feeding, or other abrasions of the skin. They can pass through unbroken mucosa.

### PATHOLOGY

The pathology of tick-borne relapsing fever closely resembles that of the louse-borne disease.

### CLINICAL PICTURE

The onset and course of tick-borne relapsing fever are much the same as those of the louse-borne disease, with the following differences. The intervals between the febrile paroxysms are usually rather shorter, being 8–12 days. The febrile periods are also slightly shorter but the fever tends to be higher; spirochaetes are less numerous in the peripheral blood during them than in the louse-borne disease. The number of relapses is usually greater, being four to six and often more. Complications are more frequent and severe; these include facial palsy, spastic paraplegia, iritis, and severe diarrhoea and dysentery. The tendency to haemorrhage is greater in the tick-borne than in the louse-borne disease. In spite of these differences the mortality of the tick-borne disease on the whole is less than that of the louse-borne; this may well be due to the epidemic incidence of the latter among very debilitated persons living under bad conditions.

Recovery from an attack of tick-borne relapsing fever is followed by substantial immunity to reinfection but this wanes and subsequent reinfection may then occur. Constant exposure of the indigenous population to infection and reinfection results in tolerance of the effects of the spirochaetes.

### DIAGNOSIS

Diagnosis is made as in the louse-borne disease, the organisms are less numerous in the blood, but laboratory animals are more readily infected with them.

### TREATMENT

The principles of chemotherapy are the same as for the louse-borne infection.

Tetracycline should be given in doses of 500 mg 6-hourly until 12 hours after the fever has subsided.

Relapses may occur, but are sometimes anticipated by giving tetracycline 500 mg 6-hourly for 2 days each week for a month.

The arsenicals are less effective in tick-borne than in louse-borne relapsing fever. Intensive penicillin treatment may terminate the febrile attack, but it does not prevent the development of subsequent relapses of the disease.

*Prophylaxis*
Avoid caves, native villages, rest-houses, and old camping sites as sleeping places. Place the feet of a bed in tins of disinfectant and use a net to avoid tick infestation at night. Repellents on the skin and in clothing may also deter tick infestation. Remove as soon as possible all ticks which may attach themselves to the body and apply iodine to the point of attachment. Ticks take some time to attach themselves firmly and begin to feed and discharge spirochaetes in the saliva, coxal, and intestinal discharges, through which the infection is conveyed.

# 23

# THE SCHISTOSOMIASES

## INTRODUCTION

Several species of blood-flukes of the genus *Schistosoma* are parasitic in man in various parts of the world. Three species, *S. haematobium, S. mansoni,* and *S. japonicum,* are common parasites of man. Other species which occasionally infect man include *S. intercalatum, S. bovis,* and *S. matthei. S. intercalatum* is found in man in the Gabon and Zäire; it produces terminal-spined eggs closely resembling those of *S. haematobium* but causes intestinal and not urinary symptoms . *S. bovis* and *S. matthei* are normally parasitic in animals but occur in man in certain localities.

All these parasites outside the mammalian host undergo a multiplicative developmental cycle in certain snails appropriate to the species. Man acquires an infection by wetting the skin with water containing the infective cercariae shed by the snail hosts. The cercariae actively penetrate the skin, find their way to the liver, and in the portal system and its ramifications develop into adult worms of two sexes. The adult mature worms live their sexual life inside the blood vessels. The gravid female worms, wrapped within the males, make their way to the terminal radicles of the portal venous system, dilating these small vessels as they ascend them against the direction of the blood flow. They then deposit their eggs one by one, retreating a little down the vessel after each egg is laid. The eggs normally are extruded from these vessels through the tissues into the bladder or the intestine, according to the location of the worms, and are voided to the exterior in the urine or faeces. They must enter fresh water or they perish; in fresh water a larva (miracidium) emerges from each of the viable eggs. The ciliated miracidia swim about for some hours until they penetrate a snail host appropriate to the species of schistosome. They actively penetrate into the snail and migrate to its liver gland. Here the miracidia undergo further development and multiply, giving rise in due course to large numbers of infective larvae (cercariae). Small clouds of cercariae are emitted by the infected snail; these swim, by means of a forked tail, in the water until they find the skin surface of man; they attach themselves, shed their tails, and penetrate. So, in due course, the cycle is repeated.

The species of schistosomes infecting man can be distinguished by the morphology of the adult worms, to a considerable extent by their sites of election in the body and the symptoms that result from the infection, and by the morphology of the eggs they produce. The snails which serve as inter-

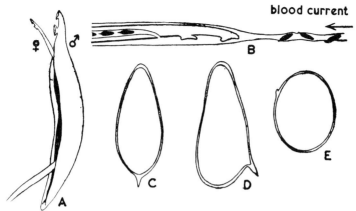

Fɪɢ. 50. A, Outline of male (length, 12 mm) and female (length, 20 mm) schistosomes *in copula*; B, Female worms retreating down venule as eggs deposited in venule; C, Outline of *Schistosoma haematobium* egg (length, 130 μm); D, *S. mansoni* egg; E, *S. japonicum* egg.

[From E.Noble Chamberlain, *A Textbook of Medicine*, John Wright & Sons Ltd., Bristol, 1951]

mediate hosts differ with the species of the worm; they are limited in geographical distribution and are specific to each of the species of schistosomes.

The schistosomiases occur extensively among people whose activities involve entry into fresh water in the endemic areas. Primitive dwellings are always within easy reach of open water or rivers; there is pollution of these with infected urine or faeces; and pools, tanks, swamps, and irrigation channels containing stagnant or slowly running water become extremely heavily infested with infected snails. The individual cercariae emerging from these in showers each survive about 2 days, but as they are constantly being renewed the water may become heavily charged with them. Children, in view of their habits, are particularly prone to expose themselves to infection. Though immersion of a part of the body in infected pools is a common means of infection, water drawn from them for domestic purposes is infective until stored for at least 3 days; on taking freshly drawn water into the mouth the cercariae may penetrate the buccal mucosa; infection equally may occur on wetting the skin.

Persons of either sex and of any age are susceptible to infection. Men occupationally are as a rule more exposed to infection than are women; male children are particularly liable to become infected. Previous infection confers some resistance to superinfection or reinfection.

The consequences of a schistosomal infection in man vary. In hyperendemic regions, with consequent heavy infections, they cause much grave disability and the complications attributable to them contribute to the mortality. In less intensely endemic areas a high proportion of the native population may be infected with *S. haematobium* or *S. mansoni* without complaining of symptoms or signs. Nevertheless, in view of the longevity (up to 20 years) of the worms, of their considerable egg production in that time, and of the histological changes due to accumulating unexpelled eggs in the tissues, the long term consequences may be serious. Detailed urological investigations have shown that the incidence of tissue damage, in the urinary bladder and ureters in young children in East and West Africa infected with *S. haematobium,* is much higher than has previously been suspected. Response to treatment at this age is usually good. Lesions may regress in time without treatment as the child becomes older and exposure is reduced.

### Imported schistosomiasis

Schistosomiasis is one of the major infections imported into countries in which the disease does not normally exist. In the absence of the vector snail there is no risk of transmission in the country to which the disease is imported but, where the snail does exist, transmission is possible. It is believed that this is the reason why the infection is so common in some Caribbean Islands and in parts of South America, to which the worm was originally carried in the slaves from Africa, and in which the appropriate snail vector already existed.

In immigrants from endemic areas it is the cause of serious illness in Europe and the U.S.A. In Europe the infection is usually caused by *S. mansoni,* sometimes by *S. haematobium.* It is seen mostly in immigrant workers from endemic areas and less commonly in travellers who have visited these areas in the Middle East and Africa. In the U.S.A., the infection is almost always due to *S. mansoni* derived from South America—especially Brazil—and certain Caribbean Islands, notably Puerto Rico.

In the East, *S. japonicum* may be exported from endemic areas into others, in individuals and immigrants. Here the other infections are very rare and come from distant geographical regions.

BASIC PATHOLOGY

There is usually some vasodilatation and round cell mobilization at the point of entry of the skin by the cercariae. This is minimal in the case of infection by the schistosomes causing the disease in man, but in infections with unadapted worms the local reaction is brisk and the cercariae are arrested by vigorous inflammatory reaction and absorbed.

As pointed out above, the cercariae of the human infections eventually reach the liver portal venous vessels and mature into the two sexes. Pairs of worms then move to the mesenteric and pelvic venous plexuses and 5–6 weeks after infection the female begins to produce eggs.

Juveniles, adults, and eggs contain antigens which form antibodies in the host. The allergic manifestations of the early clinical picture arise from resultant antibody–antigen host reactions. These reactions commonly develop before the egg laying commences. The eggs also contain antigens and the resultant antigen–antibody reactions play a part in the formation of the granulomata which develop about the living eggs which are captured by the host tissues. The living eggs themselves contain a factor which also contributes to the cellular reaction.

The ultimate pathological results of infection depend on the species of the invading schistosome and on the host response to the juvenile and adult worms and to the eggs. The major pathogenic agent is the egg containing the living miracidium. Dead (black) eggs which remain indefinitely in the tissues, and egg shells left behind by miracidia which have escaped into the tissues, do not produce granulomata but may eventually evoke a giant cell reaction.

Eggs which pass through the tissues and are discharged to the surface cause little damage. Eggs which are lodged in the tissues commonly stimulate a granulomatous reaction from which stem most of the subsequent pathological effects.

Many eggs are distributed in the blood stream and are seeded to the liver. Those that pass into the systemic circulation may set up ectopic cellular reactions when they become arrested in the tissues.

In eggs which have been arrested in the tissues the contained miracidium survives for 2–3 weeks and in that period sets up a cellular response which consists mainly of lymphocytes, plasma cells, macrophages, and eosinophils; in very heavy infections polymorphs may also be present. Later, epithelioid cells appear and a granuloma is formed similar to that seen in tuberculosis. After the death of the miracidium the egg shell may calcify and a giant cell reaction may develop.

Granulomatous reactions also develop around dying or dead worms but not usually in association with the living worm.

In the late stages of infection fibrosis may replace the granulomas and fibrotic extensions cause scarring which may determine local complications.

The pathological effects in the individual infection are determined in some degree by the anatomical distribution of the adult worms and the initial distribution of eggs in the tissues. Details are given below in the sections dealing with the individual infections.

The host response is partly determined by the intensity of infection, in terms of the numbers of female adult worms present and of their egg production. Other factors which modify the clinical effects of infection are immunological resistance acquired from long repeated exposure, the nutritional status of the patient, and regional variations in the pathogenicity of the infecting species.

Anaemia in severe cases of schistosomiasis may arise from blood loss, especially where there are bleeding venous varices, and from hypersplenism where there is splenomegaly following portal hypertension.

The eosinophil count is moderately raised in the early stages of the disease. It follows no regular pattern thereafter and is often within normal limits. In very acute heavy infections there may be practically no eosinophils in the blood and very few in the circumoval granulomas which may be composed almost entirely of polymorphs.

DIAGNOSIS OF SCHISTOSOMIASIS

Diagnosis depends on identification of the worm (e.g. in a biopsy) or its eggs (passed in urine or faeces or found in a rectal biopsy). At autopsy adult worms can be seen in the abdominal venous plexuses or in the liver; they may be extracted from the tissues by digestion.

The eggs of *S. haematobium* measure 110–170 × 50–70 μm and have a pronounced terminal spine.

Those of *S. mansoni* are about the same size, and have a single lateral spine.

The eggs of *S. japonicum* are smaller, measuring about 100 × 65 μm. There is a small lateral tubercle or hook, but no spine.

Viable eggs contain a living ciliated miracidium which moves within the shell and can be hatched out in fresh water.

In *S. haematobium* infections the eggs are found in the urine (see p. 576) and very occasionally in the faeces. They are sometimes found in rectal biopsies. In the other two infections the eggs are excreted in the faeces and may be found in rectal biopsies. Concentration methods are often necessary to demonstrate eggs in faeces.

Eggs of all species may also be found in granulomas in liver biopsies.

Egg output in excreta should be determined quantitatively by Bell's method based on sucking samples of urine or suspended faeces through filter paper. The eggs are retained on the paper and stained with aqueous ninhydrin solution. Examined by transmitted light, viable eggs containing the miracidium are stained and can be counted.

Other concentration methods for faecal samples are based on separation of the eggs by flotation or sedimentation. Common techniques are the AMS III Formol Ether method, which depends on the fixation of the eggs by formalin and the removal of fat by ether and sedimentation in 0.5 per cent glycerol in water.

Hatching of eggs in a specimen of urine is carried out by centrifuging, removing the supernatant, and reconstituting the sediment with tap water. Samples of faeces (20 g) may be emulsified in a litre of water in a flask with a narrow neck. The preparations are allowed to settle. In a few hours the eggs hatch and the miracidia can be identified in transverse lighting as minute white specks darting about in the inch of water below the meniscus.

Rectal biopsies are snipped with fine forceps from an area about 6 cm above the anal mucocutaneous junction. The material is crushed between two microscope slides and examined for eggs.

*Immune reactions*
Humoral antibodies derived from the developing worms appear in the plasma

about 4 weeks after infection, i.e. about 2 weeks before eggs are excreted. Antibodies to egg antigens are subsequently produced.

The antibodies can be detected by complement fixation, fluorescent antibody techniques and precipitin reactions, using antigens prepared from adult schistosomes or viable eggs. The tests give group reactions and are not species specific. *They are no substitute for the demonstration of eggs in diagnosis.* Other serological tests which include cercarial agglutination, the circumoval precipitin test, and miracidial immobilization are positive in many infections but are not diagnostic. Reversal of these reactions is not used as a test of cure.

Intradermal injection of antigens made usually from adult worms may be useful as a screening test of populations in epidemiological surveys. A volume of 0.1 ml is injected intradermally and the site of injection is examined in 20–30 minutes. A positive reaction is shown by the development of a wheal 2–3 times larger in diameter than that produced by the injection. Over 90 per cent of those infected for more than 6 weeks give positive results. False positive reactions occur in up to 5 per cent. The immediate reaction is a group response. Recent work suggests that specific antigens may give specific delayed sensitivity reactions similar to those in tuberculosis.

## THE TREATMENT OF SCHISTOSOMIASIS

The treatment of infections caused by all species is essentially the same. The objective is to eradicate the infection and so produce a cure, as a result of which all worms are destroyed and the laying of eggs permanently ceases. In practice it has been found that 'cure' in this sense is not easy to achieve, except sometimes in relatively light infections. The custom is therefore to define the action of a drug in terms of percentage reduction of egg excretion. Defined in this way, successful treatment can be obtained with various trivalent antimonial compounds and certain synthetic drugs which are discussed below.

### Trivalent antimonials
The drugs of this type in common use are sodium (or potassium) antimony tartrate and Stibocaptate (Astiban, TWSb).

*Sodium antimony tartrate* must be prepared to BP standards to contain less than 5 parts of lead per million. The drug is still toxic at this standard and must be given with care. It is used in some parts of the world for mass therapy.

For the individual patient it should be given intravenously slowly and well diluted and the greatest care must be taken to avoid leakage into the tissues, which is followed by painful inflammation and sometimes necrosis.

A common dosage regimen is to give it in doses of 0.5 ml of a 6 per cent solution in saline or distilled water, to a maximum single dose of 2.0 ml for persons of 60 kg and over. Children of less than 15 kg are not given the drug. The dose is diluted to 10–15 ml in saline and given very slowly. It is given on alternate days on twelve to sixteen occasions. Thus, the maximum dosage for an adult is:

Day 1:  0.5 ml of 6 per cent solution   (30 mg)
Day 3:  1.0 ml of 6 per cent solution   (60 mg)
Day 5:  2.0 ml of 6 per cent solution (120 mg)

Subsequent dosage on alternate days:

2.0 ml of 6 per cent solution (120 mg)

Oral dosage with sodium antimony tartrate is being tried with some success in mainland China for *S. japonicum* infection.

*S. haematobium* infections usually respond well to a course of twelve doses. *S. mansoni* and *S. japonicum* infections respond less favourably and may need the full sixteen doses.

In some cases a second course is needed. This should be started not less than 6 weeks after the completion of the first course.

The side-effects are unpleasant. The patient often feels pain and constriction in the chest and develops a hard unproductive cough during the injection, which should take about 10 minutes. (It is the custom in Europe to give the drug diluted in this manner. In Egypt, where it has been used extensively for mass therapy, the solution is often given undiluted and rapidly, with apparently few serious ill-effects.) Nausea is common and vomiting is frequent after the injection. The patient should be treated in bed and should if possible remain in hospital during treatment. The drug causes tachycardia and changes in the electrocardiogram, including depression of the T wave and movement of the isoelectric levels; the significance of these changes is uncertain. It may cause severe vomiting, diarrhoea, and jaundice. These are indications for stopping the administration. Death has been caused by the drug and contra-indications for its use include cardiac, hepatic, and renal disorders.

Despite these disadvantages, it is still probably the most widely used antischistosomal drug.

*Stibocaptate* (also called *Astiban* or TWSb). Many workers regard this as a better and safer drug which has the advantage of being given, if desired, by the intramuscular route. This drug is antimony dimercaptosuccinate, a trivalent antimonial which is mixed with British antilewisite (BAL). It is less toxic than sodium antimony tartrate and has fewer side-effects. Nevertheless, deaths have been reported following its usage.

Stibocaptate is usually given intramuscularly as a 10 per cent solution in 5 per cent glucose, at a dosage of 6–10 mg per kg body weight either daily or on alternate days on five occasions. The drug should be given in divided doses during the day; the individual adult daily dose should not exceed 0.5 g.

Successful results with relatively fewer toxic effects have been obtained by giving this dosage once weekly for 5 weeks. As with the sodium antimony tartrate, the patient should be treated in bed or at least receive the injection when at rest and remain in bed for at least 2 hours afterwards.

Side-effects include pain at the injection site, nausea and vomiting for several hours after the injection, muscle and joint pains, and tachycardia. ECG changes similar to those occurring during a course of sodium antimony tartrate develop usually after the third or fourth dose. Death has occurred in very rare instances at about the same time.

Stibocaptate has been used extensively for mass therapy.

Of the other antimony compounds, *Stibophen* is most commonly used. Like Stibocaptate this drug is given intramuscularly and is thus useful when intravenous therapy is contra-indicated. The drug is given as a 6.4 per cent solution in successive doses on alternate days on 10–15 occasions, as follows:

Day 1:         1.5 ml
Day 3:         3.5 ml
Day 5:         5.0 ml
Day 7 *et seq.*: 5.0 ml

Side-effects are usually mild and include pain at the injection site and some nausea. Changes occur in the ECG as above.

*Stibophen* was used for mass therapy in Egypt but has been given up because of the number of unexpected deaths that resulted, usually from shock, sometimes accompanied by hyperpyrexia, and occurring after the fourth or fifth dose.

*Antimony lithium thiomalate* (Anthiomaline) is still used in some areas, with success and a moderate degree of side-effects. The dose is 2.0 ml of the solution (1.0 ml contains 10 mg antimony) given intramuscularly on alternate days on fifteen to twenty occasions.

*Niridazole* (Ambilhar) is an aminonitrothiazole which is very active against all human species of schistosomes.

It is given orally in a dosage of 25 mg per kg body weight daily, in two divided doses for 7 days.

It usually has few side-effects but in some patients anxiety, bad dreams and nightmares, mental confusion, hallucinations, and convulsions may occur. Some deaths have been recorded. It is now believed that the toxic effects arise from raised concentration of the drug in the peripheral blood occurring in cases with severe liver damage and especially when there is some short circuit of the portal and systemic blood circulation such as may develop in schistosomal hepatic fibrosis. It is thus contra-indicated in patients with liver disorders or with a history of psychosis or epilepsy. The neuropsychiatric effects can to some extent be controlled by barbiturates, and are usually transient and subside within 24 hours of cessation of treatment. Electrocardiographical changes similar to those produced by antimony occur during treatment; their importance is uncertain.

The drug has been used successfully in all forms of human schistosomiasis and has not yet been finally assessed. At present it appears to be one of the best compounds for the treatment of *S. haematobium* infections. It has been used with great success in the ambulatory treatment of such infections in children.

*Lucanthone* (Miracil D; Nilodin) is one of a group of thioxanthones which has been given orally with success in *S. haematobium* infections. Response in the other infections has been poor. Relapse after treatment is common.

The drug has not caused death, but has unpleasant side-effects including intense nausea and sometimes diarrhoea, epigastric pain, giddiness, muscular twitchings, insomnia, and depression. Side-effects may be reduced by combining lucanthone with resin in order to slow the absorption in the intestine.

Dosage is 10 mg per kg body weight once daily for 10–20 days. The alternative intensive course of 1 g twice daily for 3 days is associated with severe side-effects.

*Hycanthone* (*Etrenol*) a metabolite of the action of *Aspergillus* spp. on lucanthone, is now under trial but has not yet been adequately assessed. The drug has been given intramuscularly in a single dose of 3 mg per kg body weight. It has been found successful in the treatment of *S. haematobium* infections and useful in light and moderately heavy infections with *S. mansoni*.

The side-effects include vomiting, which may be severe. Deaths have been recorded following the therapeutic dosage but only in cases in which many other drugs have also been given. Two were recently reported from Zäire (one *S. intercalatum*; one *S. mansoni*); in both the liver was already severely damaged before the drug was used. In some areas dosages of 1.5 or 2.0 mg per kg body weight have proved effective and have had less severe side-effects.

*Metrifonate*. See p. 383.

### TEST OF CURE

In individuals who are not exposed to reinfection, the absence of viable eggs 3 months subsequent to treatment may be regarded as 'cure'. In those reinfected immediately, new batches of eggs will appear within 6 weeks to 2 months and observation should therefore be extended to at least 3 months after treatment. Reappearance of eggs or a clinical relapse may result from the survival of worms which were not fully developed during the period of treatment. Eggs in such cases will normally appear within 3 months.

The results of treatment are expressed either as 'cure', that is, the continued absence of viable eggs from the excreta or as 'percentage reduction of egg output'. The latter is based on quantitative examination of samples of excreta and is independent of the egg output before treatment. It is now generally adopted. 'Cure' as such is usually recorded only in light infections.

Dead or 'black' eggs passed in urine or faeces at irregular intervals after treatment or found in biopsies are of no clinical significance; they do not represent the continued presence of the female worm.

## VESICAL SCHISTOSOMIASIS

### DEFINITION

Vesical schistosomiasis is due to infection of the vesical and pelvic venous plexuses with *S. haematobium*.

### GEOGRAPHICAL DISTRIBUTION

Probably originating in the Nile Valley, where it is highly endemic, vesical schistosomiasis has become established widely though irregularly around the Mediterranean littoral, throughout Africa and the adjacent islands, and in the Middle East, where suitable snail vectors exist. The disease does not occur elsewhere except for a small focus in Bombay province in India.

### AETIOLOGY

The terminal-spined eggs are passed in the urine. On getting into fresh water the eggs hatch and miracidia emerge and infect suitable snails. Man acquires the infection by wetting the skin or mucous membranes with fresh water containing the infective larvae (cercariae) discharged from the parasitized snails. The snails in which *S. haematobium* commonly develops are species of the genus *Bulinus*. *B. truncatus* is the most important in Egypt; many other species have been shown to be effective vectors of this parasite elsewhere.

Man is usually the only significant reservoir of infection. Baboons and monkeys have been found naturally infected.

### PATHOLOGY

The distribution of the egg-laying females leads to lesions developing in the early stages in the urinary bladder and the ureters and later in the prostate, seminal vesicles, uterus, vagina, and kidneys. Eggs may be seeded to any part of the body and may set up local lesions arising from granulomatous reactions about them, sometimes followed by fibrosis. In some organs, including the lungs, these reactions are usually minimal, so that eggs may be recovered by digestion of tissues *post mortem* in the absence of apparent lesions.

Eggs are deposited in the venules of the bladder wall and penetrate to the tissue, setting up very active granulomatous reactions; some of these may become necrotic, others become replaced by fibrous tissue. The shells commonly calcify.

The bladder wall becomes irregularly granulomatous and fibrotic. Elasticity is lost as the lesions may extend into the muscle tissue. Contracture and calcification result in limitation of movement and volume, leading clinically to persistent dribbling and frequency. Granulomatous nodules, polyps, and papillomas commonly form in the mucosa. Ulceration of the surface often occurs with bleeding, especially in areas where many eggs have calcified, forming the so-called sandy patches. Secondary infection leads to chronic cystitis with necrosis of areas of the wall and pus and blood in the urine. Carcinoma may develop in association with the schistosomal bladder lesions.

The ureters show similar changes. There is irregular dilatation and constriction, especially in the lower third. These changes arise from the same processes of granuloma formation, fibrosis, and calcification. Secondary infection spreads from the bladder and may ultimately involve the pelvis of the kidney. Hydronephrosis and pyonephrosis are common in the late stages.

Similar lesions develop in the pelvic organs and may lead to extensive fibrosis and, with secondary infection, to abscess formation and chronic sinuses.

Eggs are found most easily in the urine. They appear only rarely in the faeces but may be found in granulomas in the rectal mucosa, where extensive damage is most uncommon.

CLINICAL PICTURE

At the time of penetration of the cercariae, especially if the number is large, there is an itching and pricking sensation with erythema which may be followed by cercarial dermatitis. This usually lasts for no more than 2 or 3 days and is less severe than that due to the penetration of non-human schistosome cercariae.

Some 4 or more weeks later there may be a general allergic reaction with irregular fever, malaise, and muscle pains, and sometimes a generalized urticarial eruption. A temporary eosinophilia of 15–30 per cent is usual at this time. This stage lasts from 2 weeks to 2 months, and varies in its severity. It is often minimal.

Eggs appear in the urine 5–6 weeks after infection. Their appearance may not immediately stimulate any obvious clinical signs.

Usually 3–6 months, but sometimes a couple of years or more, after infection, localizing symptoms due to the presence of eggs in the tissues, and the consequent lesions, make their appearance. There is commonly some frequency of micturition and intermittent haematuria; blood may be limited to the terminal few drops of urine or be present throughout the passage of urine. Small clots are common and sometimes cause considerable pain when passed. It is not associated with dysuria, but there may be urethral and bladder pain after the act of micturition. Vigorous exercise before micturition may induce haematuria. As papilloma formation and ulceration increase in the bladder it becomes irritable and contracted; there is frequency and precipitancy; in severe cases there is dribbling incontinence with the passage of increased amounts of blood and some clots, and pus due to secondary infection, in the urine. The bladder shows areas of calcification at its base; it may become so extensively calcified that in severe long-standing cases its whole outline can clearly be seen radiologically; the volume is usually grossly limited.

With the increase in the lesions in the bladder signs of more generalized genito-urinary and pelvic involvement develop. Damage to the walls of the ureters, and obstruction of their orifices, make them dilated and tortuous; an ascending bacterial infection causes pyelitis and pyelonephrosis; the renal and

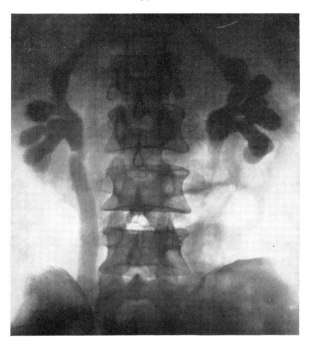

FIG. 51. Dilated renal pelves and ureters.
[Long-standing *S. haematobium* infection: Courtesy Professor H.M.Gilles]

ureteral involvement may end in uraemia. Chronic inflammatory reactions due to secondary bacterial infection, with sinus and fistula formation, cause much damage to the affected structures in the pelvis. Neoplastic changes are particularly liable to occur in the bladder. The patient may eventually die after years of increasing suffering.

The severity of vesical schistosomiasis varies very greatly. Not all those suffering from it pass through the stages described but these are commonly seen in those heavily infected and repeatedly reinfected in the hyperendemic areas such as the Nile Valley. In cases of light infection the patient may suffer a minimum of inconvenience.

The half life of the worms is reckoned at about 5 years but individual worms live for 20 or more years, and the progress of the condition is often very

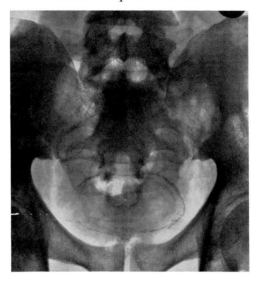

FIG. 52. Contracted bladder with calcifications in wall.
[Long-standing *S. haematobium* infection: Courtesy Professor H.M.Gilles]

slow; there may be increasing disablement when irreversible structural tissue changes have taken place.

In many endemic areas, infection is seen most frequently in children, probably because exposure to infected water is maximal in childhood and becomes less in adult life. Many children seem relatively unaffected, even though they have haematuria. Examination at this stage may reveal filling defects in the bladder and sometimes extensive damage to the ureters. These lesions often regress considerably as the child grows up and reinfection becomes rarer. Even gross lesions usually respond well to treatment. In the same geographical areas adults who give a history of haematuria as children often show minimal or no evidence of the infection and their working capacity appears unimpeded.

### DIAGNOSIS

The terminal-spined eggs usually can best be found by microscopical examination of urine taken between 10.00 and 14.00 hours. Alternatively, the sediment of a 24-hour urine specimen may be examined. An early morning specimen, after rest, does not usually contain so many eggs.

Biopsy through a proctoscope of a fragment of rectal mucosa, which is teased out and examined microscopically, will yield *S. haematobium* eggs in most cases of infection; they may be found there when none can be found at the time in the urine. Rarely, occasional eggs may be found in the faeces.

Cytoscopy will usually reveal lesions at the base of the bladder. The cystoscope when being passed grates over the 'sandy patches' of calcification and bilharzial tubercle formation. Material obtained from these lesions through an operating cystoscope contain living or dead and calcified eggs. Adults are sometimes found in biopsies.

Radiological examination will reveal evidence of calcification in the bladder wall and elsewhere. Marked calcification of the bladder is common in the late stages of severe cases. An IVP is needed for determining changes in the volume of the bladder and the ureteral lumen and the calyces of the kidneys. Signs of pyelonephrosis are common in advanced cases. As pointed out above, gross changes may be present in the bladder and ureters, sometimes with hydronephrosis, in the apparent absence of severe signs and symptoms. This situation is common in children in some endemic areas.

Serological tests using antigens prepared from adult parasites give group, and not specific, reactions. They are no substitute for the demonstration of eggs.

### TREATMENT

Infection with *S. haematobium* responds to chemotherapy better than the infection with the other species.

Probably the most used drugs for treatment are Niridazole, with Stibocaptate as an alternative.

For details see p. 375.

#### Metrifonate

In the last few years the organo-phosphorus compound metrifonate (Bilarcil®, Bager Ag) in doses of 7.5 mg per kg body weight, repeated at fortnightly intervals for 3 doses, has proved successful in the treatment of *S. haematobium* infections, especially in children. Results appear slightly better than with Niridazole or hycanthone. Tolerance is good, despite the anticipated drop in blood cholinesterases.

Recent work in Rhodesia has shown that, in doses of 7.5 mg per kg body weight once every 4 weeks, it has a prophylactic effect against *S. haematobium* infection. It is highly effective, easy and cheap to administer, and is safe.

It has no value against *S. mansoni* infections.

#### General

Surgical treatment which may be needed to deal with fistulae, abscesses, carcinoma of the bladder, etc. should be withheld if possible until after a full course of chemotherapy.

The individual patient should be treated in hospital if given antimonials or Niridazole.

## INTESTINAL SCHISTOSOMIASIS

Intestinal schistosomiasis is due to infection of radicles of the inferior mesenteric vein with the trematode parasite *Schistosoma mansoni*. The disease is characterized by dysenteric symptoms and, in severe cases, by fibrosis of the liver with enlargement of the spleen and ascites.

Like *S. haematobium, S. mansoni* probably originated in the Nile Valley and has spread thence further afield. Its present areas of distribution are rather more focalized than are those of *S. haematobium*. Though the two infections occur concurrently in many areas *S. mansoni* has not spread around the Mediterranean littoral and occurs in only a few foci in the Middle East, including Yemen and parts of Saudi Arabia. *S. mansoni* infection is common in certain areas of South America, especially in Brazil; it occurs in some Caribbean Islands (notably Puerto Rico and St Lucia), where *S. haematobium* has not established itself. The probability is that the infection was introduced to the Americas by the transport of infected African slaves.

AETIOLOGY

The adults of *S. mansoni* commonly infect the branches of the inferior mesenteric veins in the walls of the large bowel. The lateral-spined eggs escape from superficial vessels in the bowel wall into the lumen of the intestine, and are passed to the exterior in the faeces. The eggs if deposited in water give rise to miracidia; these enter snails and undergo further development and vigorous multiplication to form cercariae; the latter emerge from the snails and actively penetrate the skin or mucosae of man, so causing the infection.

The snails in which *S. mansoni* develops are species of the genus *Biomphalaria* in Africa and *Australorbis* in the western hemisphere. *B. alexandrina* is the main vector in Egypt and *B. pfeifferi* that most important in West and in most of East Africa. Man is usually the major reservoir of the infection. A high prevalence of *S. mansoni* infection in baboons in Kenya suggests the possibility of their being epidemiologically important. Other animals may also sometimes be involved.

PATHOLOGY

The adult worms reach the small tributaries of the inferior mesenteric vein from the portal vessels in the liver. Granulomas form around eggs lodged in all parts of the intestinal walls and mucosal changes result not unlike those in the bladder in *S. haematobium* infection, leading to irregular thickening, ulceration, bleeding, formation of granulomatous 'papillomas', and subsequently to fibrosis which may interfere with gut motility and narrow the lumen. With the more diffuse distribution of the parasites the individual lesions are less accessible to visual examination during life. Bilharzial tubercles, nodular submucosal thickening, ulcerations, and papilloma formation may be seen in the lowermost part of the gut sigmoidoscopically. Inflammatory tumours due to secondary bacterial infection may develop; the abdominal lymph glands are often enlarged, and many contain eggs. Carcinomatous changes may occur in association with chronic schistosomal lesions, especially in the sigmoid colon and recto-colic area.

The location of the worms, and the free drainage of the vessels in which they lie, into the portal circulation, facilitate embolism of the eggs to the liver. As they lodge there the usual cellular reactions develop with formation of granulomas. After the deaths of the miracidia in the eggs the subsequent fibrotic changes cause periportal fibrosis. Portal hypertension may result from the changes in the liver with the characteristic picture of ascites and enlargement of the spleen, which gets progressively bigger and may eventually occupy most of the left side of the abdominal cavity.

The combination of enlarged irregularly fibrosed liver and greatly enlarged spleen is commonly called Egyptian hepatosplenomegaly.

Eggs may lodge ectopically in any tissues and cause lesions. They are commonly caught up in the lungs, where they cause characteristic granulomas which may give rise to clinical bronchitic or pneumonic signs and may cause fine mottling of the pulmonary X-ray shadows. Later they cause arteriolar fibrosis and circulatory obstruction, sometimes with recanalization and shunting of pulmonary and splenic blood. Pulmonary hypertension and *cor pulmonale* result. Such a picture is usually seen in patients with advanced hepatic fibrosis and portal hypertension, in whom a collateral circulation has made access of eggs to the lungs easier. Eggs may also reach the brain or spinal cord and cause granulomatous space-occupying tumours. The central nervous system complications in *S. mansoni* infection involve the human cord more frequently than the brain.

### CLINICAL PICTURE

The stage of initial infection when the cercariae are penetrating differs little from the same stage in vesical schistosomiasis.

The stage of toxaemia, which follows a month or so later, is usually more severe than the corresponding stage of the urinary disease. In heavy infections there is fever, nausea, vomiting, diarrhoea, abdominal pain and tenderness, and a dry cough with dyspnoea. There may be marked urticaria, several crops of wheals appearing on any part of the skin, sometimes on the oral mucosa. There may be swelling and tenderness of the liver. An eosinophilia of 30 per cent or more, with a total white cell count of at least 15,000, is usual.

Two months to 2 years after the initial infection, the time being dependent on the intensity of the infection, the infiltrative stage becomes manifest. Commonly the first evidence in severe cases is colic and diarrhoea, with the passage of blood and mucus containing the characteristic lateral-spined eggs. If there are numerous lesions low in the rectum, this dysenteric diarrhoea is severe and is associated with marked tenesmus. Exacerbations of the symptoms of intestinal schistosomiasis in the early stages tend to recur at intervals of 2 or 3 weeks. There is anorexia and wasting. The colon becomes thickened, spastic and tender and many ova are carried to the lungs. An end result of the periarteritis caused by the presence of eggs and associated granulomas and subsequent fibrosis of the pulmonary arterioles is pulmonary hypertension with enlargement of the right heart (*cor pulmonale*). In this condition haemoptysis may be severe.

As the infection continues, the engorged hypertrophied mucosa of the large bowel bleeds more readily; ulceration and secondary infection cause the appearance of pus in the motions; and polypoidal tumours develop in the rectum and tend to prolapse. Inflammatory tumours can be felt within the abdomen, usually along the line of the descending and sigmoid colon or the caecum. The abdominal lymph glands become enlarged and palpable. Sinuses and fistulae commonly form in the indurated perineum and buttocks in the latest stages of the disease. Hardening and shrinkage due to fibrosis may transform the affected gut into a fibrous irregular tube largely devoid of mucosa. At this stage the patient presents with a history of intermittent diarrhoea with mucus, or with mucus and blood, and with periods of intermission, sometimes constipation. The picture may resemble that of carcinoma of the colon or of amoebic colitis.

In the early stages the liver enlarges and becomes tender and the spleen is palpable. As the disease progresses hepatic fibrosis develops and the liver at first enlarges further and then shrinks so that late in the picture it may be only just palpable.

The portal hypertension due to the hepatic fibrosis causes the spleen to enlarge and ascites may develop. There is increasing hepatic insufficiency, which may terminate within a few years or may progress over 15–20 years and be brought to an end by intercurrent infection. Portal hypertension commonly leads eventually to the development of varices in the oesophageal and gastric veins. Repeated and sometimes fatal haematemesis may result.

In the early stages pneumonic signs occur in heavy infections when the other complications of intestinal schistosomiasis are numerous. In addition to those occurring as a direct result of the presence of parturient female worms in the abdomen, eggs may be found ectopically in various organs and tissues. The lesions sometimes found in the central nervous system, in contrast to those due to *S. japonicum* infections, tend to involve the cord rather than the brain. A transverse myelitis with various forms of palsy is the usual result in this case.

The effects of *S. mansoni* schistosomiasis are dependent on the numbers of worms and on the sites of deposition and of lodgement of the eggs. In the highly endemic areas the morbidity and mortality rates due to the disease are

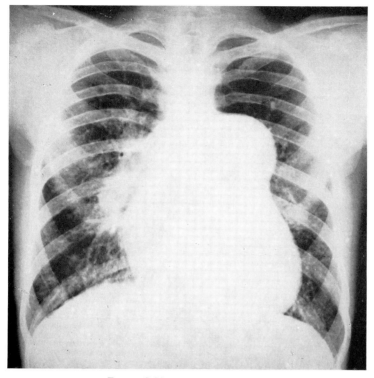

FIG. 53. Schistosomal *cor pulmonale.*

Egyptian male aged 26 years; ill 3 years. Aneurysmal dilatation of the pulmonary artery and its main branches; right ventricular hypertrophy; and fine mottling of the lung parenchyma. There was hepatosplenomegaly; ova of *S. mansoni* and also those of *S. haematobium* were found in the stools.

[By courtesy of Dr Z.Farid]

high; elsewhere many persons may harbour light infections with no apparent inconvenience and the diagnosis may be made only incidentally.

### DIAGNOSIS

In heavy infections the lateral-spined eggs can be found in the blood and mucus in the motions. Where the infection is light repeated search over many days for flecks of blood or mucus on the exterior of the formed stools may be necessary to find the eggs. Various concentration methods have been elaborated for the examination of stools in such cases.

Even with these and other concentration methods it may be necessary to examine daily specimens of stool over a month in light asymptomatic infections before the eggs are recovered.

The patient should be examined by sigmoidoscope for observation of mucosal lesions and obtaining specimens of faecal mucus for searching for eggs. Rectal biopsy is useful.

The complement fixation and other serological and intradermal tests are not satisfactory procedures for diagnosis.

A barium enema with screening may disclose filling defects, irregular constrictions, and restriction of the gut movement. The picture closely resembles that of carcinoma *or* amoebic colitis. It improves with treatment but permanent deformity may be caused by the fibrosis.

TREATMENT

*S. mansoni* infections respond less favourably to treatment than *S. haematobium* infections. The basis of chemotherapy is as described on p. 375.

*Light and moderate infections*
The choice lies between an antimonial and Niridazole.

The antimonial most commonly used is Stibocaptate, which can be given intramuscularly in fewer doses than sodium antimony tartrate, which has to be given intravenously.

Niridazole has the great advantage of being given orally. In light infections it can be used without fear of toxicity. Unfortunately, it is contra-indicated in individuals with a psychotic history or with cardiac or hepatic disability and its use is consequently restricted.

*Severe and complicated infections*
Where there is measurable hepatic damage and particularly in cases with portal hypertension and indications of collateral circulation Niridazole must not be used. The only present alternatives are Stibocaptate or sodium antimony tartrate.

The portal hypertension is dealt with in the usual way; paracentesis may be needed for relief of the ascites but should not be repeated more often than possible. Hepatic coma is treated by standard methods. Transfusion is necessary in the event of severe haematemesis, melaena, or haemoptysis. Portal hypertension may sometimes require portal venous shunt operations; surgery should not be practised until an attempt has been made by chemotherapy to control the infection. Where there is gross anaemia with a hypersplenic element, removal of the spleen may help. Splenic removal may also be necessary when the organ becomes too large and is causing physical distress.

Ectopic lesions in the brain may need operation, which should be performed only after specific chemotherapy.

Where there is already a porto-systemic shunt (sometimes provided gratuitously by surgical interference) any form of specific treatment carries the risk of embolic seeding into the general circulation of dead or dying adult worms. If the infection is heavy, the persistent and continuous damage caused by eggs lodging in the tissues, including what is left of the liver, must be controlled and this means that chemotherapy is desirable. In a given case the physician has to decide on balance whether the condition of the patient would benefit or otherwise by treatment.

## ASIATIC SCHISTOSOMIASIS

### DEFINITION

Far Eastern or visceral schistosomiasis (Katayama disease) is due to infection of radicles of the inferior and superior mesenteric veins with *Schistosoma japonicum*. The disease is characterized by visceral lesions with dysenteric symptoms, hepatic fibrosis, enlargement of the spleen, and ascites.

### GEOGRAPHICAL DISTRIBUTION

Limited to the Far East the disease is found extensively throughout the Yangtze Basin and the south-eastern part of China. It is prevalent in some Philippine Islands, including southern Luzon. Leyte, and Mindanao, in Sulawesi (Celebes), and in foci in Laos and Kampuchea. A small burnt-out focus exists in southern Thailand. It has recently been found to be endemic in Laos on Khong Island in the Mekong River near the border with Kampuchea. The infection has recently been eliminated from Japan. Animal but not human infection occurs in Taiwan.

### AETIOLOGY

The adult *S. japonicum* normally infect the branches of the superior mesenteric vein draining the mesentery and small intestine and the inferior mesenteric vein draining the large bowel.

The eggs have no spine, but there is a small tubercle on one side of them. Normally they find their way into the lumen of the bowel and are voided to the exterior in the stools. The cycle of development is similar to that of *S. haematobium* or *S. mansoni*.

The snails in which *S. japonicum* develops are species of the genus *Oncomelania*. *O. nosophora* is an important vector in the coastal area of China; *O. formosana* in Taiwan; *O. lupensis* in the Yangtze Basin; and *O. quadrasi* in the Philippine Islands.

The infection in Khong Island, Laos, is transmitted by *Lithoglyphosis* spp. at low water in the River Mekong itself. This is a most interesting example of infection being transmitted by an unusual vector snail on the banks of a great and fast-flowing river.

## PATHOLOGY

The basic histopathology of *S. japonicum* lesions is similar to that of other schistosomal infections of man. This worm is a more prolific producer of eggs than in the other species. In view of this fact, and of the distribution of the female worms in the body, the pathological lesions are more widespread and extensive. The organs involved are the small bowel and the mesentery and the upper part of the large intestine. The eggs are very readily conveyed in the portal system to the liver. The resultant fibrosis causes portal hypertension with gross enlargement of the spleen, ascites, and the development of collateral circulations with gastro-oesophageal varices. Pulmonary hypertension is less common than in *S. mansoni* infections. Ectopic lesions due to *S. japonicum* much more commonly occur in the brain than is the case with *S. mansoni* infections.

### CLINICAL PICTURE

The stage of initial infection by cercariae resembles that of the other human schistosomal infections.

The early stage of sensitivity reaction, the Katayama syndrome, is severe and may appear within 2–3 weeks of infection. There is a marked urticaria with angioneurotic oedema and fever, vomiting, diarrhoea, cramps in the abdominal muscles, and tenderness along the line of the colon, especially the caecum and sigmoid, liver tenderness and enlargement, and a dry cough with dyspnoea, physical signs of bronchitis or bronchopneumonia, and scattered soft mottling of the lung fields on X-ray. The stage lasts for some weeks, during which there is a marked eosinophilia.

The infiltrative stage may follow without intermission. The diarrhoea becomes more severe and there is frequent passage of loose bloody mucoid stools which contain the eggs. There is often a continuing or remittent daily fever. Anorexia causes wasting and there is an increasing anaemia but a diminution or even disappearance of the earlier eosinophilia. The colon is often palpable and tender; the liver and spleen are engorged, enlarged, and tender. As fibrous tissue replaces the earlier focal abscesses and bilharzial tubercles the acute symptoms diminish and the fever lessens or disappears. As the liver becomes more fibrotic it shrinks, portal tension rises, and the spleen increases in size. The mesentery and omentum become thickened and fibrotic and, by binding down the colon, may cause a constriction to appear across an otherwise swollen abdomen in the wasted subject. Ascites develops and may become progressive, with great distension of the abdomen; the superficial veins on the abdominal wall distend and become tortuous. Haematemesis often follows rupture of varicose veins in the stomach or oesophagus. Melaena may result from haemorrhage into the intestines or stomach. The lungs are involved as in mansonian schistosomiasis but less commonly.

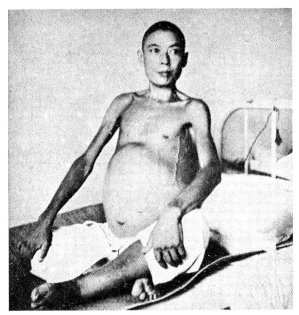

FIG. 54. Hepatic cirrhosis, portal hypertension, and ascites in a Chinese with *S. japonicum* infection. Note the prominent superficial abdominal veins.

[By courtesy of *The Lancet*]

Ectopic localization of eggs is common. In the central nervous system the lesions tend to occur in the brain rather than in the cord; schistosomal granulomata cause the clinical manifestations of an expanding tumour, with Jacksonian attacks, optic neuritis, monoplegia, hemiplegia or quadriplegia, various mental and perceptive derangements, or coma.

On the whole, Asiatic schistosomiasis, though it varies greatly in severity, is a grave disease; the morbidity and mortality resulting from it are greater than with corresponding degrees of infection with the other schistosomes.

Early and continued infections in childhood may give rise to dwarfism, probably due to hypopituitarism. *Cor pulmonale* is sometimes seen in children in hyperendemic areas.

### DIAGNOSIS

The eggs are small and have no spine; there is a small lateral tubercle or hook. They can be recovered from the stools with greater ease than in *S. mansoni* infections. The same methods of search for them are employed. Intestinal biopsy through a proctoscope, or preferably a sigmoidoscope, is a quick, effective means of finding eggs and establishing a definitive diagnosis.

The complement fixation, intradermal, and other serological tests employed are similar to those used in the other infections.

TREATMENT

Chemotherapy of this infection is difficult. Full dosage with sodium antimony tartrate or with Stibocaptate is usually regarded as the best procedure. In the Philippines moderate to good results have been claimed with Stibophen. The Chinese claim success with oral sodium antimony tartrate. Niridazole is effective in light, uncomplicated infections, but the common early liver involvement excludes its general use.

For treatment of complicated cases see under *S. mansoni* infections (p. 388).

Control is attempted in the same way as in other infections. It is much more difficult in *S. japonicum* infections, however, because the common domestic animals, including the dog, the pig and the ox, are all susceptible and are often heavily infected in hyperendemic areas. Moreover, the snail is amphibious.

## NON-HUMAN SCHISTOSOME DERMATITIS

In some parts of the world it is well known that bathing in local water is followed by dermatitis, sometimes called 'swimmer's itch'. This is caused by the penetration of the skin by cercariae of schistosomes with bird or animal hosts. Although the cercariae cause the local skin reactions, they do not develop further in the human host and are rapidly removed from the tissues by the cellular response.

Schistosomal dermatitis occurs in many areas where the human schistosomal infections are unknown; it may also be produced in sensitized individuals by the cercariae of the human schistosomes. In South-east Asia it has become an occupational hazard of some importance, causing considerable loss of working time. In this region the commonest and most active parasite is *Schistosoma spindale*. Others recently discovered in isolated areas include *Trichobilharzia maegraithi* and *Orientobilharzia harinasuti*.

In an individual who has not previously been exposed to the cercariae or has been exposed only occasionally, the penetration causes prickling or itching for an hour or so, with the appearance of small macules which may persist for some hours. In some cases there is a diffuse erythema rather than a macular eruption and occasionally there is a local urticaria. Ten to 15 hours after penetration papules may replace the macules and the appearance of these is associated with intense itching for some days. Sometimes after exposure to great numbers of cercariae the papules become confluent. The papules usually disappear within a week, leaving pigmented spots. On the second or third day vesicles may form; these are ruptured by scratching, and on bacterial infection they may become pustular.

In initial infections, both natural and experimental, schistosome cercariae may produce only a slight reaction; after repeated exposure to attack the reactions usually become much more pronounced as a result of sensitization.

In highly sensitized individuals the reaction, even to small numbers of cercariae penetrating a very limited area of skin, may be considerable; if large areas of skin are penetrated by great numbers of cercariae there may be a very severe generalized reaction with prostration. Some individuals do not become sensitized even after repeated exposures to cercariae over long periods. Others develop an irregular and persistent nodular or eczematous dermatitis which causes considerable irritation and may lead to loss of labour time.

There is no specific treatment. Antihistamine drugs bring relief applied locally as ointments or taken orally when the dermatitis is widespread. Personal protection against cercariae is afforded by wearing rubber boots, or even by wearing a moderately tightly woven cloth. A film of oil or grease on the body is ineffective; indeed it encourages the attachment of those cercariae which normally penetrate the oily skins of water-birds.

## PROPHYLAXIS FOR SCHISTOSOMIASIS

Avoidance of any contact with 'fresh' water is the ideal in the endemic areas. This is practically impossible, although contact can be greatly reduced by common sense—by avoiding swimming or wading (as yacthsmen do) in streams and lakes, by drying wet skin quickly, by drinking water that has been boiled or allowed to stand for at least 3 days (thus killing the infective cercariae).

Piping water to villages seems to have only minor effects on incidence in itself, unless the water is first treated, at least by sedimentation for several days.

Destruction of the snails by molluscicides or burning, and weed clearance in canals, streams, etc. is also inadequate, quite apart from being too costly to carry out and maintain.

As noted above, personal protection against cercarial penetration is not highly successful. Some cercaricides and repellents are useful for short periods when applied to exposed surfaces. These include the insecticides dimethylphthalate and dibutyl phthalate applied directly to the skin or impregnated in closely woven clothing. Various unguents made from wool fat and containing hexachlorophene and benzyl benzoate have also been successful.

Until the worms in the endemic areas can be completely eliminated, however, probably the best form of prophylaxis would be offered by a non-toxic drug with true prophylactic effect on all schistosomes. So far, no such drug has been produced, but in *Schistosoma haematobium* infections there is evidence that metrifonate has some prophylactic action; it has none in the other schistosome infections. In isolated communities hycanthone has been found to have considerable suppressive (? prophylactic) effect on the incidence of *S. mansoni*. In St Lucia, for instance, results of regular mass therapy alone proved considerably better than those obtained by measures limited to piping and control of water supplies to villages (including the installation of laundries, baths, etc.) or to snail control only.

# 24

# SKIN CONDITIONS, MISCELLANEOUS

DESERT SORE

A wide variety of inflammatory skin ulcerations is included in this term, including ulcers arising from pyogenic agents and others in which the principal organism is *Corynebacterium diphtheriae*. These ulcerations are seen most commonly in hot, arid countries, including parts of Africa and Australia. They appear singly or in groups on exposed parts of the body, especially the wrists and legs.

They vary considerably in size. The surrounding skin is itchy and erythematous. The edges are undermined, the ulcerated surface is yellowish and may be covered by a thin crust. There is often a profuse seropurulent discharge. The lesions are very persistent.

Pyogenic organisms are present in all ulcers; in some, *C. diphtheriae* is present. Ulcers of the latter type may represent primary diphtheritic lesions which have become secondarily infected, or vice versa. Fusiform bacilli and treponemata are absent.

Treatment consists in cleaning the ulcerated area and the application of local dressings containing sulphonamides, acriflavine, or penicillin. Indolent cases may respond to occlusive treatment as for tropical ulcer.

When *C. diphtheriae* is present, preliminary intramuscular injection of antitoxin is indicated.

## CUTANEOUS DIPHTHERIA

Skin infection with virulent strains of *Corynebacterium diphtheriae* causing ulceration is common in certain dry, hot parts of India, Africa, and the Middle East and is occasionally observed in hot, moist regions. The infection may be spread from skin to skin or from the pharynx or vice versa. It is not known whether the diphtheria organism initiates the lesion or gains entrance through an abrasion or existing pyogenic ulceration.

Diphtheritic ulcers usually appear on the exposed parts, especially the legs. They appear rapidly and tend to become chronic and indolent. The lesion commences as a vesicle and rapidly ulcerates. The ulcers are small, seldom exceeding a few centimetres across, rounded, clearly demarcated, and may be multiple.

The surrounding skin is erythematous or slightly bluish, and raised. The edges are inverted and slightly undermined. The surface is deeply ulcerated and usually covered with grey exudate or a dark crust.

*C. diphtheriae* can be demonstrated in the ulcerated tissue. Bacteriological assistance is required for identification and estimation of virulence. Pyogenic cocci and other organisms are commonly also present.

Treatment consists of a single dose of 20,000 units of antitoxin intramuscularly and the application of local penicillin compresses. Healing is rapid. Sulphonamides and bland ointments are ineffective.

Paralytic sequelae similar to those arising from faucial diphtheria have been reported.

## MYCOBACTERIAL ULCERS

Mycobacterial skin ulcers, which occur in Australia, Papua New Guinea, East Africa (for instance the Buruli ulcer in Uganda), and in parts of West Africa including Zaïre, may be difficult to distinguish clinically from tropical ulcer or tertiary yaws lesions. The lesions occur chiefly on the legs or arms and most often in children. They may be diagnosed bacteriologically by finding the acid-fast *Mycobacteria*, usually in extracellular clumps in the necrotic granulation tissue of the ulcer and in histological sections of the margins. Early lesions may appear as oedematous areas or as nodules which gradually enlarge and finally ulcerate irregularly. The ulceration may involve the underlying muscle and bone; irregular calcification may develop under the lesion. The base is covered by adherent slough through which pale red 'gelatinous' granulation tissue can be seen. The margins are raised, firm, and sometimes hyperpigmented. There may be satellite lesions. Local glands are not involved in the absence of secondary infection. The Mantoux test is usually negative and does not convert. It is thought that the lesions may result from sensitivity and violent reaction upon infection with the *Mycobacteria,* or that they appear a long time after infection, when local sensitization has developed. In some cases the ulcers have been observed to develop in areas of local trauma, such as a scratch or insect bite. Chemotherapy with antituberculosis drugs is ineffective. Excision is regarded as the best treatment; it is followed by rapid healing.

## SCABIES

### DEFINITION

Dermatitis (the classical 'itch') is caused by infestation with *Sarcoptes scabiei.*

## DISTRIBUTION AND AETIOLOGY

A world-wide complaint, especially common in some parts of the tropics and subtropics.

*S. scabiei* is very small. The gravid female burrows into the epidermis and dies at the end of the tunnel after depositing eggs. Larvae hatch in a few days and begin further burrows, eventually maturing in about 4 weeks. Mating takes place on the skin surface and the 'cycle' is repeated, the resulting lesion developing rapidly through the activities of successive generations.

Transmission occurs by direct skin contact, through contaminated under-clothing, or possibly via infested bedding.

## CLINICAL PICTURE

Intense local pruritus and dermatitis usually appear within a few days of infection. The tissue reaction may, however, be delayed for weeks. It is probably due to the burrowing, as the mite does not apparently produce noxious fluids. The first visible lesion is a reddish black line a centimetre or more in length over which the skin is slightly elevated. At one end an orifice may be visible. At the other a tiny vesicle conceals the female.

Itching is intense, especially at night, and frequent scratching and excoriation are followed by secondary infection. Unless treated the lesions persist almost indefinitely and gradually spread from area to area.

The mite can penetrate the skin everywhere, but is found most frequently where the epithelium is thin and delicate, especially between the fingers and toes, the backs of the hands, the wrist, the genitals, groin, breasts, and axillae. The head and neck usually escape.

## DIAGNOSIS

Examination of scrapings from lesions with a lens or the low power of the microscope may reveal the mite or bits of it. The parasite may be most easily found by selecting for examination the white bleb usually to be seen at the end of a linear lesion. It can often be dissected out with the point of a needle.

Scrapings are best examined on a slide after soaking them in 10 per cent potassium hydroxide and covering with a coverslip. The mite is pale, roughly globular, about 300 $\mu$m in length, has eight very short legs and numerous bristles.

## TREATMENT

Pyogenic infections must be treated as they arise.

The parts affected or, better, the whole body except the head and neck, should be scrubbed or soaked once or twice in the day with soap and water (preferably Tetmosol soap) and thoroughly dried. Sulphur ointment, **benzyl** benzoate, or tetmosol are then applied.

*Benzyl benzoate.* An aromatic oily liquid is usually made up as a lotion with equal parts alcohol and soft soap. It is rubbed in well, allowed to dry, then rubbed in again. Baths are given every 24 hours.

Benzyl benzoate may be very irritating to the skin.

*Tetmosol.* A 5 per cent solution is applied once or twice a day. Soap is now manufactured containing tetmosol (10 per cent) which may be satisfactory by itself as a therapeutic agent or prophylactic. This is relatively non-irritant.

### PROPHYLAXIS

Cleanliness and avoidance of contact with infested bodies and materials are the first essentials.

## MYIASIS

The skin may be invaded from time to time by the larvae of certain flies which burrow into the subcutaneous tissues and cause inflammatory lesions in which they mature, escaping for pupation after a variable time.

In tropical America such lesions may be produced by *Dermatobia hominis* (the bot or warble fly). Larvae are deposited on the skin by mosquitoes upon which the bot fly has placed her eggs. They penetrate vertically and produce painful boil-like swellings in 3–4 weeks. After 6 weeks the mature larva emerges. Secondary infection is usual. The larva should be extracted surgically.

The larva of *Cordylobia anthropophaga* (the Tumbu fly) causes similar lesions in parts of Africa. The infection is spread by any means which expose the human skin to the first instar larva. Dirty clothes, or clothes which have been dried on grass, may provide the opportunity for the larva to reach and penetrate the skin.

The penetration of the skin is usually unnoticed. In a day or two a papule forms and grows into a furuncular swelling in which the larva becomes active at intervals, causing severe local symptoms, and the escape of serous fluid from the 'head' of the boil at which the posterior end of the larva is presenting. The local lesion is fully developed within 2–3 weeks. It is intensely painful and there may be local adenitis and even a general febrile reaction.

A film of liquid paraffin is placed over the opening in the skin after removing any scab that may be present. The posterior end of the larvae begins to emerge. More oil is added drop by drop. The larva tries harder to reach the surface for breathing and in doing so lubricates the walls of the lesion. After a while it can be slowly expressed by pressure (often painful) on either side of the lesion.

Healing of the wound is usually rapid, but may leave some scarring.

The larvae of *Auchmeromyia luteola* (the so-called Congo floor maggot) hatch from the floor of native huts and attach themselves to those sleeping on the floors. During the night the elongated, dirty white, translucent larvae attach temselves firmly to the skin by means of spines and suck blood, changing colour during the process to bright red. When replete, they drop off the victim and continue their development.

Blow-fly maggots may infest cutaneous lesions, bodily orifices, etc. causing intensive tissue invasion and destruction, especially in the nasal cavities and the orbit. Extension to the meninges or brain may occur. Larvae may be coughed or sneezed out. The flies most commonly concerned are *Cochliomyia* spp. (*Callitroga*), the screw worm in the Americas and *Chrysomyia* in eastern and north eastern Africa. Others which sometimes cause lesions are the 'flesh' flies, *Sarcophaga* spp. and *Wohlfahrtia* spp., and the sheep bot-fly *Oestrus*.

Treatment consists of removing the larvae and dealing with the infection by antibiotics.

Intestinal myiasis is mainly accidental, resulting from swallowing eggs or larvae in infested food. Invasion of the intestinal mucosa may occur in sarcophaga infections.

Creeping eruptions somewhat similar to those due to an errant round worm larvae may arise from cutaneous infection with the larvae of certain flies, for instance, from infection with the larvae of the horse bot-fly (*Gasterophilus* spp.), each lesion containing a single minute larva which has hatched from eggs deposited on the hairs, usually of the limbs. The larva of the cattle warble fly *Hypoderma bovis* may give rise to similar lesions. For treatment see p. 555.

## VESICANT BEETLES

Beetles belonging to the families *Cantharidae* and *Staphylinidae* are known to cause lesions of the skin which may be both inconvenient and severe.

Cantharides beetles, especially the bright metallic-green Spanish fly, cause large painful blisters if crushed against the skin.

Rove beetles belonging to the genus *Paederus* are also intensely vesicant. They are bright orange except for the head, very short wing cases, and last two abdominal segments which are black. They are widely distributed and known for their irritant effects, particularly in the Amazon valley and many parts of Africa. Provided they are unmolested on the skin there is no cutaneous reaction. If irritated or rubbed into the skin deliberately or at pressure points, such as the belt or shoulder areas, small bullae, blisters, and raw tender ulcers develop after a latent period of about 12 hours. The reaction is often mistaken for fungoid infections. Particularly unpleasant results occur when the vesicant material is introduced into the eye. A severe conjunctivitis with oedema of the lids and weeping is set up. These insects have been suspected of causing blindness in young children.

As in the case of other noxious creatures, some local knowledge of the genera and species, and their habits, is required before diagnosis can be made.

## FLEAS

Fleas are small, laterally compressed, wingless, ectoparasitic arthropods with mouth parts adapted to piercing and sucking. Some have combs on the head or thorax or both; others are combless. They tend to remain on a given host but will migrate to other hosts in suitable circumstances. Eggs are dropped haphazardly and hatch in 3–4 days. The active larvae are commonly found in dust; in the resting stage the larva or the adult may remain dormant for months.

The two major families are important to man.

The *Pulicidae* include *Pulex irritanus,* the human flea, *Xenopsylla* spp. commonly found on the rat and vector of bubonic plague and various fleas of rats, mice, dogs, and cats. The *Tungidae* include *T. penetrans* (the Chigoe or Jigger flea) the female of which burrows beneath the human skin and causes serious incapacity especially when secondarily infected.

Flea bites appear as small discrete erythematous, sometimes petechial, spots, which are usually very irritating, especially in sensitized individuals.

Medically, the most important flea is *Xenopsylla cheopis,* the major vector of bubonic plague in man; other species of *Xenopsylla* may also transmit plague. Other genera of fleas may be concerned with transmission of *Pasteurella pestis* in reservoir animals.

Murine typhus (*Rickettsia mooseri*) spreads from the rat to man via the bite of *Xenopyslla* spp. and is maintained as an enzootic in rats by rodent lice.

The cysticeroid stage of the rat tapeworm *Hymenolepis diminuta* develops in the body cavity of human, rat, and mouse fleas. Human infection with the adult follows swallowing infected fleas.

Exceptionally, the dog tapeworm *Dipylidium caninum* may be similarly transmitted to man.

Dog and cat fleas can be controlled in the animals by frequent washing. DDT is used for dusting heavily infected dogs or their kennels. Toxic effects may result.

Houses may be cleared by spraying with 5 per cent DDT and rat runs by dusting DDT powder (8–10 per cent).

Protection against biting from *Xenopsylla* suspected of being infected with plague may be achieved by dusting the environment with DDT or using DDT-impregnated clothing.

Resistance to DDT and its analogues has developed in many fleas.

Gamma BHC and organo-phosphorus compounds are alternatives but resistance may also be developed against them.


## LICE


Lice are obligatory parasites of man. Those which infest man are: *Pediculus humanus corporis* (the body louse), *P. hum. capitis* (the head louse) and *Phthirus pubis* (the crab louse).

The louse has a flat body and an indistinctly segmented thorax, no wings, and 6 legs modified for grasping. The female lays up to 5 eggs (also called 'nits') in the day. These adhere to hairs and hatch in about 8 days. The nymphs mature in 14 days and the adult lives about 4 weeks.

Lice take two blood meals daily. The bite causes local irritation and small haemorrhagic lesions.

*P. hum. corporis* attaches itself to body hair and commonly migrates, especially to coarse clothing, where it will survive for as long as a week in cold conditions. *P. hum. capitis* attaches itself to the scalp hair. Both avoid light.

Lice transfer to other hosts as a result of close contact with an infested person. Migration is increased from the host during exercise or during fever.

Relapsing fever (*Borrelia recurrentis*) is transmitted by crushing infected lice and introducing infective material through skin lesions. An infected louse may remain infective for a month.

The rickettsia of exanthematic (louse-borne) typhus and trench fever (*R. quintana*) are conveyed in the faeces of infected lice in the same way.

The cysticercoid stage of the dog tapeworm *Dipylidium caninum* develops in the body louse and may be transmitted to man when the arthropod is swallowed.

The crab louse *Phthirus pubis* is broader and flatter than the other lice and has powerful claws on the second and third legs. It clings to hairs in the pubis and groin and occasionally wanders to other hairy skin. The bite is similar to that of the body louse. They are not known to transmit infections to man.

Lice can be eliminated by dusting with DDT powder (10 per cent). Three dustings at weekly intervals will remove adults and nits completely. As an alternative for head lice, liquids containing DDT (1 per cent) and various solvents and emulsifiers, including benzyl benzoate and Tween 80, may be used. In the treatment of head lice the DDT powder can be applied to the head and neck directly. The hair should be cut short and kept well washed. The crab louse is destroyed by DDT or by emulsions containing lauryl thiocyanate.

Resistance to DDT has developed in some strains of *Pediculus hum. corporis* but not in *P. hum. capitis* or *Phthirus pubis*. Gamma BHC or Pyrethrum powders are alternatives to DDT; some resistance to the former is suspected.

Some preparations of DDT, especially oil suspensions and wall sprays, may cause toxic effects in man.

Cleanliness, frequent, thorough washing and avoidance of contact with other infested individuals prevent further infection.

Louse-infested clothing is best dealt with by heat. A hot iron is useful for getting into the folds where the lice tend to congregate.

# 25

# SMALLPOX AND ALASTRIM

Smallpox is a virus infection formerly of wide distribution and of great importance to the health of the community because of its tendency to spread.

## GEOGRAPHICAL DISTRIBUTION

In the last decade mass vaccination combined with a search-and-containment policy has proved remarkably successful. Smallpox has been claimed by special commissions to have been eradicated from all main endemic areas, apart from laboratory accidents such as the recent Birmingham outbreak.

Some doubts still linger about the validity of this 'eradication' and especially about the need to sustain the expensive on-going logistics and enthusiasm involved in the programmes, something that has certainly not been the case in the time-limited malaria eradication programmes.

Smallpox is still included in the four internationally quarantinable diseases under the International Health Regulations and decisions regarding the possession of a valid vaccination certificate remain the prerogatives of individual countries concerned about possible importation.

In view of the current uncertainty, it therefore seems reasonable to continue to describe the disease in this Text. The next few years might well decide the issue beyond reasonable doubt—one way or the other

## AETIOLOGY

The causative virus is large (250 $\mu$m) and exists in two main epidemiological forms. The more pathogenic gives rise to the severe disease smallpox (variola major), the less pathogenic kind to alastrim (variola minor). A poxvirus closely related to smallpox is *vaccinia,* the cause of cowpox; this is relatively non-pathogenic and is modified by passage through the calf for use in vaccines.

The sexes are equally affected. Any age is susceptible but in an unprotected community the disease appears commonly in children.

Smallpox is normally transmitted by the introduction of the virus through the mucous membranes of the upper respiratory tract.

In the incubation period the virus is multiplying in the reticulo-endothelial cells of the internal organs and the patient is consequently not infectious. In the prodromal stage of the disease viraemia has occurred and, as the clinical picture develops, changes occur in the mucous membranes of the upper respiratory tract in parallel with those on the skin. The virus reaches the surface and the patient becomes infectious. A working rule is thus that the patient is not infectious until the rash begins. He is most infectious in the early eruptive stages and is usually no longer infectious so far as the respiratory tract is concerned by the twelfth day of the disease, by which time the lesions in the trachea and nasopharyngeal mucous membranes have healed. The skin lesions are highly infectious right up to the stage of the drying scab; the bedclothes, floor dust, and anything in contact with the patient, become contaminated. The patient who dies of overwhelming viraemia before the rash gets beyond the stage of being erythematous, even if haemorrhagic, may be relatively non-infectious since he may die before the lesions in the pharyngeal and tracheal mucous membranes have reached the point of breaking down and discharging the virus into the respiratory tract.

Although there is no doubt that the usual mode of transmission is infection via the nasopharynx, cases of smallpox sometimes develop in outbreaks in non-endemic areas, at a distance from the original source and without any obvious contact with infectious cases. The explanation of such transmission is a subject of considerable controversy. There seems little doubt that sometimes aerial convection of infected dust or particles of skin lesions is responsible. This seemed to be the case in the outbreak of imported smallpox in West Germany in the late 1960s and presumably in the 1978 laboratory episode in England.

### PATHOLOGY

The virus infects the body through the mucous membranes and enters the reticulo-endothelial cells in which it multiplies during the incubation period. It then enters the blood stream, causing the clinical prodromal stage. The viraemia is short-lived; the virus cannot usually be recovered from the blood after the second day of the overt disease. The virus reaches the skin and mucous membranes where it causes the characteristic lesions. In the skin the small blood vessels of the dermis and corium are first involved. The endothelium swells and may degenerate. The vessels become congested and dilated. Some perivascular lymphocytic cuffing occurs. This is the stage of the erythematous prodromal rash. In the epithelium, above these vascular disturbances, swelling and degeneration of the cells in the middle layer occur, giving rise clinically to the early maculopapular lesions. The cells necrose and fluid fills the space to produce the vesicle. Polymorphs now migrate from the corium and enter the fluid, giving rise to the pustule (at this stage there is *no* secondary bacterial infection). Later, epithelialization occurs beneath the damaged area and the pustule dries up and is discharged as a crust or scab. Scarring results from replacement of damaged tissues, commonly the sweat and sebaceous glands, by fibrous tissue. Haemorrhagic smallpox results from direct bleeding from the affected dermal vessels or bleeding into the maculo-papular or vesicular stages of the rash.

Typical lesions may occur in the conjunctiva. They do not develop in the avascular cornea, but where there is pannus or injured vascularized tissue, corneal ulceration may develop and the anterior chamber and iris may be involved.

Lesions in mucous membranes are similar, but the release of virus to the surface occurs much more easily and probably earlier, giving rise in the nasopharynx to a highly infectious state. Lesions are common in the mouth, the tongue, uvula, nasopharynx, and sometimes the trachea and oesophagus. In haemorrhagic smallpox bleeding may occur from any mucous membrane.

Lesions in other organs are primarily the result of the multiplication of the virus in the reticulo-endothelial cells and changes in the small blood vessels similar to those described above. In very severe cases, haemorrhages occur in many organs, especially the spleen, lungs, and gastro-intestinal tract.

### CLINICAL PICTURE: SMALLPOX (VARIOLA MAJOR)

The incubation period is remarkably constant, although variation occurs. The prodromal illness begins about 12 days after infection and the focal rash begins to develop about 2 days later.

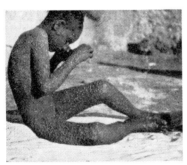

FIG. 55. Smallpox. Note centrifugal rash distribution and evidence of photophobia.
[By courtesy of Dr W.H.P.Lightbody]

The disease is sometimes toxic and rapidly fatal; death may occur before the focal rash appears. Haemorrhagic complications may develop during an otherwise 'typical' attack. On the other hand, the disease may run a mild course and may be modified by vaccination so that the illness does not get beyond the prodromal febrile stage and no focal rash develops. The vast majority of non-immune patients, however, develop the highly characteristic 'typical' smallpox, which is described here.

The prodromal illness is ushered in by general malaise and some prostration, usually headache and often backache. The temperature rises abruptly, commonly with chills, and reaches 39.4–40.6° C by the second day. The fever persists for 4 or 5 days, the temperature falling to normal 2 or 3 days after the focal rash has begun to develop. There may be an erythematous fleeting rash on the trunk and sometimes on the face in the prodromal febrile stage and this is very occasionally petechial. During the first febrile stage the patient is severely ill and becomes increasingly toxic. Prostration is out of proportion to the fever and delirium and light coma are not uncommon.

In most cases, however, there is only the characteristic focal rash, which starts on the third day after the onset of the fever.

The rash appears first on the skin of the face. Lesions may be noted in the mouth, especially on the tongue, palate, and uvula 12 hours or so before the skin becomes involved. Within a day the rash spreads to the trunk and arms, sometimes appearing first on the dorsal aspects of the hands and usually last on the legs. It is fully distributed within 2 days and shortly afterwards the temperature falls to normal and the patient feels much better for a further few days, while the lesions of the rash develop. The lesions begin as minute spots, become macules 3–4 mm across, deep-seated and firm in the skin; by the second day of development they are larger and lifted above the skin. A day later the vesicles appear and within the next 2 days pustules develop. The progress of the lesions on the face on which they first appear remains anything up to a day ahead of those elsewhere but, apart from this, in general the lesions all over the body are in about the same stage of development at any one time (this is a major distinction from the crops of lesions which occur in chickenpox). The pustules begin to dry up and separate as from the twelfth or thirteenth day of the rash, beginning on the face.

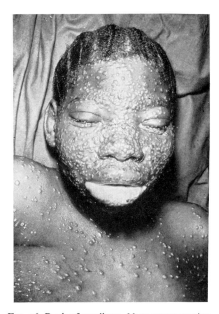

Fig. 56. Rash of smallpox. Note concentration of lesions on face as contrasted with body. The lips and eyelids are involved and oedematous.

[From Brian Maegraith and C.S.Leithead, *Clinical Methods in Tropical Medicine*, Cassell, London, 1962. By courtesy of Dr John Weir]

A secondary rise of temperature is usual, beginning within 2 days of the appearance of the pustules. The fever is commonly lower than that of the prodromal stage and lasts only a few days. This reaction is not due to secondary infection which may, however, occur as the pustules break down and may then complicate the picture, depending on the infecting organisms.

As the focal rash develops the patient may again become gravely toxic and may pass into delirium, with incontinence of urine and faeces. The toxic effects, which may be less notable in the early stages, tend to be most severe during the pustular stage of the rash, improving towards convalescence in those who will recover, but increasing in confluent, haemorrhagic, and hypertoxic cases which frequently end fatally. Death usually occurs about the tenth to the fifteenth day of the rash, but may come much earlier in complicated cases.

*The focal rash.* The rash appears first on the forehead and soon afterwards on the wrists. It spreads up the forearms and legs and appears on the back of the trunk. Its distribution is centrifugal. There are usually more lesions on the face than elsewhere, more on the legs than the thighs, on the forearms than the upper arms. Lesions are scattered over the trunk and may follow lines of pressure, for example the belt-line, or scratch marks. The hollows of the axilla are usually free but lesions may occur over the tendons. The whole rash comes out in the course of 48 hours at the most.

The first lesions are reddish macules which may be mistaken for measles. These turn into papules, vesicles, and ultimately pustules as described above. The papules are rounded, up to 7.5 mm across, hard, and deep in the skin. Many remain discrete; some become confluent. In very severe cases the lesions may become haemorrhagic and widely confluent. They are ringed by a narrow irregular zone of erythema. The vesicles are domed, not easily broken, and do not collapse completely when broken. The pustules are sometimes centrally depressed (umbilicated); they eventually desiccate, forming a crust, which drops off and leaves some pitting beneath which scarring is common. The progress from macule to pustule takes from 5 to 7 days and crusts begin to separate about the thirteenth day. In very severe cases the lesions may be confluent. In such cases the secondary infection is very severe and usually fatal.

In the palms and soles the lesions appear as deep-seated, stony hard papules which become the so-called 'brown seeds', and eventually drop out, sometimes weeks after the onset.

The mucous membranes may become involved, especially those of the mouth, the pharynx and larynx (sometimes with acute oedema and even the trachea. Mucosal vesicles usually break down into shallow ulcers. As pointed out above, mucosal lesions may appear in the mouth before developing on the skin.

Conjunctivitis and photophobia are early and severe in most cases. Pustules may form in the conjunctiva but not on the cornea unless it is vascularized from other injury or infection. The lids may be oedematous. Keratitis may develop and spread rapidly, leading to corneal ulceration and occasionally sloughing of whole cornea. Sight may be permanently impaired by these complications.

### Complicated cases

The infection may produce very toxic effects in some patients who may die in the early febrile stage before the focal rash develops. In some the rash may develop quickly, become confluent and haemorrhagic. In others the normal development of the rash may be associated with haemorrhagic complications including haemorrhages under the skin and visible mucous membranes and bleeding from all orifices, with haemoptysis, haematemesis, and haematuria. Rarely a dusky erythematous rash may appear on the trunk, with massive petechiae and haemorrhages under the skin and mucous membranes and purpuric spots and blotches. Such cases are extremely toxic and death may occur before the focal rash develops; it is said that the appearance of the latter in such circumstances may be delayed until 4 or 5 days after the onset.

## MODIFIED SMALLPOX

Vaccination may modify the toxic effects of smallpox and the appearance and extent of the focal rash.

Vaccinated persons in whom there is still considerable residual immunity may develop the primary febrile episode without the subsequent appearance of the rash. The disease in such cases may be mild, occasionally severe, but rarely fatal.

The rash is commonly modified by successful vaccination. The lesions are often small, irregularly dispersed, and few in number; there is less ultimate scarring. Occasionally the distribution may resemble that of chickenpox rather than smallpox, but the progression of the lesions usually remains typical.

### COURSE AND PROGNOSIS

In unprotected subjects, especially in children under 5 years old, the prognosis is bad with a death rate as high as 50 per cent. The severity of the disease is much lower in vaccinated individuals. Vaccination in infancy will protect until about puberty.

Severe early toxic symptoms usually herald a severe attack. The more severe the skin lesions the worse the outlook.

Absence of remission between the primary and secondary fevers is a bad omen.

When smallpox is severe foetal death and abortion are practically certain. Live birth may occur when the patient is in the third trimester; the child may be born with smallpox or develop it after birth.

### DIAGNOSIS

The body must be examined in a good light and the type and distribution of the rash carefully determined. The early severe toxaemia is often suggestive in an endemic area, especially during a known outbreak. This is absent in chickenpox, which is perhaps the commonest source of confusion. In chickenpox the skin lesions tend to come out in succcessive crops so that several stages of development are present at any one time in any one area. They are irregular in size and shape; unlike the deep seated lesions of smallpox they are very superficial. The vesicles are easily ruptured and empty completely. Surrounding erythema is distinct. Vesicles mature in 24 hours. The whole cycle from macule to scab takes only a few days and is often complete in 2 days. There are fewer lesions on the extremities than on the trunk, on which the lesions first appear; the axilla is invaded; there are few lesions on the hands and feet.

The history of successful vaccination or otherwise should always be ascertained. Successful vaccination less than 3 years previously is a strong point against the diagnosis of smallpox. The early stages of the rash may be mistaken for measles or typhus, the papulo-vesicular stages for urticaria or drug rashes. Centrifugal distribution of the rash and a fall rather than rise of temperature at the time of its appearance are in favour of a diagnosis of smallpox.

The rapid diagnosis of smallpox is very important. It depends on interpretation of the clinical picture and on laboratory examinations which include the detection of elementary bodies in smears from lesions, the demonstration of viral antibodies and antigens, and the culture of the organism.

Elementary bodies are present in petechial lesions, papules, and the bases of vesicles. Scrapings of these lesions should be collected after removal of the superficial epidermis with a scalpel. Smears fixed in methyl alcohol and stained with methyl violet will show the bodies, which are also present in chickenpox; those in smallpox are bigger and much more numerous. Culture on the chorio-allantoic membrane of the chick embryos is made from the scrapings and from scales from the second day of the disease; colonies develop in 48–72 hours. Using the electron microscope the diagnosis can be made in 24 hours.

Viral diagnosis depends on identification of antigens from ground-up material collected as above and on the complement fixation reaction in serum taken not earlier than the well-developed pustular stage.

Great care must be exercised in collecting and transporting such samples, which are highly infectious.

### TREATMENT

There is no specific treatment for the stage of viral infection. General nursing, feeding, etc., is of tremendous importance.

The secondary infection of the pustules can be much modified by the early use of antibiotics, especially tetracycline.

All cases must be isolated and kept under fly or mosquito netting. All secretions, scabs, etc., should be regarded as highly infectious and dust should be controlled as much as possible.

Patients must be regarded as infectious until all lesions are healed and scabs separated.

### CLINICAL PICTURE OF ALASTRIM (VARIOLA MINOR)

This form of the disease was once common in some areas of central and southern Africa and in South America, especially Brazil. In these areas it has now apparently been eradicated. There was a small imported outbreak in Britain in the late 1960s. It causes only mild constitutional effects and the mortality rate is very low. It resembles the abortive form of the major disease which occasionally develops in individuals who have been successfully vaccinated. There is cross-protection, but the two forms of the disease are distinct in that variola minor does not become classical smallpox. Outbreaks of alastrim do not reach epidemic proportions. Infection occurs in the same manner as smallpox.

The general reactions to the infection are seldom severe; there may be none. The rash appears on the third or fourth day or later, first on the face and soft palate, then on hands and arms and legs. The individual lesions in the eruption are essentially the same as in smallpox, but are often more superficially placed on the skin. There is usually only one crop. Mortality is low.

Methods of diagnosis are the same as in smallpox, but antibodies develop later and the strain of virus causing variola minor grows in the chick allantoic membrane at a slightly lower temperature than the strain causing variola major.

### PROPHYLAXIS OF SMALLPOX

Prevention of spread in an outbreak should be attempted by vaccination of all contacts and other non-vaccinated persons. Contacts should be quarantined for 16 days. Vaccination may protect or lead to modification of the disease if performed within 4 or 5 days of exposure.

Control of smallpox in a community is largely still regarded a matter of mass vaccination. However, Methisazone (Marboran) has been used successfully as a prophylactic in smallpox contacts, in doses of 1.5–3.0 g twice daily for 4 days. Administration is started as soon as possible after exposure. The drug has not been found of any value in treatment of an established case of smallpox but has some action on alastrim.

People exposed to smallpox in endemic areas should be vaccinated. Where vaccination is inadvisable, as in eczema, congenital deficiency of lymphocyte production, or in pregnancy, a certificate should be provided explaining the reason, this will usually be accepted internationally. In some countries, valid certificates of vaccination are still required for international travel. In view of the very successful 'eradication' campaign, many, including the U.S.A., no longer demand certificates except in those coming from areas where there is a known outbreak, for example, from Birmingham, U.K. (in 1978). A certificate of successful vaccination or revaccination is usually valid for 3 years. An individual coming from an area where there there is an outbreak may be required to have a certificate not more than 1 year old. It should be remembered that a vaccination certificate *per se* is no guarantee of immunity, especially after revaccination, when the development of a 'take' at the vaccination site is seldom checked.

*Complications of vaccination*

After primary vaccination there is usually some reaction which gives rise to fever and malaise. The vaccinated area is often erythematous and swollen and there is some local adenitis. If the latter involves the cervical glands following vaccination high in the arm it may be mistaken for stiffness of the neck and meningitis.

The vaccinia may be spread from the vaccination site by the fingers and lesions are not uncommon on the nasal mucosa, the eyelids, the cutaneous–mucosal junction of the anus, etc. Occasionally a vaccinia viraemia may cause the development of lesions distant from the site. Vaccination must be avoided in eczematous individuals, especially children, in whom widespread and sometimes generalized or confluent lesions may develop.

The most serious complication is post-vaccinial encephalitis or encephalopathy. This is rare after vaccination in infants and after revaccination, and is more likely to occur after primary vaccination of schoolchildren and young adults. The mortality is greatest in infants under 6 months. In countries, including the U.K., in which the present risk of smallpox infection is negligible, it is generally held that the overall risks of acquiring infection are less than those of complications from vaccination, which is therefore not advised except in a local outbreak.

The complications of vaccination are probably reduced by the administration of $\gamma$-globulin but opinions on this point are divided.

# 26

# SNAKE BITE AND OTHER VENOMOUS
# BITES AND STINGS

## (Contributed by H.A.Reid)

The medically important poisonous snakes all have fangs in the front of the upper jaw and may be classified as follows:

*Elapidae*. Land snakes with relatively short fixed front fangs. These include cobras (Asia and Africa), mambas (Africa), kraits (Asia), coral snakes (Asia and the Americas), tiger snakes, and the taipan (Australia).

*Hydrophiidae*. Sea snakes with small heads, long thin bodies, and prominent flattened tails. They are common in Asian coastal waters.

*Viperidae*. Land snakes with long erectile fangs which are often the only teeth in the maxillary bone. They are usually concealed in a mucosal sheath when retracted against the palate. The body is often short and relatively fat. In most, but not all the viperidae, the triangular or spade-shaped head is covered with many small scales and there is a distinct neck.

Vipers are divided into two classes; the pit or *crotaline* vipers, which have a thermosensitive pit between the eye and the nostrils, and the *viperine* vipers, without such pits. Both classes occur in Asia where, for example, Russell's viper and the saw-scaled viper are viperine; the Japanese Habu, the Malayan pit viper, and the Taiwan bamboo viper are crotaline. Only viperine vipers are found in Europe and Africa and only crotaline vipers in the Americas. Vipers do not naturally exist in Australia and adjacent islands. (The so-called 'death adder' in Australia is an elapid.)

Snake bite is mainly a rural and occupational hazard. The incidence of snake bite varies widely from region to region. In many districts, in spite of the large population of poisonous snakes, bites and fatalities are relatively uncommon. In others bites are frequent and the annual mortality is considerable, though surprisingly low considering the lethal potential of most venomous snakes.

Most bites occur in daylight and on the foot or ankle because the victim treads on or near the snake.

The effect of the bite depends mainly on the amount of venom injected. *Snakes frequently bite without injecting venom.*

### VENOMS

Envenoming in man involves multiple toxic reactions occurring simultaneously or sequentially; also, autopharmacological substances may be released by activation of the kinin system, complement system, and so on. Most viper venoms are predominantly vasculotoxic in man, causing a rapidly developing swelling of the part bitten. This swelling is often misinterpreted as due to venous thrombosis or to inflammation (or both) but necropsy in such cases has revealed patent veins and no evidence of inflammation. The swelling is presumably due to venom diffusing through the tissues and affecting vascular permeability from the outside. Local necrosis in viper bites is mainly ischaemic, thrombosis blocking local blood vessels and causing 'dry gangrene'. Local necrosis in cobra bites is clinically different, more like 'wet gangrene', an early feature being a characteristic putrid smell. Presumably it is mainly due to direct cytolytic venom action. Shock is a main cause of death in viper bites and the cause is multifactorial, including hypovolaemia, acidosis, cardiac, and pulmonary effects. Haemorrhage into a vital organ, especially the brain, is the usual cause of death in many viper envenomings and can be delayed until several days after the bite. The bleeding is mainly due to direct endothelial damage by a venom component, haemorrhagin, which does not affect coagulation. Non-clotting blood due to defibrinogenation develops in some viper envenomings and can aggravate bleeding.

Most elapid venoms are principally neurotoxic, producing a selective neuromuscular block affecting mainly the muscles of the eyes, tongue, throat, and chest, and leading to respiratory failure in severe poisoning. Sea-snake venoms are primarily myotoxic and damage skeletal muscle with release of myoglobin and potassium into the plasma and urine. Hypotension, electrocardiographic abnormalities, and raised serum enzyme levels can occur in serious elapid and viper bite poisoning and may be due to a direct cardiotoxic effect. Acute renal failure may follow serious poisoning by all types of venomous snake; the pathogenesis includes decreased renal blood flow, pigmenturia, and a direct nephrotoxic effect of venom.

Although the effects of snake envenoming in man may be conveniently though arbitrarily classified into vasculotoxic for vipers, neurotoxic for elapids, and myotoxic for sea snakes, there are notable exceptions to such a classification. Thus, vipers such as *Bitis atropos* and *Crotalus durissus terrficus* have mainly neurotoxic, not haemorrhagic, effects. Some Pacific-Australian elapids are myotoxic rather than neurotoxic; others can cause significant haemorrhage and clotting changes. Many viper venoms such as *B. arietans* and *Causus* do not affect clotting in human victims.

CLINICAL FEATURES OF SNAKE BITE

Fright, especially the fear of rapid and unpleasant death, is the most common symptom following snake bite. It is important to distinguish emotional symptoms such as faintness, stupor, cold clammy skin, feeble pulse, and rapid shallow breathing, from those of systemic poisoning. Emotional symptoms come on rapidly within minutes of the bite whereas systemic poisoning symptoms rarely start until $\frac{1}{2}$ to 1 hour after the bite. Emotional symptoms resolve dramatically following a placebo injection. However, early collapse with hypotension is sometimes due to venom effects and not to fright; it usually resolves spontaneously within $\frac{1}{2}$ to 1 hour.

Local swelling with variable pain follows viper bites if venom is injected. It is a valuable clinical sign because if it is absent and the snake responsible for the bite is known to be a viper, systemic poisoning can be excluded since local swelling starts within a few minutes of the bite. The amount of swelling in viper bite is roughly proportional to the venom dose—if it extends above the knee or elbow, after a bite on the foot or the hand, for instance, systemic poisoning is likely. Blisters extending up the limb are a sign of high venom dose.

Swelling in cobra envenoming develops more slowly than in viper bites, taking 1 or more hours; it is usually not so marked. In bites by other elapid snakes or by sea snakes there is no local swelling regardless of the amount of venom injected.

Local necrosis, sometimes extensive, in the region of the bite may occur in viper bites, especially in rattlesnake bites or when the injury has occurred on a finger or toe. It also occurs in Asian and African spitting cobra bite, usually appearing a week or more after the bite.

Signs of systemic poisoning differ according to the type of snake responsible. Vomiting is an early warning sign of both elapid and viper bite poisoning.

Ptosis is usually the earliest sign of systemic neurotoxic poisoning such as occurs in cobra bite. It is followed within some hours by glossopharyngeal palsy, intercostal muscle paralysis, variable limb, and diaphragmatic paresis. The latter results in respiratory failure; but inhalation of vomit or secretions can cause sudden death by respiratory obstruction many hours before the diaphragm is weakened. A significant early clinical sign of developing respiratory failure is mental confusion.

An early sign of systemic viper bite poisoning is blood-stained spit (which may become blood-stained within 15 minutes of the bite). Non-clotting blood and other haemorrhagic signs (oozing from injection sites, bleeding from gums, ecchymoses, positive tourniquet test, and so on) follow in 1–3 hours; in severe cases shock develops.

In systemic poisoning following sea-snake bite, myalgia starts $\frac{1}{2}$ to 1 hour after the bite. Limb, neck, or trunk movements then become very painful. A few hours later the urine is discoloured brown or red by myoglobin. The later stages are similar to those of neurotoxic poisoning; but even if respiratory failure is prevented by tracheostomy and artificial respiration, death may still occur from hyperkalaemic cardiac arrest, or several days after the bite, from acute renal failure.

Recovery from haemorrhagic and neurotoxic poisoning is rapid and usually complete within a few days. Without specific antivenom, natural recovery from severe sea-snake poisoning may take months, since skeletal muscles are extensively damaged. The local swelling of viper poisoning resolves within 1–3 weeks as a rule and in the absence of necrosis or meddlesome local measures, such as incision or application of dressings, secondary bacterial infection is unusual.

### DIAGNOSIS

Of human victims seeking medical help following snake bite, more than one-half will have minimal or no poisoning. Only about one-quarter will develop severe systemic poisoning: this group will benefit from specific antivenom. Clinicians must decide: (i) Was a significant amount of venom injected? (ii) Is systemic poisoning present? (as a general rule, this is the only indication for antivenom therapy); (iii) If so, is it of elapid, sea-snake, or viperid type? (iv) How severe are the systemic symptoms, particularly in terms of antivenom requirement?

The decision on the amount of venom injected can often be made on examination of the bite wound. Thus, in many countries where vipers are the only common snakes, absent or minimal local swelling 2 hours after the bite indicates that no significant amount of venom was injected.

Early evidence of systemic poisoning includes (a) blood-stained spit and non-clotting blood in viperine bite, (b) ptosis after an elapid bite, and (c) myalgia and later myoglobinuria in sea-snake bite. A polymorph leucocytosis exceeding $20 \times 10^9/l$ indicates serious poisoning in all three types of bite.

In most cases those receiving a venom dose large enough to cause systemic poisoning will already have signs by the time they reach medical help. In the rare cases seen soon after the bite—within the latent period between bite and onset of systemic symptoms (usually 1–2 hours but occasionally up to 10 hours)—the patient should be admitted after a placebo injection and carefully observed every half hour by the doctor for these early systemic signs.

Viperine poisoning is severe if, within 1–2 hours of the bite, swelling has extended above knee or elbow (if the bite is on the foot or hand respectively), signs of shock are evident or haemorrhagic signs besides haemoptysis develop. The latter do not usually appear for 5–6 hours.

Severe elapid poisoning is indicated by the onset of neurotoxic signs within 1 hour or less of the bite and by their rapid progression to respiratory failure. Mental confusion strongly suggests developing respiratory failure; ptosis and glossopharyngeal palsy may make assessment of mental awareness difficult. Severe sea-snake bite poisoning is shown by myoglobinuria 1–2 hours after the bite; ptosis develops later than in cobra neurotoxic poisoning but there is rapid progression of signs in a few hours to final respiratory failure.

## IMMEDIATE TREATMENT

Reassurance of the patient is most important.

A firm but not tight tourniquet should be applied just above the bite. The application of a tourniquet is useful psychologically in the distressed patient. Some authorities consider this the primary value. In any case, tourniquets should be removed as soon as more effective measures become available. The bitten limb should be moved as little as possible because movement can spread the venom even when a tourniquet has been applied.

The bite wound should be wiped to get rid of any venom which may have spilled from the fangs at the time of biting.

Incisions or suction over the area of the bite should be avoided. Indeed, some of the worst effects of non-lethal bites have resulted from inexpert incisions involving local nerves, tendons, and vessels.

The local application of chemicals such as the time-honoured permanganate crystals is useless and may aggravate the injuries sustained during biting or enthusiastic incision.

## MEDICAL TREATMENT

The patient should be treated in hospital as soon as possible. Adequate reassurance is most important in the general medical treatment of snake bite. A placebo injection should be given promptly unless signs of systemic poisoning are already evident. In the latter event specific antivenom is given. If a tourniquet has been applied it should be released. The patient should be admitted and carefully observed by the doctor every half hour for the first few hours. If further signs have not developed within 12 hours the patient can usually be discharged.

Cases which show signs of systemic poisoning require antivenom. If some hours have elapsed since the bite the antivenom may be less successful, but should nevertheless be given. Good responses have been obtained from antivenom injected 2–3 days after the bite.

### Antivenom

Antivenom should NOT be given as a routine in all cases of suspected snake bite. In the small proportion of cases in which sufficient venom has been injected to cause systemic poisoning, the signs will usually be evident by the time the patient reaches hospital. In rare cases the signs will not develop until after admission. Careful and frequent observation for the few important diagnostic signs is essential; for example during the night ptosis may easily be mistaken by a nurse for sleep.

If antivenom is correctly used, systemic symptoms improve within an hour and often resolve completely within 24 hours. Its efficacy in preventing or lessening local necrosis is uncertain. But, since necrosis can be so disabling, if a patient presents within 3 hours of a bite reliably attributed to a necrotizing snake such as a spitting cobra or puff adder and shows swelling spreading from the bite, and if funds permit, antivenom should be given.

Antivenom should be diluted with isotonic saline and administered by intravenous drip. Infusion is much safer than bolus injection which often causes reactions through activating complement. Specific antivenom is desirable but if there is no information regarding the species of snake, polyvalent serum may be given.

Information should be available regarding local poisonous snakes and the antivenoms available. An indication of the specific antivenom to be used in a given case may be obtained from the clinical signs: Haemorrhagic signs indicate viper poisoning. Neurotoxic signs with local swelling at the bite indicates cobra, and without swelling, mamba or krait, etc. Myotoxic symptoms and the circumstances of the bite indicate sea-snake antivenom.

The effective dose depends on the potency of the antivenom but, as a general guide, is 50–100 ml (usually contained in five or ten ampoules) administered by intravenous drip taking about 30 minutes. If clinical improvement is not distinct within an hour the dose should be repeated.

Recent work has shown that, if antivenom remains clear, potency has been retained—regardless of the date of manufacture. But if the antivenom is turbid or discoloured it should not be used.

Serum sensitivity tests are not advocated as they can be very misleading. Reactions have occurred despite negative test results, and in some severe cases with a positive test reaction intravenous antivenom was subsequently infused without any reaction. A known 'allergic' history contra-indicates antivenom, unless it seems very likely the victim will die from envenoming. In that event, two intravenous drips should be set up, one with antivenom and the other with adrenalin. Small amounts of adrenalin are infused first, then antivenom; according to progress antivenom is increased, adrenalin decreased. Steroids should be used in delayed serum reactions.

### GENERAL TREATMENT

Treatment of general effects is very important. Blood transfusion may be needed for haemorrhage or shock. Heparin is contra-indicated in snake bite because it may aggravate bleeding from damaged endothelium. Neurotoxic venoms, such as those injected by cobras, lead to respiratory failure; tracheostomy and artificial respiration may be essential. Acute renal failure can complicate all types of snake bite poisoning—sea snake, elapid, and viperine. Peritoneal dialysis may be needed.

The site of the bite should be left alone. If the lower limb has been bitten it should be rested on the bed; upper limbs can be rested in a sling. No coverings or dressings should be applied as they greatly increase the incidence of secondary bacterial infection. Similarly blisters should be left alone. But as soon as local necrosis is obvious, sloughs should be excised. Physiological saline is the best dressing. Broad spectrum antibiotics will minimize the risk of local infection and administration of anti-tetanus serum is advisable in cases with local necrosis. Skin grafting may be needed at a later stage if necrosis is extensive.

Local pain may be relieved by rest or elevation and analgesics when necessary.

The fangs of certain cobras, particularly *N. nigricollis* in Africa, are so designed that venom can be ejected at right angles to the length. The snake instead of striking, 'spits'. The stream of venom squirts for up to 5.5 m and may strike the victim's face and eyes. Painful conjunctivitis with rapidly developing palpebral oedema results.

Treatment consists of washing thoroughly with water or bland solutions such as boric acid.

## SCORPION STINGS

Many genera and species of scorpions are found in the tropics and the degree of toxicity of the venom varies widely from region to region.

Scorpions shelter by day in warm dry areas under stones, in crevices in rocks, in wood piles, inside shoes and cupboards, etc. They are most active at night.

Stings are largely the reward of the careless and unwary and should be few and far between with reasonable care. The poison is injected by a sting in the terminal abdominal segments usually with the tail bent forward over the body.

In many parts of the world the incidence of stings is high, the mortality rate low. In some districts there may be considerable mortality amongst children. Scorpion stings should be regarded seriously in children.

The signs of stinging are similar in all parts of the world, but vary greatly in degree. Local reactions are prominent in most cases. General effects may come on rapidly or may be delayed for some hours after the sting. The general effects of the venom are essentially neurotoxic, probably stimulating the autonomic nervous system, and are displayed at their worst in young children.

The sting leaves a single puncture. It occurs most commonly in the legs and feet. The local reaction is immediate and may be extremely painful. A red weal appears at the site, the surrounding tissues become oedematous and there may be some oozing of blood. In systemic poisoning the pulse may be slow and lachrymation, nasal secretion, and repeated sneezing are common. Sweating may be profuse. The skin is pale. There may be salivation, nausea, and vomiting. The pupils are sometimes widely dilated. The patient complains bitterly of the local pain, is often dizzy and trembling, and has intense headache and restlessness. Coma and respiratory depression may develop in severe and fatal cases within a few hours of the sting. Cardiovascular collapse is a common terminal event in children after stinging by certain species.

## TREATMENT

Information regarding the local species of scorpions and the availability of antivenom is important in a given district. If possible, the scorpion should be killed and kept for examination.

Rapid local relief is often obtained by the subdermal injection of 2.5 ml of 1 per cent lignocaine around the site of the sting, repeated after an hour if necessary.

General treatment consists in dealing with complications such as shock and by administration of specific antivenom intravenously.

## SPIDER BITES

Most spiders have poison fangs but few are powerful enough to inject the venom through the human skin. The bites of certain genera are, however, known to cause serious toxic symptoms and even death. Details of poisonous spiders should be sought in the localities concerned, and only the briefest mention is necessary here.

The best known poisonous spider is the Black Widow, *Latrodectus mactans,* which is found in many parts of the world, including the United States, and parts of South America. As in most arachnid poisonings man is bitten only by the female. The body is round and about 1.0 cm long, the abdomen large and shiny black, marked ventrally with a characteristic red hourglass pattern. The male is much smaller.

The web is coarse and irregular and contains a tube in which the spider lurks. It is frequently found in corners and holes in barns and outbuildings. Biting often occurs in outdoor privies.

The effects of the bite vary considerably. In many cases bites probably occur without notable symptoms but they may be followed by severe local and general reactions, the development of which has been watched experimentally by observers who have subjected themselves to biting.

There may be local stinging pain, erythema, and oedema. Severe pain spreads rapidly from the bitten area to local muscles and eventually to the chest, abdomen, and limbs. Muscular spasms, especially of flexor muscles, cause the patient to double up. Tremors and convulsions are common and severe. Constricted pupils, sweating, and excessive salivation are common. Vascular collapse may appear within a few hours of the bite. There is frequently severe epigastric pain accompanied by abdominal rigidity. The temperature rises, the pulse rate is fast, and there may be profuse sweating.

Deaths occur as a rule only in very young children.

*Treatment*
Antivenom has been prepared and used successfully by the intravenous route.

Intravenous administration of 10–20 ml of 10 per cent calcium gluconate or 10 mg diazepam and subcutaneous injections of atropine are said to relieve the muscular spasm. Hot baths may also relieve the spasms.

*Loxosceles* poisoning has been reported from Australia, Chile, the U.S.A., and the Middle East. The bite is followed by a severe painful erythematous, oedematous local reaction sometimes associated with widespread oedema of the limb. Within a week blisters appear at the site and are followed by a black gangrenous patch which sloughs off, leaving an ulcer which may be several inches across. Healing leaves a scar. Haemoglobinuria and acute renal failure may occur.

## POISONOUS COELENTERATES, SHELLFISH, AND FISH

Jellyfish can cause stings in man, usually producing superficial but painful skin lesions, and sometimes shock. Those commonly involved are *Physalia* spp. (Portuguese Man-O-War), *Cubomedusa* spp. (sea wasps), and *Cyanea* spp.

*Physalia* has a crested sausage-shaped bell and submerged finger-like processes with one main blue tentacle covered with poisonous nematocysts and up to 30 m long when extended. When the skin is hit by the tentacle a long line of discontinuous wheals is caused with surrounding flare. Pain and discomfort is severe, but systemic reactions are rare unless there are many stings. No fatalities have been reported.

The *Cubomedusae* are a few inches across, cuboid, colourless, and transparent with trailing tentacles armed with nematocysts. They are found in calm water and move by jet propulsion. Several species are known to cause severe stinging, which may be fatal within a few minutes of the sting from acute heart failure. If victims survive the first few minutes recovery is the rule. Multiple stinging results in the lines of contact with the tentacles appearing on the skin as bright red streaks dotted with wheals. Oedema follows and the whole thickness of the affected skin may slough and be replaced ultimately by scar tissue.

*Cyanea* is found in deep waters. It is a slimy jellyfish up to 25 cm across, with hundreds of tentacles falling from the body. Contact results in local severe burning pain, erythema and whealing. General effects are sometimes severe.

In an average jellyfish sting only a small proportion of nematocysts discharge venom. Treatment consists of applying alcohol or 10 per cent formalin to kill the undischarged nematocysts. If alcohol or formalin are not available dry sand should be sprinkled on. In severe cases with collapse, tourniquets should be applied to delay venom absorption; external cardiac massage and mouth-to-nose artificial respiration may be needed. Sea wasp antivenom is now available in Australia as an adjunct to treatment.

Toxic substances have been found in the poisonous sea anemone *Rho-*

*dactis* and in mussels and clams on the North Pacific coast. Poisoning after eating shellfish has been reported from other areas including South-east Asia. The toxin, which is apparently derived from dinoflagellates on which the shellfish feed, causes neuromuscular paralysis, sometimes ending fatally in respiratory failure. It is not inhibited by anticurare drugs.

A variant of this form of poisoning, called *Ciguatera,* occurs in the South Pacific as a result of eating fish which have fed on small herbivorous fish which have in turn been eating poisonous algae. The fish most commonly involved are snappers, groupers, barracuda, eels, and the surgeon fish. The clinical effects come on soon after a meal of fish and include prostration, nausea, vomiting, profuse sweating, numbness of lips and throat, abdominal cramps, muscular weakness, and incoordination. Death may occur from respiratory paralysis. The toxin works at the nerve muscle junction.

Venomous marine snails of the genus *Conus* may, when handled, inject neurotoxin through a hollow, needle-like radula tooth.

There are many venomous fish usually found inshore from reefs, often buried in mud or sand. These include the stone and scorpion fish found on coral reefs and in shallow, sandy waters. The injury is caused by penetration of venomous spines when the fish is trodden upon or detached from a fish hook. In some waters the stingray causes injury and intoxication by barbed spines which are situated near the base of the slender active tail.

There is usually an immediate reaction about the puncture wound in poisoning from venomous fish with marked pain and sometimes oedema, and erythema. The most effective treatment for the local pain is hot water. The part stung is immersed in water as hot as the patient can bear (and only the patient can decide how hot this is). The pain is relieved within seconds and the part stung must be quickly removed from the water to avoid blistering. It should be reimmersed as pain recurs (within seconds at first, later within minutes). This procedure should be continued until the pain no longer recurs (usually about half an hour). It is important to explain details of this simple but highly effective treatment to the patient who should be given a can of water recently brought to boiling point. This should be added to the immersing water to keep it as *constantly hot* as he can bear. If the water is not hot enough, the treatment is not effective; if the stung part is immersed too long in very hot water, blistering will result.

If the part stung is unsuitable for immersion in hot water (for example, the face or trunk), intramuscular or intravenous pethidine should be given, 100 mg for an adult, 2 mg per kg body weight for children. Alternatively, the area should be infiltrated through the puncture wound with 2–5 ml of 1% lignocaine hydrochloride.

# 27

# SPRUE, TROPICAL AND OTHER
# MALABSORPTION SYNDROMES

Tropical sprue is a primary malabsorption syndrome of unknown aetiology. The classical case is characterized by steatorrhoea, glossitis and stomatitis, dyspepsia, abdominal distension, gross emaciation, and megalocytic anaemia.

There are many variants in which certain features of the classical picture may predominate, while others may be absent.

The malabsorption syndrome must be distinguished from very similar events resulting from infection with *Giardia lamblia* (see p. 24), with *Capillaria philippinensis* (see p. 558), or with *Strongyloides stercoralis*. Malabsorption also occurs as a secondary phenomenon in Crohn's disease, Whipples' disease, coeliac disease, and intestinal lesions, including tuberculosis, diverticulosis and blind (surgical) intestinal loops.

## DISTRIBUTION

The sprue picture is found in parts of the tropics, subtropics, and the New World; the distribution is regional rather than climatic. It occurs most frequently in parts of India, Pakistan, Bangladesh, Sri Lanka, Burma, central and southern China, Hong Kong, Singapore, Malaysia, Vietnam, Indonesia, and the Philippines. It has been described also in the U.S.A., Central America, the Guianas, the Caribbean, especially Puerto Rico and Haiti, and the Fiji Islands. Isolated cases have been reported in Mauritius, Malta, southern Italy, and the Middle East. It has very seldom been described in central or southern Africa.

## AETIOLOGY

Tropical sprue may have a very localized distribution in a given area. It may, for instance, occur in several occupants of the same house, or in several members of one family. A variant of the syndrome, the so-called hill diarrhoea, was sometimes seen in high-altitude stations in India and is very like the same syndrome seen in Hong Kong.

Continued subsistence on inadequate diet is a prominent factor in the clinical history of certain forms of sprue. On the other hand, the classical syndrome tends to develop commonly in an economic group accustomed to apparently well-balanced and adequate diet.

The individual subject commonly gives a history of having lived for some time, usually for years, in a recognized endemic area. Occasionally he may have resided in the region for only a few weeks. Sprue may develop some time, even years, after the patient has left the endemic region for a more temperate climate.

The classical picture was regarded at one time as primarily a disease of Europeans and those of mixed blood. This is not the case. It occurs commonly in local native inhabitants of India, Burma, Pakistan, and Bangladesh for instance, sometimes in almost epidemic form.

Sprue is most commonly seen in people of 20–40 years of age. It rarely occurs in children. Women, especially when pregnant, are said to be more susceptible than men, except when the latter are under circumstances such as those of military service.

### PATHOLOGY AND PATHOGENESIS

There is no convincing evidence of the existence of any specific infective agent. Previous or contemporaneous amoebic or bacillary dysentery or other dysenteric disturbances do not predispose to the appearance of sprue.

Certain features of sprue may be explained to some extent on the assumption of primary dietary deficiencies of one kind or another. It has been suggested, for instance, that the megalocytic anaemia of sprue arises from deficiency in extrinsic haemopoietic factor. The anaemia, however, often develops in cases in which there is no evidence of the exclusion of this factor, and the picture of nutritional macrocytic anaemia and not of sprue is the usual sequence of such deficiency.

On the whole there is little evidence that deficiencies of vitamins, especially those of the B group, *per se* are a constant feature of the genesis of sprue. Unquestioned vitamin deficiencies do, however, develop in the syndrome and it is often difficult in a particular case to decide whether these are primary or not. The balance of the evidence suggests that they are not. The clinical picture of vitamin B deficiency differs from that of sprue. It appears wherever the deficiency exists and is as common in Africa, where sprue is very rare, as in India, where sprue is endemic. Furthermore, the patent vitamin deficiencies in sprue can be restored without appreciable effect on the prevailing basic deficiencies in intestinal absorption.

It has been suggested that the vitamin deficiencies of sprue arise from interference with intestinal biosynthesis of the vitamins, resulting from redistribution of intestinal bacteria, which have been shown in some cases to flourish in the small intestine. This is unconfirmed.

There is no evidence of primary endocrine dysfunction in sprue. The low serum calcium and tetany which is sometimes present, and the flat glucose tolerance curve, are due to absorptive defects. The sodium and chloride deficiencies seen in late cases result from fluid and electrolyte loss and are not related to adrenal insufficiency.

The primary disturbance in sprue seems to be defective intestinal absorption, involving particularly fat and certain carbohydrates.

It appears to be mainly the particulate absorption of fat which is at fault. The intestinal juices contain their normal complement of enzymes and the splitting of triglycerides proceeds normally. Because of the incomplete absorption of triglycerides, however, the quantity of free acids produced in the intestine is increased. Unsaturated long chain fatty acids are absorbed in unusual amounts, possibly accounting for the excessive secretion of intestinal mucus which is believed to be responsible for the so-called 'deficiency' pattern seen in the barium meal. The more saturated acids are less well absorbed and cause intestinal irritation and diarrhoea. Insoluble soaps are formed with calcium, leading to abnormal loss of that mineral. Bacterial invasion of the disturbed small intestine takes place and may lead, as mentioned above, to secondary avitaminosis.

There is at present no good explanation of the origin of the absorptive defect. There seems to be in some cases a temporary or inherent jejuno-ileal insufficiency of unknown origin similar to that arising in post-operative gastrocolic fistula. It may be that the primary cause of the defect varies from case to case. Dietary faults such as the ingestion of rancid animal fats, deficiencies, disturbances in intestinal enzyme metabolism, and changes in the intestinal flora may be concerned in the individual case. The syndrome does not respond to a gluten-free diet.

Although it appears that the basic defect in sprue is failure of intestinal absorption, the genesis of the full clinical syndrome is much more complex. Thus, apparent clinical recovery under treatment often proceeds without immediate change in the absorptive defects and in some cases the latter may disappear before there is any notable clinical improvement.

### Morbid anatomy
In the advanced case there are atrophic changes in the skin, atrophic glossitis and gastritis. The intestinal walls are thin and may be perforated in the terminal stages. Biopsy of the jejunum in fully developed sprue reveals a decrease in absorptive surface, with leaf-like, ridged or convoluted villi, and increase in numbers of goblet cells. There may be a subepithelial cellular infiltration with plasma cells, lymphocytes, and sometimes eosinophils. Oedema is common. These changes differ from the flat, featureless, villous atrophy seen in idiopathic steatorrhoea. The red bone marrow may be increased diffusely or largely replaced by pale fat-free and practically acellular tissue. Megaloblastic changes are obvious in many anaemic cases. Involvement of the spinal cord such as seen in pernicious anaemia is rare.

### Laboratory findings
*Fat absorption.* The stool usually contains excess total fat. Individual specimens may, however, have normal fat content. The rate of absorption of

fat can therefore be determined best by a fat balance test. An estimate of fat absorption may also be made by collection and analysis of two or more consecutive daily faecal excretions.

The normal subject excretes about 5 g of fat per day; the sprue case excretes 10–15 g or more.

Faecal fat is present as free fatty acids and soaps (split) and triglycerides (unsplit). The ratio of split to unsplit fat is high, i.e. 3 : 1 to 6 : 1 (normal about 2 : 1).

A simple alternative to the fat absorption test is the estimation of the absorption of vitamin A, which is depressed in sprue.

*Blood fat.* The resting total fatty acid content is about normal. The total blood fat curve after a meal is low. The chylomicrograph (indicating particulate absorption) is flat in cases of sprue with diarrhoea; it may be normal in non-diarrhoeic cases.

*Xylose excretion.* This test is routinely used in most laboratories. The bladder is emptied after fasting overnight. Twenty-five grammes of xylose in 500 ml water is given and all the urine passed over the next 5 hours is collected and the xylose content determined. A normal person should pass not less than 4 g xylose in this time. Low excretion indicates malabsorption.

*Blood sugar.* The fasting glucose concentration is often low. The post-absorptive curve for glucose is flat; the curve for fructose is normal.

The disappearance of glucose from the blood-stream after intravenous injection is normal or slightly delayed.

*Jejunal biopsy* may reveal the patterns of villi described above.

### Blood electrolytes

*Serum sodium chloride and potassium* tend to remain within normal limits until the late stages which may be associated with dehydration and shock. Under these circumstances the serum sodium values are low, the chloride also low but less reduced in proportion. Potassium concentrations may fall or remain unchanged despite the overall loss of potassium from the gut.

*Plasma calcium* concentration may be low, especially in cases with tetany. Normal calcium values may exist in some tetanic cases, in which the magnesium concentration is low.

*Blood protein.* In very advanced cases or in patients who have been living on diets deficient in protein the blood protein levels may be very low. The albumin content is principally affected.

*Prothrombin.* In severe cases the prothrombin index is often low and can be restored by the parenteral administration of vitamin K.

### Blood cells and marrow

*Erythrocytes.* In the developed case anaemia is present. The cell count usually ranges between 2 and 4 million erythrocytes per mm$^3$. It varies considerably from time to time in individual cases.

The blood picture is one of megalocytosis, which may be pronounced, and some degree of aniso- and poikilocytosis. The Price–Jones curve resembles that of pernicious anaemia. The mean cell volume is raised above normal and the cell haemoglobin content is high.

The anaemia is thus megaloblastic. It may be dimorphic, with an added element of iron deficiency.

*Leucocytes* show no characteristic changes.

In the anaemic case the marrow smear reveals mixed megaloblastic and normoblastic hyperplasia. In advanced cases the marrow may be very hypoplastic.

### Gastric juice
Free hydrochloric acid may be absent. Achlorhydria is seldom histamine fast. Occasionally there may be hyperchlorhydria. The enzymes are normal.

### Duodenal juice
Enzymes, pigments, bile salts are normal. Emulsification of fat is normal. Intestinal bacteria may be present in large numbers. For a time this was regarded as having some significance in pathogenesis but there is now considerable doubt that this is the case.

### Faeces
The stool of classical sprue is bulky, soft, porridgy, greyish-white, greasy, gaseous, and extremely offensive. Microscopic examination reveals fatty acid crystals, fat globules, and undigested food particles. With successful treatment and in remission the stool becomes normal in size, consistency, and colour; in remission the fat content may nevertheless remain high.

### Urine
The diastase content is normal. The nicotinic acid content is low in clinically deficient cases. When salt and water deficiency has become established the usual changes in urinary chloride occur. In severe cases there may be no chloride. Urobilin, urobilinogen, and porphyrin may be present in severely anaemic cases.

### CLINICAL PICTURE
The description given here is that of classical tropical sprue.

There are many primary malabsorption syndromes which are now regarded loosely as sprue. These include mild to moderate diarrhoea with some steatorrhoea and few other signs or symptoms, such as described in recent years in Hong Kong, and variants of the classical theme, sometimes called the sprue syndrome, which appeared commonly in expatriates and indigenous residents and troops in Burma and India during the Second World War and which occur sporadically today in the same areas. These cases do not present the full classical picture, but defective intestinal absorption of fat and glucose is a constant feature. The relative emphasis and order of appearance of signs and symptoms varies widely in individual subjects. Outbreaks in troops on subsistence rations were so common and geographically localized during the war that they were described as 'epidemic'. Some cases proceeded after some months into the classical picture of tropical sprue. Others recovered spontaneously. Most responded well to treatment.

The clinical history reveals present or past sojourn in an endemic region. There may or may not be evidence of sustained subsistence on a deficient diet.

The beginnings of the syndrome may be so indefinite as to be missed altogether. Frequently, however, there is an initial short afebrile attack of watery diarrhoea, or a series of such attacks with intervals of remission. At this stage a mistaken diagnosis of food poisoning or dysentery is common.

The motions during the diarrhoea are at first urgent, watery, pale, frothy, and offensive. A few motions only are passed in the day, commonly in the morning. Immediate relief is usually obtained by rest in bed and a high protein diet. With or without such treatment remissions are to be expected, alternating with further periods of diarrhoea or looseness lasting a few days or weeks.

Gradually the looseness or diarrhoea becomes a constant feature and the character of the stool changes slowly to that of the classical sprue stool: greasy, bulky, gaseous, soft, pale, and foul-smelling. Remissions frequently occur even at this stage, in which the diarrhoea and the appearance of the stool improve. Eventually the condition becomes one of habitual looseness or mild diarrhoea. Several stools are passed in the day, chiefly in the morning. The desire for stool is urgent and the motion is passed explosively with accompanying large volumes of gas. Defaecation is painless, but is commonly preceded by abdominal colic.

This development of the syndrome from early diarrhoea is the commonest form of its appearance, but in some subjects the diarrhoea may not develop until other features of the syndrome have appeared. Thus loss of weight, dyspepsia, or sore tongue may be the first indication of the onset.

Dyspepsia at some stage is a constant feature. It usually comes on after the diarrhoea and varies in intensity from one case to another and from time to time in the same case. The patient complains of flatulence and abdominal discomfort, especially after food. Abdominal distension becomes marked, especially in the lower half of the abdomen, due to distension of the small intestine. The dyspepsia and distension develop in severity during the day, becoming commonly more acute until the passage of the early morning stool. In the later stages the abdomen is distended, especially in its lower half. It feels doughy and peristalsis may be visible through the thinned abdominal wall. (The 'sprue abdomen'.)

Examination of the gastric juice may reveal achlorhydria at any stage. This is frequently inconstant, and responds well to histamine. In some cases the juice acidity is normal or high. In the dyspeptic case a barium meals shows delayed gastric emptying and irregular clumping of the barium in the small intestine, instead of the normal feathering. This is the so-called 'deficiency pattern', which appears to be caused by the presence of excess mucus in the gut. In a few cases the large intestine may show some dilatation and loss of pattern due to mural atrophy. Megacolon, such as seen in coeliac disease or non-tropical sprue is very unusual.

The appetite is one of the many inconstant factors in sprue. In the early stages there may be no change but, as dyspepsia develops, periods of anorexia become common. The patient may show a distaste for certain foods which experience has taught him exacerbate his symptoms. Painful deficiency lesions in the mouth and oesophagus may emphasise his anorexia. Later, the appetite may return and the patient may become ravenous and make his condition worse by overeating and bad choice of food. The appetite often recovers very early in treatment before any real clinical improvement is established.

The establishment of diarrhoea or looseness and dyspepsia is usually followed quickly by changes in the tongue and mouth. Occasionally these may precede the gastro-intestinal signs.

The tongue becomes sore and sensitive to spiced foods, alcohol, and tobacco. The appetite suffers correspondingly.

The tongue is abnormally clean and small, red, inflamed patches and ultimately vesicles and ulcers appear irregularly at the sides and on the frenum. Similar lesions develop in the mouth on the floor, cheeks, and lips. The palate is infrequently affected. The severity of the lesions varies from day to day but in the untreated case tends to progress, with irregular remission, until the filiform papillae are eventually lost and the tongue becomes smooth, shiny, and fissured. In severe cases there may be persistent and inconvenient salivation and dribbling. Sometimes the lesions may involve the oesophagus and lead to dysphagia and severe retrosternal discomfort on swallowing.

Secondary deficiencies of the vitamin B group give rise to other changes in the mouth, which are commonly seen in advanced cases but may be absent. These include cheilosis and angular stomatitis. In cheilosis the lips, especially the lower, are inflamed and swollen, the mucous membrane is cracked and peeling, covered with small dark curled flakes of epithelium. Angular stomatitis occurs as cracks and fissures at the angles of the mouth, which are irritating and easily secondarily infected. Eye changes due to ariboflavinosis, including mild conjunctivitis, photophobia, and lachrymation may appear in some cases.

Throughout the progress of the syndrome weight is rapidly lost and the patient becomes increasingly emaciated. The skin eventually becomes dry, flaky, and wrinkled and the subcutaneous fat disappears. Irregular patches of light brown pigment may appear over the forehead and malar regions and on the back and buttocks. The nails are ridged and brittle.

In some cases the skin changes may superficially resemble those of avita-minosis, especially when they become prominent over the shin bones and scrotum. The symmetrical lesions of pellagra, however, never develop in sprue. Occasionally, an irritating dry eczema may appear, especially in the flexor areas of the limbs. Pre-existing fungal infections also tend to spread, and produce 'ids' (see p. 120).

The appearance of anaemia is erratic. It may develop early; occasionally it may be the presenting sign. Most often, however, it develops after the diar-rhoea and dyspepsia have become established. It is commonly of medium severity, varying considerably from time to time. There may be haemolytic crises associated with considerable loss of red cells and haemoglobin in the severe case. The megaloblastic hyperchromic anaemia characteristic of the well-developed case is similar to that of pernicious anaemia and indicates a defect in production rather than excessive blood loss. It is now considered that such anaemias may be additional to the syndrome arising from extraneous factors and are not essential to the basic picture of sprue. In some cases there may be some iron deficiency and occasionally the anaemia may be predo-minantly hypochromic.

Anaemia is seldom severe enough in itself in sprue in the East to cause the patient to present himself for that reason. It is usually the gastro-intestinal symptoms or the loss of weight and development of lassitude or the mouth changes which impress him most. In sprue, as seen in the Caribbean, megalo-cytic anaemia may be a very important and sometimes presenting feature.

During the development of classical sprue personality changes tend to occur. The patient becomes increasingly querulous and irritable. He is diffi-cult and unreasonable over his food and treatment and becomes very intro-spective, especially over his abdominal condition.

Tetany with carpopedal spasm may appear irregularly, especially during periods of exacerbation of the gastrointestinal symptoms. It is normally associated with a low serum calcium concentration, sometimes a low mag-nesium concentration.

Central nervous changes are very uncommon. Subacute combined degen-eration does not occur. Spastic paraplegia and peripheral neuritis arising from vitamin deficiency have been reported. Neuritic pains and hyperaesthesia and tingling in the arms and legs, with tenderness in the calf muscles, are not uncommon. Impotence is common in the male.

The final stages of tropical sprue appear months or years after the onset. The progress of the condition is seldom continuous; there are usually irregular periods of remission of variable length during which the signs and symptoms may almost completely subside, only to reappear often more severely in successive stages of exacerbation.

Eventually some vascular dysfunction develops, the blood pressures fall, there may be some right-sided dilatation of the heart and medical shock.

Serious dehydration resulting from mixed water and salt loss may dominate the closing stages. The patient shows the clinical features of dehydration, with inelastic skin, hollow eyes, and tight drawing of the skin over the malar bones. The state of dehydration may be confused with that of emaciation but examination will reveal a reduction in plasma sodium and chloride and often the absence of chloride in the urine. It is most important to demonstrate the dehydration since it can often be readily corrected and yet be fatal if missed.

Vascular failure, with rising pulse rate, falling blood pressures and loss of circulating plasma volume and associated haemoconcentration is common in the advanced case. It may be accompanied by oliguria, or anuria and acute uraemia.

Secondary infections are common in severe sprue, particularly bronchopneumonia. These require specific antibiotic therapy. If overlooked, they may be fatal.

### DIAGNOSIS

The clinical diagnosis in the individual subject is made on the history (sojourn in an endemic region at some period is essential) and the demonstration of intestinal absorption defects.

Conditions likely to be confused with sprue are other steatorrhoeic states, macrocytic anaemias, and vitamin-deficiency syndromes.

In children, coeliac disease resembles sprue in some ways. The steatorrhoea is of the same type, but the anaemia is mild and usually hypochromic and response to liver treatment is poor.

In non-tropical (idiopathic) steatorrhoea the endemic history is missing. The calcium metabolism is grossly affected and osteoporosis is common. Bone changes are rare in sprue. Megacolon is much commoner than in sprue. The anaemia and megalocytosis are generally less pronounced. Many cases respond to a gluten-free diet. The glucose absorption curve in idiopathic steatorrhoea is of the 'flat' type.

Infection with *G. lamblia* often results in steatorrhoea which recesses after treatment of the infection. Other parasitic infections which may induce steatorrhoea include strongyloidiasis and capillariasis (in which a full-blown malabsorption syndrome may develop). *Diphyllobothrium latum* may cause megaloblastic anaemia.

The effects of obstruction of the lacteal flow may closely simulate sprue. The typical sprue abdomen is developed and the biochemical picture is similar. Diagnosis is made by discovering the aetiological factor involved, especially enlargement of the mesenteric glands due to tuberculosis, cancer, or Hodgkin's disease. Short-circuit intestinal operations may have similar effects. These conditions are all, however, accompanied by hypochromic anaemia and normoblastic marrow responses.

In chronic pancreatitis the faeces contain a high percentage of neutral fat and the split fat content is low—the reverse of the situation in sprue. The enzyme content of the duodenal juice is reduced and glucose absorption is normal or diabetic in type.

The anaemia may be confused with that of pernicious anaemia or tropical megaloblastic anaemia. Steatorrhoea is absent, however, in these conditions. Moreover, in pernicious anaemia profound central nervous changes may occur, the achlorhydria is persistent, the abdominal signs are absent, and the glucose curve is normal.

Changes in the tongue and mouth, similar megaloblastic anaemia, and diarrhoea are often present in pellagra, but there is no steatorrhoea, and the classical pellaginous symmetrical dermatitis is absent in sprue. Other vitamin deficiency syndomes are also unaccompanied by steatorrhoea.

### COURSE AND PROGNOSIS

Sprue progresses after the onset by a series of remissions and relapses. Great emaciation with dehydration and vascular failure are common in the late stages. Intercurrent infection is often fatal. In rare cases intestinal ulceration and perforation may occur. In untreated classical sprue the mortality may be as high as 25 per cent. Spontaneous cure is common in all forms of the syndrome. This makes assessment of treatment methods sometimes difficult.

Response to treatment is usually rapid. With co-operation from the patient clinical cure is usual. The order of disappearance of signs and symptoms varies from case to case. Diarrhoea usually clears quickly. The blood is often very slow to regenerate fully. The defect in fat absorption is frequently the last sign to disappear.

Relapse may occur at any stage, even after apparent full recovery. Cure should not be predicted for at least 3 years after treatment. The subsequent histories of treated cases indicate a high recovery rate. Prognosis, however, deteriorates with age.

In some cases the 'syndrome' may go on to the full picture of sprue. It responds well in the early stages to chemotherapy.

### TREATMENT

The patient should be put to bed and transferred as quickly as possible to hospital for investigation and confirmation of the diagnosis.

Long-term treatment is complicated and tedious. Immediate treatment is often a matter of urgency.

*Immediate treatment*
*Diarrhoea.* The relatively insoluble sulphonamides, such as sulphaguanidine, are often effective in controlling diarrhoea in the early stages. A course of antibiotics such as tetracycline or penicillin may be equally successful.

Drugs such as opium, codeine, belladonna, kaolin, or bismuth may also be given by mouth; atropine and codeine intramuscularly. In the later stages diarrhoea may respond dramatically to administration of liver, vegetable extracts, folic acid, or vitamin $B_{12}$.

### Effect of antibiotics on malabsorption

The most commonly used antibiotic is tetracycline (250 mg 6-hourly). In subjects who have acquired sprue in Hong Kong this has resulted in clinical improvement, return to normal stool, reduction of steatorrhoea, and increase in sugar and $B_{12}$ absorption.

In other geographical areas, notably India, results have not been so good.

Long-term treatment with tetracycline lasting several months has been successful in Puerto Rico and is now under trial elsewhere.

*Complications.* Complications must be treated immediately before attempting to adjust the diet and attend to the basic syndrome.

*Dehydration* is indicated by the appearance of the patient. Mild degrees can be corrected by oral therapy, by keeping up the supply of water and salt in the form of soft drinks, soups, etc. or 'normal' saline diluted 1 in 5 with water. More severe cases require intravenous infusion of saline. The degree of dehydration can be estimated clinically by the methods used in cholera (see p. 60). When dehydration is severe oral administration is unsuccessful and may be dangerous, since absorption from the gut may be delayed and the fluid may merely accumulate in the intestinal lumen. Inattention to dehydration may be fatal. The management of dehydration is discussed elsewhere (p.60).

In severe cases acidosis may be present and must be adjusted (see p. 61).

*Anaemia.* The administration of folic acid may have immediate effect on the anaemia (see below) and general condition of the patient but not on the fat absorption. If the haemoglobin is below 8 g or PCV below 12 per cent transfusion is required. Half a litre given over 4 hours is usually sufficient in the first instance. Where there are signs of cardiac overloading, the transfusion may be given by partial exchange, the rate of infusion is one arm being matched to the rate of withdrawal from a vein in the other. Where there is iron deficiency, ferrous sulphate 200 mg thrice daily is adequate. Parenteral iron is rarely needed.

*Shock* is indicated by low blood pressure and haemoconcentration. Treatment is described on p. 280.

*Tetany.* Calcium lactate, 325 mg thrice daily may be given and continued until the plasma calcium concentrations can be checked.

*Vitamin deficiencies.* Local cleansing and oral hygiene may help the lesions in the mouth but relief in severe cases requires parenteral use of nicotinic amide and riboflavine (for details see below).

### General treatment

*Diet.* Whatever the immediate treatment, the patient must at the earliest moment be placed on a diet suitable to him. This will vary from patient to patient and there is little virtue in the use of standardized dietary regimes.

If marked hypoproteinaemia is present, a high protein diet is naturally of great value, similarly if fat or milk intolerance occurs these substances should be avoided. In severe cases, all oral feeding may have to be stopped, while in mild cases the patient may be able to continue on his usual diet.

The addition of lightly cooked liver to the diet, or the administration of liver extracts, orally or parenterally, speeds up the process of recovery. Liver should not, however, be regarded as a substitute for proper dieting, but as an adjuvant.

*Tropical sprue does not respond to a gluten-free diet.*

*Folic acid.* Folic acid may have a dramatic effect in certain anaemic cases and very little in others. In severe cases 10–20 mg may be given intramuscularly daily for the first week, followed by an oral dose of 5 mg daily, continued for several weeks. Milder cases may be given 20 mg orally twice weekly.

*Vitamin $B_{12}$.* This may be given sometimes in addition to the folic acid. Primary $B_{12}$ deficiency is rare but, if there is suspicion of deficiency, the vitamin should be given intramuscularly as 1–2 mg cyanocobalamin immediately, followed by 0.25 mg once weekly for up to 3 months.

*Other vitamins.* Nicotinic amide and riboflavine are very effective in controlling the tongue and mouth lesions. In most cases deficiencies are multiple and it is sufficient to give a vitamin B complex preparation orally, or intramuscularly if necessary in the early stages of treatment. Vitamin C is rarely deficient but it is advisable to see that the diet contains fresh fruit juice.

The administration of vitamins will not check the advance of the syndrome or improve the absorption defects.

*Corticosteroids.* These normally have no place in the treatment of sprue. Occasional cases in which the adrenal is affected excrete very small amounts of 17-oxogenic steroids and in these cases, according to Baker, hydrocortisone, dexamethasone, or prednisone in the usual doses may be life-savers.

# 28

# TOXOPLASMOSIS

## DEFINITION

A disease resulting from infection with the intracellular protozoal parasite *Toxoplasma gondii.*

## GEOGRAPHICAL DISTRIBUTION

The infection is world-wide. It has been found in parts of Europe, the Middle East, Sri Lanka, South-east Asia, Australia, the Pacific islands, and the Americas.

## AETIOLOGY

The causative organism is a protozoon which was regarded as one of the sporozoa but which has now been shown to be a coccidian parasite related to the genus *Isospora.* As seen in man, it is an intracellular parasite usually lying within endothelial cells and mononuclear leucocytes, but occasionally found in free-living forms in tissue fluids. The parasite is small (about 5 μm in length) and crescentic with one end rounded. Intracellular forms are usually oval or rounded. The nucleus is large and lies near the rounded end of the parasite; a paranuclear body is present in the pointed end. It multiplies by longitudinal fission within the invaded cells, which rupture and set free the parasites which invade adjacent cells. Multiplication may be very rapid. Less virulent strains multiply more slowly and may gradually fill the cytoplasm of the host cell, eventually losing their nuclei and remaining as cyst-like structures, packed with parasites and known as pseudocysts.

*T. gondii* can be cultivated in living tissue cells, as on the chorio-allantoic membrane of the chick.

The many animal reservoirs include cats, pigs, cattle, sheep, dogs, and rodents.

The mode of transmission to man is not yet certain, but incidence is often high in slaughter-house operators and veterinary workers. In the latter, transmission may result from direct contact with infected animal tissues. In other circumstances infection may be transmitted on food, especially vegetables, or by the respiratory tract. Laboratory workers have been infected. Transmission may also result from air-borne infection from coughing of individuals whose lungs are involved.

Congenital transmission is relatively common. The disease may be fatal in early infancy and older children are often blind and hydrocephalic and mentally retarded.

It has been shown that pathogen-free domestic cats, infected by feeding with mouse brain containing cysts of *T. gondii*, produce oocysts in the faeces and schizogonic and gametogonic stages in the epithelial cells of the small intestine. Isolated cysts introduced intraperitoneally into mice produce toxoplasma infections. On this evidence it is concluded that *Toxoplasma* is, in fact, a coccidian similar to *Isospora* (see p. 24).

Toxoplasmosis may thus be acquired by the ingestion of oocysts (which are very resistant) in the faeces of the cat and probably of other domestic and wild feline animals. The asexual and gametogonic cycles occur in the intestinal mucosa. The parasite develops in cells on the tips of ileal villi in cats. Oocysts are passed in the faeces and are resistant and long lived. They remain highly infective even in earth and dust. Man is presumed to ingest oocysts via cat faeces. This may be the common mode of infection. Gametogony does not occur in man, who does not pass infective oocysts.

## PATHOLOGY

After ingestion the oocyst develops in the intestinal mucosa and releases parasites into the blood-stream. These are taken up by the reticulo-endothelial cells in which they multiply to form 'pseudocysts', containing about 20 endocysts, which are ultimately discharged into contiguous cells or systemically into most organs, where they proliferate, invading many other cells in the same way—including parenchymal cells—and in some cases forming large 'cysts', containing masses of inert cytocysts. Where the parasite is proliferative, serious lesions occur, with focal areas of necrosis and infiltration with lymphocytes, monocytes and plasma cells.

In congenitally acquired infections the lesions predominate in the brain, spinal cord, and retina or choroid. In the brain characteristic necrotic foci occur and minute granulomata are found, which commonly calcify.

## CLINICAL PICTURE

Toxoplasmosis is often described in terms of the concentration of the clinical features in relation to certain organs, but the simplest differentiation is (a) congenital and (b) acquired infections.

### Congenital toxoplasmosis
This is predominantly neurological, resulting from encephalomyelitis, the effects of which are evident at or soon after birth. Few infants survive the first few weeks of life but some survive to adult life.

When the mother is infected early in pregnancy the usual effect on the foetus is hydrocephalus which commonly causes obstructed labour. Microcephalus may also occur. Infants who survive to childhood are mentally deficient and frequently suffer from epileptic convulsions. Ocular lesions, including vitreous opacities and choroidoretinitis, are common and are associated with nystagmus. The characteristic retinal lesions are usually bilateral and lead to blindness; they are occasionally unilateral.

Micro-ophthalmia may present in striking contrast to the enormous hydrocephalic head. Infection of the mother in the first trimester may also lead to abortion. The infection of the mother does not usually affect the foetus in subsequent pregnancies.

### Acquired toxoplasmosis
This is usually divided into various clinical types, which are not separate entities but merely patterns determined by the site of the active infection.

*Lymphatic toxoplasmosis* is probably the commonest form of the infection. It is seen in patients of all ages, especially those concerned with domestic animals which may be reservoirs, such as pigs, cattle, dogs, and rabbits. There is commonly generalized glandular enlargement, some groups of glands being more affected than others. The cervical, neck, axillary, and inguinal glands are usually involved. The glands are discrete, moderately enlarged, firm but not tender, except during the febrile episodes which occur from time to time. The overlying skin is not involved. Mediastinal and pulmonary hilar glands are sometimes involved and the picture may be mistaken for Hodgkin's disease.

The glandular enlargement persists for months, sometimes for years. The spleen and liver are usually palpable.

Irregular moderate fever occurs in the early stages in many cases, usually starting before the appearance of the adenitis, and may persist for weeks, recurring at irregular intervals. Some cases are febrile throughout. The constitutional symptoms are commonly moderate, but may be severe.

The lymphatic syndrome is nearly always benign. The enlargement may last for years in children.

*Cerebrospinal toxoplasmosis* is commoner in children than in adults. The clinical picture is that of an acute or subacute meningo-encephalitis. The onset is acute and in adults may be accompanied by a rash. There are fever, severe headache, cerebral vomiting, disorientation, delirium, and sometimes maniacal attacks. Convulsions occur commonly in children. The patient often complains of rapidly advancing deafness and focal choroidoretinitis, which often involves the macula and eventually leads to scarring, visual disturbances, and eventual blindness. Occasionally the attack is fulminating and death may occur in a few days from the onset. The course is usually a matter of months and in some cases, especially in adults, there are bouts of clinical signs of the meningo-encephalitis with intervals of quiescence, sometimes extending over months or even years. Some patients recover without sequelae. Others have persistent headache and irregular explosions of maniacal or psychotic behaviour. In children the meningo-encephalitis is usually fatal. In adults, recovery is common but there may be persistent neurological and psychotic sequelae. In some cases, the onset may take the form of suddenly developing abnormal behaviour and motor activity.

The syndrome has to be differentiated from the effects of similar meningo-encephalitis caused by arbovirus infections. The cerebrospinal fluid is often xanthochromic, the protein content is considerably raised, and leucocytes are present in large numbers.

*Exanthematous toxoplasmosis* occurs mainly in adults, usually individuals such as cattlemen, closely concerned with reservoir animals. There is sudden onset with moderate to high fever, sometimes rigors. A generalized maculo-papular, erythematous rash develops after some days resembling the rash of tick typhus but absent from the palms and soles. Myalgia is present from the onset, with scattered small areas of acutely painful, localized tenderness, which persist after the acute phase has subsided and may become palpable in the muscle substance.

There is commonly tachycardia and sometimes abnormal rhythms and cardiac dilatation. Pneumonitis develops in severe cases, with dyspnoea and sometimes respiratory failure. The syndrome may be complicated, especially in adults, with the signs of meningo-encephalitis. Death may occur in the acute attack, or the disease may slowly devolve over some months.

Toxoplasmosis often exists without clinical expression and is discovered by laboratory tests, as explained below.

In endemic areas such evidence of infection is often considerable, although the overt disease is relatively uncommon.

### DIAGNOSIS

Congenital toxoplasmosis is strongly suggested in new-born infants with hydrocephalus or microcephalus, choroidoretinitis with blindness, and calcified foci in the brain detected radiologically or at autopsy. In older children serious disturbances of vision or blindness due to choroidoretinitis, associated with mental deficiency, with or without hydrocephalus, also indicate toxoplasmosis.

In adults with acquired toxoplasmosis the clinical diagnosis is often extremely difficult as the signs are largely non-specific and differentiation has to be made from other causes of lymph gland enlargement, pneumonitis, and encephalomyelitis.

Biopsy material from bone marrow, spleen, lymph glands, or centrifugates from the cerebrospinal fluid may reveal the organisms which can also be cultured by intraperitoneal passage in mice, hamsters, or guinea pigs.

Laboratory diagnosis is made by examining the patient's serum for specific complement fixing antibodies (using antigen made from duck embryo *Toxoplasma* cultures) and for neutralizing antibodies. The dye test is also commonly used, in which the patient's serum is mixed with a suspension of *Toxoplasma* parasites and methylene blue; if antibodies are present, the parasites do not stain; otherwise, they do. Skin tests are made by intradermal inoculation of 0.1 ml antigen; a positive reaction occurs when a large wheal with pseudopods and a surrounding arteriolar flare develops in 20–30 minutes.

For diagnosis of active infection a titre of 1 in 8 or more in the complement fixation test and 1 in 128 in the dye test is usually demanded.

Complement-fixing antibodies develop later in the disease than those responsible for the positive dye test. They disappear sooner. A positive complement–fixation reaction thus usually indicates active disease.

Indirect haemagglutination tests and the indirect fluorescent antibody reaction test also become positive in the serum during the infection. The latter may be used to identify cysts in tissue sections.

### TREATMENT

Pyrimethamine with or without sulphonamides is usually effective in acquired toxoplasmosis. The neurological sequelae resist treatment.

A short course of treatment may be successful in mild infections. Relapse is possible after some months, so it is probably better to give the longer course.

*Pyrimethamine* 50 mg orally at once, followed in 6 hours by 25 mg. A dose of 50 mg is given daily for the next 13 days.

*Sulphadiazine* is given concurrently in doses of 1.0 g 6-hourly for 14 days.

Some authors advise much longer treatment in severe intractable cases, continuing for several months on the same dose of pyrimethamine and 1–2 g sulphadiazine daiy. This course puts a good deal of pressure on the bone marrow. Frequent white cell counts are necessary and the treatment should be interrupted for 2–3 weeks at intervals. The treatment is stopped if signs of bone marrow involvement appear.

Broad spectrum antibiotics including tetracycline and chloretracycline have been used successfully, alone or with concurrent pyrimethamine, especially in heavy infections.

Folic acid (5 mg thrice daily) and vitamin B are given concurrently. Thyroxin is sometimes given in addition. Corticosteroids have no effect on the acute stages of the disease but may be given to relieve the neurological and psychotic effects: they have also been given for treatment for the choroido-retinitis, with equivocal results.

Active infection in a women in the first 5 months of pregnancy should be treated (short treatment). At this stage the infection may be stopped in the mother and congenital transmission may be prevented. If active disease is diagnosed later in pregnancy, the woman must again be treated, but the chances of congenital transmission may not be affected. A positive serum test before pregnancy without subsequent rise in titre indicates that treatment is unnecessary.

# 29

# TRACHOMA

A granulomatous chronic keratoconjunctivitis caused by a virus-like organism and leading to serious complications involving the cornea and eyelids.

### DISTRIBUTION AND AETIOLOGY

Trachoma has a world-wide distribution. It is especially common in the poverty and dirt of certain hot dry areas of the tropics and subtropics.

The causative organism has recently been named as a TRIC agent, which is considered intermediate between a virus and a bacterium. The disease has been successfully transmitted to man and apes. The infective agent is transmitted in nature from eye to eye by direct contact with fingers, fomites, etc.; the role of flies has not been determined. Filthy living conditions, malnutrition, and pre-existing bacterial conjunctivitis predispose to its spread. In an endemic area the prevalence varies widely. It is higher in rural areas than in urban, but adjacent villages may show great differences in prevalence.

### PATHOLOGY

The infection in trachoma primarily involves the conjunctival epithelium. The more superficial cells change to pavement type and may exfoliate; the deeper cells proliferate as ramifying columns into the subepithelial tissue. At this stage many cells contain inclusion bodies which lie in the cytoplasm close to the nucleus. The corium is vascular and densely infiltrated with lymphoid cells which may localize to form scattered follicles. In the later stages so-called trachoma bodies or granules develop, consisting of a central mass of mononuclear macrophages and large cells containing cytoplasmic inclusions and a peripheral collection of lymphocytes. Irregular scarring eventually develops, especially in the upper lid.

Involvement of the cornea appears very early in the form of lymphocytic infiltration and vascularization nearly always in the upper limbus. The pannus so produced extends and is often complicated by ulceration of the corneal epithelium.

At any stage the picture may be complicated by the effects of secondary bacterial infection.

## CLINICAL PICTURE

The onset is usually insidious. In experimental trachoma it may occur within a few days of inoculation of infective material.

The first signs of the disease are often missed because they are so mild as to cause no appreciable symptoms. The earliest indication is the appearance of a number of small, pinhead-sized, pale follicles beneath the epithelium over the tarsal plates, especially in the upper lid. These follicles can be clearly seen against the hyperaemic background after everting the lid. There is often practically no discomfort, but there may be some itching, smarting, and excessive lachrymation.

Sometimes the lymphoid infiltration is generalized, so that follicles as such are not formed and the mucosa appears reddened and velvety. This occurs especially in the presence of other bacterial conjunctival infection, and is usually accompanied by acute symptoms of irritation, including some palpebral oedema, lachrymation, and mucopurulent discharge.

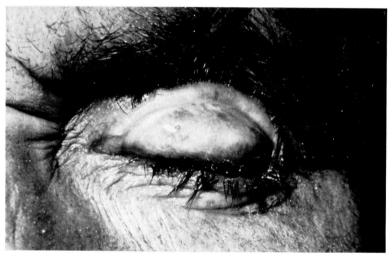

FIG. 57. Trachoma. Note scarring and vascularization of upper lid and matting of eyelashes.

[Iran. Courtesy of Dr Ch. Mofidi]

The inflammatory reaction invades the cornea in the earliest stages. Infiltration with lymphocytes and increased vascularization of the conjunctiva superior to the cornea is followed by similar changes in the cornea itself and a pannus is formed in the upper limbus. The symptoms and signs become more severe and the patient often now appears for the first time for treatment.

The lesions develop especially in the upper lid, almost always in both eyes. On inspection of the tarsal conjunctiva after eversion, pathognomonic small granules may be seen protruding above the general level of the surface. These measure a millimetre or more across. They closely resemble boiled sago grains and contain mucoid material which can be easily squeezed out by pressure. There may be only one or two or there may be large numbers. There is usually an accompanying papillary hypertrophy which is displayed as a red, rough, or shaggy background almost invariably secondarily infected. Symptoms are often severe. The eyes itch and irritate. There may be thick gluey or mucopurulent discharge. Lachrymation and photophobia may be intense. Repeated attacks of acute bacterial conjunctivitis often occur and exacerbate the condition. In untreated cases corneal complications are very common. The pannus intensifies. Small ulcerations appear at the advancing edge or within it. The ulcers are small, shallow, only slightly infiltrated, and very irritating and painful. They easily become secondarily infected and may lead to permanent corneal scarring and opacity.

Trachoma tends to heal by scarring, leaving fine white cicatrices, mainly in the upper lids just inside the lid margin and over the tarsal plate. Scarring may be excessive in the region of the Meibomian glands and eventually leads to distortion of their orifices and to inversion of the edge of the lid (entropion), so that the eyelashes point inwards and rub against the cornea (trichiasis). These are common complications. Where oedema of the lid is excessive (usually a sequel to heavy secondary infection) the edge may evert rather than invert (ectropion). The lower border of the upper lid is frequently distorted.

When pannus is severe the upper lid is often carried well down over the eye, giving the patient a sleepy appearance. This ptosis is a very characteristic clinical sign of the disease.

In the late stages of untreated trachoma the deformity of the lids, especially the upper, may be extreme. Damage to the cornea from pannus, ulceration, secondary infection, and scarring may lead to permanent blindness.

### DIAGNOSIS

Scrapings (stained with Giemsa or iodine) from early cases, but not always from later ones, may reveal the cytoplasmic inclusion bodies, which appear as red acidophilic granules against a circumscribed bluish background of inclusion material, the whole forming a small mass lying close to the nucleus and somewhat smaller than it. Similar inclusions are found in other conditions, including non-gonococcal conjunctivitis of infants and follicular conjunctivitis.

Clinical diagnosis in the early stages depends on inspection of the conjunctiva and the detection of characteristic follicles. Early invasion of the cornea is important. Some authorities suggest that a clinical diagnosis should not be made unless upper limbus pannus is present. Appearance of sago granules is diagnostic. By this time pannus is usually well developed.

### TREATMENT

Therapy concerns treatment of the active infective stages and repair of the tissue damage done to the eyes and lids.

### Active treatment

The infection responds to sulphonamides and various antibiotics including the tetracyclines, erythromycin, and penicillin. The agent is resistant to streptomycin.

### Systemic treatment

This may be given where the circumstances permit, or where local treatment cannot be supervised or is apparently unsuccessful. Examples are:

### Broad spectrum antibiotic

Tetracycline: 500 mg 6-hourly for 3–5 days. Children in proportion to weight.

### Soluble sulphonamide

Sulphadimidine: 2 g immediately, followed by 1 g 6-hourly for 10 days.

### Long-acting sulphonamide

Sulfadoxine: 1 g given once at intervals of 14 days for up to 3 months. (This regimen has been used for mass therapy.)

### Local treatment

Tetracycline ointment 1 per cent, applied to the eyes twice daily (including once at night) for 1–3 months, or twice daily for 3–6 consecutive days (whichever is possible under the circumstances) for up to 6 months. This will also control most local secondary infections. This technique is extensively used in mass campaigns where the people themselves are taught to use it (schoolchildren are used to deal with their own families).

An alternative is sodium sulphacetamide as a 6 per cent ointment or a 10 per cent solution, applied as above. This technique requires trained personnel.

### Combined therapy

In hospital the combination of tetracycline orally and locally gives the best results. Sulphonamides are cheaper; at clinics the long-acting sulphonamide plus tetracycline ointment is successful under proper supervision.

Clinical improvement is usually rapid, largely because of the early elimination of local bacterial infection. The effects of the trachoma, such as follicular lid reactions and keratitis, disappear more slowly but should clear in a few months.

*Repair of tissue damage*
Scarring and deformity of the lids: surgical interference is required. Bilateral tarsectomy is often successful in combination with chemotherapy.

Corneal ulcers require careful treatment aimed at minimizing secondary infection. Early ulcers respond well to antibiotics.

*Control*
The basic factors are improvement in living conditions, reduction of poverty and filth, and the corresponding rise in the desire and demand for personal hygiene. Overcrowding may not in itself be a primary factor in transmission since the disease is commoner in the country than in the overpopulated towns.

There is no effective vaccination.

# 30

# TROPICAL ULCER

### DEFINITION

Superficial skin ulceration of uncertain aetiology found extensively in the tropics and usually associated with the presence of *Bacillus fusiformis* and *Treponema vincenti.*

### DISTRIBUTION

Tropical ulcer is common in certain districts of tropical South America, Central America, the West Indies, Africa, India (Naga sore), Assam, Sri Lanka, Vietnam, south China, Malaysia, Thailand, Indonesia, the Philippines, Melanesia, Papua New Guinea, Northern Australia, the Solomons and other islands.

It has occurred in 'epidemics' at various times in North Africa, Melanesia, and Assam.

### AETIOLOGY

The aetiological factors concerned in the appearance of tropical ulcers have been summarized in the phrase, 'filth, food, friction, and fuso-spirillosis'. To these must be added local trauma.

Tropical ulcer is seen most frequently in low-lying, hot, moist regions; it may occur, however, in areas as high as 558 m above sea level. It is particularly common in open-air workers whose work is sweaty and who are exposed to local injury, especially about the legs. It is more common in males than in females, and in adolescents and young adults than in children or the aged.

It is associated with filthy, overcrowded living conditions and appears particularly in those who wear little clothing and go barefoot. Malnutrition and dietary deficiencies, especially of protein, predispose to ulceration, as was demonstrated in European prisoners of war in the Far East. Concomitant debilitating diseases, especially malaria, are frequently present.

It is not known how the ulceration is established but it is generally accepted that direct contagion from ulcer to skin is important. It is possible that flies may spread the condition by passing from feeding on an active ulcer to bites, cuts and abrasions on the new victim. Local injuries, especially cuts and abrasions, are probably necessary for successful inoculation. Ulcers have been observed in parts of the body which have been pricked or cut by instruments used for the surgical excision of known lesions.

In freshly developing ulcers two organisms are practically always present, i.e. *B. fusiformis* and *T. vincenti*. It is not certain whether these are true causal agents or secondary invaders, but their association with this form of ulcer is so close as to permit the working hypothesis that they are concerned in its genesis. Other organisms including various pyogenic cocci are also present, but inconsistently and in relatively small numbers.

*B. fusiformis* is a sausage-shaped, straight or curved rod of variable size. The ends are tapered and, in stained preparations, the body is characteristically banded or beaded. The organism is an obligatory anaerobe. It is usually non-motile but some motile strains have been observed. It is Gram-positive, but decolorized by long exposure to alcohol. It is found in enormous numbers in active ulcers. It is less prominent in and may be absent from more established lesions. It disappears during healing and may return in a relapse.

*T. vincenti* is an actively motile, anaerobic treponema with several loose spirals. It is found in the necrotic material covering the ulcer surface and for some depth in the granulation tissue beneath. It is believed to be the same organism as that found in Vincent's stomatitis.

Both *B. fusiformis* and *T. vincenti* are found in the buccal cavity under normal conditions. It is not known whether spread from the mouth is concerned in any way with the pathogenesis of ulceration.

Material from ulcers containing both these organisms is capable of transmitting fresh ulceration both to animals and man. Intradermal injection of cultures of either organism separately does not readily produce ulcers, although mixed injection is sometimes successful. Filtrates from ulcer slough or tissue are non-infective.

Transmission by means of injection of material from fresh ulcers is usually successful only if the recipient tissues are bruised or injured in some way.

The role of other organisms, including the pyogenic cocci is also uncertain. It is believed that they may be important pathogenic agents in some cases, secondary invaders in others.

### PATHOLOGY

*The active ulcer*

Examination of the slough or of the scrapings from the granulation tissue beneath will reveal multitudes of both *B. fusiformis* and *T. vincenti*. There will usually also be staphylococci and streptococci but in much smaller numbers.

At the growing edges of the ulcer the epithelium is raised and thickened and deep papillary processes project into the corium. The surrounding skin and corium is often oedematous and irregularly infiltrated with polymorphs.

In the ulcerated area the surface tissues undergo coagulative necrosis and merge with a loose pseudomembrane consisting largely of fibrin, necrotic cells, masses of fusiform bacilli, and spirochaetes.

The deeper tissue is infiltrated with lymphocytic and plasma cells and with foci of polymorphs. The lesion extends into the surrounding connective tissues and there is usually a considerable mobilization of fibroblasts beneath the ulcerated area. In severe rapidly progressive cases the deeper underlying tissues may be affected; especially bone, which may become necrotic. Muscle is usually not attacked.

In rare cases large blood vessels may be eroded.

*The established ulcer*

After its early rapid growth the ulcer tends to remain more or less stationary, sometimes for many years. The acute inflammatory reaction subsides and the base becomes filled with indolent granulation tissue. New epithelium is formed at the periphery and grows slowly in towards the centre of the ulcer. Hypertrophy and downgrowth of the epithelium at the edges is prominent. In long-standing ulcers there is often extensive dense fibrosis in the tissues beneath and proximal to the ulcer.

Healing eventually occurs and the ulcerated area becomes thinly epithelialized from the edges inwards. The epithelium over the healed ulcer is often thin and easily damaged and relapses are common. In long-standing lesions or in those in which there has been extensive necrosis healing may occur with gross scarring.

Carcinomatous changes may occur in long-standing indolent ulcers.

### CLINICAL PICTURE

Tropical ulcer appears most frequently on exposed parts of the limbs and body. It does not appear on the face. It is commonest on the lower third of the leg, involving the ankle or dorsum of the foot, and sometimes the phalanges. It also occurs infrequently on the arms and fingers. It is believed to arise as a rule in the region of bruising, cuts, abrasions, bites, and other damage to the skin and subcutaneous tissues.

There is usually only one ulcer at a time in a given patient. Occasionally there may be a group suggesting autoinfection. Relapse of ulceration is fairly common in the scars of old ulcers. No immunity is produced; fresh ulcers may develop in other parts of the body after the healing of an ulcer.

Opportunities for watching the early development of tropical ulcer are rare, since the patient usually seeks advice for the first time long after the ulcer has developed. In those cases which have been observed, however, and in experimental inoculation, the lesion begins as a vesicle, which ruptures and leaves an ulcerating sloughing surface, or as a papule which enlarges rapidly, becomes inflamed and breaks down into ulceration.

The active ulcer once formed at first spreads rapidly. It may measure 5 cm across in a few weeks, but it is commonly smaller. It is very itchy and sensitive in this stage, causing considerable pain and annoyance.

The skin near the lesion is swollen, reddened, and oedematous. The margin is slightly raised and the edges, which sometimes may be a little undermined, slope sharply down to the ulcerated surface. The surface is covered with a foul-smelling, grey-green, sometimes bloody slough forming a false membrane, attached firmly to the underlying tissues. The slough covers the ulcer and separates with some difficulty, revealing soft pulpy granulation tissue beneath. There may be a covering purulent, greyish discharge.

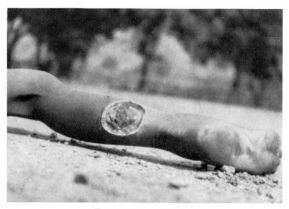

FIG. 58. Tropical ulcer.
[Courtesy of Dr H.Peaston]

The ulcer may stop growing in a few weeks or may continue to spread slowly in width and depth, coming to involve surrounding and underlying tissue. In the chronic stage the edge is pale, heaped up and hard, forming a raised ring round the ulcerated area. The base is composed of firm, pale, granulomatous tissue which does not bleed easily, and is free from slough.

After a variable period, sometimes of years, the ulcer heals. Epithelium grows in from the edges and in the absence of heavy secondary infection may remain thin and delicate, so that further ulceration may result from trauma. Healing is not always complete. Parts of the original ulcerated area may be covered with epithelium while other parts remain florid and active or are penetrated by discharging sinuses, especially if bone is involved. Where there has been massive formation of deep fibrous tissue there is usually notable scarring and deformity. Serious incapacity may result from the involvement of joints and subsequent ankylosis.

The majority of cases are ambulant throughout. Some general reaction, including fever, may accompany the developing stages of the ulcer but, on the whole, the general effects are much less evident than might be expected from the appearance of the ulceration.

There is no leucocytosis unless from other causes. Some patients may show a relative lymphocytosis.

Even in the acute stages local lymphangitis and lymphadenitis are uncommon, except when there is obvious secondary infection. Local gland abscesses practically never occur and generalized septicaemia is very rare.

The active ulcer is sensitive to pressure, the surrounds are itchy and may become secondarily infected by scratching. As the ulcer becomes more established, local tenderness and pain tend to become less pronounced and may be absent. Some depigmentation or hyperpigmentation in light skins often occurs after healing.

### DIAGNOSIS

The existence of severe usually very chronic local ulceration without pronounced general symptoms is suggestive of tropical ulcer. The appearance of the ulcer, with raised edges and a covering of grey, bloody pseudomembrane, is usually diagnostic. Examination of the slough usually reveals an enormous variety of organisms including *B. fusiformis* and *T. vincenti*. The latter are present in practically all fresh ulcers and in many established lesions. Preparations for examination should be made from the ulcerated surface after removal of the slough with saline or dry gauze. Organisms are often found deep in the ulcerated tissues. *T. vincenti* is conveniently observed with dark-ground illumination in wet preparations. It stains well with Gram's stain (positive) or methylene blue and best with Giemsa.

Other ulcerative conditions may have to be excluded. Desert sore, cutaneous diphtheria, leishmaniasis, and mycoses should be identified by examination and are usually accompanied by other evidence of the disease. Syphilis produces serpiginous, penetrating, irregular ulcers in which *B. fusiformis* is usually absent; there is likely to be other evidence of infection, including a positive Wassermann reaction. This reaction is negative in tropical ulcer. The primary lesion of yaws may be confused occasionally but it is slower in development, the surface of the ulcer is different, being pale and shot with strands of epithelial tissue, and without the characteristic slough; the Wassermann reaction is positive. The multiple lesions of secondary yaws should present no difficulty. Tertiary yaws ulcers are irregular, less well-defined and have not the characteristic bacterial content. Mycobacterial ulcers may be difficult to differentiate (see p. 395).

Ulceration arising from varicose veins in the leg is uncommon in the tropics. The pathogenesis of such ulcers should be obvious on inspection.

### TREATMENT

Careful attention to local cuts and abrasions will greatly reduce the incidence of tropical ulcer in a population, especially in labour personnel.

Whenever possible the affected part should be rested. If the ulcer is on the leg, the limb should be elevated.

The patient should be given a well-balanced diet containing adequate protein, and intercurrent infections, especially malaria, should be treated.

Removal of the patient from tropical to temperate surroundings is often followed by rapid healing.

### Treatment of the ulcer

Many methods of local treatment have been recommended, most of which are fairly successful in early cases but less so in long-standing ulcers.

The early growing, sloughing ulcer responds better to treatment than the later, more chronic, stages.

### The early ulcer

Before any local application is made the ulcer should be thoroughly cleaned and as much of the necrotic material as possible removed. This is best done mechanically with soap and water. Gauze soaked in peroxide may be used to loosen adherent slough. In difficult cases gauze compresses of saturated magnesium sulphate or copper sulphate (1 in 200) may be applied daily until the slough separates. These may be painful.

When the ulcer is clean, gauze dressings soaked in various substances may be applied daily, or the surface may be dusted with sulphonamide powder and covered with gauze. Substances successfully employed as compresses include acriflavine 1 in 1000, cod-liver oil, bismuth iodoform paraffin paste (BIPP) or zinc iodoform paraffin paste (ZIPP), penicillin, or penicillin oitment.

When healing has commenced after any of the above, a bland ointment such as zinc and castor oil or boric acid should be substituted and continued until epithelialization is complete.

The best treatment is the administration of antibiotics, combined with local bland or antiseptic dressings.

The combination of penicillin orally or intramuscularly and applied locally has proved successful. Tetracyclines are effective administered orally in a dosage of 500 mg 6-hourly for 5 days.

Healing begins in a few days and proceeds rapidly. Relapse is uncommon.

The advantages of antibiotic treatment in mass campaign are obvious.

### The chronic ulcer

The established ulcer is indolent and may respond poorly to local treatment or oral antibiotics. A few cases have been successfully treated with tetracyclines.

One satisfacory method of dealing with indolent chronic ulcers of the leg is the occlusive technique. One of the great advantages of this technique is that the patient is kept ambulatory and long periods of enforced rest are avoided.

### Occlusive techniques

(i) *Adhesive tape.* The whole leg below the knee is shaved, washed, and dried. The ulcer is cleaned and covered with gauze.

Adhesive tape about 2.5 cm wide is then applied on the long axis of the limb or slightly obliquely. Successive strips are applied so as to overlap slightly and cover the ulcer for 7.5 cm above and below and at least 2.5 cm on either side. As far as possible the edges of the ulcer are drawn towards each other during the application of the adhesive. A circular bandage is finally applied to cover the strapping. The dressing and strapping are changed once a week, or if there is much discharge.

Tetracycline therapy should be combined with this local treatment.

Healing takes some weeks.

(ii) *Plaster*. The ulcer is cleaned or scraped, washed, and powdered with sulphonamide powder. It is then covered with a single layer of sterile gauze cut to the shape and size of the ulcer. Over this is laid a larger layer of gauze smeared with sterile petroleum jelly or BIPP, so that the ulcer is covered for several centimetres all round. A 7.5-cm plaster bandage is then applied. Alternatively some form of elastic sticking-plaster bandage may be used.

The patient is encouraged to return to work and is told to report at regular intervals. Secretion that oozes through the plaster is removed with soap and water and the casing is left untouched for a month or more if possible before being removed and replaced.

Healing should take place in about 3 months.

(iii) *Radical treatment* may be needed, especially when the underlying bone is affected. Total excision followed by skin grafting has been employed with success. Resort to such methods should be made only after the simple procedures have been given an extended trial.

# 31

## TRYPANOSOMIASES

### AFRICAN TRYPANOSOMIASIS

#### DEFINITION

Sleeping sickness. A condition caused by *Trypanosoma gambiense* and *T. rhodesiense* transmitted by *Glossina* (tsetse) flies.

The trypanosomes give rise to two distinct clinical entities, gambiense and rhodesiense trypanosomiasis.

Gambiense trypanosomiasis develops slowly and is characterized by weakness, wasting, lethargy, fever, lymph-glandular enlargement, and eventual involvement of the central nervous system. Rhodesiense trypanosomiasis develops more rapidly, glandular enlargement is uncommon and death may occur before the central nervous system is seriously involved.

#### DISTRIBUTION

Trypanosomiasis occurs within a wide belt of territory in Africa lying between latitudes 10° N and 25° S, stretching from Senegal and southern Sudan in the north to Angola and Mozambique in the south. The distribution inside this area is patchy. Regions of very high endemicity occur in Guinea, Ghana, Nigeria, Gambia, Sierra Leone, and Zaïre.

Gambiense trypanosomiasis is much more widely distributed than rhodesiense, which is largely limited to areas in East Africa, including Tanzania, Uganda, Zambia, and Zimbabwe Rhodesia. Neither is found at elevations beyond 7000 feet above sea level.

Epidemics may arise occasionally as the result of spread of infection from endemic to previously uninfected areas. There are many historical examples of such new distribution of the disease. The disease may be acquired by tourists on 'safari' tours who have gone into the endemic areas with no warning of the risk. Several deaths from *T. rhodesiense* infection have been recorded in this group.

#### AETIOLOGY

*Causative organism*
Trypanosomes are protozoa belonging to the family Trypanosomidae. They undergo metacyclic development in the intermediate insect host. In the human

450

host the metacyclic forms are converted into trypanosomes which divide by longitudinal fission.

In man *T. gambiense* and *T. rhodesiense* are morphologically identical. In the blood and tissue fluids, they appear as thin slender flagellates, varying in length from 10 to 30 $\mu$m, with a finely pointed anterior end and blunt posterior. Short stumpy forms are also seen. There are no tissue leishmanioid forms such as occur in *T. cruzi* infection. In Giemsa or Leishman preparations the cytoplasm stains blue, there is a large, oval, centrally placed, reddish nucleus and a posteriorly placed kinetoplast. In the short, stumpy forms the nucleus may lie posteriorly. The undulating membrane projects beyond the anterior end of the body as a free flagellum. In some individual parasites the flagellum may be absent. The organisms are free moving.

They may be found at various stages of the disease, in the plasma, lymph and cerebrospinal fluid, and in tissue spaces, for example in the heart and brain.

Although morphologically indistinguishable *T. gambiense* and *T. rhodesiense* cause clinically different diseases in man and are commonly transmitted by different species of glossina fly. They are thus conveniently considered as distinct. It is believed by some that they are in fact identical and are the same as *T. brucei* which infects herbivorous animals.

Occasional human infections with other trypanosomes, for example *T. rangeli,* have been recorded.

*Life cycle in the fly*

When ingested by the right species of glossina fly, trypanosomes undergo cyclical development, multiplying by longitudinal fission in the mid and hind gut, eventually becoming converted into infective metacyclic forms which reach the salivary glands and ducts and are injected into the human tissues at biting.

The fly becomes infective 18–34 days after feeding on blood containing trypanosomes.

*The vector*

Only a few species of glossina fly are known to transmit trypanosomiasis.

The most important species are: *G. palpalis, G. pallidipes, G. tachinoides,* and *G. morsitans.*

All will transmit *T. gambiense; G. morsitans* is the principal vector of *T. rhodesiense.*

Other flies may be of local importance, for example *G. swynnertoni.*

Glossina flies have very special requirements for their multiplication. They need shade and moisture and are found in the region of shady trees and scrub near lakes and rivers. The optimal temperature for their breeding is 24–30° C. Hot, dry conditions are unfavourable. Flies do not normally travel widely from their breeding grounds. The distribution differs with the species. Thus *G.*

*palpalis* and *G. tachinoides* are very dependent on shade and moisture and are never found far from them. Their distribution and that of gambiense infection which they carry may thus be locally limited. *G. morsitans* is hardier and less dependent on moisture and consequently ranges much wider.

The flies bite by daylight. Both sexes carry the infection. They are attracted by moving objects and the disease may be spread by the carriage of flies from one area to another in motor cars and trains.

*Glossina* flies produce single larvae. Their numbers are thus relatively limited. The infection is not transmitted to the fly's offspring.

*Transmission*

Trypanosomiasis is usually transmitted to man by the injection by the fly of metacyclic forms at the time of biting.

Transmission may occasionally result from mechanical transference of infective blood on the biting parts of other flies, including *Tabanus* and *Stomoxys*.

Transmission in a given area depends on man–fly contact. It should be appreciated that man–fly contact may be of high degree even when the fly is scanty. There must be suitable vectors in sufficient numbers, reservoirs of infection, and non-immune human recipients. In some regions it is believed that certain wild or domestic animals, notably the large antelope, may act as reservoirs of infective trypanosomes. In general, however, the only reservoir of importance is man.

All ages and either sex may be infected if exposed to the same conditions. In many districts, however, the disease may predominate in one sex because of its particular occupation. For example, fishing may lead to much greater exposure to infection.

The European is likely to be affected more severely than the African. The native population may acquire some form of resistance to infection with local strains of trypanosomes. Resistance is more prominent after spontaneous recovery than after chemotherapeutic interference. Its nature has not been defined.

### PATHOLOGY

In gambiense trypanosomiasis pathological changes develop at the site of the injection of the parasite, in the blood-stream, in the lymphatic and connective tissues, in certain visceral organs including the heart, and at a later stage, in the central nervous system, especially the brain and to some extent the cord with accompanying changes in the cerebrospinal fluid.

In rhodesiense trypanosomiasis the pathology is essentially the same but involvement of lymphatic glands is much less common and by the time of death the involvement of the central nervous system is frequently not as fully advanced as in gambiense infection. In rhodesiense infections, serious effusions are more common and lesions in the heart more frequent and severe.

In both infections the development of the disease in the late stages is often complicated by emaciation, malnutrition, and mineral deficiencies. Malaria and other diseases also often complicate the pathological picture.

### The pathology of gambiense trypanosomiasis
In what follows the pathological changes seen in gambiense infection are described. Points of difference in rhodesiense infection are mentioned in the section on that disease.

*Local reaction.* The pathological changes at the point of biting develop very early. A firm, tender, reddened nodule may develop in the course of a few days composed of tissue infiltrated with lymphocytes and plasma cells and containing rapidly dividing trypanosomes; the smaller blood vessels are often cuffed with small round cells.

*Lymph glands and other tissues.* The enlarged glands contain considerable numbers of parasites in the connective tissue and in the sinuses, which are packed with round cells and macrophages. There is a general proliferation of the lymphatic tissue, oedema, and vascular congestion. The trypanosomes are active in causing inflammatory reactions in the connective tissues, as they are in other parts of the body. The inflammatory phenomena seen in the lymph nodes represent merely general, largely non-specific reactions to the presence of the parasites within tissue spaces. Similar reactions occur, for instance, in the supporting tissues of the heart muscle.

Eventually the inflammatory reaction subsides and is replaced by fibrosis which is assisted by an obliterating endarteritis of the smaller vessels. Perivascular infiltration may be pronounced. Trypanosomes are rarely found in this stage.

*Central nervous system.* The leptomeninges are congested; there may be oedema and small haemorrhages; the vessels are infiltrated with round cells. Trypanosomes are scattered through the substance. The distribution of the lesion is mainly vertical.

The brain tissue is oedematous in some cases, with flattening of the convolutions. The lesions are most pronounced in the pia mater. The basic change is a meningo-encephalitis in which perivascular cuffing with round cells and microglial cells is often pronounced. There may be scattered minute haemorrhages. Changes in the blood vessels are independent of the local presence of parasites.

Occasionally there may be some endarteritis of the smaller vessels. Neuronal changes are late and secondary. The are rarely severe. In the substance of the brain, especially in the cerebral cortex and in the frontal lobe, the pons, and the medulla, there may be accumulations or 'nests' of trypanosomes, often surrounded by small glial cells, forming granulomata.

The choroid plexus is often severely congested and infiltrated with lymphocytes. It may harbour large numbers of trypanosomes in active stages of division.

Scattered irregularly through the brain substance and especially near the infiltrated blood vessels there occur large eosinophilic mononuclear cells with eccentric nuclei known as morular cells (of Mott). These are believed to be macrophages. There are frequently similar but less clearly developed changes in the upper reaches of the cord.

*The cerebrospinal fluid.* Changes in the spinal fluid occur early. The pressure is moderately raised and the numbers of cells increased; the cells are chiefly lymphocytes. Occasionally plasma cells, eosinophils and morular cells may be present. The fluid is clear as a rule but occasionally the cellular content may be high enough to produce some milkiness.

It early contains protein the concentration of which increases as the disease progresses. With the rise in protein, which may reach 100 mg or more per 100 ml, there is a coincident fall in chloride and glucose.

Trypanosomes are commonly but not invariably present in the late stages.

### CLINICAL PICTURE OF GAMBIENSE TRYPANOSOMIASIS

Gambiense infection may take the classical form but in populations of endemic areas it is often clinically mild, although it may end fatally by sudden exacerbation. Fulminating cass resembling rhodesiense infection may also appear, in which the cerebrospinal system is affected early, or there may be acute severe septicaemia and death within a few weeks or months from the onset.

The description of the disease which follows will concern first, the classical form, and secondly, the mild or apparently mild forms.

#### Classical gambiense trypanosomiasis

The classical picture of trypanosomiasis can be divided into several stages. First, there is the tumour at the site of the bite. Then follows the stage of invasion, starting as a septicaemia succeeded after a variable interval by invasion of the lymph glands. This in turn is followed by nervous system involvement.

The progress of the disease occupies anything from 9 months to 3 years or more from the first appearance of symptoms.

*The bite reaction.* A red swelling, sometimes capped by a wheal, may appear within minutes of the bite. This subsides in a few hours and may be followed in about a week by a firm, tender, slightly reddened or violet nodule, over which the skin may be oedematous. This tumour may become as much as 2–3 cm across, raised above the surface, and painful or itchy. It is sometimes surrounded by a diffuse erythematous plaque-like area. Scratching may lead to ulceration and secondary infection; pus is not produced otherwise. The ulcerated lesion is often referred to as a 'chancre'. The acute reaction commonly lasts only a few days, although the swelling may persist for 2–3 weeks. Fluid aspirated from it contains actively dividing trypanosomes. Further development of the infection can be stopped at this stage with suitable drugs. The bite tumour is more often seen in Europeans than in natives of the endemic areas. It is not usually associated with any general reaction.

### The stage of invasion

*Incubation period.* In those few cases in which it has been possible to estimate the time elapsing between the infection and the appearance of symptoms the incubation period varies from 10 days to 3 weeks. It may be very much longer. Two or more years may elapse between the bite or a visit to an endemic area and the appearance of symptoms.

*Onset.* The attack starts with fever accompanied by malaise, lassitude, insomnia, and headache. The latter is the commonest of all early symptoms and the most persistent. Trypanosomes appear in identifiable numbers in the peripheral blood.

*The fever.* The fever may occasionally start with a rigor. It is irregular in intensity and duration, usually highest in the evening. There may be severe sweating, especially at night. The initial fever seldom lasts more than a few days. It is followed by an apyrexial interval of variable length, usually some weeks.

Pyrexial and apyrexial periods succeed one another at irregular intervals for months, the fever eventually subsiding completely or becoming low grade and 'grumbling'.

The fever is invariably accompanied by a fast pulse, which persists into the apyrexial periods and sometimes throughout the disease. Prolonged tachycardia may be easily brought on by exercise or excitement. The respiratory rate during the fever is high; anorexia is common and there may be some nausea and vomiting. The urine frequently contains a small quantity of protein in the febrile period: sometimes this persists. There may also be casts.

*Rash.* A rash may appear soon after the onset of fever. It is usually found on the trunk, especially the chest and back, but may appear on the face and limbs. The eruption develops as irregular or circinate areas of transient erythema, with indistinct margins and a clear centre, often giving an annular appearance. Individual patches vary in size; they may be several inches across. Sometimes the affected skin is oedematous and may be very itchy. Fading occurs in a few hours; there is no desquamation. The rash appears at irregular intervals. It may sometimes be brought out by heat, for example after a hot bath. It is difficult to see on a dark-coloured skin.

*Oedema.* Some cases may develop scattered areas of firm subcutaneous oedema, localized commonly in the eyelids, the sheath of the penis, or in the ankles, hands, and feet. The oedema in a particular area may subside in a few days or weeks. Several regions may be affected simultaneously or in succession.

In the course of the first few weeks of the disease a generalized puffiness of the face usually develops.

*Involvement of lymph glands.* This usually occurs early and may be the first sign of the disease. The distribution of enlarged glands is roughly symmetrical. Any gland may be involved. Enlargement is often most obvious in the posterior cervical region (Winterbottom's sign). The affected glands are moderately enlarged and firm; they may continue to enlarge for months or years, tending to become softer as they get larger. They often appear as obvious discrete tumours, unattached to the skin. Eventually fibrosis takes place and the gland becomes a small, hard, discrete mass.

Glands suppurate only if secondarily infected, as they may be following interference by native 'doctors'.

Glandular enlargement occurs in the majority of cases; it may occasionally be absent even in the presence of intense blood infection.

*Blood.* Trypanosomes are present soon after infection but are not commonly found by ordinary examination until the third week after the bite, i.e. towards the end of the incubation period. In most cases there are relatively few; only one may be seen in several oil immersion fields in a thick film. Occasionally, they are numerous. They remain in the blood-stream for months after the onset. In the later stages, however, they become very scanty, except during exacerbations. It is usually easier to find them in the gland juice.

There is frequently a mild secondary anaemia in early infections. In the late stages deficiencies and malnutrition complicate the blood picture and severe macrocytic anaemia may develop.

The white cells show no special changes.

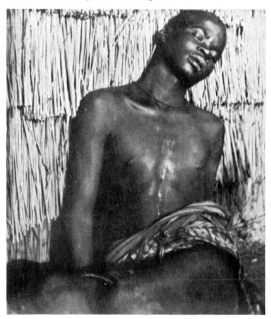

FIG. 59. Early gambiense trypanosomiasis. Falling asleep during feeding.

*General symptoms.* The spleen and liver may be enlarged.

Serous effusions, sometimes containing parasites, have occasionally been reported in joints and in the pleural and pericardial spaces in gambiense trypanosomiasis, but are more common in rhodesiense infection.

Lassitude and asthenia develop progressively as the disease advances. The patient often becomes drowsy during the day and unable to sleep at night. The appetite is not usually affected, but malnutrition is common in the more advanced stage, when the 'sleeping' patient may have to be roused to take food.

### The stage of central nervous system involvement

The clinical picture results from a continuous process of infection which eventually leads to a fully developed meningo-encephalitis and which frequently gives some indications of central nervous involvement at an early stage. Central nervous system lesions usually predominate in the late stages of the disease, and may appear sufficiently distinctive to constitute a separate phase of the disease, known as 'sleeping sickness', which commonly develops 6–12 months after the onset.

The first indications of the development of central nervous system changes are often to be seen in exacerbation of already existing symptoms, particularly lassitude and apathy, which grow progressively worse. Changes in character and personality also become prominent. Neurological signs commonly develop late.

The general condition of the patient deteriorates. He is increasingly asthenic and easily fatigued. Unless under supervision, he becomes progressively emaciated and develops signs of malnutrition and food deficiencies of one kind or another. He complains when awake of severe and persistent headache. Apathy increases; he loses interest in his surroundings, is unable to concentrate on even minor matters and has to be roused for feeding. Intellectual degeneration may be advanced. A worsening confusional state is common. Somnolence increases during the day, but there may be insomnia and restlessness at night. Eventually the patient may pass into the inert so-called 'sleeper' stage and finally become comatose.

The face becomes puffy, especially around the eyelids, producing an effect of dull, surly indifference, 'the swollen, stupid, rather sad look'. This facial puffiness may persist throughout the disease and in striking contrast to the thin emaciated body.

As the time goes on sensory and motor disturbances appear. These vary considerably in degree from patient to patient, one aspect often being especially pronounced in a given individual.

The sensory changes commonly affect the joints. Pressure on deep tissues, for example in the palm of the hands or over the ulnar nerve, is followed by severe pain a short time after the pressure has been relieved (Kerandel's sign). Muscular cramps and neuralgic pains in the long bones and joints are common. The patient complains of tingling sensations on the lips, the soles, and the palms; sometimes there may be intolerable generalized pruritus. There may be loss of spatial sensation.

The patient grows irritable, melancholic, emotional, and depressed. His memory fades, his intelligence degenerates and his character disintegrates. As the meningo-encephalitis spreads neurological changes become increasingly obvious. There may be incoordination of movements, convulsions, meningismus, hemi- or paraplegia, delirium, mania, epileptiform convulsions, coma and, in the final stages, incontinence of urine and faeces.

Among the earlier motor signs are fine tremors and fibrillary twitchings of muscles, particularly those of the face, lips, and fingers. Tremor and incoordination of the tongue cause changes in speech, which becomes slow, slurred, and indistinct and is often made worse by paresis of the lips, especially the lower, which may project forward. Paresis of the facial muscles leads to dribbling of saliva and excessive lachrymation which may be intensified by local eye changes.

Inco-ordination and emaciation of the skeletal muscles commonly leads to a slow, unsteady, swaying, shuffling gait. Knee jerks are usually lost late.

In most cases the progress of the central nervous system lesions is continuous, but occasional cases are met in which the development is spread over a year or more, sometimes 2 or 3 years, with intermittent remissions and exacerbation of the signs and symptoms.

Changes may develop in one or both eyes. Conjunctivitis with excessive lachrymation is common. Corneal opacities may develop associated with interstitial keratitis and a painless iridocyclitis. The retina may ultimately become oedematous. The changes other than those in the retina are generally benign and resolve readily; they are not common, but must be looked for, in view of the necessity of arsenical treatment. Retinal changes may lead to optic atrophy and permanent blindness.

During the whole course of the nervous stage general symptoms, especially headache and glandular enlargement, may still be evident. The state of the glands varies. Some may be enlarged and contain trypanosomes; others may be fibrosed and inactive.

The appetite is usually unaffected but the patient may go to sleep in the middle of eating, so that half-chewed food joins the saliva dribbling from his mouth. He soon becomes incapable of looking after himself and will pass rapidly into severe malnutrition and associated deficiencies unless properly nursed and fed.

Mineral and fluid deficiencies also tend to appear as the disease progresses and the patient may pass into profound and fatal dehydration resulting from combined water- and salt-deficiency. In this state oliguria occurs and the urinary chlorides are grossly reduced or absent.

Changes in the heart muscle may sometimes lead to dilatation and inadequacy. This is more common in rhodesiense than gambiense infections.

Males become impotent and, although there is no similar impotence in women, if they conceive during the disease abortion is common.

In the uncared-for case trophic sores are common. Intercurrent infection, particularly pneumococcal pneumonia and the dysenteries, are very frequent and may prove fatal. Death occurs also from acute flare-up of the infection, with overwhelming trypanosome septicaemia, from cardiac or vascular failure, or from malnutrition and deficiencies.

### MILD AND APPARENTLY MILD CASES

The classical case is seen in local inhabitants mainly during epidemics, or in non-immune individuals such as Europeans. The full picture is uncommon in the indigenous population of endemic areas, where the disease appears most frequently in a clinically mild form which exhibits few symptoms. These forms may be truly mild or slowly progressive. The usual picture is one of mild general symptoms, including fever, and glandular enlargement, particularly obvious in the neck. There may be some wasting and, at a later stage, muscular tremors and slurring speech are common, together with swollen expressionless facies and personality changes. In some patients central nervous system signs eventually become advanced. Trypanosomes can usually be found in the blood but are more easily detected in the gland juice. Occasionally the glands may be relatively unaffected and the blood infection heavy. In a group of such cases observed in Sierra Leone, involvement of the cerebrospinal space was early but did not progress.

Although the signs and symptoms may be mild at the time of examination in a given patient, this may be no indication of the prognosis. It is impossible to tell, except by serial surveys, whether the condition is, in fact, mild or not.

In some areas the cases undergo spontaneous cure; elsewhere many of them prove fatal. There is some disagreement over the cause of death in these apparently mild cases. In some the full development of nervous system involvement may occur. In others there is sudden exacerbation of the infection and death in septicaemia. Others probably die from intercurrent infection.

In the early stages of some epidemics it has been observed that most cases are apparently mild and do not progress. During the declining stages of the epidemic, however, an increasing proportion of cases develop classical sleeping sickness.

It is presumed that the milder cases seen in indigenous populations in endemic regions are the result of the development of some form of resistance to the organism acquired by previous infection. Variations in the virulence of the trypanosomes may also be a factor in modifying the clinical picture.

### PROGNOSIS

The prognosis in untreated, well-developed severe cases is bad, especially if there is a high protein content in the cerebrospinal fluid. Early cases respond well to treatment and usually recover.

The clinical assessment of an apparently mild case will depend upon some knowledge of the virulence of the local strain of trypanosomes.

DIAGNOSIS

The certain diagnosis of trypanosomiasis depends on the discovery of the parasite. Search for the organism may be made in the blood, glandular juice, and cerebrospinal fluid. Fluid from the bite tumour taken within 2 days of infection usually contains parasites.

In individual cases the diagnosis should rest on the discovery of the parasites but in mass examination of large groups of population in endemic areas a tentative diagnosis can often be made from the clinical history, the presence of enlarged glands, and the general central nervous system picture. In doubtful cases the effect on the erythrocyte sedimentation rate of a single dose of suramin or pentamidine is often a useful lead (see below). If the diagnosis in an individual case is strongly presumed and the blood and gland juice do not reveal trypanosomes, examination of the spinal fluid is advisable. In an endemic area a raised cell count and protein concentration are sometimes regarded as diagnostic even if parasites cannot be demonstrated in the fluid. In the final resort where the diagnosis of trypanosomiasis is still likely, although not proved, therapy is advisable.

### Blood
The parasite is most easily seen in a wet film made by covering a drop of blood on a slide with a coverslip. The trypanosomes move actively about causing commotion among the red cells and are easily visible under the high power of the microscope. For final identification dried thick or thin blood films should be stained and examined by the same methods as for malaria parasites.

If the parasites cannot be detected by the wet drop or thick film about 5 ml of blood may be withdrawn, citrated, and centrifuged at 10,000 rev min$^{-1}$ for 10 minutes. The supernatant fluid is removed and recentrifuged at the same speed for the same time. The supernatant from this fluid is centrifuged at 2500 rev min$^{-1}$ for a further 10 minutes and the deposit is finally examined as a wet film or dried smear.

### Lymph gland juice
Trypanosomes can usually be found in material aspirated from the glands while they are soft; they cannot be recovered from fibrosed glands. The gland is lifted between the finger and thumb and pressed up against the skin. A medium-sized, thoroughly dry hypodermic needle is inserted into the gland substance and the gland is massaged gently. A syringe is attached to the needle and suction applied. The juice in the needle is ejected on to slides and

examined either as wet or stained preparations, as for blood. In *T. rhodesiense* infections it may be difficult to find parasites in the glands; they should be sought in the blood.

### Cerebrospinal fluid
The fluid is examined for the presence of trypanosomes, cells (mostly lymphocytes) and excess protein. Trypanosomes are looked for in the centrifuged deposit by the wet film technique. The number of cells present is calculated by the usual method, the protein is estimated by various flocculation methods.

### Other diagnostic points
Certain other tests may help the diagnosis. The erythrocyte sedimentation rate over 10 minutes is calculated and the patient is given a single dose of suramin (0.5–1.0g) or pentamidine (150–200 mg). One month later the ESR is again measured. If there is a significant fall in the rate a presumptive diagnosis may be made.

There are very considerable increases in the IgM immunoglobulins, which are not specific to the infection but are significant as the rise occurs early after the infection, and a history of exposure makes this important since a low level of IgM may help to exclude the infection. The test can be carried out on dried blood samples.

Autoagglutination of the red cells is common in trypanosomiasis but has no specific importance. The formalin serum flocculation reaction is usually positive early. There may be considerable reduction in total serum protein, mainly in the albumin fraction.

Guinea pigs or rats may be inoculated intraperitoneally with 0.5 ml of blood or the final sediment from blood centrifuged as described above. Trypanosomes appear in the blood of these animals after some weeks. Initial infection of animals is easier with *T. rhodesiense* than with *T. gambiense*.

### Mass diagnosis
Examination of large population groups for evidence of trypanosomiasis should start with a census. This is followed by systematic examination of gland juice or blood or both, for trypanosomes. It is usually more economic to concentrate on examination of gland juice. In certain areas it may be necessary to examine the blood, particularly where glandular involvement is not very obvious. Lumbar puncture in mass surveys should be made only in the exceptional case and should not be carried out until the blood has been sterilized by either suramin or pentamidine.

#### RHODESIENSE TRYPANOSOMIASIS

Rhodesiense trypanosomiasis is usually a rapidly developing fatal disease. The organism is largely resistant to arsenicals and treatment is effective only in the early stages.

This form of trypanosomiasis follows the same general course as gambiense infection. There are certain points, however, which require special notice.

The distribution of rhodesiense trypanosomiasis corresponds in East Africa to the distribution of its main vector, *G. morsitans*. The disease is found in Zimbabwe Rhodesia, particularly in the north-east, Tanzania, Mozambique, Malawi, and in certain areas of north Uganda.

The pathological processes involved are similar to those of gambiense infection but the visceral effects are more obvious. For instance, serous effusions containing parasites are common and myocardial involvement may be severe. The latter arises from inflammatory cellular infiltration of the connective tissue of the cardiac muscle, usually associated with the presence of trypanosomes, which ultimately leads to fibrotic replacement of the muscle, and corresponding loss of efficiency.

In rhodesiense infection the local reaction at the bite is often severe. The incubation period may be shorter than in gambiense infections. The disease may start with rigor and severe fever. The lymph glands are commonly little involved although there may be some enlargement in the glands of the posterior triangle of the neck. Trypanosomes appear earlier in the blood and in larger numbers than in corresponding gambiense infections. Scattered fleeting firm oedematous subcutaneous swellings may occur. There is acute loss of weight and emaciation. The clinical signs of cardiac involvement appear early. The pulse is fast from the onset and remains so even in remissions; cardiac dilatation and incompetence are common. The central nervous system is involved early, sometimes within 4–5 weeks of the onset, but the meningo-encephalitic processes are seldom as advanced at death as those of gambiense trypanosomiasis, possibly because of the shorter duration of the disease. Mental symptoms, especially progressive delusional states, are usual.

Diagnosis is made as in gambiense infection.

In endemic areas an increase in cells and protein in the spinal fluid should be regarded as positive evidence of trypanosomiasis until proved otherwise.

### PROGNOSIS

In the first few weeks after the onset the prognosis with treatment is good. It gets worse the longer treatment is delayed. If the disease is diagnosed late, treatment will probably fail.

The untreated case usually dies within 9 months or a year from the onset. In some areas mild forms of the disease occur in the native population and spontaneous recovery takes place.

### TREATMENT OF TRYPANOSOMIASIS

Treatment is general and specific. The general treatment of the advanced case consists of nursing, prevention of bed sores, adequate feeding, resoration of deficiencies in the diet, treatment of cardiovascular collapse and dehydration.

## Chemotherapy

The aim of chemotherapy is to eradicate the trypanosomes (i) from the blood and tissues and (ii) from the central nervous system and cerebrospinal fluid.

### Drugs active in the blood and tissues

*Suramin* (Antrypol, Germanin). An organic urea substitute given as a 10 per cent watery solution intravenously. The drug may affect the renal epithelium—for this reason a small dose of 0.1 or 0.2 g is given first and the patient is watched. If albumin, casts and blood cells appear in the urine within 48 hours after this injection or during subsequent dosage, no more of the drug should be given. It is contra-indicated in individuals with renal disease. If there is no renal effect the adult dose is 1 g every 5–7 days, up a maximum total of 10 g. The dose for children is calculated on the basis of equivalent body weight.

*Pentamidine.* A diamidine compound given as a watery solution (usually of the isethionate) intravenously or intramuscularly every day for 10 days in doses of 3–4 mg base per kg body weight. The dose for children is calculated according to body weight. The drug is useful only in gambiense infections. Pentamidine may occasionally cause faintness, hypotension, and collapse. Adrenaline should be available and the patient should rest after injection, which should be given when he is recumbent.

*Melarsoprol and Trimelarsan.* These drugs are active in the blood and in the central nervous system (see below).

*Other drugs.* The antibiotic Puromycin has been tried with success in early cases of gambiense infection in doses of 0.5–1.0 g daily for 10 days. In more advanced gambiense cases and in rhodesiense infections good results have also been claimed with *Nitrofurazone* (see p. 466).

These drugs cannot be regarded as a substitute for melarsoprol or trimelarsan in severe infections.

### Drugs active in the central nervous system

*Toxicity.* The drugs which are most active in the meningo-encephalitic stage of the infection are listed below. They are all pentavalent arsenical compounds and consequently may be very toxic. Encephalopathy with psychoneural signs may follow their use. Peripheral neuropathy, exfoliative dermatitis, and severe diarrhoea may also occur. Considerable skill and experience is needed in their administration, the response being determined by the clinical reactions of the patient and changes in the cerebrospinal fluid. The choice in the individual case may lie between the dangers of arsenical poisoning and the certainty of death from the infection. A serious risk in the administration of tryparsamide is damage to the optic nerve with ultimate atrophy and complete blindness.

*Tryparsamide.* An organic pentavalent arsenical given intravenously as a 20 per cent solution in water in doses of 30 mg per kg body weight to a maximum single dose of 2 g. The initial dose is 1 g. Subsequent doses of 2 g are given at intervals of 5–7 days for a total of 9–20 g. Children should receive doses in proportion to body weight.

Tryparsamide resistance has been met in both gambiense and rhodesiense infections. The resistance persists through cyclical transmission in the flies. Melarsoprol is active against resistant strains. Tryparsamide is of little value in severe gambiense infections with central nervous involvement and is ineffective in advanced rhodesiense infections.

*Melarsoprol* (Mel B., Friedheim). This organic trivalent arsenical combined with dimercaprol (BAL) has replaced tryparsamide in the treatment of severe gambiense and in rhodesiense infections. It is made up as a 3.6 per cent solution in propylene glycol, given intravenously; maximum single dose 180 mg.

*Trimelarsan* (Mel W., Friedheim). This compound is similar to melarsoprol but is water soluble. It is given intramuscularly; maximum single dose 200 mg.

### TECHNIQUE OF TREATMENT

As a general rule suramin and pentamidine are both successful in clearing the blood-stream of trypanosomes in gambiense infection; in rhodesiense infection only suramin is effective.

Arsenical drugs are used to treat the central nervous system involvement. Advanced cases of gambiense infection and cases of rhodesiense infection respond to melarsoprol. Trimelarsan is usually successful in gambiense infections but not in rhodesiense infections. In the treatment of the individual case these two drugs have now largely superseded tryparsamide which may still have to be used in epidemics as the other drugs are too toxic. Dose: a course of suramin, followed after a week by tryparsamide 1 g, then 2 g weekly for 4–5 weeks.

### TREATMENT OF GAMBIENSE AND RHODESIENSE INFECTIONS

(A) *Early stage with normal cerebrospinal fluid*

1. *Pentamide:* 3–4 mg (base) per kg body weight intramuscularly daily for 10 days.
2. *Suramin* (Antrypol): test dose 0.1 or 0.2 g intravenously then, 24 hours later, 20 mg per kg body weight on days 1, 3, 7, 14, and 21. (Maximum single dose: 1 g.)

Both drugs are effective in gambiense infections; for rhodesiense infections, however, suramin is the better drug.

(B) *Intermediate and late stage with abnormal cerebrospinal fluid* (i.e. CSF containing more than five cells per mm$^3$ and/or a raised protein or trypanosomes).

*Melarsoprol* (Mel B) is the drug of choice for advanced *gambiense* and established *rhodesiense* infections. Dosage is 3.6 mg per kg body weight daily—maximum single dose 180 mg. It is made up in 5 ml ampoules containing 180 mg.

The drug is given intravenously. *Dry* syringes and needles must be used, as the solution is unstable in water.

Melarsoprol is given intravenously, with the needle accurately within the vein, since it is intensely irritant to tissues. The injection must be given slowly. Too rapid injection may cause retrosternal and abdominal pain and sometimes vomiting.

Courses of treatment should start with half the full dose, working up rapidly to the full dose. This gives the physician a chance to watch the reaction of the patient. If the dose is raised too slowly, it is believed that resistance may develop to the drug which may make relapse more likely and more difficult to treat.

Common regimens are as follows: three groups of three daily injections, each group of injections separated from the next by at least a week, or two groups of four daily injections, the second group separated from the first by a week.

A typical schedule is:

Day 1: 2.5 ml (90 mg).
Day 2: 3.0 ml (108 mg).
Day 3: 4.0 ml (144 mg) or 5.0 ml (180 mg).
Interval of 7 days.
Daily injection of 5.0 ml on each of 3 days.
Interval of 7 days.
Daily injection of 5.0 ml on each of 3 days.
*Total* of nine injections in three groups of daily injections, separated by a week.

The major toxic danger is encephalopathy, which may appear suddenly or come on slowly, usually shortly after, or during, the first group of injections. Recovery is gradual and the syndrome does not usually appear or worsen after subsequent groups of injections. Clinically, encephalopathy shows as confusion, excitement, tremors, irregular limb movements, and sometimes coma.

*Note.* A preliminary course of suramin often helps the very ill patient, especially if he is febrile and has a high parasitaemia, by clearing the blood of trypanosomes. The usual dose is 0.5 g intravenously on alternate days for three injections.

*Trimelarsan* (Mel W) is seldom used, although it is water soluble, much less irritant, and can be given intramuscularly. The dose is 4 mg per kg body weight, with a maximum of 200 mg, given as daily injections on each of 4 days, followed after 7–10 days by a further group of four injections. The consensus is that melarsoprol is to be preferred.

In cases resistant to melarsoprol or trimelarsan, *nitrofurazone* is indicated (see below).

*Response to treatment.* Except in the very late stages, treatment is usually successful in relieving signs and symptoms in both gambiense and rhodesiense infections and leads to recovery. The trypanosomes disappear from the blood-stream within a few days. They are slower to go from the spinal fluid. The progress of an individual case may be checked by periodic examination of the spinal fluid. The cellular count usually falls faster than the protein concentration.

*Toxic effects.* Toxic reactions may be counteracted by the use of dimercaprol (BAL) which unfortunately also neutralizes the therapeutic effect of the drug.

### Other drugs

In both early and late gambiense and in rhodesiense infection where arsenicals appear to be contra-indicated or have failed, nitrofurazone has been successful in doses of 500 mg given orally once daily for 2 days, then thrice daily for 5–7 days, with a maximum dose of 1500 mg daily for adults. Severe polyneuropathy may follow its use, and haemolysis may be precipitated in patients with G-6-Pd deficient erythrocytes. Fever should be controlled with suramin before nitrofurazone is used. Thiamine should be given concurrently, in doses of 20–25 mg.

#### PROPHYLAXIS

Both suramin and pentamidine are excreted slowly from the body. The concentration of the drugs in the tissues will thus remain sufficiently high to prevent infection for a considerable period after injection. Injection of 1 g suramin in an adult protects against infection with both organisms for 6–12 weeks. A single dose of 200–250 mg pentamidine protects for 3–6 months against *T. gambiense* infection, but is ineffective against *T. rhodesiense*.

## AMERICAN TRYPANOSOMIASIS

#### DEFINITION

Chagas' disease. An acute, subacute or chronic condition caused by the pleomorphic *Trypanosoma cruzi*, transmitted by certain large bugs. The acute disease occurs mainly in children. It is characterized by fever; tumour at the point of infection; transient tissue oedema, especially of the face; local lymphadenitis, and various cardiac disturbances including myocardial insufficiency. Involvement of the cerebrospinal system is occasionally severe. The chronic disease appears in adolescents and young adults, some of whom may have a history of an acute attack in childhood, and is chiefly notable for myocardial involvement.

### GEOGRAPHICAL DISTRIBUTION

The disease is scattered irregularly in Central and South America, in a wide area stretching from Mexico in the north to the Argentine in the south. The distribution of the vectors and animal reservoirs is very much more extensive than that of the human disease, which is limited to certain areas within this wide belt. It is found in various parts of Venezuela, Brazil, west Argentine, Uruguay, northern Chile, Peru, and Ecuador. It has been reported in Guatemala, Panama, and Mexico. Two cases have been reported from Texas. The disease has not otherwise been reported elsewhere in the U.S.A., although vectors and reservoir animals are common in some States, including southern California and Arizona.

It may be acquired by visitors to endemic areas, especially those who live rough and accept village living conditions.

### AETIOLOGY

#### Causative organism
The disease is caused by *T. cruzi* which closely resembles the trypanosomes of African trypanosomiasis. In the blood the organism is found as slender or stumpy trypanosomes 15–20 μm in length, with the usual undulating membrane and anteriorly placed flagellum. The nucleus is central and the large oval kinetoplast posterior. *T. cruzi* propagates in the tissue cells, not in the blood.

#### The vector
The disease is transmitted by large biting reduviid bugs belonging to the family *Triatomidae,* particularly by *Panstrongylus megistus* and *Triatoma infestans.* The larva, nymph, and adult bugs all transmit the infection; the latter is the most important.

The bugs are found under dirty, unhygienic conditions associated with either humans or animals. They are active only in darkness, so that transmission usually occurs at night. It is possible to convey infection artificially through other insects, including the bed bug, but it is doubtful whether any of these is important in natural transmission.

#### Life cycle in the vector
Trypanosomes ingested by the vector multiply by longitudinal division in the

mid and hind gut, becoming converted in 3–4 weeks into metacyclic forms resembling small trypanosomes which are infective to man. Once infected, the bug remains infective for life.

### Reservoirs of infection

Both wild and domestic animals may be infected naturally and act as important reservoirs for the infection of bugs. These include cats, dogs, pigs, many rodents, including rats, and the armadillo.

In some areas infection with *T. cruzi* is considered primarily a disease of animals transmitted accidentally to man. In other areas, especially in villages, man is the important reservoir.

### Transmission

Although the trypanosome present in the blood of human cases or of reservoir animals is infective to man, transmission in nature occurs almost always through the metacyclic forms, passed in the faeces of the bug during biting. The infective faeces is rubbed into cuts or abrasions or through the intact skin or mucous membrane. Infection through the latter occurs most frequently in the lips or the conjunctiva. The bite of the bug is important only in so far as it causes a break in the skin surface and thus facilitates the entry of the parasite.

The high incidence of transmission in children is probably the result of the greater ease with which the parasites can penetrate the delicate skin, and the greater risk of exposure to biting.

Infection is said to occur occasionally across the placenta, or by way of infected mother's milk. Metacyclic forms survive for days in dead bugs and may cause infection if the latter are accidentally eaten.

The disease occurs mostly amongst the lower economic groups living in poor squalid conditions in small villages. The appearance of the disease in a given community is highly erratic. Children are most commonly affected. The sexes are affected about equally.

There is no clear correlation between either the incidence of the infection in accessible reservoir animals or in bugs. Even when the latter show a very high rate of infection in a particular village, for instance, the known case incidence may be very low.

There is no seasonal incidence and no explanation for the very irregular distribution in relation to reservoirs and vectors. It is possible that more careful investigation will reveal a much wider distribution than is a present suspected.

#### PATHOLOGY

The tissues into which the infective metacyclic forms penetrate react vigorously. In the course of a few hours local oedema, with some cellular infiltration, causes a small subcutaneous swelling. The infection spreads rapidly along lymphatics to local lymph glands which become enlarged, congested, oedematous, and infiltrated with lymphocytes and plasma cells. Invasion of the blood-stream with trypanosomes occurs within a few days and gives rise to the early septicaemic signs of the disease. The spleen and liver eventually both enlarge.

The more severe lesions of the various organs in the later stage of the disease arise primarily as a result of the further leishmanioid development of the parasite within the tissue cells.

The trypanosomes immediately enter local reticulo-endothelial cells at the site of inoculation. Within the cells they undergo a leishmanioid stage of development and later return to the tissue spaces and blood as trypanosomes, re-entering other tissue cells and repeating the cycle. In this way the cells of many tissues become invaded and destroyed. This process is particularly notable in the macrophages of the spleen, the Kupffer cells of the liver, and in striated muscle cells, especially those of the heart. It is the damage caused in this way in the myocardium which is responsible for the most serious clinical consequences of the infection.

In the acute progressive form of the disease, which constitutes about 20 per cent of the infections in infants, massive myocardial involvement results in death within a few weeks or months. All grades of myocardial damage are met. In the less extensive heart lesions, proliferative repair takes place with replacement by fibrous tissue of areas damaged during the leishmanioid cycle. Where there has been extensive involvement of the heart, signs of myocardial damage may appear in later life.

Leishmanioid organisms may appear in the cells in other organs, including the thyroid and suprarenal. Goitrous changes in the thyroid gland are common in some districts; these are not direct effects of the disease but are due to local mineral deficiencies.

Meningo-encephalitis may occasionally develop. The meninges and brain tissue are oedematous, congested, and infiltrated; there are scattered neuro-glial and round cell infiltrations, especially about vessels. Small granulomata may develop around trypanosomes or leishmanioid forms lying in the brain substance in the region of the small vessels. Cerebral lesions are most commonly seen in the 'chronic' disease, involving the cerebellum and the frontal lobes in particular.

*T. cruzi* may remain in the blood for long periods. In the ordinary course of events during the acute attack trypanosomes are present in the largest numbers during the early stages. In mild cases or in the 'chronic' stage they may be difficult to demonstrate in the blood, except by indirect biological methods such as xenodiagnosis.

It is believed that *T. cruzi* trypanosomes as such are in some way responsible for the fever. Trypanosomes are found in considerable numbers in the blood during the acute stages of the disease. The occasional attacks of fever seen in the 'chronic' picture are also associated with discharge of trypanosomes into the blood from the leishmanioid-invaded tissue cells.

Unfortunately, the degree of parasitaemia in a given case is no real measure of the damage progressing in the tissue cells invaded by the leishmanioid forms.

CLINICAL PICTURE

American trypanosomiasis may appear in acute or in subacute or chronic forms.

### THE ACUTE DISEASE

The acute disease is commonest and most severe between the ages of 1 and 5 years. It may occur occasionally in adolescents or adults, usually in milder form.

The incubation period is usually 1–3 weeks.

The outstanding clinical pattern after onset is one of severe and intensifying myocardial damage. In heavy infections in which the damage to heart muscle is extreme, a fatal issue is certain during the first acute attack. In milder cases in which the myocardium is less damaged, recovery from the initial febrile illness occurs after some months and the condition passes into a more chronic state in which the final picture is decided by the ultimate pathological damage to the cardiac muscle. Such cases may survive to adult life with irregular intermittent febrile attacks. A proportion of infections may not produce an initial severe febrile episode and may not be detected for years. These cases are usually diagnosed during routine examination by the discovery of some degree of myocardial damage.

The onset of the febrile attack is commonly preceded by local reactions to the original inoculation of the parasite. In a single infection these reactions, when on the face, are often unilateral (as described below) but infection may occur at frequent intervals especially under the prevailing social circumstances in which infants become involved, so that bilateral facial reactions are common.

*The chagoma reaction.* The first sign of infection is usually the appearance within a few hours of a swelling at the site of entry of the metacyclic infective trypanosomes. This rapidly becomes a hard, elastic, oedematous, slightly raised, flat plaque which is hot and red and surrounded by a variable area of hard oedema. It is found most frequently on the face, on the eyelids, cheek, forehead, lips, or the conjunctiva. It may occur also on the abdomen and limbs, especially the thighs. Occasionally other swellings develop, especially in older children; for instance, they may appear on the face or arms following actual infection in the legs. If untreated the swelling may become very large and intensely painful.

The chagoma reaches its full size in a few days and may last as long as 2 or 3 months. It may have faded by the time the general signs of infection have developed.

The skin over the plaque and at its edges becomes hard and may desqua-mate. Suppuration does not occur unless there is secondary infection. The lesion usually disappears completely but in some cases, especially on the abdominal wall or thigh, there may be slight scarring or some depigmentation. In hairy parts healing may be followed by alopecia.

The glands draining the point of in-fection are usually palpable by the third day and may become considerably enlarged and remain so for weeks. The glands are firm, mildly tender, and dis-crete. The skin over them is often ery-thematous and oedematous. In a group of glands there is often one which is much more enlarged than the others.

In a few cases there may be no local reaction and the first sign of infection may be the glandular enlargement.

When the face is involved, the glands most commonly affected are the pre- and post-auricular, and the sub-maxil-lary.

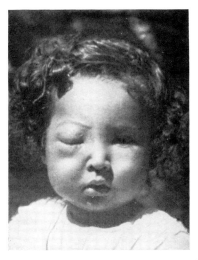

FIG. 60. Chagas disease in child of two. Note unilateral facial and palpebral oedema.

[Courtesy of *British Encyclopaedia of Medical Practice*, Butterworth & Co. London. Photograph by Dr Mazza]

*Local oedema:* The appearance of localized areas of oedema is very com-mon in the first few days of the disease. The oedema develops suddenly. It may persist for months or subside in a few days, sometimes before any general signs develop.

Unilateral involvement of the eyelids is the commonest finding (*Romana's sign*). Both lids are swollen with a hard, elastic, non-potting oedema. The oedema may remain confined to this area for some time, but more commonly spreads down into the cheek and sometimes to the neck. The eyelids of the other side may become involved; sometimes oedema may develop bilaterally.

The skin over the oedematous areas is often erythematous and blotchy, giving the appearance of bruising.

Oedema of the eyelids is accompanied by swelling and injection of the local conjunctiva. The lachrymal glands are frequently affected, becoming enlarged and tender; they can often be seen by forcing the eyelids apart with the patient looking down and inward. The lachrymal canals may be swollen and obstructed, leading to excessive lachrymation, and the eyelashes may be glued together with coagulated serous exudate. In the absence of secondary infec-tion the condition is not purulent.

From time to time during the early stages of the disease local areas of hard oedema may develop in any part of the body, particularly in the scrotum, the legs, the lower abdominal wall, and the pubis. The appearance of oedema in the limbs is sometimes accompanied by a spread of the oedema of the face and even by generalized anasarca in young infants.

*General reactions*

The general signs and symptoms commonly appear 4–14 days after infection and the appearance of local signs. The patient is restless and sleepless. He suffers from malaise, increasing exhaustion, chills, and bone and muscle pains. There is often epistaxis. Convulsions are common in young children; they are usually infrequent and severe and may be fatal.

Trypanosome forms of *T. cruzi* appear in the blood in about 10 days and may be present throughout the acute stage.

With the invasion of the blood-stream the general reaction develops. The local lesions described above persist for varying periods, often for months.

*Fever.* The general symptoms usually start with a moderate remittent fever, which may continue for several weeks. Sometimes, in infants, the initial fever is very high and continuous. In other cases it may be mild and of short duration. During the fever the pulse rate is fast (110–150 beats per minute) and there may be soft mitral bruits. In severe cases in which there is intense myocardial damage acute cardiac failure develops often within a few days of the onset of the fever. The respiration rate is fast and there is frequently some minor bronchial involvement with cough, which may tend to mask the condition. The spleen becomes palpable in the first few weeks but is seldom prominent. The liver enlarges early and may be palpable for several finger-breadths below the costal margin.

A moderate degree of general glandular enlargement is present in most cases within a week of the appearance of the local signs of infection. The glands are only slightly enlarged, not very tender, and in the early stages contain trypanosomes.

There are no characteristic changes in the erythrocytes. The white cell count is raised. In infants the increase is seen mainly in large mononuclears; in older children, in lymphocytes, which may represent as much as 70 per cent of total white cells.

In a small proportion of cases there may be fleeting morbilliform, papular or urticarial rashes. Later there is often depigmentation or hyperpigmentation of the skin over the site of the healed chagoma or in areas which have been oedematous.

*Cardiovascular system:* A very fast pulse is an indication of serious myocardial lesions resulting from repeated invasion of the muscle cells and the repetition within them of the leishmanioid cycle of the parasite. In the active stage, especially during the first week in infants, sudden dilatation of the chambers of the heart may lead to failure. The muscle lesions may also lead to various changes in cardiac rhythm, including fibrillation and heart block with corresponding changes in the electrocardiogram; the Stokes–Adams syndrome has been reported.

Cases in which cardiac involvement is extensive from the beginning will probably die within weeks or months. In less severe infections the cardiac involvement may subside spontaneously or pass on to the later fibrotic stages which are seen commonly in older children or adults.

Occasionally local or general cardiac symptoms may appear without any other previous indications of the infection. Cases in which this occurs are usually seen later in life.

### Nervous System

Involvement of the central nervous system is commoner in infants than in older children. Suckling infants may die in a few days from the meningo-encephalitis, before the cardiac changes develop. The symptoms are mainly cortical. Conclusions are severe and death occurs during them or in deep coma. Meningismus may be present.

The majority of cases show a minimum of nervous involvement and pass through the acute illness without evidence of it.

As a result of damage to the autonomic plexuses and involvement of the intestinal wall, large and sometimes enormous dilatations of the oesophagus and large intestine occur. Motility and muscular hypertrophy lead to gross dilatations of these tubular organs resulting clinically in so-called *mega-oeso-phagus* and *megacolon,* which persist into later life, or develop after the original acute episode. Such lesions have been described in most endemic areas, particularly in Brazil.

In those in which the cerebrospinal system is involved the fluid is at high pressure and contains excess lymphocytes and proteins. *T. cruzi* may sometimes be found in the centrifuged deposit.

*The duration* of the acute stage is variable. Severe cases may terminate fatally in a few days, especially in infants. More commonly the illness continues for weeks or months, the issue depending on the severity of the myocardial involvement. When this is severe, death results. When it is only moderate, recovery occurs and the patient passes into a subacute or chronic state in which febrile episodes may appear at long intervals and in which fibrotic cardiac lesions become slowly established.

SUBACUTE AND CHRONIC STAGE

The subacute disease is seen as a rule in older children from 5 to 10 years of age. There is commonly a history of an acute attack followed by a period of remission with or without mild fever and sometimes with occasional exacerbations of severe symptoms. There may, however, be no history of an acute attack.

In the subacute stage local signs such as facial oedema, if present in the acute phase, have usually subsided. If in a period of remission, the patient is listless, often mildly feverish, and has a persistently fast pulse. Arrhythmias are common.

The condition progresses to slow recovery but remissions occur subsequently from time to time. This goes on for years. The late stages are commonly associated with some permanent myocardial insufficiency.

Trypanosomes are difficult to demonstrate in the blood-stream even during the fever, except by biological methods.

In the chronic stages of the disease the dominating factor is usually some degree of myocardial fibrosis. Chronic trypanosomiasis is usually diagnosed in cases presenting with a clear earlier history of the acute or subacute disease, or with demonstrable parasites in the blood or detectable by xenodiagnosis. It is not clear how far the latter diagnosis is justified, since it is possible that at this stage a state of tolerance has been achieved between host and parasites.

In some endemic areas myocardial involvement is more frequent amongst adolescents and young adults than elsewhere and there is a tendency to include in the diagnosis of trypanosomiasis even cases without a history of infection or circulating parasites.

Cases present with all stages and types of myocardial involvement. In severe cases sudden death may occur and is often blamed on the disease.

### PROGNOSIS

The prognosis is bad in infants, especially when cardiac damage is severe. Early dilatation of the heart, persistent severe arrhythmia or pericardial effusion are unfavourable signs. It is bad in any case in which the nervous system is obviously involved.

In the subacute and chronic stages the prognosis depends entirely on the extent of myocardial involvement.

Malnutrition and coincident infective conditions, especially malaria, are serious complicating factors.

### DIAGNOSIS

Clinical diagnosis in an endemic area is usually easy in young children. Unilateral oedema of the face, especially of the eyelids, together with non-purulent conjunctivitis; the presence of a chagoma and locally involved lymph glands are all indicative of the disease. Meningo-encephalitic signs in infants and young children and persistent tachycardia, arrhythmia, or cardiac dilation, especially when associated with fever or any of the local signs above are highly suggestive.

Megacolon and megaoesophagus in individuals from endemic areas indicate present or former infection.

Definitive diagnosis requires the demonstration of trypanosomes.

### Laboratory diagnosis

*Blood.* Wet and stained thick films should be examined as in African trypanosomiasis. The trypanosomes are fragile and easily damaged. For this reason it is better to examine fresh films.

Trypanosomes are not usually present in large numbers except in very young children during the early acute disease. In older children and adults they are present only during remissions and may be missed by direct blood examination; indirect methods may be necessary.

Identification of the species of trypanosomes is important, since *T. rangeli* (which produces no clinical effects) may be present in the blood of individuals in many areas in which Chagas' disease is endemic.

*Lymph gland juice.* Trypanosomes may be present in the juice of the glands draining the area of the original infection.

The enlarged glands of the stage of general adenitis may also contain trypanosomes and leishmanioid forms.

*Blood culture.* Trypanosomes may be cultured on NNN medium. Cultures should be examined after 21 days.

*Cerebrospinal fluid.* The deposit after centrifugation of the cerebrospinal fluid may rarely contain the trypanosome in cases in which there is evidence of meningo-encephalitis. The preparation of material for examination is the same as for *T. gambiense.*

*Biopsy* of an enlarged gland, with examination of smears and histological sections stained to reveal leishmanioid parasites, may be helpful in some cases but is not usually needed.

### Biological techniques

*Xenodiagnosis.* Bugs raised in the laboratory and known to be uninfected are allowed to feed on the forearm of the suspected case for 15 minutes. The faeces are examined for metacyclic forms after 30–60 days. Infected bugs should be killed and examined in groups at intervals up to 60 days after feeding. Control groups of bugs are similarly examined for infection with *T. rangeli.*

*Animal inoculation.* Mice, puppies, and the armadillo are readily infected by *T. cruzi.* Citrated or fresh unclotted blood from the patient is injected into the animal subcutaneously or intraperitoneally (or into the conjunctiva). The blood of the animal is examined daily for trypanosomes over a period of 5–25 days after injection. The animals are finally killed and a search is made for leishmanioid parasite forms in the tissues, especially the heart. Those may be present in animals in which parasites were not found in the blood. The organism will survive for hours in citrated blood. The armadillo is used as a reservoir animal for research purposes.

*Serological tests.* Serum from the suspected case may be used in a complement fixation reaction (the Machado test), in which the antigen is an extract of organs, usually the liver, from an animal dead of the disease, or an extract of cultures of the trypanosome. A positive result is of presumptive diagnostic value. Weak positive reactions are given by sera from cases of cutaneous leishmaniasis.

The test should always be associated with other diagnostic methods. Some authors regard the complement fixation as more reliable than xenodiagnosis.

Indirect fluorescent antibody tests are sensitive and correlate well with the complement fixation tests.

### TREATMENT

Treatment of the infection is unsatisfactory. Drugs successful in African trypanosomiasis are ineffective.

Certain synthetic compounds have been found to have some action against the trypanosome form of the parasite but these and all other drugs so far tried are inactive against the leishmanioid forms responsible for the major tissue damage.

The use of present trypanosomicidal drugs is ineffective once the leishmanioid invasion of cardiac muscle, etc., has become extensive. They may be helpful if given very early in mild infections or during remissions.

Some control of blood trypanosomes has been demonstrated with various drugs. Nitrofurazone given over a long period has provided some promising results in acute cases. The nitrofuran Lampit (Bayer) is now under trial in a dosage of 5–15 mg per kg body weight daily for up to 120 days. It has the disadvantages of the other nitrofurazones. The 8-amino-quinolines have some effect on animal infections and are being tried in human cases.

The treatment of the cardiac failure is non-specific and is concerned with the emergency treatment of pulmonary oedema and standard improvement of cardiac function with lanoxin, etc., plus the rapid promotion of diuresis.

### CONTROL

Improvement in hygienic conditions, especially housing, is the first essential. Bugs can be dealt with by DDT or Gammexane. Chemotherapy of known cases helps to reduce the infectivity of local bugs.

Attempts are being made to produce a vaccine.

# 32

# THE TYPHOID FEVERS

Typhoid and paratyphoid fevers (the enteric fevers) are caused by infection with bacilli of the genus *Salmonella*.

Typhoid fever is characterized by fever, toxaemia, abdominal signs, and symptoms which may lead to intestinal haemorrhage or perforation, enlargement of the spleen, and commonly a sparse cutaneous eruption. Paratyphoid fevers are usually milder and may present a similar clinical pattern or cause an acute enteritis. Other species of *Salmonella* cause acute enteritis or food poisoning.

## GEOGRAPHICAL DISTRIBUTION

Typhoid fever is world-wide in distribution and occurs irrespectively of climate. Failures in personal hygiene, and particularly in public health precautions, may result in the appearance of typhoid even in well sanitated communities. Nevertheless, with improved water supplies and sanitation in the better developed temperate world, the incidence has steadily decreased and the disease is much more prevalent in the warmer than in the colder parts of the globe.

## AETIOLOGY

*Salmonella* organisms are motile Gram-negative bacilli which usually produce acid and gas from dextrose but not from lactose. *S. typhi,* the cause of typhoid fever, produces acid but not gas from dextrose and is non-lactose fermenting. The cultural and antigenic properties of the organisms are used in their laboratory differentiation (see Diagnosis).

The only reservoir of *S. typhi* is man and the only source of infection is infected human excrement harbouring the organisms. This is probably true of the paratyphoids, but other *Salmonellas* spp., for example, *S. typhimurium,* infect many animals which may act as reservoirs.

Excretors are thus the most important factor in the epidemiology of the typhoid fevers.

Every person who becomes infected with enteric organisms will excrete them at some time or other. Where no clinical signs or symptoms develop, the individuals are classified as 'symptomless excretors'. If they continue to excrete the bacilli they become 'carriers'. The same applies to persons who have become ill after infection and continue to excrete the organisms subsequently. Most individuals who have had clinical typhoid stop excreting the organisms within 3 months of onset. Those who continue to excrete after 3 months are usually classified as 'carriers'. About 3 per cent excrete the bacilli after a year. The situation is much the same in the paratyphoids. *S. typhi* is exceptionally persistent and the carrier state may continue in an individual for 20 years or more. The proportion of infected persons who become carriers after clinical typhoid is unaffected by modern successful treatment of the acute attack with chloramphenicol.

Faecal carriers are the commonest and most important. The condition is most often seen in middle-aged persons and is commoner in women than in men; it is rare in children. The carrier rate in proportion to the population in a given geographical area depends on the hygienic situation. In the United Kingdom it is said to be about 1 in 100,000. It is much higher in areas where hygiene standards are low.

Excretion of the organisms is intermittent but the epidemiological importance of a carrier depends finally on the prevailing hygienic environment and possibilities of spread of infection.

The health of the carrier is usually unaffected but clinical autogenous typhoid fever may occasionally develop in individuals who have been known carriers for years. The organism is most commonly retained in the gall bladder, which may or may not show evidence of involvement, or may contain stones which are themselves infected. As in the disease itself, it is believed that the infection of the gut, from which the carrier excretes the bacilli, comes from the bile or via the gall bladder. Cholecystectomy may be successful in curing the carrier state.

Urinary carriers are uncommon. Bacilli are excreted intermittently in the typhoid case for the first 2 months. If excretion continues, some abnormality of the genito-urinary tract, such as chronic pyelonephritis or schistosomal vesical or ureteric lesions, may be present and should be dealt with.

Detection of carriers is a matter of isolation of the relevant organism from the faeces or urine by the usual methods (see under Diagnosis). The Widal reaction and especially the Vi test may be of some value in tracing persons for further bacteriological study in relatively non-endemic areas, but are of little help in highly endemic areas where large numbers of people may give positive reactions.

The organisms discharged in faeces and urine are disseminated into water, milk, or other foodstuffs. Infection follows ingestion of the contaminated material.

Typhoid and paratyphoid organisms will remain alive in water for days. When the water is clean they will not multiply but oxygenation and the presence of organic matter will assist their growth. The organisms persist for 2–3 weeks in sewage. Typhoid bacilli have been recovered from sea water.

Outbreaks of typhoid are often water-borne, although the organism is usually present in small numbers, except in gross infections. Outbreaks will develop where pollution with infected faeces is heavy and persistent. They are commonly explosive, since groups of people partake from the same infected water at the same time. Although bacilli may survive in sea water, they exist therein in very small numbers and are not known to have led to outbreaks in a normal environment. However, shellfish, which concentrate water in the process of feeding, may become heavily infected and act as sources of human infection even in sea water.

Many outbreaks result from the ingestion of milk and cream products. These foodstuffs are sterilized by pasteurization but the bacilli are added later by the carrier who prepares the food. Cold and tinned meats may be similarly infected and cause serious outbreaks. Tinned meat in itself is extremely safe unless infection is introduced by dirty fluid used for cooling the occasional faulty tin during processing. Where sanitary conditions are bad and typhoid is endemic, flies may be important in transmission, carrying the bacilli on the feet and proboscis.

Infection rarely spreads from patients under treatment except through gross carelessness and then only by direct contamination of food or drink.

### PATHOGENESIS AND PATHOLOGY

The organisms enter the body through the mouth. It is not known where or how they penetrate the mucous membranes. There is some evidence that the bacilli may penetrate into the lymphoid tissue of the pharynx or oesophagus. Some are probably destroyed in the stomach; others reach the intestine and are absorbed into the lymphoid tissue, where they invade the reticulo-endothelial cells in which they multiply. Small numbers reach the blood-stream at this stage and settle in the reticulo-endothelial cells of the liver, spleen, and other organs without causing a persistent septicaemia. It is possible that this process takes place during the incubation period, which comes to its end after the reticulo-endothelial cells discharge the bacilli into the blood-stream. The organisms now invade the tissues afresh via the blood, and the spleen, the gut, and the gall bladder. In the spleen there is further invasion of the reticulo-endothelial cells in which the bacilli multiply; the tissue hypertrophies and the organ enlarges and becomes palpable (an important clinical diagnostic sign). In the intestine the reticulo-endothelial cells of the lymphoid accumulations also become infected and hypertrophy; the infection probably comes mainly from the blood-stream at this stage, although some bacilli may enter the gut lumen from the gall bladder, which is early and invariably involved. (As pointed out above, chronic infection of the gall bladder and its contents is the usual pattern in the faecal carrier.) Bacilli from the gall bladder are the main source of the infection of the intestinal contents.

The primary lesions in typhoid are the infection of the reticulo-endothelial cells, the multiplication therein of the bacilli and the proliferation of the cells with the development of local inflammatory reactions which lead to their degeneration and necrosis. Histological preparations of the lesions, especially in the intestine, disclose many hypertrophied and actively phagocytic, mononuclear, reticulo-endothelial cells which contain erythrocytes, damaged lymphocytes, and multiplying bacilli. The interstitial spaces contain very few organisms.

The lesions occur most commonly in the spleen, the mesenteric lymph nodes, and the lymphoid tissue of the intestinal wall. In the latter, the so-called Peyer's patches are involved.

At autopsy the patches in the lower reaches of the ileum are usually most affected. The upper colon and caecum may also be involved. The mucosa is normal except in the region of these lymphoid accumulations, over which large ulcers may develop, covered in sloughs, which may separate, disclosing a bleeding surface. The ulcers may extend right through the thickness of the wall, causing perforation, with local or general peritonitis. In some cases the ulcers may be superficial. When the ulcers heal, the epithelium is replaced but without restoration of the glandular tissue or scarring. Some cases may show a more generalized enteritis; others, even with serious clinical features, may present with a macroscopically normal-looking intestinal wall.

The ulcers arise from necrosis of the infected reticulo-endothelial lymphoid tissue and are responsible for the two most serious intestinal complications, haemorrhage, and perforation. Bleeding may merely be oozing; it may be sudden and severe where larger vessels are eroded. Perforation may be small, with localized fibrinous peritonitis, or large, with leakage of the gut contents freely into the abdominal cavity; the latter is usually associated with general peritonitis and paralytic ileus. In patients on chloramphenicol treatment leakage may still occur but is usually sterile.

Necrotic foci centred round infected and degenerate and necrotic reticulo-endothelial cells may sometimes be found in the mesenteric lymph glands, which are always involved. They are also common in the spleen and liver and may occur in the kidneys. The mucosa of the gall bladder is corrugated and may be papillomatous; it contains bacilli in reticulo-endothelial cells in the lymphoid tissues, often contiguous to the small blood vessels.

The abdominal symptoms of the typhoid case can be explained to some extent by the pathological findings described above. The characteristic toxic prostration is thought to be due to some form of endotoxin produced by the multiplying organism or its products and lysis. There is some experimental evidence that endotoxins may also be involved in the hypertrophy of the lymphoid and recticulo-endothelial tissue which occurs in the liver, spleen, and mesenteric glands as a prelude to necrosis.

*S. typhi* may cause inflammatory lesions in other tissues including the lungs, the myocardium and endocardium, and the bones, which give rise to complications during the acute attack, in convalescence or later. In such complications the toxic effects of the endotoxins may also be involved. Essentially the pathological processes are similar to those described above and the complications will be considered with the clinical picture.

In paratyphoid infections the pathological changes may be similar but milder and less extensive. In other salmonella infections the picture is more commonly one of a general enteritis, an acute inflammation of the intestinal mucosa which may be very extensive but is usually transient, in keeping with the clinical picture and which suggests a direct intestinal infection.

## CLINICAL PICTURE

The clinical picture of classical typhoid fever is described below. The disease is now usually modified by chloramphenicol treatment and is often reduced to a 4–5-day febrile illness, instead of the long and exhausting condition that occurs in the absence of treatment. The classical disease still appears in many rural areas where specific treatment is not available, or where the diagnosis has been missed in the early stages, as is often the case in sporadic infections, and in infections introduced in travellers infected abroad and returning to countries where the disease is uncommon.

The incubation period varies. It is usually 10–14 days. In water-borne infections, because of the light infection of the source, the incubation period may extend to 3 weeks or longer. Where the original infection is heavy or continuous the incubation period may be as short as 3–5 days.

Typhoid fever is a febrile condition in which the oral temperature reaches a plateau in 3–5 days from the onset and continues at about the same level throughout the illness. The onset is usually insidious. The patient over several days becomes anorexic and suffers from a moderate but nagging frontal headache and muscle and joint pains. Abdominal discomfort is present but often without pain or localized tenderness. Diarrhoea at this stage is uncommon. The patient is usually constipated. This is an important point to note. Typhoid in its early stages *is not one of the classical diarrhoeal diseases* (Christie).

There may occasionally be severe abdominal pain, usually on the right side, which may be mistaken for acute surgical conditions, including appendicitis. Vomiting may occur rarely.

For the first few days there is often a sharp cough, sometimes with a little sticky sputum which may contain typhoid bacilli. There may be signs of bronchitis. The patient sometimes complains of sore throat and there may be some epistaxis; in such persons the nasopharynx is infected but seldom ulcerated.

In the ordinary progress of the disease the patient is severely ill by the end of the first week after the onset. He is toxic and confused and usually complains of persistent headache. His tongue is thickly coated and breath unpleasant; sordes tends to collect at the corners of his mouth. He feels abdominal discomfort but there are few localizing signs. The abdomen may be distended and feels full and slightly doughy but without tenderness. The tip of the spleen can now be felt, again without tenderness.

The fever is seldom accompanied by chills or rigor.

The oral temperature may reach 38.3–38.9° C in the evenings for the first few days, the maximum rising a little each day until 39.4–40° C is attained by the third to fifth day. Thereafter the temperature may remain at about this level without much variation through the day. Sometimes the temperature swings widely, a feature which is likely to be missed unless the patient has the fortune to be in a hospital bed on a 4-hourly chart. In many cases the pulse rate is fast to begin with but falls to 80–90 beats per minute irrespective of the fever; in others it remains fast and more in keeping with the rate expected for the fever.

A characteristic feature is the quick development of toxic signs. The patient's consciousness becomes blurred and he may eventually become stuporose and quite out of touch with his surroundings. This toxic mental state and general prostration increases as the disease proceeds.

The onset may be abrupt rather than insidious and the patient may become desperately ill in a few days with high fever and severe prostration. The early development of high swinging fever and sweating may suggest acute tuberculosis. In some patients there may be diarrhoea from the onset, usually due to other organisms. Cough and chest pain may suggest acute bronchitis or may be associated with the signs of lobar pneumonia. On rare occasions the bacilli may early invade the cerebrospinal spaces and the patient develops the signs and symptoms of acute meningitis, with cloudy fluid containing organisms. In some cases the mental signs may predominate from the start, with rapid development of stupor and coma. In very severe septicaemic cases there may be early haemorrhagic signs and occasionally moderate jaundice.

These variants are uncommon. In the usual severe case the onset is insidious and the disease builds up during the first week to the picture described above.

By the end of the first week the classical rose spots may appear and may continue to appear irregularly over the next week or longer as the disease develops.

The spots are macular, about 2 mm in diameter, seldom raised above the surface, and easily fade on pressure. Each lasts only 2–4 days. They are characteristically sparse in typhoid, more numerous in the paratyphoid fevers. They are usually found on the abdominal wall, the lower thorax, and on the back of the trunk. In very severe cases in the later stages of the disease they become petechial and purpura may develop.

In mild cases the condition reached in the first week may persist for a further 1 or 2 weeks and is followed by lysis of fever and convalescence. In most cases the fever persists for 2 or more weeks and the patient becomes progressively worse.

By the third week the patient has deteriorated into the *typhoid state* with increasing toxaemia and prostration, loss of awareness, and confusion. The state of the patient at this stage is vividly described by Christie.

The patient 'is now completely out of touch, dull, disorientated, and stunned with toxaemia, stupid and unanimated, torpid yet sleepless, confused and muttering, not unconscious but conscious of nothing. . . . His face reflects the profound toxaemia; sunken, sallow, but with a flush over the cheekbones that tends to spread as the illness worsens, his eyes glistening and perhaps injected, but expressive of nothing but inexpressible insensibility'.

At this stage diarrhoea may develop with the passage of the so-called pea soup stools; the constipation, on the other hand, may persist. Blood may appear in the stool at any time after the middle of the second week as the result of erosion of the lesions in the intestinal wall. When haemorrhage is severe there may be large amounts of blood and sometimes clots passed but occasionally the blood remains in the intestinal lumen. Moderate bleeding may continue for days, during which considerable volumes of blood may be lost. Severe haemorrhage is usually indicated by a rapid increase of pulse rate, a fall in temperature and collapse, with air hunger.

Perforation may occur over the same period. It is the most serious complication which was frequently fatal until the introduction of chloramphenicol treatment. With treatment the mortality has been considerably reduced, but the liability to perforation remains, although under chloramphenicol the perforation is usually localized and sterile.

Perforation may occur in a case which appears to be going well, but more often in the severe case. There may be sudden acute abdominal pain, rigidity and guarding of the abdominal wall, and vomiting, with loss of abdominal sounds due to development of paralytic ileus. In the severely toxaemic individual the signs of the development of perforation may come on more slowly, taking a day or two to develop, and are often masked by the patient's dullness and apathy and may easily be missed unless the patient is under constant observation. In small perforations there is usually evidence of increasing distress, some abdominal pain and guarding with tenderness on the right side, over the terminal ileum. There is usually a rise in pulse rate and fall of temperature. The patient breathes with his thorax rather than with his distending abdomen which may fail to move with respiration. Signs of free fluid may be detected and there may be reduction in liver dullness.

Gross perforation produces rapid and profound collapse.

Myocardial involvement often becomes evident in cases which survive in profound toxaemia into the third week or longer. The pulse becomes fast and thin, the heart sounds weak and the blood pressures fall. Signs of venous congestion develop and the patient may die from cardiovascular failure.

Other complications are mentioned above. Most are uncommon and all are now rare in chloramphenicol-treated patients. Thrombophlebitis, especially of the veins of the legs, sometimes developed, especially in elderly patients in early convalescence after a long toxic illness; it was probably associated with prolonged lying in bed and is now uncommon in treated patients. Periostitis, especially in the tibia and the lower ribs and sometimes with abscess formation with *S. typhi* present in the pus, occasionally develops in late convalescence in untreated cases, but very rarely after chloramphenicol treatment.

The complications may cause death or the patient may succumb to the toxaemia without obvious complication. Death occurs commonly in the third or fourth week. The death rate in untreated cases is high.

The patient who recovers does so slowly. The fever subsides by lysis and convalescence is long. In patients diagnosed soon after onset and treated with chloramphenicol the disease is commonly limited to 4–5 days of fever and the abdominal picture and complications do not develop. The longer the treatment is delayed the nearer the picture approaches to the classical typhoid described above.

Relapse may occur, sometimes after an afebrile period of only a few days, sometimes after some weeks. The relapse is clinically similar to the primary attack. It usually lasts only 7–10 days but may continue for several weeks. Complications may develop during the relapse. It is to be noted that chloramphenicol does not affect the possibility of relapse, despite its dramatic effect in limiting the primary clinical attack.

In children the disease is usually milder than in the adult, with a short febrile attack and relatively less toxaemia. The clinical picture may more closely resemble an acute enteritis and the diagnosis may be missed. The mortality up to the age of about 10 years is low. Leucopenia may not be present; the organisms are usually recoverable from the blood.

### DIAGNOSIS

Diagnosis depends on the recovery and identification of the causative organisms, the classification of which by cultural methods, bacteriophage typing, etc., must be determined by the bacteriologist.

The organisms can usually be isolated from the blood in the acute stages of the disease. They are most easily found in the first 7–10 days of the febrile illness, but are commonly present in the late second and the third week and may persist throughout in prolonged illness. The bacilli may be recovered from the blood during the febrile period in a relapse.

In the suspected case 5 ml of the blood should be withdrawn aseptically from an arm vein. Half is added to bile salt or other specific broth medium and half to glucose broth for growth of other organisms. Serum contains factors which are lytic to *Salmonella* and must therefore be adequately diluted by the medium (not less than 1 in 5). For this reason, better results may be obtained by seeding clot after removal of the serum.

Culture from the faeces is possible in about half the cases of typhoid during the first week of the clinical disease. In the second and third weeks of the classical case the number of organisms excreted in the faeces increases enormously and culture is proportionately easier. Organisms may continue to be excreted in the faeces for 2–3 months. If infection persists beyond this point the patient should be regarded as a 'carrier'.

Culture should be attempted from faeces, not from rectal swabs. The latter are often satisfactory in bacillary dysentery and cholera but are not in typhoid.

Culture from the faeces must be repeated on several occasions whatever the clinical state of the patient or the length of his illness. One negative result means nothing, especially in light infections.

The organisms may be cultured from midstream specimens of urine, but much less frequently than from the faeces. The culture may be erratically positive in the first few weeks. The bacilli disappear from the urine long before they go from the faeces, except in cases where there is some genito-urinary abnormality, such as hydronephrosis, when they may continue to be excreted.

*S. typhi* can sometimes be cultured from bile obtained by duodenal intubation even when it cannot be cultured from the faeces. This method may be valuable in identifying carriers but is not used in the diagnosis of suspected typhoid.

Serological evidence of infection depends on the host reaction to the somatic O antigen and the flagellar H antigen of the organisms. The identification of antibodies is usually made by the Widal agglutination test in which serial dilutions of the suspect serum are incubated with suspensions of *S. typhi* and of *S. paratyphi* A and B, and occasionally C, treated to agglutinate with either O or H antibodies. A *Salmonella* group suspension is often included in this test; this usually contains *S. typhimurium* H antigen.

There is substantial antigenic overlap in the typhoid and paratyphoid O antigens so that the Widal test commonly shows considerable cross-agglutinations. Nevertheless, the O titre of the infecting organism is usually distinct. H antigens are specific. A titre of 1:40 for H or O antibodies is suspicious in an unvaccinated individual living in a normally non-endemic area and 1/80 is often regarded as diagnostic. The titre in some infections may be much higher.

The test should be repeated at intervals. A rising titre is significant. The test usually becomes positive by the tenth day of the overt illness and the titres may continue to rise until convalescence. In some patients antibodies may not be produced or may never reach high titres throughout the infection.

In endemic areas the test is much less valuable since antibodies will be common in the population as a result of past infection. In febrile patients in such areas a high and rising O titre may be of some significance. The same thing applies in patients who have previously been vaccinated with TAB vaccine. In the latter case, antibodies to all H and O organisms will be present, not just to the antigens of the suspected infecting organism. A further complication in interpreting the agglutination results is the anamnestic reaction, which affects only the H antibodies, which frequently rise in titre during a febrile illness not related to salmonella infection, or some other stimulus. The evidence for such reactions is not convincing and it is reasonable to hold that a clear rise in H titres must be regarded primarily as an indication of fresh salmonella infection.

In any case, the Widal test is no substitute for the culture of the bacilli from the blood or stools.

*S. typhi* and *S. paratyphi* C sometimes contain an additional Vi antigen which, in organisms possessing O antigen, increases the virulence, probably by protecting the O antigen against agglutination by O antibody. The Vi antigen usually stimulates the production of Vi antibody which can be detected at about the same time as other antibodies in the acute disease. The antibody may be present in the serum of people harbouring the bacilli: its detection is thus of some value in detecting carriers in normally non-endemic areas, but not in endemic areas.

The leucocyte count in the blood in the uncomplicated *S. typhi* infection is usually low in the first 7–10 days of the illness. The leucopenia is moderate, with a total cell count of 3000–5000 per mm$^3$; there is a severe granulocytopenia and relative increase in lymphocytes and polymorphs. As the disease progresses, the cell count may rise and a polymorphonuclear leucocytosis may develop as the intestinal lesions become secondarily infected; it may become considerable in cases with pneumonic or abdominal complications.

In some cases there is leucocytosis from the beginning, with considerable increase in polymorphs. This is the usual picture in meningitic typhoid.

### TREATMENT

The diet should be nourishing and readily assimilable; it should be given in small quantities at frequent intervals; it should be as liberal as possible and free from indigestible and fermentable matter. The fluid intake must be adequate to compensate for that lost from the bowel and as a result of sweating. The temperature when it mounts over 39° C should be reduced by sponging. The strictest precautions must be taken to disinfect or destroy all linen soiled with infected excreta; and the latter must be promptly disinfected, flies being denied access to them.

*Chloramphenicol.* Chloramphenicol exerts a powerful bacteriostatic action on *S. typhi*. It controls the multiplication of the organisms and the progress of the infection until the natural defensive mechanism overcomes them. Relapse may follow its use. The drug is equally effective in *S. paratyphi* infections in which the disease has taken an enteric course; it is not so successful in acute enteritis.

A loading dose, as originally recommended, is not advisable, since it may precipitate toxic crises and shock. In desperately ill patients the first few doses may be given intramuscularly. Otherwise the drug should be given by mouth.

*Dosage.* 500 mg 4-hourly (3 g daily) until the temperature has settled (usually 3–5 days), thereafter 500 mg 6-hourly for up to a total of 10 days. There are many alternative regimens.

*Toxicity*. Rare instances of aplastic anaemia have been reported during treatment with chloramphenicol. There is sometimes a degree of leucopenia due largely to neutropenia. On the whole, these effects have been somewhat exaggerated in the medical press and most physicians have little trouble with the drug. Nevertheless, the blood should be examined daily during treatment.

*Resistance*. Resistance to chloramphenicol has developed in some parts of the world, including Burma. This was apparently not transferable by the R factor (see p. 35), but some strains in Mexico are now known to be multi-resistant and transferable via the R factor. Resistance in this case may have originated in a non-pathogenic bowel commensal. Some recent visitors have brought this resistant strain to Britain—a nice illustration of the dangers of disease importation by modern travel.

*Corticosteroids*. These are useful in the highly toxic case in which their effect on immunity production can be ignored. An intramuscular injection of 200 mg hydrocortisone may be followed by prednisone 20 mg for a further 3 days. Marked abdominal signs, especially those suggesting haemorrhage, contra-indicate the use of steroids.

*TAB vaccine* has sometimes been given during an attack of typhoid to stimulate the immune response of the patient which is needed to supplement the bacteriostasis induced by the chloramphenicol. There is no evidence that this procedure has any value either in the progress of the disease or in preventing subsequent relapses.

*Other antibiotics*. No other antibiotics have the specific effects of chloramphenicol. Tetracyclines have been used in moderately ill cases in conjunction with chloramphenicol in half the dosage quoted above but it is not clear whether they have helped. Ampicillin, which is bacteriocidal against *S. typhi*, is sometimes successful in clearing infection in carriers but is not effective in treating the disease. It is now being tried concurrently with chloramphenicol.

*Septrin (co-trimoxazole)* is a useful alternative to chloramphenicol in the treatment of typhoid, especially where drug resistance has developed. Tablets contain 80 mg trimethoprim and 400 mg sulphamethoxazole. Two are given every 12 hours for 14 days. The drug is prepared as a suspension for children. There have been several reports of resistance in which the bacilli were, however, sensitive to chloramphenicol. Neutropenia and thrombocytopenia have occurred occasionally with this drug.

### Treatment of complications

Complications such as typhoid pneumonia will respond to the chloramphenicol being used for treatment.

When perforation occurs in patients receiving chloramphenicol, the associated peritonitis is usually confined and operation is seldom necessary. The situation is consequently less serious than in untreated patients in whom operation and drainage may be needed with a consequent mortality rate of about 80 per cent. In the latter patients chloramphenicol should be given in high doses until the condition improves. In all patients in whom perforation has occurred an intragastric tube should be passed and aspiration performed regularly to relieve distension; no food should be offered by mouth and saline infusion should be given intravenously.

Haemorrhage results from the erosion of vessels in the intestine. If the vessels are small, there may be little more than oozing. If they are large, alarming quantities of blood may be lost and must be quickly replaced by transfusion. For this reason, all typhoid patients should be blood grouped immediately on admission. Feeding by mouth should be stopped in the event of haemorrhage and the patient should be sedated.

### TREATMENT OF CARRIER INFECTIONS

Cholecystectomy is advisable if lesions or stones are detected in the gall bladder. Treatment with chloramphenicol is unreliable. Ampicillin is probably the most successful drug given over a long period in doses of 1 g orally 6-hourly for 4 weeks. Septrin is at present under trial.

### PROPHYLAXIS

Inoculation with killed typhoid organisms provides strong but not absolute protection against infection and the disease. Vaccines give protection against small doses of the bacillus, but not against massive doses.

Vaccines previously in general use consisted of suspensions of killed *S. typhi, S. paratyphi A,* and *S. paratyphi B* (TAB), to which tetanus toxoid was often added (TABT).

Injection of TAB subcutaneously is followed by severe local and general reactions and is now seldom used. TABT can be given intradermally, with minimal reactions.

Although both these vaccines protect well against typhoid, there is little evidence of protection against the paratyphoids, certainly A.

Modern practice is therefore to use a monovalent T vaccine, containing *S. typhi* only, in a single dose of 0.2 ml intradermally or in two similar doses 14 days apart. The prophylactic effect is as good as with the other vaccines and local and general reactions are minimal. Tetanus toxoid, if required, is given independently.

Vaccination is advisable, but not compulsory, for people going to endemic areas. Typhoid is one of the commoner 'imported' disease seen in short-term travellers.

The means of avoiding infection, in addition to cleanliness, protected water supplies and proper sewerage, are of general application. Caution in the consumption of foods or of fluids which may be contaminated; an attack on fly-breeding places in the vicinity of dwellings: the detection of carriers and their exclusion from food-handling occupations.

All patients suffering from the disease must be strictly segregated and linen and utensils used by them must be placed in disinfectant before cleansing or destruction. All discharges must similarly be dealt with and nurses and attendants must wear protective clothing.

# 33

# THE TYPHUS FEVERS

INTRODUCTION

The typhus fevers are diseases of man due to infection with one or other of a number of species of rickettsial organisms which are small pleomorphic bodies intermediate between bacteria and viruses. With the exception of *Rickettsia prowazeki*, which causes louse-borne typhus, *Rickettsia* normally infects rodents and other mammals and infection of man is incidental and sporadic. They are conveyed from one host to another by arthropods; certain lice, fleas, ticks, and mites transmit the various types of typhus fevers to man. The diseases in man are characterized by a short incubation period and an acute course of about 2 weeks is associated with sustained fever, severe toxaemia, a rash which appears on the fifth or sixth day, and marked nervous symptoms. The mortality varies with the type of infection; in some forms of the disease it is very high.

The main types of typhus fevers are usually described in terms of the vectors. They include louse-borne (Epidemic, Brill's disease, Trench fever), flea-borne (Endemic, Murine), mite-borne (Scrub typhus, Rickettsial pox), and tick-borne (American spotted fever; Bullis fever; African tick typhus; Fièvre boutonneuse). Another rickettsial disease of man is Q fever, which is primarily an enzootic in certain wild and domestic animals, spread by ticks.

The most important of these infections are discussed below.

*The rickettsias*
The rickettsias appear as rounded forms 0.3–1.0 μm in diameter and rods from 1.5 to 2.5 μm in length, but they vary considerably in form in differing environments. They are Gram-negative and stain well with the Romanowsky dyes when water adjusted to pH 7.4 is used as a diluent. Most small laboratory animals can be infected with the rickettsias which infect man, but the degree of their susceptibility to the different organisms varies. In laboratory animals, as in man, the rickettsias live intracellularly and attack chiefly the endothelial cells lining the smaller blood vessels. They can be cultured in living tissue culture media, and on the yolk-sac membrane of developing chick embryos. As a rule they do not survive for long at room temperature or at 37° C and are quickly killed by heat and most antiseptics; but in infected louse faeces *R. prowazeki* remains viable for months if the temperature and humidity are kept low. *R. (Coxiella) burneti*, the cause of Q fever, is unusually resistant to heat,

to drying, and to chemical disinfectants. If subjected to quick freezing in a sealed ampoule and stored in dry ice ($-76°$ C) the organisms remain viable for several years, provided that they are rapidly thawed from the deeply frozen state: slow thawing after a deep freeze kills them.

*R. prowazeki* is the organism responsible for epidemic louse-borne typhus; it is the only one of these organisms which can maintain itself in man and his own ectoparasites; it requires neither non-human ectoparasites nor other mammals for its survival. *R. mooseri*, which causes murine typhus, is a closely allied species, morphologically and antigenically similar to *R. prowazeki*; it shows certain biological differences from it, in that it is normally a parasite of rats and mice and is conveyed by the rat louse *Polyplax spinulosus* and the rat flea *Xenopsylla cheopis*; it gains entry only incidentally and accidentally into man. It is not normally transmissible by the human louse or the human flea although both have been infected with it artificially. *R. orientalis* (or *R. tsutsugamushi*), of which there are several antigenic types, is the organism responsible for scrub, or mite-borne typhus; in nature it is a parasite of wild rodents, being conveyed from one to another by mites of the genus *Trombicula*. Probably several species of these mites serve as vectors; the two held to be chiefly responsible for human infection are *T. akamushi* and *T. deliensis*. The infection is maintained from one generation of mites to the next by trans-ovarial passage; as each mite takes only a single meal on warm-blooded animals during its lifetime, a female mite can infect another mammalian host only through its offspring.

The rickettsias of the tick-borne typhus group are of three species, *R. rickettsi*, *R. conori*, and *R. australis*. *R. rickettsi* normally infects small mammals and occurs in man only as an accidental infection. The species includes a number of varieties all conveyed by ticks. Man is attacked by ticks in search of a blood meal and is infected by the bite. These organisms are not transmissible by lice, by fleas, or by mites. The diseases in man caused by these organisms have been called the 'spotted fever' or tick-borne group of typhuses. The ticks responsible for their spread vary with the locality and the disease shows clinical variations from one region to another. Rocky Mountain spotted fever, of which there are several varieties, is commonly conveyed by the wood tick *Dermacentor andersoni*.

*R. conori*, which causes Fièvre boutonneuse, is morphologically indistinguishable from *R. rickettsi*. It has long been known to be transmissible by the common dog tick *Rhipicephalus sanguineus*, which is of world-wide distribution. The dog appears to be the usual reservoir of the infection, but *R. conori* var. *pijperi*, the cause of an endemic tick typhus in South Africa and East Africa, has been recovered from local wild rodents and their ticks.

*R. australis* occurs in bandicoots and rodents in Queensland, Australia, where it causes sporadic cases of North Queensland tick typhus.

*R. (Coxiella) burneti* which causes Q fever is an enzootic of wild and domestic animals (including cattle) naturally transmitted by ticks. It is usually conveyed to man by the inhalation of infected dust or by drinking infected milk.

Certain strains of *Bacillus proteus* agglutinate in the presence of serum from patients suffering from rickettsial infections. The reaction results from inter-action of the somatic (O) antigen of the bacilli with agglutinins in the serum. In some forms of typhus the agglutinins are relatively specific, so that the species of infecting *Rickettsia* may be identified by testing the serum of the patient against syspensions of the proteus bacilli. For this purpose suspensions of *B. proteus* OX 19, OX 2, and OXK are added separately to serially diluted samples of serum from the patient, in the so-called Weil–Felix test.

In the following table are summarized the results obtained in Weil–Felix tests using the three standard strains of *B. proteus*, i.e., OX 19, OX 2, and OXK and sera from cases of the various forms of typhus. From this table it will be seen that mite-borne is the only form of typhus in which the test is specific. Nevertheless, in the great majority of cases of louse-borne and flea-borne typhus OX 19 is agglutinated to a high titre; and in the majority of cases of tick-borne typhus OX 19 and OX 2 are agglutinated, though at a low titre. The test is therefore of considerable help in the diagnosis and differentia-tion of rickettsial infections. After the tenth day of the disease agglutinins are present in significant titre in the serum; the titres thereafter continue to rise for 7–10 days then gradually diminish over a period of months. It is the rising titre which is of particular help in diagnosis, and therefore the test should be repeated at intervals during the development of the disease.

| Disease | OX 19 | OX 2 | OXK |
|---------|-------|------|-----|
| Louse-borne<br>Flea-borne | + + + to − | + + to − | − |
| Tick-borne | − to + + | − to + + | + to − |
| Mite-borne | − | − | + + + |
| Q Fever | − | − | − |

Means of identifying with some precision the strains and types of rickettsial infections include the agglutination by sera of suspensions of rickettsias and cross-absorption tests; a complement fixation test, using as antigen extracts or suspensions of rickettsias; the passive protection of animals by hyperimmune sera; and a number of special neutralization and antitoxic tests performed on experimental animals after a strain of organisms has been recovered and maintained in culture. By these tests the antigenic relationship of differing and of closely allied types of rickettsias are gradually being determined, but a great deal of work has still to be done in this field.

### ANIMAL INOCULATION

Animal inoculation offers a means of differentiation of rickettsias. Blood taken from patients early in the febrile period, about the time of the appearance of the rash of louse-borne typhus, and inoculated intraperitoneally into a male guinea pig causes fever after about 10 days. This is due to infection with *R. prowazeki*. Blood from cases of murine typhus (*R. mooseri*) injected into guinea pigs causes fever and an inflammatory reaction in the tunica vaginalis of the testis, from which the organisms can be recovered (tunica or Neill-Mooser reaction). Blood containing *R. rickettsi* on injection into guinea-pigs causes no general reaction but a local reaction involving the testes and the scrotum (scrotal reaction). Blood from cases of mite-borne typhus (*R. orientalis*) inoculated intraperitoneally into guinea-pigs causes no fever or reaction but mice so inoculated die in a few days; at autopsy there is a white peritoneal exudate with numerous *R. orientalis* in the peritoneal cells (peritoneal reaction).

## EPIDEMIC LOUSE-BORNE TYPHUS

### DEFINITION

Typhus exanthematicus is due to infection with *R. prowazeki*. The organism is conveyed from man to man by the human louse *Pediculus humanus*. The course of the disease is characterized by a sudden onset, sustained fever, severe toxaemia, a generalized rash which appears about the fifth day, and marked nervous symptoms. Its duration is about 16 days and the mortality is high, especially in some epidemics.

### GEOGRAPHICAL DISTRIBUTION

Wherever the climatic conditions and state of hygiene favour infestation with the human louse epidemic typhus may appear. Such conditions mostly prevail in the colder parts of the globe, but they are by no means limited to these regions. Outbreaks have occurred recently in Ethiopia and the Sudan.

### AETIOLOGY

Throughout the febrile stage of the disease *R. prowazeki* is present in the blood of a patient suffering from it. The louse *P. humanus* feeds exclusively on man. Lice feeding on a patient suffering from epidemic typhus become infected with the causative organism and after 8–10 days excrete it in their faeces. *R. prowazeki* in the intestine of the louse enters and multiplies very freely in the cytoplasm of the epithelial cells of its mid gut. The infected cells become swollen and rupture, liberating the organisms into the faeces, in which they escape to the exterior in large numbers. Inunction of the infected faeces through abrasions of the skin or mucous surfaces, or their inhalation, are the means by which they enter a fresh host.

Lice tend to leave the body of persons suffering from high fever and they also leave the cooling or cold skin of the dying or dead. This tendency to migrate favours the dissemination of the disease. Inhalation of the dried faeces of infected lice in the dust from linen and clothing of the sick or dead can result in transmission of the disease in the absence of migration of the infected lice. On occasion it has been suspected that the organism may remain viable and infective in clothing kept under suitable conditions for many years.

The only known reservoir of the infection is man.

*R. prowazeki* can be introduced by inoculation or by insufflation of the lungs into laboratory animals including monkeys, guinea pigs, rats, and other rodents. In them it usually causes a febrile illness and during this illness the organism can be recovered from them.

Typhus exanthematicus is one of the greatest epidemic diseases of history. It has been associated with nearly every great war and famine since the fifteenth century. Few diseases can spread through a community or ravage a continent with greater rapidity than epidemic typhus. It is a disease of poverty, filth, human distress, and overcrowding. In the tropics, where clothing is scanty or absent, louse infestation is unusual. In the very cold climates where clothing is worn for long periods without removal, and people huddle together to keep warm, louse infestation is very prevalent.

In children epidemic typhus can be a relatively mild disease; it increases in severity with rising age, until at and over 40 years of age the mortality from it is extremely high. One attack of typhus exanthematicus affords a substantial life-long immunity to reinfection, although this is not invariably absolute. It is believed that the infection usually clears completely but occasionally it may persist at low levels for prolonged periods producing a state of 'premunization'. It has been claimed on epidemiological and other grounds that *Brill's disease* is a recrudescence, with mild symptoms, of the infection some years after clinical recovery from an attack of classical louse-born typhus.

PATHOLOGY

*R. prowazeki* parasitizes the endothelial cells lining the blood vessels of the skin, the central nervous system, the skeletal muscles, and myocardium and, to a lesser extent, those of the kidney, testis, and other organs. The affected cells become swollen and there is a vigorous proliferation of the vascular endothelium in which mitotic figures can be seen. Around the affected vessels circumscribed groups of proliferating cells appear. These are the typhus 'nodules' of Fraenkel; they are composed of mononuclear phagocytic cells probably of endothelial origin. A diffuse perivascular infiltration of mononuclear cells, lymphoid and plasma cells, mast cells, and some polymorphonuclear cells is also evident in the skin. The vascular damage leads to thrombosis, and to haemorrhage from the vessels; both these are constant features of the pathology of typhus exanthematicus. They are also invariable in the central nervous system. Commonly there are bronchopneumonia and myocardial lesions similar to those described above. The spleen is usually enlarged. At times there are gangrenous patches of skin and deep sloughs in the subcutaneous tissues and even muscles. In some epidemics gangrene of the extremities is common.

### CLINICAL PICTURE

The incubation period can range from 5 to 23 days; usually it is between 8 and 14 days.

The onset is abrupt, with the usual manifestations of a very severe febrile toxaemia. It is initiated by rigors, headache, and muscular pains and a fever which mounts steadily, with occasional remissions, to 39.4° C and then remains continuous, with relatively small fluctuations. The headache and pains in the back and limbs become more severe. The face is flushed and congested; the conjunctivae are suffused; the tongue is furred and tremulous; and the mouth becomes dry and sores form on the lips. There is nasal catarrh, with reddening of the nasopharynx and of the fauces, pharynx, and tonsils. Epistaxis is common. The respiration rate is increased, and there are signs of bronchitis. There is abdominal discomfort, with constipation and not diarrhoea. The spleen is palpable by the third day. From the patient may issue a distinctive mouse-like odour. Deafness is a common symptom. After the third or fourth day there is marked torpor, often associated with delirium; the condition now resembles that seen in severe typhoid in the third week.

The rash appears about the fifth day of the disease; it shows first on the shoulders and axillae and soon spreads to the abdomen, chest, back, and extremities; it rarely occurs on the face or on the palms and soles. The rash consists of rose spots; these are not unlike those of typhoid, but they are much more numerous and widespread. They fade on pressure for the first day or so; but later they become dull red in colour and no longer fade on pressure. By about the tenth day of the disease they are brownish red and beginning to disappear. In addition, there is a blotchy eruption, or 'subcuticular mottling'; this also first appears on the shoulders and axillae, and then extends to the chest, abdomen, back, and extremities. In very severe cases there may be purpuric patches which sometimes attain a large size. Haematemesis, melaena, and haematuria all may be evident in the gravest cases.

Nervous symptoms are pronounced; they take the form of dreams of a frightful nature, of tremors and twitching of the muscles (subsultus tendinum), of tremors of the tongue, and of stupor and delirium; they develop during the first week of the disease and are of diagnostic significance. In severe cases coma may supervene on the sixth or seventh day, or maniacal symptoms may develop. The knee jerks may disappear about the fifth day. Incontinence of urine and of faeces may occur on the sixth or seventh day and persist into convalescence. Cerebral involvement is more marked in typhus than in any comparable febrile disease; the mental power often is not fully restored for 6 months or more after an attack of even moderate severity. In some cases head retraction, delirium, and meningeal symptoms may simulate cerebrospinal fever; lumbar puncture is then advisable to differentiate between the two.

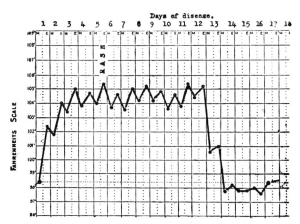

FIG. 61. Temperature chart of case of louse-borne typhus.

[From E. Noble Chamberlain, *A Textbook of Medicine*, John Wright & Sons Ltd., Bristol, 1951]

The respiratory system is always involved to a greater or less extent. Bronchitis is often followed by bronchopneumonia, and sometimes by pleurisy or empyema. The condition may terminate by abscess or gangrene of the lung.

In favourable cases the temperature begins to fall by rapid lysis on the twelfth or thirteenth day; it reaches normal between the fourteenth and sixteenth days, when the attack ends.

In fatal cases death usually occurs during the second week and most frequently between the tenth and twelfth days. Acute renal failure with anuria and uraemia is a common cause of death. A rising blood urea nitrogen is of bad prognostic significance.

Signs of acute myocardial involvement are common. Gangrene of areas of skin frequently occurs. In some epidemics symmetrical gangrene of the extremities may occur in a high proportion of cases. Suppurative parotitis is a common complication.

### DIAGNOSIS

The Weil–Felix test is usually positive.

A titre of 1 in 25 with OX 19 at the end of the first week is suggestive and a titre of 1 in 100 by the second week is highly significant. A rise in titre can be expected over the period of the illness. Agglutinins disappear about 6 months after recovery.

The serum of the patient may be set up in serial dilutions against suspensions of specific rickettsiae grown in tissue culture. The results are more specific than those recorded in the Weil–Felix test. The reaction is positive by the end of the second week of the illness.

Complement fixation tests may also be made, using antigens prepared from specific organisms or tissues of infected animals. These tests are less reliable than the agglutination tests for diagnosis of acute louse-borne typhus. They are seldom positive before the end of the third week.

For diagnosis by animal inoculation, see above (p. 493).

### TREATMENT

The patient should be washed thoroughly on admission and his clothes disinfested by heat. The patient should be dusted with 10 per cent DDT powder (see p. 346).

Nursing is of great importance. Attention must be paid to rehydration when necessary and an input:output fluid record must be kept. Each specimen of urine passed should be examined. The onset of serious oliguria or anuria can be detected in this way.

*Chemotherapy.* Nearly all types of human typhus have been shown to respond most satisfactorily to chloramphenicol treatment by mouth. The tetracyclines have proved equally effective.

Chloramphenicol is given by the mouth. The initial dose is 2–3 g; this is followed by 500 mg 6-hourly for 24 hours; 250 mg 6-hourly is then given until the temperature has been normal for 2 days. Unless the case is moribund, there is rapid clinical improvement; the fever vanishes, usually within 2 days; the patient soon becomes convalescent and recovers. The immediate side-effects of chloramphenicol treatment are negligible but fatal aplastic anaemia has on occasions followed its use.

The tetracyclines are given in similar dosage. The side-effects are minimal.

Steroid treatment during the first day or two of a very severe attack of typhus may ease the patient until the specific treatment takes effect.

Prednisone 40 mg is given immediately, then 20 mg 6-hourly for two doses.

Renal failure, dehydration, and shock are treated by standard methods (see p. 281).

All patients and contacts must be completely freed of lice. Clothing and bedding should be immersed in a solution of disinfectant before being sterilized. Disinfestation of the surrounding population as a whole, by the use of DDT and other insecticides, should be undertaken promptly and vigorously at the outset of a suspected epidemic. By these means epidemic typhus has on several occasions been stamped out before it properly gained a foothold and flared up on a grand scale.

Personal prophylaxis for those at risk, including travellers going into the rare endemic areas, requires precautions against louse infestation, for example by employing insect repellents such as dimethylphthalate, the use of DDT, and the wearing of protective clothing.

*Vaccination*

Vaccines prepared from cultures of *R. prowazeki* and *R. mooseri*, and from the hyperinfected tissues of animals, such as the lungs after infection by insufflation, have been used successfully. The best vaccine is Cox's, made from killed cultures of strains of the two organisms grown on the yolk-sacs of developing chick embryos. The vaccine is given subcutaneously in doses of 1 ml on two or three occasions at 10-day intervals; reinforcing doses should be given at 6-monthly intervals during the period of risk of infection. A satisfactory, though not absolute, protection is afforded against louse-borne and flea-borne typhus by this vaccine immunization. If an attack of either develops in spite of the vaccination, its severity is much modified as a result of it. The vaccine affords no protection against mite-borne or tick-borne rickettsia infections.

An avirulent living culture of a strain of *R. prowazeki* (Strain E) is under trial as a vaccine. It affords a more efficient and lasting protection against challenge with virulent strains of organisms than do vaccines of the Cox type (up to 5 years). This reduces the local incidence of the disease and reduces the mortality of an infection to practically zero. It is given as two subcutaneous doses of 1 ml, separated by 10–14 days, followed by a booster dose as required.

# FLEA-BORNE (MURINE) TYPHUS

### DEFINITION

Murine typhus is due to infection with *R. mooseri*. The organism normally infects rats, from one to another of which it is conveyed by rodent lice and fleas. The rat flea *Xenopsylla cheopis* may infest man and convey the infection to him in its excreta. The resultant disease is clinically indistinguishable from typhus exanthematicus; but it is much milder and its mortality is low.

### GEOGRAPHICAL DISTRIBUTION

Flea-borne (endemic) typhus is world-wide in distribution. Various names were applied to it before its aetiology locally was appreciated. These include tarbardillo in Mexico, Toulon ship fever, urban tropical typhus or shop typhus in Malaysia, and Manchurian typhus, among others. Wherever the rat lives in close association with man, irrespective of climate, flea-borne typhus may occur.

### AETIOLOGY

Strains of *Rickettsia mooseri* have been recovered from wild rats in many parts of the world. In them the infection is enzootic and symptomless. It is conveyed from one animal to another by the rat louse *Polyplax spinulosus*, and by the rat flea *X. cheopis*. In these ectoparasites the infection is an intestinal one, and the faeces contain the organism. The rat flea *X. cheopis* in default of its normal host may temporarily infest man and take a blood meal from him. Infection of man is the result of entry of the *Rickettsia* excreted in the faeces of an infected flea through abrasions of the skin; alternatively man may be infected by inhalation of the organism in dust containing infective rat flea or louse faeces. *R. mooseri* is also passed in the urine of infected rats; it has been suggested that Toulon ship fever is acquired by contamination of food with infected rat urine, as well as by the agency of the rat flea.

Flea-borne typhus thus occurs as sporadic infection of man. As the human ectoparasites, *Pediculus humanus* and *Pulex irritans*, are at best inefficient vectors of *R. mooseri*, flea-borne typhus does not spread from man to man and therefore does not become epidemic. As already stated, it has been postulated that occasionally *R. mooseri* becomes adapted to effective transmission by the human louse and that this may be the genesis of an epidemic of louse-borne typhus.

*R. mooseri* is very closely related to *R. prowazeki*; it is similar in size, shape, staining properties, and its resistance to chemical and physical agents. Its antigenic structure is also very similar to that of *R. prowazeki*, though some minor differences have been demonstrated by detailed antigenic and serological studies. In human cases of flea-borne typhus the Weil–Felix reaction is identical with that in louse-borne typhus; the histopathological lesions are identical; and an attack of one of these diseases immunizes against an attack of the other.

On intraperitoneal inoculation of *R. mooseri* into male guinea-pigs the tunica or Neill–Mooser reaction results and the animals develop a more pronounced febrile reaction than after injection of blood containing *R. prowazeki*. The human louse, *Pediculus humanus*, can be infected with *R. mooseri* by intra-rectal injection but not by experimental feeding.

## PATHOLOGY

There is no essential difference in the histopathology of *R. mooseri* infections from that seen in *R. prowazeki* infections.

## CLINICAL PICTURE

The clinical picture is that of epidemic louse-borne typhus, except for the mildness of the disease, the infrequency of severe complications, and the correspondingly low mortality.

## DIAGNOSIS

See under louse-borne typhus.

## TREATMENT

The specific treatment is that of the epidemic louse-borne typhus disease. Specific personal prophylaxis lies in the protection afforded by Cox's vaccine. This is sometimes advised for travellers, but is not usually necessary.

# MITE-BORNE TYPHUS

## DEFINITION

Mite-borne or scrub typhus is due to infection with *R. orientalis* (or *R. tsutsugamushi*). The organism normally infects small bush-dwelling rodents and other mammals, and is conveyed from one to another by trombiculid mites in which it is transmitted hereditarily. The larval mites may attack man and convey the infection to him by their bites. In general the resultant disease clinically resembles epidemic louse-borne typhus but in some details differs from it. The mortality may be high.

## GEOGRAPHICAL DISTRIBUTION

Scrub fever, tsutsugamushi or Japanese river fever, Sumatran mite-fever, Malayan rural typhus, and other names have been applied to diseases all now recognized as mite-borne typhus. The disease occurs in jungle and bush country in South-east Asia, Australasia including Queensland (Australia), Papua New Guinea and New Britain, and the Western Pacific. It is endemic in Japan, south China, Taiwan, Laos, Thailand, Malaysia, Indonesia, the Philippines, and Vietnam. It occurs also in many parts of India, Burma, and Sri Lanka.

## AETIOLOGY

Strains of the causative organism, *R. orientalis*, have been recovered from many rodents and small mammals and from several species of trombiculid mites in the enzootic and endemic areas. The areas in which man acquires the disease are usually very sharply demarcated regions in bush country, where there is sufficient ground moisture for the mites to flourish in association with a suitable population of small mammals. Such conditions are found in uncultivated areas of vegetation along river courses. The mites principally responsible for conveying the disease from one mammalian host to another are *Trombicula akamushi* and *T. deliensis*. These mites take a single meal on mammals during their lives; this meal of blood, lymph, or tissue juice is engorged during the six-legged larval stage. A septicaemic infection of the mite with *R. orientalis* follows. The female transmits the infection transovarially to its offspring, which infect further mammalian hosts by biting. The larval mites show a catholic taste in search of this meal, and will attack man as well as other mammals of all sizes. Man is a rare and sporadic host of the infection unless engaged in large numbers, such as during war or agricultural clearing operations, in the jungle foci of infection. In the Second World War some thousands of troops engaged in jungle warfare were infected with *R. orientalis* and suffered from scrub fever. The infection does not spread from man to man directly or through the agency of his normal ectoparasites, the human louse and the human flea. Air-borne infections with *R. orientalis* may occur among laboratory workers.

*R. orientalis* is rather less pleomorphic than the other species of rickettsias which infect man. It lives within the cytoplasm of endothelial cells, appearing as bipolar-staining bodies. It can be cultured in living tissues and, with some difficulty, on the yolk-sac of the developing chick embryo. It can be readily established in laboratory animals; in mice it causes a fatal infection with fever and ascites (peritoneal reaction) when injected intraperitoneally; in rats it produces a symptomless infection unless introduced intravenously in large dosage, when it causes death.

Antigenically *R. orientalis* is distinct from *R. prowazeki* and *R. mooseri*, and from the tick-borne species of rickettsiae. In the Weil–Felix test Proteus OXK only is agglutinated. Cross-immunity tests, complement fixation tests, neutralization tests, and toxin–antitoxin techniques show not only its clear differentiation from other species of *Rickettsia*, but the existence of antigenically different strains. This antigenic variation between strains of *R. orientalis* contrasts with the antigenic homogenicity of strains of *R. prowazeki*.

## PATHOLOGY

The histopathology of scrub fever is broadly similar to that of epidemic louse-borne typhus. The lesions of the small vessels as a rule are less pronounced than in epidemic typhus. A specific rickettsial toxin is formed by *R. orientalis*. The action of this toxin on the peripheral capillaries, together with the characteristic capillary and vascular pathology, is thought to be responsible for the peripheral circulatory collapse which contributes to death in a high proportion of fatal cases.

## CLINICAL PICTURE

The incubation period is 6–18 days. The onset resembles that of epidemic typhus but there is a primary lesion or eschar at the site of the infective bite. This appears before symptoms develop. This eschar is a small necrotic ulcer covered with a blackened scab and is commonly situated on the trunk. The lymph glands draining it may be enlarged; not uncommonly there is general lymphatic glandular enlargement. The presence of this lesion is of clinical diagnostic importance and it should always be carefully sought. It is by no means invariably found and is more commonly seen in some endemic areas than others. It persists for about 3 weeks, that is, until the disease has run its course.

The rash appears between the fifth and eighth days of the disease as a macular eruption on the sides of the chest and the abdomen; it soon spreads to the extremities. It persists for some days before fading; it may then fade rapidly over a few hours.

The fever lasts about 2 weeks; the temperature then falls to normal by slow lysis over several days. The symptoms and signs are those usual in epidemic typhus. Death in fatal cases takes place about the end of the second week; commonly it is attributable to myocardial involvement, secondary pneumonia, encephalitis, or circulatory failure. The mortality ranges from 2 to over 60 per cent.

## DIAGNOSIS

The clinical picture, the circumstances and locality, and the presence of a typical eschar, are highly suggestive of the condition. The Weil–Felix reaction is of much value; agglutinins for Proteus OXK, but not for Proteus OX 19 or OX 2, begin to appear in the patient's serum about the tenth day of the disease. They rise in titre to a maximum by the end of the third week and thereafter decline to a low level by the sixth week, when they may disappear. Repeated tests are advisable to demonstrate a rising titre. The maximum figure reached may not exceed 1 : 160 but a steady rise to this figure is highly suggestive of the diagnosis. Other forms of typhus do not give a positive Weil–Felix reaction with Proteus OXK. Leptospirosis and louse-borne relapsing fever may occasionally do so.

Diagnosis can be made by agglutination of specific rickettsial suspensions or by complement fixation.

Blood or crushed tissue from an infective active case, or suspensions of crushed larval mites taken from rodent hosts in endemic areas, will infect many laboratory animals. The material is injected intraperitoneally. In white mice a fatal infection results in a characteristic peritoneal inflammatory reaction.

### TREATMENT

As for typhus exanthematicus with chloramphenicol or tetracyclines. Patients with evidence of myocarditis, including inversion of the T wave in the ECG, should be given long convalescence and rest. Digitalization may be needed.

### PROPHYLAXIS

Vaccines have been made from *R. orientalis,* but none so far produced has afforded adequate protection of man against scrub typhus.

Communal prophylaxis takes the form of avoidance or destruction of those clearly defined areas of vegetation where the disease is acquired.

Personal prophylaxis, when the areas cannot be avoided, lies in active movement through them and the wearing of protective apparel drenched with insect repellents such as dimethylphthalate.

Chloramphenicol in oral dosage of 3 g once weekly will not prevent infection but will abort the clinical attack.

## TICK-BORNE TYPHUS

### DEFINITION

The tick-borne typhuses are due to infection with *Rickettsia rickettsi, R. conori* or *R. australis.* These organisms are normally enzootic in a wide variety of animals. They are conveyed from one animal to another by a number of ticks of different genera and many species. Man is infected sporadically by ticks seeking a blood meal on him. The course of the resultant diseases in general resembles that of epidemic louse-borne typhus, but differs from it in details. The mortality varies with the local variations in the disease; in some it is high.

### GEOGRAPHICAL DISTRIBUTION

Various forms of tick-borne typhus have been identified in each of the continents of the world. These include the Rocky Mountain spotted fevers of North America, the spotted fevers of South America, and African and the

Indian tick-bite fevers, North Queensland tick-typhus, and Fièvre boutonneuse of the Mediterranean regions.

### AETIOLOGY

*R. rickettsi*, the causative organism of the various types of Rocky Mountain
spotted fever and the spotted fevers of South America, in nature infects a very
varied assortment of small wild mammals in which it usually causes a symptomless infection. A large number of ticks of various genera and species have
been found to serve as efficient vectors of the organism. In these when taken
up in a blood meal it causes a generalized infection; the ticks after a period can
infect by their bites; and the female ticks transmit their infections to their
offspring. The organisms, like all the rickettsias, are very small; they frequently are seen in lanceolate pairs surrounded by a clear zone or halo, as
though encapsulated, and so look like pneumococci. Like other rickettsias
they can be grown on living tissue cultures and on the chorio-allantois and
yolk-sac of the developing chick embryo. An outstanding feature of these
tick-borne species is their predilection for the nuclei of the cells they parasitize;
they are not confined to the cytoplasm, as are the other species of *Rickettsia*.
This intranuclear invasion is seen not only in cells in artificial cultures but also
in the tissues of animals infected with the organisms.

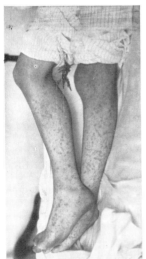 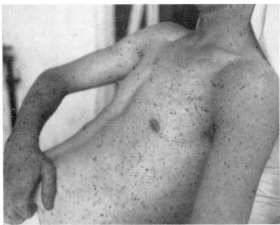

FIG. 62. (a and b). The rash of tick-borne typhus.
[Courtesy of Col. B.Blewitt, R.A.M.C.]

The tick typhus due to *R. rickettsi* in the Americas affects chiefly rural populations, especially those whose outdoor work brings them into contact with wild life and with tick-infested stock or pastures. Hunters, trappers, campers, and others often acquire it when following their pursuits; but women and children largely confined to the precincts of a house may be infected by ticks on dogs and other household animal pets including rabbits.

*R. rickettsi* var. *pijperi* is the name given to a similar organism which causes 'tick-bite fever' in Africa south of the Sahara, in West Africa, Sudan, Somalia, and Ethiopia. This is a mild form of sporadic typhus with a low mortality. The animal reservoirs are wild rodents; the domestic dog may also become infected and act as a reservoir. Clinically the disease resembles Fièvre boutonneuse which is found in the Mediterranean littoral. There are antigenic differences between *R. rickettsi* var. *pijperi* and *R. conori* and the relationship of the former to the *R. rickettsi* of the Americas appears to be a close one.

Tick typhus is also found in Iran, Siberia, and north-east India.

### PATHOLOGY

In tissue culture and in the tissues of infected animals *R. rickettsi* can be found sparsely in the cytoplasm of the infected cells and in great numbers in their nuclei. There may be solid masses of the organisms which often entirely fill and greatly distend the nuclei.

The histopathological lesions produced by *R. rickettsi* are similar to those of typhus exanthematicus. There is endothelial proliferation of capillaries, arterioles, and venules but Fraenkel's typhus nodules are less pronounced. In addition, thrombo-necrotic lesions are prominent and are characteristic of these infections. These lesions are due to the presence of fibrinous thrombi in arterioles and venules, which may be partially or wholly occluded by them. In late lesions the vessel wall is infiltrated with endothelial cells and polymorphonuclear leucocytes, and numerous organisms can be seen in the smooth muscle cells as well as in the endothelial cells of the vessel wall. The pathology in this disease is a destructive panangeitis of peripheral vessels in contrast to the purely proliferative endangeitis of typhus exanthematicus.

At autopsy extensive haemorrhages, and gangrenous sloughing of the scrotum, prepuce, vulva, fingers, toes, or lobes of the ears, are common in the severer forms of the tick-borne typhuses.

### CLINICAL PICTURE

The severity of attacks of the tick-borne typhuses ranges from mild attacks in ambulatory patients to fulminating attacks with early death. Most cases fall between these extremes and their general progress much resembles that of classical louse-borne typhus. The main differentiating features are the duration of the fever, the time of appearance of the eruption, and its distribution. American tick typhus is a serious disease; high mortality rates have been recorded in some outbreaks.

The incubation period ranges from 2 days to 2 weeks, but commonly is about 1 week. The onset is similar to that of the louse-borne disease. The marked remittent fever steadily mounts into the second week of the diseases; it continues until about the end of the third week when, as in the louse-borne disease, it declines by rapid lysis.

A rash which resembles the mottling of early measles appears on the third or fourth day. This fades and is succeeded by a rose-spot eruption which appears first on the wrists and ankles and then extends rapidly over most of the body including the palms and soles, the scalp, and sometimes the eyelids and mucosae of the mouth and throat. The abdomen and face are the areas last and least affected. The spots at first are less pronounced during the morning periods of remission of the fever, but they become progressively more prominent until they are petechial. In severe cases they become a purplish red and confluent and then they often become necrotic.

Sloughing and necrotic lesions of the skin, of the genitalia, and of the extremities are common in the severer forms of Rocky Mountain spotted fever.

Fièvre boutonneuse, the result of infection with *R. conori*, is characterized by the presence of a primary sore (tâche noire) at the site of the infecting tick bite. The rose-spot eruption in this disease extends to the palms, the soles, and the face. This form of tick typhus is comparatively mild, and the mortality from it is low. The tick involved is usually from the dog.

### DIAGNOSIS

This is apparent on the history and clinical findings in the known areas of endemicity of these diseases. In regions where other forms of typhus also occur their differentiation on clinical examination is difficult. The Weil–Felix test may be of help in distinguishing them, but it is not specific and may be misleading. The complement fixation test is of greater value in identifying the spotted fevers. Recovery of a strain of the organism by guinea-pig and other animal inoculation and serological studies, where these can be performed, are of specific value in diagnosis and identification.

### TREATMENT

Chloramphenicol or tetracyclines, used as in other forms of typhus, act dramatically and specifically. Prednisone, given as for epidemic typhus, will modify severe effects in desperately ill patients. Shock and dehydration are treated by the usual methods (see p. 60).

In the regions of endemicity the destruction of ticks by burning infested vegetation, dipping stock, and destroying the wild animal hosts of the tick lessens the risk of infection. The early removal of ticks from the body and cauterization of the site of the bite is of much value in forestalling infection, as ticks do not infect usually until attached for some hours. Vaccines prepared from the tissues of infected ticks have been in use for some years. The injection of these affords a substantial protection against infection with *R. rickettsi*. Vaccines prepared from growth of the organism on the yolk-sac tissues of developing chick embryos are now available (Cox's method) and are of equal value to those made from ticks for personal prophylaxis. The vaccines are given subcutaneously or intramuscularly in doses of 1.0 ml on three occasions at about weekly intervals. The inoculations should be repeated annually in the spring, before the time of greatest activity of ticks, as the protection they confer does not last more than a year.

## Q FEVER

### DEFINITION

An acute febrile illness caused by *Coxiella* (*Rickettsia*) *burneti*, characterized by sudden onset, general signs, and commonly interstitial pneumonitis.

There is no rash and agglutinins to *Proteus* do not develop.

### GEOGRAPHICAL DISTRIBUTION

The disease was first described in Australia. It occurs in many parts of the world, including the U.K., Spain, Italy, Greece, the Middle East, north, tropical, and southern Africa, and the U.S.A.

### AETIOLOGY

The organism is small and pleomorphic. It is present in the blood in the febrile stages of the illness and usually in the sputum. It may be present in the urine and in tissues from infected animals, especially in the spleen.

The disease is an enzootic in many wild and domestic animals, transmitted by certain ticks in which the infection can be continued transovarially. It is commonly transmitted to cattle. The organism is discharged in the tick faeces. It is resistant to desiccation and is transmitted to man by inhalation of infected dust or milk, very occasionally directly by the ticks. Infection also occurs in those handling infected tissues, secretions, etc. It is easily spread to man in the laboratory and can be experimentally transmitted by intranasal instillation of infected material.

## PATHOLOGY

There are few reports of autopsies in man. Patchy consolidation of the bases of the lungs has been the commonest finding, with infiltration and thickening of the alveolar walls and perivascular spaces by macrophages and lymphocytes. There is sometimes necrosis of the alveolar septa. In other organs including the testes, kidneys, the brain, and spleen, foci of macrophages and round cells have been observed. The organism can be found in smears of these tissues, especially the lungs. Vegetative endocarditis has been found in a few cases.

## CLINICAL PICTURE

The incubation period is 2–3 weeks. Onset is usually sudden. The severity varies greatly, ranging from mild fever lasting a day or two, to the classical picture of rapidly developing, moderate remittent, or swinging fever (39.0–40.0° C). The fever persists for a few days up to 3 weeks. General symptoms include severe headache and muscular pains. Shivering, as a result of subjective feelings of cold, is common; rigor is rare. Nocturnal sweating may be severe. Insomnia, anorexia, and nausea are usual. A slight dry cough develops about the fourth day, with pain in the chest, often localized to the bases, or only one base. Sputum is mucoid or mucopurulent and may be blood-streaked. In severe cases there may be dyspnoea and cyanosis. Physical pulmonary signs at this stage are localized reduction of intake of air, occasional scattered rhonchi and crepitations, usually over one or both bases. The signs vary from day to day but usually show as 'atypical' pneumonic patches involving small areas, usually in the bases. These may persist into convalescence.

Rarely, the liver may enlarge and mild jaundice and other signs of disturbed hepatic dysfunction occur. Occasionally, valvular lesions in the heart may be detected.

Convalescence is slow. In a small percentage of cases, there may be relapses, occurring after some months, with fever and pulmonary signs.

Complications are uncommon. They include meningo-encephalitis and orchitis. A fatal issue is rare.

## DIAGNOSIS

Clinical diagnosis is helped by knowing the patient's occupation, especially association with live-stock.

The organism can be recovered in the febrile stages by injection of blood or urine intraperitoneally into guinea pigs in which splenic enlargement occurs; the organism can be recovered from the spleen.

Agglutinins appear in the blood by the end of the second week and increase over the next 2 weeks. They are identified by using killed suspensions of C.

*burneti.* A titre of 1:16 is considered suspicious. Complement-fixing bodies may be present in the first week and are in high titre by the third or fourth week. A titre of 1 : 20 is significant. This may rise much higher.

The Weil–Felix reaction is *negative*.

### TREATMENT

Tetracyclines, or chloramphenicol, in the usual doses are highly effective. The former are most widely used.

Prophylaxis of individuals likely to be exposed may be achieved by immunization with a vaccine made from *C. burneti* grown on chick yolk-sac then formalized. Animals may be equally successfully vaccinated. Milk from infected herds must be pasteurized.

Avoidance of transmission from patient to patient is easy; it needs only sterilization of sputum and excreta. Isolation is not necessary but vaccination may be desirable.

# 34

# VIRUS FEVERS, INCLUDING YELLOW FEVER

INTRODUCTION

Febrile illnesses of short duration due to virus infections are common throughout the tropics. In some instances the clinical picture is reasonably identifiable and the causative agent known, in others there is clinically little more than fever and the agent has not been identified. Accounts are given below of some of the better-known infections. It should be remembered that many other virus infections may occur in both temperate and tropical regions. Thus, influenza may appear anywhere, sometimes in pandemic form. Hepatitis is common and may occur in epidemics. Poliomyelitis is very common in many tropical emergent countries and is a risk to the unvaccinated adult, especially caucasians living in close contact with the indigenous population, a high proportion of whom possess immunity from early childhood. Other entroviruses of world-wide distribution are also common in the developing world, where hygienic conditions are usually bad, including Coxsackie and Echo viruses, both of which cause febrile illnesses and aseptic meningitis. In investigating the cause of any acute febrile illness these more cosmopolitan infections must always be considered, since abortive attacks may present without signs other than fever.

Many of the viral agents producing short-term fevers and other signs are transmitted to man by arthropod vectors and are known as *Arboviruses*. The majority are zoonoses; they occur as diseases of mammals or birds which may be transmitted only accidentally to man via an arthropod vector, either sporadically or in epidemics. A few arboviruses, for example yellow fever and dengue, once established in the human, can be transmitted from man to man via the appropriate arthropod vector. Three main groups of arboviruses have been serologically defined, i.e. Groups A, B, and C. Many viruses still remain unclassified. About fifty arboviruses are known to produce clinical symptoms in man.

The diseases most important to man usually result from infections with Group B arboviruses, which include yellow fever, certain forms of encephalitis including Japanese B encephalitis, and the dengue fevers.

Group A viruses cause febrile illnesses and sometimes myelo-encephalitis in many parts of the world. An example of a Group A arbovirus is Chikungunya, which is mosquito transmitted (usually *Aedes* spp.) in East and West Africa, India, and South-east Asia. In Africa the disease is characterized by

510

short fever which may be biphasic, very severe joint pains, and a late developing itchy maculopapular rash. In Asia, the virus is one of the causes of haemorrhagic fever.

Group C viruses are widespread in tropical Central and South America. Nine are known to cause human disease, largely short-term fevers.

With a few exceptions, the clinical syndromes resulting from arbovirus infections are mild and of short duration. Their chief significance lies in the loss of labour they cause and in their frequent misdiagnosis as malaria (particularly important in assessment of antimalarial drugs used for suppression).

It is not possible to deal here with more than a few representative examples of the virus fevers. Yellow fever, dengue, sandfly fever, the haemorrhagic fevers, Japanese B encephalomyelitis, Lassa fever, Marburg and Ebola fevers are discussed.

## YELLOW FEVER

### DEFINITION

An acute infectious disease caused by a Group B arbovirus transmitted by certain genera of culicine mosquitoes. It is endemic in parts of tropical Africa and America. Severe cases exhibit fever, with relatively slow pulse, early and progressive albuminuria, vomiting, some jaundice, and varying degrees of hepatic, renal or vascular failure.

The disease has special provisions relating to it in the International Health Regulations (1969).

### DISTRIBUTION

The usual vector mosquito *Aedes aegypti* is much more widely distributed than the disease, which occurs irregularly over wide areas of Africa and South and Central America, and in a few Caribbean Islands, but has never been reported in Asia. The reason for its failure to reach Asia, where *A. aegypti* abounds and is a good vector, is not known.

Yellow fever has appeared in most of the northern areas of South American states during this century, including Venezuela, Bolivia, northern Peru, the interior of Colombia, and particularly Brazil. It is enzootic in monkeys in the forests of the Amazon valley, spreading thence to man from time to time. It is now rarely met in Central America, but a few cases have been reported in Trinidad, in which there has been one rural case in the last few months (1979). It has been reported in many parts of West and Central Africa, within an area ranging from Senegal to Zaïre. Immunity surveys have disclosed that the disease is much more widely spread than was formerly realized. Indications of fresh infection have been reported in the last decade in Kenya, Uganda,

Ethiopia, Somaliland, Eritrea (including the coast of the Red Sea), and Zambia. Tanzania appears to be free. In Uganda a permanent focus of infection exists in the Bwamba forest. The disease in Africa is also primarily an enzootic in monkeys.

Yellow fever is caused by a small virus measuring about 20 $\mu$m. The virus is present in the blood for 1–2 days before onset of clinical signs. It remains in the blood in the first 4 days, occasionally longer. It can be transmitted by blood inoculation to rhesus monkeys in which it causes a condition similar to the human disease. It can be successfully passaged intracerebrally in mice. After repeated passage it eventually becomes changed so that although it will continue to cause encephalitis in mice it will no longer reproduce the disease in monkeys or man. This altered neurotropic virus is the basis for the production of living attenuated vaccines, which can be grown in tissue culture (see later). It is killed rapidly at room temperature but survives for long periods if frozen and desiccated.

The African and American viruses are identical. The disease was probably introduced into America by infected African slaves.

### Immunity

A very powerful and long-lasting immunity is set up after an attack of yellow fever or successful vaccination, which affords protection against further attacks.

There is some cross-immunity to yellow fever engendered by certain other viruses which may exist in a community in which yellow fever is endemic. Infection with some of these viruses may also lead to stimulation and acceleration of the production of immune bodies on infection with yellow fever. Factors such as these probably account for the mildness of yellow fever attacks in individuals, especially children, living in endemic areas.

### The vectors

Females of several culicine mosquitoes can transmit the virus under laboratory conditions. The most important natural vectors are *A. aegypti, A. africanus,* and certain species of *Haemagogus.*

The vector becomes infected by sucking infective blood from a human or animal case.

The mosquito does not become infective until 12 days to 3 weeks after ingesting the virus-containing blood (the so-called extrinsic incubation period). It subsequently remains infective for the rest of its life. The life span of the vector is about 3 months, so that the maximum period of infectivity in individual insects is unlikely to exceed 2 months. This is an important factor in the epidemiology of the disease.

*Epidemiology*

Yellow fever is divided epidemiologically into urban and jungle varieties, which immunologically and clinically are the same but which differ in regard to vector and source of infection.

In urban yellow fever the maintenance host of infection is man and the vector is almost always the domestic breeder, *A. aegypti.* In a recent epidemic in Ethiopia, however, the vector was *A. simpsoni.* In jungle yellow fever the maintenance host is not man but certain forest animals, notably primates, and the vectors are various species of *Aedes* (other than *A. aegypti*) and *Haemagogus* mosquitoes.

*Transmission*

The successful transmission of urban or jungle yellow fever depends on a constant supply of active vectors, the existence of infective reservoirs, and the presence of suitable non-immune hosts.

When conditions are favourable and the latter are in good supply, epidemics may develop. Unless the supply of non-immunes is kept up, however, the epidemic will die out as the survivors become immune.

In endemic areas the infection is kept going mainly through young children or non-immune visitors. Infants are not easily infected, possibly because of some immunity acquired from the mother. Adults native to the endemic areas are commonly protected as a result of modified infection during childhood.

The vector of urban yellow fever, *A. aegypti,* is found in and about human dwellings. It breeds in small collections of water lying in artificial containers, tree holes, etc. In warm, moist conditions breeding and transmission will continue the year round. Where rains and dry seasons alternate, transmission is seasonal and at its maximum in the rains. The mosquito is killed by cold or desert conditions but probably survives from one season to the other as eggs or adults. It is to be found in association with immunes as high as 1200 metres above sea level. Control is relatively easy and has greatly reduced the incidence of urban yellow fever.

Jungle yellow fever occurs in dwellers or workers near or in forest regions and is transmitted to man by accident, probably during epizootics. In Uganda, for instance, the disease is passed from monkey to monkey by *A. africanus,* which normally exists only at high levels in the trees and is thus not very likely to transmit the infection to man. The spread to humans probably occurs as a result of the accidental infection of some other vector infesting the forest margins, such as *A. simpsoni,* from an infected monkey descended from the forest. In other forest regions, for example in Brazil, the disease is transmitted from animal to animal by mosquitoes which during the day are found chiefly in the treetops but which may descend at night to ground level and transmit direct to man. Once the disease has become established in humans it can be transmitted cyclically by *A. aegypti* and may become epidemic.

*Morbid anatomy*

There is nothing specific about the macroscopic appearance of the body. Rigidity and *livor mortis* appear early. The blood is fluid. The skin becomes yellower as the dissection proceeds and blood drains from the body. Jaundice may be minimal; it is more obvious in the more prolonged cases and may be intense in fulminating cases. The subcutaneous fat is very bright yellow. There may be petechial haemorrhages beneath the skin and mucous membranes and under the pleura, peri- and endocardium, and peritoneum. The lungs are often oedematous and may be shot with small haemorrhages, many of which lie beneath the plura. The abdominal organs may show few macroscopic changes. The liver is often normal in size and yellow-brown in colour. Occasionally, in very acute cases it may be enlarged and palpable. The cut surface is often bloody and greasy and the lobular pattern is usually exaggerated. The kidneys are sometimes tense and swollen, with scattered medullary congestion.

The gastric and intestinal contents frequently contain altered blood and the intestinal mucosa is peppered with petechial haemorrhages most prominent in the upper duodenum and stomach.

*Histological changes*

The changes in the liver tissue are of diagnostic importance. They are essentially non-inflammatory although there may be a small degree of cellular infiltration of the parenchyma. Coagulative degeneration of the cytoplasm of the polygonal cells occurs early and may involve the greater part of the lobule except the most peripherally and centrally placed cells. The degeneration is scattered over the whole lobule but is often most pronounced in the midzonal region; it is usually well developed in the central zone, but in the region of the central vein there are often a few less affected cells which have escaped the coagulative changes and have undergone fatty degeneration. The vessels of the lobule may be considerably congested; there are rarely haemorrhages.

The cytoplasm of the degenerating cells is acidophil and stains pink with eosin. Sometimes rounded masses of coagulated material appear in the cytoplasm before it is completely disintegrated. These have been called *Councilman bodies,* and are often incorrectly regarded as specific; they do in fact occur in other forms of coagulative degeneration. As the disease progresses the degeneration becomes more extensive, necrosis occurs and the cells disintegrate. In the late stages practically the whole lobule may become involved.

Changes also occur in the nuclei. The chromatin concentrates against the nuclear membrane and in some cases nuclear inclusions called *Torres bodies* becomes visible. These are composed of irregular masses of minute eosinophilic dots occupying the bulk of the nucleus.

Coagulative degeneration occurs in most cases. The nuclear inclusions may or may not be present. In some outbreaks they may appear in a high proportion of cases; in others they may be few or absent. They are a characteristic feature of the pathological picture in laboratory yellow fever in rhesus monkeys. The virus is found in the cytoplasm and not in the nucleus of the infected liver cells.

In surviving cases resolution appears to be rapid and complete. No permanent hepatic insufficiency is left and there is no residual cirrhosis.

### CLINICAL PICTURE

*Incubation period*
The intrinsic incubation period, that is the time elapsing between the infection and the onset of the disease, varies from 3 to 10 days.

*Mild cases*
In endemic areas most cases are clinically mild, especially in native children. Severe and fulminating cases are usually seen in epidemics in areas of usually low endemicity and in non-immune visitors.

The mild cases may pass practically unnoticed. There is, however, usually severe headache and some fever, conjunctival infection, and sometimes epistaxis. Some nausea and bilious vomiting are common. Albuminuria is present from the outset. There is complete recovery in 3 or 4 days.

In more severe cases the fever starts abruptly, sometimes with rigor, reaching 39.5–40° C and falling to normal in 3–4 days. The temperature falls more slowly than the pulse, which is initially fast.

The patient complains of severe frontal headache, backache, and bone and joint pains. The conjunctivae are often intensely injected and there may be epistaxis. There is nausea almost from the beginning and often severe bilious vomiting. The liver is not usually palpable but epigastric tenderness and discomfort may be severe, some mild icterus may develop by the fourth day, fading rapidly in convalescence.

Protein appears in the urine on the first day and increases in amount until recovery. The urinary volume is reduced and there are usually tubular casts.

The whole syndrome lasts only a few days, after which the temperature falls to normal and recovery is rapid and complete.

*The classical picture*
In previously unexposed subjects the disease is much more serious. It develops in two main phases, separated by an interval of comparative calm.

The first phase is very similar to that described above, but more severe.

The onset is abrupt. The temperature rises, frequently with rigor, to 38.9–40° C and remains at about this level for 1 or 2 days, subsequently falling slowly to normal or near it about 3 or 4 days from the onset. The pulse rate is high at first but drops rapidly so that a discrepancy between pulse and temperature develops. Occasionally the temperature may rise after the onset without much corresponding change in pulse rate. The increasing slowness of the pulse rate relative to the temperature (called Faget's sign) is of some clinical diagnostic value although it also occurs in other acute virus infections.

Peripheral congestion is pronounced, giving the face a blotchy appearance. Conjunctival injection and photophobia develop early. Bleeding from the gums and nose may occur. Headache, backache, and limb pains are severe. The patient is restless and considerably more prostrated than might be expected from the fever. Gastro-intestinal disturbances are the rule and appear early. There is severe epigastric discomfort and tenderness, anorexia, nausea, and vomiting. The vomit contains excess bile and sometimes altered blood. Watery bilious diarrhoea or melaena may develop.

Jaundice becomes visible about the fourth day. It is usually not pronounced and may be no more than an icteric tinge in the conjunctivae. The yellow colour can sometimes be recognized after blanching the skin with pressure. In some epidemics, cases have been described in which jaundice was intense and developed rapidly, resembling the picture of fulminating infective hepatitis.

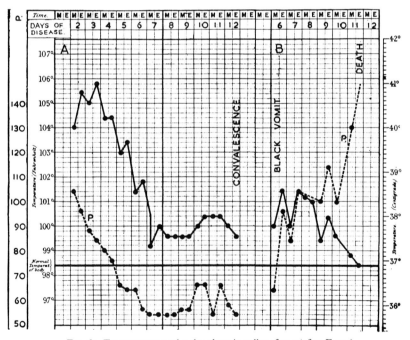

FIG. 63. Temperature and pulse chart in yellow fever (after Faget).

A. Case which recovered. Note falling pulse and high temperature (Faget's sign).
B. Fatal case. Note the rising pulse and falling temperature—a bad prognostic sign.

Protein appears in the urine on the first day and increases steadily in amount. Tubular casts appear and the urinary volume falls to oliguric levels. The temperature now falls to normal or thereabouts as a remission occurs.

With the fall of the temperature the patient feels better and the signs and symptoms subside. The vomiting stops, the epigastric discomfort diminishes, and recovery may now take place.

In the more serious cases after a few hours to 2 days of remission the fever returns and the patient passes rapidly into a state of severe intoxication and prostration.

The temperature rises rapidly but seldom reaches the level attained in the primary febrile period. The pulse at first quickens a little but remains slow in proportion to the fever, and often continues to fall until by the tenth day it may be as slow as 40 beats per minute. After usually not more than 3 or 4 days the temperature again falls. In fatal cases the pulse rate frequently rises sharply towards the end, at a time when the temperature is falling.

Most of the signs present in the early febrile period become exaggerated. Epigastric discomfort, nausea, and vomiting become very severe. Bleeding from the mucous membrane of the gut leads to vomiting of changed blood, sometimes in large amounts—the so-called black vomit. Blood also appears in the stool.

In the classical case, jaundice increases slightly. In a few cases it may become considerable but it is usually much less evident than the name of the disease would suggest. Bile appears in the urine. Fulminating cases may present with large liver and intense deepening jaundice.

Albuminuria increases. Oliguria sets in and renal failure with anuria, rising blood urea, and acute uraemia is likely to develop. It is the commonest cause of death.

Petechial haemorrhages appear in the mucous membrane and sometimes under the skin. Bleeding from the nose and lips may become more severe and fresh blood may appear in the vomit.

In the late stages there is often intractable hiccup.

Death also commonly occurs from vascular failure. It may be sudden or heralded by rapid fall of blood pressures with haemoconcentration, rapid fall of body temperature and quickening pulse rate.

The overall picture of the second febrile stage may be dominated by signs of hepatic, renal or vascular failure separately or together.

Throughout the disease the patient is usually conscious, anxious, and restless. Delirium or coma occur only terminally and are not common. In a few cases there may be late central nervous system signs including meningismus, probably arising from vascular accidents.

Fulminating cases are occasionally seen, especially in epidemics, in which there is no period of remission and death occurs in a few days from the onset. There is usually a very high fever with the signs of acute hepatic failure including deepening jaundice.

The severe attack of yellow fever is over one way or another by the eleventh or twelfth day. Death occurs most commonly between the fifth and eighth days. The great majority of clinically mild cases recover completely in 3 or 4 days. Prognosis must be guarded in severe cases. The clinical appearance in the early stages is not a good guide to developments since desperate signs may appear very rapidly. A rise of temperature with return of symptoms following the remission is unfavourable. Deepening jaundice, severe haemorrhage from the gut, falling blood pressure, and rising pulse rate associated with rapidly falling temperature or the onset of anuria with rising blood urea nitrogen concentration are all grave portents.

The overall mortality rate of yellow fever is low. There is, however, a high mortality amongst the severe cases which develop in non-immunes.

*The blood*

Severe loss of blood by haemorrhage may be reflected in the later stages by some secondary anaemia. If vascular failure develops, the anaemia may be temporarily masked by haemoconcentration.

Leucopenia develops rapidly in most severe cases. It may be evident from the onset, but is occasionally preceded by a transient leucocytosis. By the third or fourth day the white cell count is usually about 3000–4000 cells per mm$^3$ with a relative lymphocytosis and granulocytopenia with a shift to the left. Eosinophil numbers are reduced. The normal count is restored slowly during convalescence. These changes are common in other acute virus infections.

The electrolyte content of the blood changes in accordance with losses arising from vomiting, bleeding, and diarrhoea. The blood urea nitrogen and non-protein nitrogen concentrations rise considerably, especially in cases in which there is severe oliguria or anuria and uraemia. The bilirubin content of the plasma rises and increases progressively as the jaundice develops.

*The urine*

The urinary volume is usually low from the beginning, especially when vomiting is severe. The chloride content is also low. Protein appears on the first day and increases steadily in amount. Tubular casts are common in practically all cases; they may be present in large numbers in oliguric cases. Red blood cells may appear, especially in the second febrile period as the result of haemorrhage into the urinary tract. Bile is present in the late stages. Acute renal failure is the commonest fatal complication. Anuria develops with rapidly rising blood urea concentration, associated with clinical uraemia.

*The vomit*

In the early days of the disease the vomit is watery or mucous and contains bile, sometimes in considerable amounts. Unaltered or swallowed blood from buccal or nasal bleeding may be present. In the later stages the vomit contains brown or black altered blood—the so-called black vomit—arising from haemorrhages in the mucosa of the stomach.

DIAGNOSIS

The clinical diagnosis of yellow fever in the isolated mild case is extremely difficult.

The diagnosis in the severe case can be suspected in an endemic area on the grounds of sudden fever, conjunctival injection, severe prostration out of proportion to the fever, epigastric discomfort and vomiting, jaundice appearing over several days in the absence of enlargement of the liver, the slow pulse in relation to the fever, and progressively increasing proteinuria.

The clinical diagnosis is greatly helped by the existence of a known outbreak of yellow fever.

Yellow fever may have to be distinguished from a variety of other conditions, including *infectious and serum hepatitis, blackwater fever, complicated falciparum malaria, leptospirosis,* and *relapsing fever.*

*Laboratory diagnosis*

*Specific antibodies.* Antibodies capable of protecting mice from the neurotropic virus are present in measurable quantities by the fourth day of the human disease and increase rapidly in strength to reach full titre in about 10 days. *In order to make a diagnosis it is necessary to demonstrate an increase in these antibodies over a period of days.* Single examinations are not directly helpful, since immune bodies remain permanently in the blood after an attack, and a positive finding will merely indicate that an attack has at some time occurred in a given (unvaccinated) individual. The presence of a high titre of antibody at the beginning of a severe illness suspected of being yellow fever would, of course, rule out the diagnosis.

The mouse protection test is also valuable for surveying endemic areas. The immune content of sera taken from random samples of the population will thus indicate whether the disease has occurred in the district. The immune content of serial samples from young children taken over an interval of a year or more will indicate further whether the disease is still active in the locality. The overlap of immunity with that induced by other viruses must be taken into account in making these assessments.

*Identification of the virus.* Blood taken within the first 3–4 days of the disease contains the virus and can be used to infect rhesus monkeys. The identification of the virus is a highly technical procedure which can be carried out only by specially equipped and screened laboratories.

*Histological examination of the liver.* Coagulative midzonal degeneration of hepatic cells, and possibly nuclear inclusions, can be demonstrated in early cases in sections of liver tissues fixed in formalin and stained with eosin and haematoxylin. In fulminating or late cases there may be so much tissue destruction that identification is difficult. On the whole, however, a firm diagnosis can usually be made from histological material if the observer is sufficiently experienced. Other existing lesions of the liver, such as fibrosis, may obscure the mid-zonal pattern.

In endemic areas examinating of liver tissue should be carried out as a routine in all fatal febrile illnesses of short duration. The tissue samples may be removed from the cadaver by an instrument called a viscerotome; they are fixed in formalin and examined subsequently.

## TREATMENT

There is no specific treatment for yellow fever. Convalescent serum, penicillin, and sulphonamides are ineffective.

The patient must be carefully nursed in bed. He should be kept as quiet as possible and not moved unless absolutely necessary. The patient must be nursed under a mosquito net.

Treatment is largely symptomatic. Small frequent drinks containing glucose should be administered. If vomiting makes this impossible glucose drip infusion should be given intravenously. Isotonic glucose saline should be substituted if there is notable dehydration. The appearance of shock calls for immediate infusion of plasma.

A fluid intake–output balance must be kept. All specimens of urine passed should be measured and examined in order to keep check on the appearance of anuria. Renal failure must be treated as described elsewhere (see p. 280).

Procedures designed to lessen the liver damage, such as the administration of vitamin K, have provided equivocal results. It is possible that in some cases the intravenous infusion of protein hydrolysates may be helpful.

## PROPHYLAXIS

*Entomological control*

Urban yellow fever can be effectively controlled by eradication of the vector *A. aegypti* by destruction of breeding places and spray killing of adults. Continuous control by such measures has largely terminated transmission of the urban disease. Jungle fever is not amenable to entomological control.

*Vaccination*

Protection of individuals and communities may be afforded by the use of vaccines prepared from the attenuated living virus. Travellers to endemic areas, or coming from endemic areas, especially so called 'receptive' areas (*A. aegypti,* but no virus infection) must be vaccinated.

Two living attenuated vaccines are available. The 17D vaccine is made from the virus originally isolated in West Africa, attenuated by growth in tissue culture, and prepared in chick embryos. The vaccine was originally prepared in a vehicle of human serum but this led to outbreaks of serum hepatitis. Albumin is now used. A French (Dakar) vaccine is prepared from neurotropic virus grown in mouse brain.

The 17D vaccine has to be kept in the cold and is normally given by subcutaneous injection. It has also been given by scarification. The French vaccine, which is much less sensitive to heat, is given by scarification.

The risk of encephalitis is small but somewhat greater with the French vaccine.

Mass vaccination with both these vaccines has been extensively carried out in endemic areas in Africa, with very good results.

Antibodies demonstrable by the mouse protection test are present in the blood of most individuals 10 days after inoculation with the vaccine; they remain in the blood in undiminished strength for years. It is considered that protection against the disease is assured in vaccinated persons for at least 10 years after successful vaccination. The international vaccination certificate is valid for this period.

# VIRUS HEPATITIS

## INFECTIOUS HEPATITIS: SERUM HEPATITIS

### DEFINITION

Diseases involving the liver, caused by at least two distinct, but not yet fully identified, virus groups. Both are distributed widely and the signs, symptoms, and sequelae are very much alike. Clinical manifestations vary considerably in severity, from anicteric trivial illness to rapidly fatal, complete liver failure with deep jaundice. Some cases are caused by unidentified viruses which produce clinically similar pictures but are antigenically unrelated to the infectious and serum hepatitis viruses. Such 'unspecified' viral hepatitis in some areas is the commonest form of transfusion hepatitis.

### EPIDEMIOLOGY AND DISTRIBUTION

#### HEPATITIS A VIRUS: HAV

The virus of infectious hepatitis is now usually referred to as HAV, i.e. hepatitis A virus. It is a small, cuboidal virus measuring about 25–28 nm, without an envelope or subunits. It may be empty or full and is best identified by immune electrophoresis. It is found in the faeces and in the liver cells of the infected individual.

HAV is relatively resistant to heat, acid, non-ionic detergents, and cold but is inactivated by dilute formaldehyde and chlorine.

Antibodies to HAV can be detected in infected human serum and in certain wild animals, including the chimpanzee.

The virus will not grow in cell culture, but can be passed orally or intravenously to colony-born, infection-free chimpanzees and certain species of marmoset monkeys which develop clinical, biochemical, and histological evidence of infection, with the appearance of anti-HAV in the serum in convalescence. At this stage, primate infection is a useful research tool, but much limited by the few colony-bred animals available. It has no place as yet in diagnosis.

*Distribution*

Infection with HAV has a world-wide distribution, which is not clearly defined, because of difficulties of surveillance and differing clinical and sub-clinical patterns. Epidemics occur and there are numerous endemic tropical and subtropical areas.

More than half the infections are found in children under 15 years of age. There are probably many more which are subclinical and remain undetected. All ages may be infected. On the whole the incidence seems to be declining and a greater proportion of clinical cases is appearing in adults. There are patterns of incidence. Peaks of infection occur in temperate endemic zones every 5–20 years. There is also some seasonal variation in these areas with maximal incidence in late autumn and early winter, and minimal in midsummer.

*Mode of transmission*

Despite the high incidence of antibody in wild chimpanzees and marmosets, there is no record of human infection resulting from contact with these or other animals.

It is believed that the virus infection is most commonly maintained by the intestinal–oral route in man, especially in families and in conditions of over-crowding and bad sanitation. Transmission also seems to be maintained in institutions and in conditions of temporary overcrowding—the disease was very prevalent in the desert campaigns of the Second World War.

In poor sanitary conditions, water-borne epidemics often occur. Out-breaks involving local water supplies may also arise in highly developed countries in Europe and the U.S.A. Outbreaks may also be food-borne, sometimes arising from infected food-handlers who are in the incubation period and following the ingestion of uncooked or incompletely cooked food, commonly shellfish.

There is little evidence that infection can be transmitted by the respiratory route, by urine, or by sexual contact. Syringe transmission has been recorded. The disease is not congenital.

# I SERUM HEPATITIS

## HEPATITIS B VIRUS: HBV

The virus is a double-shelled, roughly spheroidal organism about twice the size of HAV. It may be full or empty and consists of a small core (called 'c' or HBc) and a lipoprotein polypeptide outer envelope (called the surface 's', or HBs).

The identification of the virus followed the discovery of the so-called 'Australia' antigen in the serum of Australian Aborigines, which had a very clear association with virus B hepatitis and was relatively easy to detect. The antigen (HBsAg) is now used to evaluate the epidemiology of HBV infection by serological surveys.

The antigen carrier rate is highest in tropical and temperate endemic regions, higher in males than females, higher in young children than in adults, and considerably higher in urban than in rural communities.

Antibodies (anti-HBsAg) can also often be detected, though not in all known cases of past hepatitis. Their incidence increases with the age of the individual.

Both antigen and corresponding antibody show the highest prevalences in overcrowded and unhygienic conditions such as occur in developing countries.

### Distribution

Various subtypes (phenotypes) are found in different geographical areas.

One—*ayw*—occurs in most of Africa, the eastern Mediterranean areas, the Middle East, Pakistan, Bangladesh and India. A second—*adw*—occurs in Europe and the Americas and, together with a third—*adv*—in Indonesia, Malaysia, Thailand, and Papua New Guinea. The latter appears alone in the rest of South-east Asia and the Far East.

Injection with HBV is followed by the appearance in the serum of an antigen related to the surface (HBsAg). The homologous antibody (anti-HBs) appears later in the disease. Antibodies related to the core substance (anti-HBc) also appear later.

The presence of HBsAg in the serum is a specific indicator of infection. The antigen first appears some weeks after exposure, at a time when deviations of the 'liver function' tests are developing and usually some clinical signs of hepatitis have become apparent. After the attack, the antigen usually disappears, but it may persist for years.

The majority of patients develop anti-HBs in the serum during convalescence. In carriers of the antigen, the antibody is often present, but in very low titre.

The two antigenic components, the surface and the core antigens, are found in the hepatocytes, not only in obvious clinical cases, but in a proportion of apparently 'healthy' persons with HBsAg in the blood. This suggests that the effect of the virus on the liver cell may not be direct, so much as involved, with immunological processes arising from the formation of complement–antigen–antibody complexes.

HBsAg appears in most patients in the incubation period, 4–6 weeks after infection and 2–8 weeks after onset of jaundice or elevation of the serum transaminases. It persists in the acute illness and clears in convalescence. The antibody response in acute cases occurs later, but a secondary or anamnestic appearance of the antibody may occur after the antigen is no longer detectable in the serum and persists from 6 months to 3 years.

The core antigen does not appear in the serum but its antibody does, 2–10 weeks after the HBsAg first becomes detectable.

High titres of antibody to the core antigen (anti-HBc) are found in chronically infected individuals, who usually carry detectable amounts of the surface antigen.

Cell-mediated immunity to HBV develops in the acute stages of the disease, persists into convalescence, and disappears on recovery. It cannot be detected in the chronic asymptomatic antigen carrier. It is presumed to be concerned with terminating the infection and also promoting the liver cell damage.

In acute hepatitis the fall of titres of HBsAg, coinciding with the rise of antibodies and fall of complement suggests the elimination of the antigen by the formation of immune complexes which may abort the infection and also be involved in the pathological changes in the liver. At the moment, the pathogenic significance of immune complexes in the characteristic liver damage is unknown.

Further studies are required. There is no good animal laboratory model. Mild disease has been induced with several phenotypes in infection-free chimpanzees. The *adw* phenotype has been successfully transmitted to *Macacca mulatta*—this infection is apparently enhanced by previous malaria infection.

*Mode of transmission*

Infection is usually parenteral, during blood or plasma-serum infusion. Any kind of syringe usage could be effective.

The very high carrier rates in tropical areas also suggests that blood-sucking insects could be involved. The antigens have occasionally been identified in pooled wild mosquitoes of several species, but artificial feeding of insects has not been successful. It is possible that infection could be transferred by mechanical transmission by biting insects but there is no evidence of this.

The virus seems to be transmitted primarily by parenteral means, but other methods may exist and should not be ignored. Non-parenteral transmission may occur. Thus, carriers tend to appear in several members of families, so that body fluids and excretions may be involved such as urine, saliva, milk, faeces, and even semen. Infection by the oral route has been demonstrated experimentally, but this seems unlikely in man, except as enteric or faecal–oral spread—the major mode in hepatitis A infection. There is evidence of an antibody-blocking substance in faeces and the intestinal mucosa.

Perinatal transplacental transmission has been occasionally demonstrated in babies born of asymptomatic carriers. A point of interest is the high incidence of antigen or antibody in family contacts of patients with a history of clinical hepatitis B.

*Transfusion*

The use of blood, plasma, and serum from antigen carriers is a very common method of transmission. It should be avoided by not using the blood of possible carriers but these are always difficult to detect, even after an obvious previous attack of hepatitis.

Infection may result from using blood containing the antigen–antibody complex in which the antibody is in excess, so that the antibody tests are positive and antigen tests negative. If this were so, the use of antibody positive blood should be excluded, amounting to 20 per cent of available blood donors in some areas. Fortunately, the general view seems to be that blood containing anti HBs but without detectable free antigen is safe.

Certain groups of people are at special risk of acquiring HBV infection.

These include doctors, dentists, nurses, blood bank technicians, and anyone involved with processing blood. Hepatitis is a major problem in patients and staff of haemodialysis units.

PATHOLOGY

The liver parenchymal cells may show no obvious signs of damage even in cases with clinical jaundice. In most case, however, there is some evidence of cellular damage and necrosis.

Hepatocytes may develop changes, beginning as gross eosinophilic stippling of the cytoplasm. The nucleus later becomes pyknotic and may disappear. The cell shrinks and may be extruded. Some cells undergo rapid autolysis of both cytoplasm and nucleus; such autolysis predominates in fulminating cases.

The cellular lesions are usually distributed irregularly through the organ, but tend to be most pronounced in the central zones of the affected lobules. In fulminant cases practically all the cells of the lobule may be damaged except for a few peripherally placed.

Intralobular tissue and the portal tracts are infiltrated. The infiltration is most pronounced in the tracts, but the lobular substance is also involved.

The cells are mostly mononuclear and include lymphocytes, histiocytes, and plasma cells. Eosinophils are sometimes present in small numbers, but rarely polymorphs. The portal tracts are tightly packed with cells, which may appear to spill over into the peripheral regions of the lobule. The Kupffer cells are swollen and may contain bile pigment granules. There may also be small plugs of bile in the canaliculi of the parenchymal cells.

Regeneration appears to go on in parallel with the cellular damage. It is first indicated by the appearance of giant cells. It may be profuse but irregular. In mild cases the structure of the lobule is restored, or there may develop isolated amorphous masses or regenerated hepatocytes with no lobular structure and apparently separated from the functioning organ as a whole, usually by layers of fibrous tissue.

The late stages of recovery are sometimes accompanied by gross, irregular liver fibrosis, in which the portal tracts remain infiltrated with mononuclear cells. Portal hypertension may develop with the usual serious consequences.

The incidence of such fibrosis varies from place to place. It is usually uncommon.

### CLINICAL PICTURE

The clinical effects of infection with HAV and HBV are very similar. In this text the features of infectious hepatitis HAV will be detailed and a few of the minor differences in HBV infection noted.

### INFECTIOUS HEPATITIS: HAV INFECTION

There may be no clinical evidence of infection, although the biochemical 'liver function' tests become abnormal. Some patients who do not develop jaundice (and these probably represent the majority) feel mildly ill, with headache, generalized muscle and joint pains, and complain of abdominal discomfort. Most become anorexic, actually taking a dislike to food of any sort, accompanied by nausea at the sight of it. This condition, which affects young children and middle-aged women in particular, may resolve in a week or so without further developments, or linger on for weeks or months. In the more severe cases, although there is no bile in the urine, the stools become very pale, resembling those passed by icteric patients. Not surprisingly, the milder cases are often missed clinically.

Some patients develop jaundice, which may be the first sign of trouble. Usually there are several days of pre-icteric malaise, with an increasing dislike for food—*all* food, not just fatty dishes. Nausea is usual and persistent but vomiting is rare at this stage. Vague upper abdominal discomfort is the main complaint. Occasionally, there may be acute abdominal pain. There is usually headache, sometimes severe, and generalized muscle and joint pains.

The body temperature rises over the pre-icteric phase to about 39° C with chills and occasionally rigors. Children may be severely ill at this stage. After 2–3 days jaundice begins to appear, first noticed in the sclera of the eyes, and deepens rapidly. The urine becomes dark from discharge of bile and the faeces become pale yellow.

The fever now subsides in the usual case, as the jaundice appears and deepens. The skin becomes itchy and, in about half the patients, the edge of the liver can be palpated, soft but not tender.

In mild cases the patient may remain jaundiced for some time but begins to feel well in a few days and can soon be allowed out of bed. In more severe reactions, which occur especially in older people, the feeling of illness and nausea continue and the dislike of food persists. In most patients, the worst is over within a fortnight and the appetite returns, irrespective of whether there is still jaundice or not. In fact, at the point when the patient begins to feel better, the colour may be at its deepest. Inside a month the jaundice disappears and the colour of the urine and faeces returns to normal.

In some individuals the jaundice may deepen to bronze and remain for several months, usually accompanied by notable skin itching. Despite the colour, however, the patient feels well and the prognosis is good.

Occasionally, the outlook worsens and the disease becomes fulminant, with rapidly deepening jaundice, vomiting, and the development of hepatic coma. Cerebral disturbances precede the coma and the temperature rises rapidly to 40–41° C. Haemorrhages appear under the skin and mucous membranes, with bleeding into the stomach and intestines. Death occurs in a few days. This pattern may develop from the beginning of the illness, or appear during an apparently mild attack. Death may also terminate severe cases in whom the signs of hepatitis persist for some months.

Relapses may occur months after apparent complete recovery. These are usually severe but seldom fatal.

SERUM HEPATITIS: HBV INFECTION

The clinical pictures are similar to those described above, but the incubation period, estimated from the time of transfusion, etc., is much longer. In infectious hepatitis it is 15–40 days. In serum hepatitis it is 60–160 days or even longer. The disease is uncommon in children, who tend to receive less parenteral treatment.

The onset is insidious, without prolonged prodromal signs. The usual first indication is the appearance of slowly deepening jaundice.

The disease on the whole is more serious than infectious hepatitis and has a higher death rate.

The prognosis in infectious hepatitis is good. Many infections are mild, even when jaundice appears. Post-hepatitis liver fibrosis may occur and lead to portal hypertension but this is probably a rare sequel.

In serum hepatitis the prognosis is worse. Whereas the death rate in infectious hepatitis is about 1 in 2000, it may be as high as 1 in 5 in serum hepatitis in elderly people.

### DIAGNOSIS

The well-developed clinical picture is characteristic, but the viral infections have to be separated from other causes of jaundice by standard diagnostic techniques, including the so-called 'liver function' tests, and the identification of the viruses.

Deviations of the 'liver function' tests vary to some extent with the cause of the hepatitis but are not definitive in diagnosis. For example, blood alkaline phosphatase is raised in the viral infections but is usually very much higher in obstructive jaundice. Blood transaminases SGOT (glutamic-oxalo-acetic transaminase) and SGPT (glutamic-pyruvic transaminase) are raised and are usually higher in viral than obstructive jaundice. A rise in these transaminases may be a useful diagnostic pointer in the non-icteric patient, or during the incubation period.

The detection of the virus in the faeces and the hepatocytes is a very specialized procedure which should be left to experts. The same applies to the detection of the antigens and antibodies. Serial measurement of the latter may be useful in that a rising anti-HAV antibody is regarded as indicating genuine infection.

Such techniques are useful in institutional outbreaks and in limited areas where the outbreak results from infected water or food, especially shellfish, in which the virus may be concentrated.

Measurement of antigens and antibodies in the population in most areas, including the developed world, shows a high correlation of positives with age. Thus, in some parts of the U.S.A., the evidence of infection or past infection in children under 4 years of age was 13 per cent; in people over 50 years of age it was 50 per cent.

Liver biopsy is not usually called for. During the active disease the risk of bleeding from this operation is high. However, when it is performed, the tissue may show the typical monocellular infiltration of portal tracts and lobules. Because of the interference with blood coagulation mechanisms which are usual in hepatitis, biopsy is carried out only when some parasitic cause, such as *Opisthorchis,* is suspected or when the patient is in an active yellow fever endemic area and is not protected from the latter by vaccination.

### TREATMENT

There is no specific therapy.

Bed rest is usually demanded by the patient. When he feels better, he should be allowed to get up and walk about.

Diet should be decided by the patient. To begin with, *all* food is distasteful to him, not only fat. When his appetite returns there is no need to restrict anything, including fat, unless he wishes it. In long-continued cases protein intake should be kept low, because of the possibility of hepatic coma.

Itching may be relieved by antihistaminic drugs or calamine lotion. Corti-costeroids may help, but there is no indication for their use in the ordinary case.

Convalescence is slow.

Alcohol is usually prohibited, largely on the grounds that a damaged liver cannot metabolize it properly and that fibrosis may be stimulated. There is very little evidence to support these views. Where the decision is left to the patient he often decides against drinking or greatly reduces his intake.

### CONTROL

There seems little doubt that the spread of both HAV and HBV is enhanced by bad hygiene and crowded living and is commoner in the poorer parts of the world.

Spread of HAV can therefore be limited to an extent proportional to effort, by improvement in hygiene, better sanitation in latrines and cooking and eating vessels, and bed linen—where it exists.

Good, clean drinking water is very important.

In the spread of HBV vital factors are careful use of apparatus used for parenteral treatment, such as syringes and needles. Disposable equipment, used only once, is the ideal. Equally important is the preparation of the material to be injected—blood, serum and plasma, drug solutions and suspensions, etc.

There is some risk in vaccination, especially mass vaccination, in which blood may be accidentally passed from one person to another. Drug taking by syringe has high personal and communal risks.

There is no satisfactory vaccine for any form of A or B hepatitis virus.

Partial protection can be achieved in the individual by the use of normal pooled human $\gamma$-globulin. This can be given to those at special risk, or in local outbreaks in which it controls the clinical severity and allows some immunity to develop.

Protection with $\gamma$-globulin lasts only a few months. A single dose is 250–500 mg. Where an individual is constantly exposed to infectious hepatitis in an endemic area regular injections of $\gamma$-globulin at 6-monthly intervals have sometimes been used. Most authors are not in favour of this technique, in view of the possible side-effects of giving the globulin and the uncertainty of its protective effects except over a short interval of a few months.

$\gamma$-Globulin in the above dosage is sometimes recommended for travellers visiting highly endemic areas.

$\gamma$-Globulin is less effective against HBV infection, even when given at spaced intervals after the transfusion or injection. It has also been added to the transfusion but without effect.

Some method of killing the HBV in the injected fluid will have to be found before protection against the infection can really be claimed.

# DENGUE

## DEFINITION

Breakbone fever. An acute non-fatal disease caused by Group B arboviruses (Dengue viruses) transmitted by the mosquito *Aedes aegypti*.

The same group of viruses may cause South-east Asian haemorrhagic fevers, with high mortality (see p. 573).

## GEOGRAPHICAL DISTRIBUTION

Dengue occurs in most of the subtropics and tropics, especially in coastal areas. It appears in southern North America, South America including Brazil, the West Indies, the Mediterranean seaboard, Egypt and the Middle East, north, central and South Africa, Greece, southern Russia and Turkey, India, Pakistan, Bangladesh, China, South-east Asia, many Pacific Islands, the Solomon Islands and New Hebrides, and northern Australia.

## AETIOLOGY

*Causal agent*

Dengue is caused by a Group B arbovirus. There are at least four, and possibly six, antigenically overlapping strains so far identified by passage in mice.

An attack induces immunity against the homologous strain of the virus lasting about a year and affords protection against other strains for a variable period of months.

*The vector*

The females of numerous species of *Aedes* mosquitoes are capable of transmitting the disease. By far the commonest natural vector is *A. aegypti*. In Asia *A. albopictus* is also a vector.

*Transmission*

The virus is present in the blood of the human patient for as long as 3 days after the onset and possibly for a short time before. The mosquito becomes infective 8–12 days after ingesting blood containing the virus. It remains infective for the rest of its life and injects the virus during biting.

Breeding and activity of the vector are maximal in hot, moist conditions and minimal in the cold. The disease is therefore often seasonal in its incidence occurring in the wet season in the tropics or summer and autumn in the subtropics.

Man is the usual maintenance host of the infection; certain monkeys which can be infected by laboratory strains may also act as such.

Non-immunes of any race and age and of either sex are susceptible.

Transmission may be kept up by the reinfection of local inhabitants who have lost or are losing immunity acquired in previous attacks, or by infection of visiting non-immunes.

When the latter are numerous, or when the local community has been free from the disease for over a year, explosive epidemics appear, which burn themselves out after involving the majority of susceptible individuals.

### PATHOLOGY

There is no information available.

### CLINICAL PICTURE

The clinical picture varies widely from individual to individual in the same outbreak and from epidemic to epidemic; this is also true of cases artificially infected under laboratory conditions. The disease lasts anything from 1 to 10 days.

The incubation period varies from 5 to 9 days. There are often prodromal symptoms including malaise, headache, and mild shivering, which come on 2 or 3 days before the onset.

The onset is abrupt. The patient can often recall the time almost to the hour. The temperature rises sharply to 39–41° C, frequently with rigor. Many of the other signs and symptoms begin equally suddenly. The most impressive are headache and intense agonizing pains in the joints, long bones, and back, which may be so severe as to prevent sleep.

The headache is diffuse, sometimes concentrated in the post- and supra-orbital regions. The eyeball and muscles about the eye become tender to touch and movements of the eyes are painful.

The bodily pains are shooting in character and accompanied by considerable soreness on pressure over muscles and tendons. The joint pains are centred in the muscle insertions.

The appetite is lost completely. Nausea is common and vomiting may be frequent and severe. There is usually epigastric discomfort and tenderness.

A blotchy congestion of the peripheral circulation, particularly notable in the face, develops early producing an effect which is sometimes referred to erroneously as the primary rash.

Epistaxis is common. Photophobia is often pronounced and may be accompanied by puffiness of the eyelids, severe conjunctival injection, and excessive lachrymation.

There may be a slight cough in the early stages but respiratory symptoms are minimal and the nasopharynx is not involved.

The patient is restless and anxious; there is acute depression and often unreasonable fear regarding the outcome of the illness. Insomnia is the rule, sleep occurring in short spells often broken by disturbing dreams.

The pulse is fast at the onset. It may fall despite the high temperature, reaching a rate of 40–60 beats per minute within the first 4 or 5 days, persisting at that level throughout the course of the illness, and often for several days into convalescence.

The fever is initially high and remittent and tends to be continuous, falling to normal after the first 3 or 4 days, usually by crisis associated with sweating and often diarrhoea.

In many cases the temperature now remains normal and the patient passes into convalescence. In others there is a remission lasting a few hours to 2 days, during which the symptoms almost completely subside. This is followed by a secondary febrile period which lasts 2 or 3 days, ending by lysis. The temperature rises suddenly, usually to a somewhat lower level than in the primary fever but occasionally exceeding it.

The primary and secondary febrile phases separated by an afebrile remission constitute the classical saddleback fever. Experience has shown that this is no more common in dengue than is simple continuous remittent fever.

With the reappearance of fever the pulse rate rises for a short time, then falls to the level obtaining at the end of the initial febrile stage. The signs and symptoms return with the fever, but are usually not so severe as in the first stage.

### The rash

The true dengue rash seldom develops before the fourth or fifth day. In cases in which the fever is saddlebacked, the rash nearly always appears during the second febrile phase, commonly within a few hours of the reappearance of the fever.

Many cases never show a rash. In others it may be fleeting or become a dominant feature. In some districts the majority of cases develop a rash, in others the minority. The rash may be characteristic of a particular epidemic and absent in others.

It is morbilliform, fades easily on pressure, and is very bright red, contrasting with the bluish tinge of measles. It may be complicated by petechial haemorrhages.

It appears first on the dorsal surface of the hands and the feet; it spreads rapidly to the arms and legs and often includes the trunk; it sometimes involves the face. It comes up very rapidly and begins to fade as the temperature subsides. Fine desquamation associated with some brown pigmentation usually occurs. The eruption is intensely itchy, especially during desquamation, and scratching may lead to secondary infection. The pruritus may be the overriding concern of the already depressed sufferer.

Leucopenia develops immediately, sometimes before the fever, and rapidly becomes severe, the white cell count reaching 2000–3000 cells per mm$^3$ by the fourth to sixth day, independent of the fever. Recovery of the cell count is slow and takes place a week or more after the fever has subsided. There is a reduction in all forms of leucocytes, most notable in the granulocytes in which there is a pronounced shift to the left. The proportion of lymphocytes present is of the order of 60–65 per cent.

*Lymph glands*

Moderate enlargement of lymph glands, which may be general and symmetrical or confined to certain groups, is a striking feature of the disease in some districts and in certain outbreaks. It is not, however, a constant finding.

The glands are palpable, only slightly tender, and remain discrete. Enlargement starts early and is evident by the second day. Subsidence in convalescence is slow. Suppuration does not occur without secondary sepsis.

### PROGNOSIS

Dengue is a non-fatal disease. The most serious complication is profound depression which may continue for several weeks after the subsidence of the active disease and is often aggravated by the intense pruritus. Despite this depression there is little evidence to support the firmly held view that suicide is common after the disease. Complete recovery is the rule, although convalescence may be very slow.

### DIAGNOSIS

During a known outbreak the diagnosis is usually easy, particularly if certain features are present, including the very abrupt onset, severe headache and bone pains, the saddleback fever, bradycardia, the rash, and rapidly developing leucopenia and shift of the Arneth count to the left.

The individual case may present considerable difficulty and confusion may arise with almost any acute febrile illness, especially measles, malaria, yellow fever, phlebotomus and other similar fevers, and influenza. In measles distinguishing features are the early coryza, Koplik spots, and the widespread bluish rash first appearing on the face. It is often impossible to separate phlebotomus fever from atypical dengue, unless there is good evidence regarding the vector.

Influenza also causes difficulty at times but can usually be distinguished by the acute upper respiratory involvement and the absence of rash, changes in the leucocytes or lymph glands.

Laboratory methods of diagnosing dengue depend on isolation of the virus and the detection of virological immune bodies in the serum.

### TREATMENT

Treatment is entirely symptomatic. Calamine lotion or antihistaminics may relieve the pruritus.

# SANDFLY FEVER

## DEFINITION

Sandfly fever: Papataci fever: Three-day fever. An acute non-fatal virus disease transmitted by the sandfly *Phlebotomus papatasi*.

## GEOGRAPHICAL DISTRIBUTION

The distribution depends on that of the fly. The disease is common in many parts of the tropics and subtropics, appearing mainly in the hot dry weather. It occurs in Portugal, the Balkans, Italy, the Aegean Islands, most of the Mediterranean littoral, Egypt and the Middle East, East and North Africa, India, Pakistan, Bangladesh, Burma, China, and parts of South America as far south as northern Argentina.

It has been reported in communities living 1500 metres above sea level.

In most areas where antimalarial residual insecticide spraying has been used the vector has disappeared, and with it the disease. Recent failure of antimalarial campaigns has been followed in former endemic areas by return of the vector and the disease.

## AETIOLOGY

The causal agent is a very small unclassified virus which exists in several closely allied antigenic strains.

During the disease the virus is present in the patient's blood for 1–2 days before the onset and for about a day afterwards.

The maintenance host of infection is man.

### The vector
Females of several species of phlebotomus flies (sandflies) can transmit the infection. The commonest is *P. papatasi*. These insects are most active and voracious at night, resting during the day in cool, shady, dry places such as cracks in stonework. They never fly far from their breeding grounds. The limit of flight is usually 15–30 metres.

### Transmission
The fly becomes infective 6–8 days after ingesting human blood in which the virus is circulating. It remains infective for life. The disease is transmitted by the bite of the infected fly. It can be passed experimentally from man to man by injection of infective blood.

### Epidemiology
The disease is highly seasonal in its incidence, occurring in most districts in the

late spring and sometimes becoming epidemic in the summer. It disappears in the autumn and winter.

No race is immune. Both sexes are freely attacked at all ages.

All non-immunes are highly susceptible and will almost certainly become infected on entering any residual active endemic area at the right time. In an epidemic the natives of the area are usually unaffected, indicating the presence of considerable resistance to infection, probably acquired by repeated past infection. Immunity is strongly developed for the homologous strain but appears to be of short duration. Fresh attacks can develop within a few months of an infection. There is some cross-immunity between various strains of phlebotomus virus but none with dengue.

### CLINICAL PICTURE

An attack of phlebotomus fever closely resembles one of dengue without the rash, saddleback fever, or glandular involvement. The whole affair seldom lasts more than 3 or 4 days.

The incubation period varies from 3 to 7 days.

The onset is very sudden. There is a rapid rise of temperature to 39.4–40.6° C, often associated with rigor. Thereafter the temperature remains elevated for 1–3 days, rarely longer. The fever is remittent and ends by crisis accompanied by intense sweating and sometimes epistaxis. In a few cases there may be a short remission followed by a few further hours of fever, the temperature chart thus resembling the saddleback fever of dengue.

The signs and symptoms appear as abruptly as the fever, usually without any marked prodromata. The conjunctivae are injected; photophobia and lachrymation are common. There is very severe headache and pain especially at the back of the orbit. Long bone, joint pains, and backache are very troublesome and may be severe enough to cause insomnia. The patient is deeply depressed. Anorexia may be complete. Nausea is common and there may be some vomiting. The pharynx is injected and sore and there is usually some mild bronchitic involvement which results in an unproductive cough; there may be a few scattered râles. The pulse is often slow in relation to the fever; it may be very fast. Leucopenia develops immediately after the onset. The total count may fall as low as 3000 cells per mm$^3$. There is an absolute reduction in neutrophils, with considerable shift to the left. The lymphocytes and other cells are reduced much less in proportion. There is no rash and no glandular involvement. The erythrocyte sedimentation rate is seldom affected.

The disease is non-fatal in spite of the fact that it is very severe while it lasts. The depression is relieved only slowly and convalescence may be a matter of weeks.

There is no laboratory method of making a certain diagnosis.

The clinical picture should be recognized during an epidemic, but may be easily confused with atypical dengue, and with influenza.

Diagnosis depends on clinical and epidemiological evidence. Treatment is entirely symptomatic.

## HAEMORRHAGIC FEVERS

### DEFINITION AND GEOGRAPHICAL DISTRIBUTION

Acute fevers, presumed to be of viral origin, with headache, general and localized pains, prostration, and haemorrhagic signs occurring in many parts of the world, including South and Central America, eastern and southern U.S.S.R., India, Pakistan, Bangladesh, Korea, South-east Asia, and Africa. Yellow fever is dealt with separately above.

Most haemorrhagic fevers are caused by arboviruses transmitted by mosquitoes, ticks, mites, and other vectors. Some are zoonoses, with special animal reservoirs. In some areas the viruses and vectors have been identified; in others they have not. In Africa transmission may occur via the discharges and secretions of animal reservoirs, usually rodents. (See Lassa, Marburg, and Ebola fevers later.)

For convenience, a few of the major haemorrhagic fevers are considered here separately as they occur in Asia and Africa. Some American fevers are mentioned with the African infections.

## ASIAN HAEMORRHAGIC FEVERS

### AETIOLOGY

Probably the most important current form of haemorrhagic fevers are those occurring in South-east Asia, transmitted by *Aedes* mosquitoes. These are caused by Group B viruses, including dengue Types II, I, III, and IV and the Group A virus chikungunya. Similar fevers have been reported from southern India. Haemorrhagic fevers transmitted by ticks occur in India and Russia and by mites in the Argentine.

Another Group B virus, in this case conveyed by ticks, which causes a haemorrhagic syndrome is the Kyasanur Forest virus. A closely related Group B virus conveyed by ticks causes a haemorrhagic fever in Omsk, USSR. Crimean haemorrhagic fever is conveyed by ticks; the causative agent is one of the ungrouped viruses. Group C viruses so far have not been found to cause haemorrhagic syndromes (see also p. 511). Neither the cause of the Korean form of haemorrhagic fever nor its vector has yet been identified; but there is every reason to believe that an arthropod-born virus was responsible for it. The vector is thought to have been a tick.

*South-east Asian haemorrhagic fever*

Autopsies on over 100 cases of South-east Asian mosquito-borne haemorrhagic fever between the ages of 5 months and 14 years with 75 under 5 years of
age have been described from Thailand. All were Thai, Chinese, or Thai–
Chinese.

Gross macroscopic pathological findings were non-specific and included
petechial haemorrhages in the stomach, jejunum and ileum, and in the endocardium, epicardium and, less frequently, the myocardium. Petechiae in the
lungs were mostly subpleural. Subcapsular haemorrhages were present in
some livers. Effusions into serous cavities were common, especially the pleural
cavity. The liver was enlarged in more than half and fatty changes and focal
necrosis were common. The spleen was slightly enlarged, congested; subcapsular haemorrhages were present in some.

The most significant microscopical findings were evidence of vascular
damage and haemorrhage and increased reticulo-endothelial activity.
Changes in the liver included fatty degeneration, acidophilic necrosis of liver
cells (mostly focal), and Kupffer cells. In some specimens there were cytoplasmic coagulative changes resembling the 'Councilman bodies' of yellow fever
and infiltration of the periportal areas with lymphoid cells, proliferation of the
Kupffer cells, and mononuclear concentrations in the sinusoids. Some lesions
may have arisen from the shock, in which sinusoidal congestion and central
necrosis of liver cells occurs; others may have been specific to the infection.
Liver necrosis of more extensive type has been reported (in a case in which
dengue virus was isolated).

Degenerative changes in the renal proximal convoluted tubules were
present but no frank tubular necrosis such as occurred in the Korean outbreak. (The children in shock from Thai haemorrhagic fever did not develop
the acute renal failure characteristic of Korean haemorrhagic fever in adults.)
Generalized vascular damage was probably the most important factor in the
disease; it showed essentially as diapedesis of erythrocytes around the blood
vessels in the skin, intestinal mucosa, and visceral organs. Necrosis or thrombosis of blood vessels was rare. Thrombocytopenia was a consistent finding.

*Korean haemorrhagic fever*

In this outbreak the vascular damage described in the South-east Asian
disease was again the prominent feature. Large haemorrhages were sometimes
present in the liver, spleen, and kidneys in which there were also scattered
areas of focal coagulative necrosis and sparse cellular infiltration, mostly
lymphocytes. A major difference from the South-east Asian disease was the
frequency of kidney lesions of the renal anoxia type with necrosis and degener-
tion of the epithelium of the distal and proximal convoluted tubules and
Henle's loop, with dilatation and plugging of the lumina with blood and

hyaline casts and debris. The glomeruli showed little change except that some were ischaemic; the cortical vessels were ischaemic and the medullary irregularly congested. These findings were to be expected in an illness in which the principal cause of death was renal failure with anuria and uraemia.

CLINICAL PICTURE

*South-east Asia mosquito-borne haemorrhagic fever*
Mosquito-borne haemorrhagic fever occurs in the Philippines, Thailand, Malaysia, Singapore, Indonesia, and Vietnam, in areas in which endemic dengue has been previously reported or occurs concurrently. Outbreaks also occur from time to time in parts of India.

The clinical picture varies from one geographical region to the other but a common pattern is clearly seen in Thailand, where it is primarily a disease of children up to 14 years of age with a peak incidence at 4–5 years. Cases have been very occasionally recorded in individuals as old as 20–21 years. The disease is practically confined to indigenous children (in Thailand, to Thais and Chinese). It is extremely rare in expatriate European children.

The severity varies from mild to fatal.

The onset is usually abrupt, with high fever which may become remittent or intermittent. There is general malaise and often a sore throat with infected pharynx and sometimes epistaxis. Headache and muscle and joint pains develop and there is usually some gastro-intestinal discomfort, nausea, and maybe some vomiting. The liver is commonly enlarged and palpable. The situation worsens progressively and by the second or third day in a serious case there may be bleeding from the gums, abdominal pain becomes more severe, and haematemesis and melaena appear. Extensive purpuric spots and petechiae may develop in the skin or there may be intracutaneous or subcutaneous haemorrhages and large ecchymoses. The patient becomes increasingly restless as the temperature now begins to fall. About the fourth or fifth day, especially when haemorrhagic manifestations are severe, shock may develop rapidly, with cold blotchy skin, low blood pressures, and sometimes convulsions.

Jaundice occurs in a few patients. Renal failure is rare.

The fatality rate after the appearance of shock varies from 15 to 50 per cent. Convalescence in cases which did not develop shock or which recover from it is usually rapid and uncomplicated.

In the Philippines the picture is somewhat similar but milder. Towards the end of the febrile period there may develop a scattered morbilliform rash principally on the extremities, chest, and back; there is no pruritus or desquamation such as is seen in dengue fever. Liver enlargement is uncommon in the Philippine disease, but is common in cases in Singapore and Penang.

*Other forms of haemorrhagic fever*

The clinical picture in other forms of haemorrhagic fever is often similar to the above, although in some episodes adults may be commonly involved. In some, acute renal failure with increasing uraemia may develop as the fever subsides. In such cases there is a high mortality rate. This was a common complication in the Korean outbreaks seen in expatriate troops in 1952–53.

*Korean haemorrhagic fever*

This disease, up to 1952, was divided into three clinical stages: febrile, toxic, and oliguric.

The febrile stage began suddenly with rigor and severe headache, retro-orbital pain, backache, and muscle pains. An irregular remittent fever of moderate intensity developed, which lasted for about 6 days. The patient was prostrated; nausea and vomiting were common. Petechial haemorrhages appeared on the skin and mucous membranes about the third day; haemorrhages into the skin were easily induced by trauma. Slight general lymphatic gland enlargement was common but the spleen and liver were not usually palpable. Heavy proteinuria developed from the third or fourth day and the output of urine was reduced. Erythrocytes and hyaline casts appeared in the urine at about the same time.

Throughout the illness there was usually a moderate leucocytosis and lowering of the platelet count.

The fever subsided by rapid lysis about the sixth day and the toxic phase developed. The symptoms, especially the backache, became more severe and the blood pressures fell notably. In some patients shock developed in the next 2 days.

Skin petechiae became more pronounced and sometimes haemorrhages appeared under the skin following slight injury. Bleeding from the nose and into the stomach and intestines occurred; haemorrhages developed in the lungs; there was sometimes visible haematuria. Oedema in the face and orbits, involving the conjunctivae, was common at this stage. In most cases the signs of shock then diminished and the haemorrhages stopped. Signs of renal failure then appeared. The output of urine diminished rapidly and within a day or two in the most severe cases anuria developed, with rising blood urea and the clinical picture of acute uraemia. Patients who reached this stage seldom survived. A few, however, did pass from oliguria into diuresis and recovered; evidence of damage to the renal epithelium persisted well into convalescence in the form of the passage of large quantities of dilute urine.

## DIAGNOSIS

In epidemics or outbreaks in endemic areas the clinical diagnosis is usually obvious.

The white cell count is low in most cases but there may be a moderate leucocytosis in others. There is marked thrombocytopenia and the bone marrow commonly shows arrest of the production of platelets from the megakaryocytes. Bleeding times are prolonged. The tourniquet test is positive early in the disease.

Urine contains protein. There is usually some oliguria and, where renal failure develops, anuria.

In South-east Asian haemorrhagic fever it is possible to isolate the virus from the blood in some cases. In Thailand the commonest agent isolated has been dengue Type II; this has also been isolated in the Philippines, Vietnam, Singapore, Malaysia, and in similar cases in Calcutta and Vellore in India. All dengue types have been recovered. In some areas in milder forms of the disease the Group A virus chikungunya has been isolated.

Serological diagnosis is commonly employed to determine a rising titre of viral antibodies. Identification of the serotype is difficult since the disease occurs in areas in which dengue virus infection is endemic.

### TREATMENT

There is no specific treatment.

The measures employed are those used to counter haemorrhage, thrombocytopenia, shock, dehydration, and renal failure when it occurs.

Blood transfusion is often necessary to replace blood lost in the haemorrhagic phase and platelet transfusion has been tried.

## AFRICAN AND AMERICAN HAEMORRHAGIC FEVERS

### A. Lassa fever

#### DEFINITION AND GEOGRAPHICAL DISTRIBUTION

Lassa fever is the fourth of the *Arenaviruses* known to affect man. These viruses derive their name from the 'sand sprinkled' appearance under the electron microscope. The type virus is lymphocytic chorio-meningitis. The disease has a world-wide distribution. The animal reservoirs are rodents, including hamsters and mice. Laboratory workers are thus at particular risk and frequently become infected. The disease is apparently often mild, occasionally meningitis or meningo-encephalitis may develop. The overall death rate is usually low in people living in endemic areas, but may be very high in some isolated outbreaks.

The two arenaviruses causing haemorrhagic fever in South America appear in restricted rural areas. Argentinian (Junin) haemorrhagic fever occurs in annual outbreaks in the maize-growing areas around Buenos Aires and the Provinces of Cordoba and Santa Fe. Farmers are most often attacked and outbreaks occur at harvesting time, when the reservoir hosts are most abundant. The mortality rate varies from 3 to 15 per cent.

Bolivian (Machupo) haemorrhagic fever occurs sporadically in rural areas of the northern provinces of the country.

Transmission of these diseases is nearly always from animal to man in bad living conditions where the reservoir animal's faeces and urine can contaminate food and water. Man-to-man infection is uncommon.

The transmission of Lassa fever depends on a rodent reservoir, which does not itself become ill, but which transmits the virus through its faeces and urine by contamination of food and water, or by blood and tissue fluids in those, such as laboratory workers, who are in contact with the reservoir animals. Man-to-man transmission occurs in conditions of close contact, where the individual concerned is dealing with urine, faeces, autopsy material, etc. The modes of transmission in 'outbreaks' in rural areas are not known.

The disease was first described in 1969 in a European missionary nurse in Lassa, North Eastern State, Nigeria. She and one of her nurses died. A second nurse who had been in attendance developed the disease and was flown to the U.S.A., where the virus was recovered from urine and blood and a laboratory infection occurred. A year later there was a small outbreak in the same area of Nigeria, with thirteen deaths in twenty-eight recorded cases. Serological evidence shows the infection to be widespread in Nigeria. Lassa fever also occurs in Liberia and Sierra Leone and there is serological evidence of its presence in Guinea, Mozambique, and the Central African Empire, in which no outbreaks with high fatality have been reported. Thus, infection in the local population must generally be mild or asymptomatic, and the serious clinical effects are seen in relatively few, as in yellow fever. This is illustrated by the much higher death rate seen in hospital patients (about 35–40 per cent) as compared with that in the general community (about 2–3 per cent). Gilles has reported a high incidence of subclinical and mild cases in rural populations in Sierra Leone, with low death rate; more serious cases are few and treated in hospital, where the death rate is much higher.

### AETIOLOGY

The epidemiology is still not fully understood. In the first outbreak in Nigeria, all cases were Europeans; in the second, all except one were Nigerians. The rodent maintenance host in Nigeria is the multimammate rat *Mastomys natalensis* and transmission occurs usually via urine and excreta infecting water and foodstuffs in insanitary conditions; or from patients by aerosol transmission or by direct contact with blood or other tissue fluids, for example during sampling of blood, or while doing an autopsy.

### CLINICAL PICTURE AND PATHOLOGY

The onset is gradual over a few days of malaise, chills, headache, muscle, and joint pains, and sometimes increasing nausea. The illness begins with fever.

Lassa fever should be suspected in any febrile patient from a known infected area, especially if prostration is greater than would normally be expected from the height of the fever. Sore throat, with white patches on the fauces is a common early sign followed by ulcerative pharyngitis with enlargement and tenderness of local glands. There is sometimes a rash which develops early and may become petechial. Vomiting is frequent as are severe muscular thoracic and abdominal pains. A cough develops, with signs of pneumonitis. The toxicity increases and serous effusions appear, especially in the pleural cavities. The pleural effusion is usually blood-stained. There may be facial and ankle oedema. Bleeding from mucous membranes with haematemesis, malaena, and haematuria and other haemorrhagic signs, may develop. The patient becomes progressively disorientated and may pass into coma. Death occurs in about 50 per cent of severe cases within a fortnight of the onset. It is caused by acute myocardial failure, shock, or pneumonitis. In the patients who recover, the illness recedes after 2–3 weeks and convalescence is slow.

As pointed out above, most cases in endemic areas are mild or asymptomatic and do not go on to develop the whole picture.

At autopsy, the usual findings are patchy pneumonitis, sometimes haemorrhagic, haemorrhagic pleural effusion, and acute mycocarditis with round cell tissue infiltration. In the early stages there is acute pharyngeal inflammation with ulceration.

### DIAGNOSIS

Certain diagnosis can be made only by isolation of the virus (from excreta, blood, tissue fluids, etc.) in tissue culture carried out under the strictest supervision in properly organized laboratories.

The flourescent antibody technique is the most rapid serological diagnostic method. Complement-fixation tests are slower to become positive, usually by the fourteenth day, using Lassa virus antigen. These tests are useful diagnostically only if serial serum specimens are obtained from the beginning of the illness onwards. Otherwise, they are valuable tools for mapping endemic areas.

### TREATMENT AND MANAGEMENT

There is no specific treatment. Shock, dehydration, etc., are dealt with by standard methods. In one case it has been shown that plasma from a recently convalescent patient appeared to be effective in limiting the infection and aborting the clinical effects. At present, it is believed that this transfer of passive immunity may be the only specific way to help the patient. As blood containing immune bodies is likely to be available only in the endemic areas, the patient should be treated on the spot.

Known or suspect cases have recently been flown by aeroplane out of the endemic areas to Europe and the U.S.A. This could be a dangerous health hazard. Fortunately, Lassa fever does not appear to be highly infective except under special circumstances, including direct contact with tissues, secretions and blood. Thus, a case was flown to the U.K. from Sierra Leone on a scheduled flight, severely ill, and within 4 days of onset. The patient, who recovered, was treated at home and later in a general hospital. No fellow passengers, family, or laboratory or medical personnel became infected.

The excreta of acutely ill patients is highly infective; so are the vomit and pharyngeal secretions and saliva. The virus is present in the blood throughout the illness and for at least a fortnight afterwards. It may be present over an even longer period in the urine. Air-borne infection has not been demonstrated.

Contacts must be watched over a period of at least 3 weeks and regarded as suspect if they become febrile.

### B. The Marburg group of viruses: Ebola fever

Cases of fever associated with haemorrhagic features appeared sporadically and as an epidemic in southern Sudan between July and September 1976. At about the same time similar diseases broke out in the neighbouring areas of Zaïre. An epidemic developed which involved the rural community and many of the staff of hospitals dealing with severe cases, suggesting possible person-to-person transmission.

The clinical pictures seen in this epidemic closely resembled those seen in the outbreak in Germany in Marburg and Frankfurt in 1967—from which the infecting agent (a virus) received its name, the 'Marburg' virus. This infection was reported again in 1975 in South Africa in a few people who had passed through Rhodesia on the way to the Cape.

In the epidemics in Sudan and Zaïre in 1976, the illness began with a sudden high fever, sometimes with rigors, but usually with little prodromata, sore throat with characteristic erythema, and later small areas of yellowish exudate, chest pains, a dry cough, and vomiting and diarrhoea, which was sometimes profuse. Anorexia and dysphagia were common. There were acute muscle and joint pains. Dehydration was rapid and severe. Haemorrhagic signs developed after a few days. There was acute epistaxis, with subconjunctival haemorrhages, haemoptysis, haematemesis, melaena, and haematuria. In some cases a generalized body rash developed, including the palms and soles, more easily seen in white than black skins, and followed by itchy desquamation. Leucopenia was common and there was usually a notable reduction in the thrombocyte count. There were no characteristic changes in other coagulation factors.

In all, there were over 500 notified cases, with more than 300 deaths by the end of November 1976. The death rate outside hospital has not been calculated. It may well have been low, as many cases were probably mild or even subclinical.

The epidemics eventually came under control, following the efforts of a combined Sudanese–WHO team and of a joint international Commission in Zaïre.

The organism was isolated. It was morphologically indistinguishable from the Marburg virus—a large rod-shaped RNA virus—but was antigenically totally different. The virus has been labelled 'Ebola', after a small stream in Zaïre flowing near a village from which the first isolate was recovered.

The Marburg and Ebola viruses share no antigenic relationship to one another or to any other known virus.

The Marburg outbreak was reported first in 1967 in Marburg and Frankfurt. It occurred in people who had been working on the blood, tissues, and tissue cultures of *Cercopithecus* monkeys recently imported from Uganda, or on the blood and secretions of patients. It did not develop in those that handled whole monkeys.

The clinical picture was much as described above and of the 29 persons infected 7 died. Autopsy revealed necrotic cellular lesions in the liver and other organs, including the kidneys, with transformation of lymphoid tissue to plasma calls and monocytes. Liver damage was accompanied by signs of tissue regeneration, as in hepatitis.

Diagnosis was confirmed by inoculation of blood on tissue suspensions into guinea-pigs or hamsters in which the infection is fatal (also in Rhesus monkeys). Paired sera were also examined, using a complement fixation test.

It was at first thought that the *Ceropithecus aethiops* monkey from Uganda was the probable natural reservoir of the infection but this is now considered unlikely and the animal reservoir is unknown. Nevertheless, the disease was for some time called 'the green monkey disease'. That the disease is African, and not something accidentally picked up in transit via airports, is shown by the recent appearance of cases in a small group of individuals who reached South Africa after passing through Zimbabwe-Rhodesia.

The need for monkey and other animal tissue for tissue culture and the production of vaccines, such as the poliomyelitis vaccine, is such that, as the developed world demands more and more animals for biological materials and research, collectors will have to plunge deeper into untapped areas for supplies and may from time to time come up against infections to which man has not previously been exposed. The Marburg viruses are examples, since the natural reservoirs have still not been determined.

*Movement of febrile passengers by air*

Marburg, Ebola, and Lassa fevers well illustrate the dangers and uncertainties of air transport of febrile patients suffering from unknown infections.

In the U.K. special isolation facilities have been prepared for reception of suspected cases and the diseases are now notifiable. Surveillance of contacts is also carried out. Until there is more certain evidence of the modes of transmission, the present high security measures should rightly be enforced in all countries.

In the course of time it is likely that more diseases of this kind will be uncovered. They illustrate the significance of removing 'the evil at source' by eradication in endemic areas.

The panic Lassa fever and Marburg and Ebola fevers have caused in Europe and U.S.A. has, in fact, greatly helped the growing campaigns against export/import of exotic disease, especially by air, and has emphasized once again the vital significance of obtaining a geographical history from every patient and of providing more rigorous international measures for movement of febrile patients.


## VIRUS MENINGO-ENCEPHALITIS

Meningo-encephalitis is commonly caused by arboviruses, which often have a typical geographical distribution. Syndromes include St Louis encephalitis, the reservoirs of which are chickens and other birds; Western, Eastern, and Venezuelan equine encephalomyelitis, the reservoirs of which are horses, mules, and sometimes birds; Russian spring–summer encephalitis spread by ticks from wild rodents, and Japanese B encephalitis. The diseases caused by these viruses vary in severity but the clinical features are essentially the result of involvement of the brain and cord.

Japanese B encephalitis may be taken as an example.

This disease, which is endemic in some regions and sometimes epidemic, is caused by a Group B arbovirus transmitted in various geographical areas, including Japan, Thailand, Malaysia, the Philippines, Burma, and India, by certain species of *Culex* especially *C. tritaeniorhynchus* and *C. gelidus* mosquitoes. There is some evidence that one of the principal maintenance hosts in Asian areas may be pigs.

The incubation period is about a week. Onset is acute, with moderate remittent fever usually with bradycardia and subsiding after a few days, muscular rigidity and exaggerated tendon reflexes. There is a headache, mental disturbance, disorientation, and in the severe cases coma may develop. In the acute stage there is pronounced lethargy but the muscle tone is high. All degrees of spasticity may occur and there may be clonic contractions or general convulsions. In some cases, signs of meningeal irritation may dominate the picture and lead to errors of diagnosis. Rigidity of the neck and back muscles and sometimes the masseter muscles is common. Muscular tremors occur especially in the facial muscles and hands. There may be inco-ordination. In some serious cases paralysis occurs as a result of extension of the lesions to the cord. The eye muscles are not usually involved.

The acute clinical state may be fulminating, with death in 24–48 hours. Commonly, the disease lasts 7–10 days and recovery is slow. Neurological sequelae are uncommon but the mental symptoms often clear slowly and the muscular tremors may persist for weeks or months and raise the question of the diagnosis of disseminated sclerosis.

In some outbreaks the mortality rate in severe cases is as high as 50 per cent. Serological studies have indicated that infection without clinical effect is very common in endemic areas.

Diagnosis is often indicated by a knowledge of the endemic areas or during an epidemic. It may be confirmed serologically, by complement fixation, haemagglutination, or mouse-protection tests.

The cerebrospinal fluid usually indicates the presence of a non-specific inflammatory reaction. It may be under moderate increased pressure. Mono-cytic cells are increased in number, but the fluid is seldom cloudy. The protein content is usually raised only moderately but may be over 300 mg per cent.

There is no specific treatment.

Mouse-brain and kidney vaccines are under trial for protection of exposed populations.

Mosquito control is at present impracticable. Spread of infection is often worsened by socio-economic developments involving water conservation.

# 35

# WORM INFECTIONS, MISCELLANEOUS

In this chapter various infections or infestations with nematodes, cestodes, and trematodes are discussed.

Hookworm infection is described in Chapter 11; Filariasis and Dracontiasis in Chapter 7; Schistosomiasis in Chapter 23.

## ASCARIASIS

### DEFINITION

Ascariasis is the condition of infection with the large round-worm, *Ascaris lumbricoides*. Light infections rarely cause clinical signs; heavy infections may result in symptoms and signs due to the mechanical effects of the presence of the worms.

### GEOGRAPHICAL DISTRIBUTION

This parasite occurs ubiquitously, irrespective of climate. It is a dirt disease and is most prevalent where cleanliness and sanitation are defective or absent.

### AETIOLOGY AND CLINICAL PICTURE

The adult worms are large, ivory-white, and cylindrical with pointed ends. They are of two sexes; the males, which have coiled tails, measure about 15 cm and the females about 22 cm in length. The adults inhabit the lumen of the small bowel, where they are unattached and move freely. They possess an alimentary tract and gain their nutriment from the intestinal contents. The females, whether impregnated or not, extrude numerous eggs which are passed in the stools of the patient. In the fertilized eggs, after passage to the exterior, there develops a vermicule. The egg is then infective if swallowed. The eggs are extraordinarily resistant to environmental change and even to antiseptics; they survive for months or even years in a viable state in the open; and they may be blown about in dust. Infection with occasional worms is explained by these facts. Infection with numerous worms is the result of gross faecal pollution of food or drink.

547

On swallowing eggs containing vermicules the latter emerge, bore into the wall of the small intestine, and are carried in the circulation to the lungs, where they lodge. The vermicules penetrate into the alveoli, are expelled via the bronchioles, bronchi, and trachea, are swallowed, and then pass through the stomach to the small bowel, where they become adult males and females.

The migration of large numbers of larvae at one time may cause a severe verminous pneumonitis. There is a cough, with blood-stained sputum in which larvae may be found on microscopical examination. In certain susceptible persons, under these conditions, there may be generalized allergic manifestations, with an eosinophilia. When the number of migrating larvae is small their passage usually escapes notice.

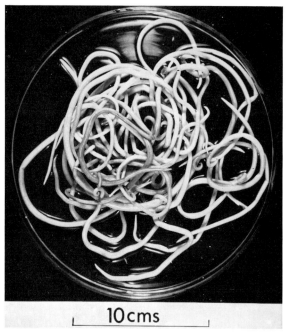

10cms

FIG. 64. *A. lumbricoides.* Worms from patient after treatment.
[Courtesy Mr J.Brady]

A few adult worms in the small intestine do not usually give rise to any symptoms. A worm or worms may be passed in the stools. When a worm wanders from its normal site of election into the stomach it may be vomited. Sometimes it may ascend the oesophagus and pass through the nasopharynx to emerge from a nostril.

Numerous worms, and they may number as many as two hundred, in the small bowel cause abdominal discomfort and distension. A small child with a heavy ascaris infestation will have a protruding belly. Intestinal obstruction, perforation, or volvulus may be a result of the infection. Occasionally worms ascend the common bile duct or pancreatic duct and cause obstruction or rupture.

If mature female worms are present, eggs will be found in the stools on microscopical examination. These eggs may be infertile if female worms alone are present, or fertile if both sexes are represented.

Adult worms may be passed in the faeces, vomited, or occasionally appear in the nasopharynx.

As pointed out above (p. 172), where ascaris and hookworm infection are present in the same patient, drugs should be employed which are active against both infections.

Eosinophilia, except when there is an allergic reaction to the worms, is unusual.

Caution should be exercised when treating children with large loads of ascarids; if all the worms are affected simultaneously a tangled mass of them may cause intestinal obstruction or even rupture. Repeated dosage, with small amounts of a drug and the removal of a few worms at a time, is wiser under such circumstances.

Piperazine salts (the citrate, adipate, or phosphate) when given as a single dose are effective ascaricides. The dose is 4 g; this should be followed next day by a saline purge to evacuate the affected worms. Prepared in the form of a syrup the drug is acceptable to children and given in a single dose does not cause toxicity.

Mebendazole in tablet form in a dosage of 100 mg twice daily for 3 consecutive days is safe and very effective in ascariasis in children. No side effects have been reported.

Bephenium hydroxynaphthoate (Alcopar) which is effective against hookworms is also active against *Ascaris*. The dose for adults is a single one of 2.5 g (base); that for infants under 2 years of age is half this. When there is diarrhoea treatment should be continued for 3 days. Neither fasting nor purging is necessary, and the treatment is devoid of toxicity.

# ENTEROBIASIS

Threadworm or pinworm infection is due to the presence in the intestine of the small nematode *Enterobius vermicularis*. The emergence of the gravid female worms from the anus on to the surrounding skin causes irritation. Scratching may cause a severe dermatitis.

World-wide and uninfluenced by climate.

*E. vermicularis* is a strictly human parasite. The worms are small, white, and thread-like; the sexes are distinct; the males, which have coiled tails, measure about 5 mm, and the females 15–20 mm in length. The insignificant males are rarely seen, as they perish within the bowel. The adult worms live unattached and free in the lumen of the lower small and the large intestine. They have an alimentary tract and obtain their nutriment from the intestinal contents. The parturient female worms emerge from the anus on to the perianal and perineal skin. Here they die and disintegrate, liberating many eggs, which are colourless, transparent, and asymmetrical, flattened on one side; each fertilized egg contains a single coiled larva. The eggs are sticky and adhere to skin or clothing; they are readily transferred to towels and other linen. Embryonated eggs are infective. On being swallowed the larvae develop into adult male and female worms within the small intestine. The male worm dies after fertilizing the female, which migrates to the rectum.

The worms within the intestine rarely cause symptoms, though their presence in the vermiform appendix may precipitate an attack of appendicitis. The migration of the parturient female worms through the anus, particularly at night, to the surrounding skin causes severe itching, which may become intolerable and seriously interfere with sleep. The consequent scratching may result in septic dermatitis. In the process of scratching the fingers and finger nails become contaminated with embryonated eggs, which can thus readily be conveyed to the mouth. This is especially the case with children, who tend thus to reinfect themselves to an increasing degree. Cross-infection by contamination of linen and towels readily occurs and when one member of a household becomes infected with threadworms sooner or later the remainder are likely to acquire the infection. It is therefore advisable to ensure that no more than a single person of a family is infected before undertaking only his treatment.

In cases of heavy infestation the patient may notice female worms on his finger tips after scratching the perianal region.

Occasionally a worm may be seen in the stools. Eggs are not passed in the faeces. They are found on the perianal skin. A scraping may be made with a knife blade, preferably on rising from the night's rest. Better, a swab consisting of a small piece of cellophane on the end of a wire, glass-rod or stick can be rolled over the area. The eggs adhere to the cellophane, which is opened out, moistened, and examined microscopically under a cover-slip.

TREATMENT

First, if possible, the cycle of self-reinfection must be controlled or broken. This is attempted by scrupulous cleanliness, the wearing of occlusive clothing (drawers and gloves) to prevent scratching, and the daily boiling of all possibly infected linen. If completely successful this measure alone may result in freedom from threadworms within 2 months.

Mebendazole, given as a single dose of 100 mg, irespective of age, is the drug of choice. Piperazine salts (the citrate, adipate, or phosphate) are effective and have negligible side-effects. The dosage is 300 mg of the citrate for each year of age up to a maximum of 1.8 g given in two doses daily by mouth for a week.

Pripsen granules contain 4 g of piperazine phosphate and standardized senna laxative. The dose for children up to 6 years is 7.5 g ($\frac{2}{3}$ of a sachet); above that age, and for adults, it is 10 g (4 teaspoonsful); the granules are swallowed in milk or water in the morning by children and usually at bedtime by adults. A single dose treatment is effective but retreatment after 2 weeks is desirable.

Viprynium (Vanquin) suspension, containing the equivalent of 10 mg of anhydrous base per millilitre, in a single dose, is effective for this infection and devoid of toxicity. For children under 2 years, 5 ml is given by mouth; for those of 2–4 years, 7.5 ml; 4–7 years, 10–15 ml; 7–13 years, 15–20 ml; and over this 25–30 ml. The stools are stained red.

Thiabendazole (Mintezol), 25 mg per kg body weight twice daily for 2–3 days or 50 mg per kg body weight on two occasions with a 12-hour interval is also very effective.

STRONGYLOIDIASIS

DEFINITION: LIFE CYCLE

A widely spread condition due to infection with *Strongyloides stercoralis,* especially common in parts of China, South-east Asia, South America, Africa, and other areas which are suitable for development of the worm. The life cycle of the worm varies according to the environmental circumstances. The basic cycle involves a free-living adult stage in warm, moist, faecal soil. Rhabditiform larvae are passed in human faeces and after three moults develop in the soil into free-living adults. This cycle may be repeated indefinitely in the right conditions. When conditions are bad, fine delicate filariform larvae are formed. These pierce the human skin, reach the right side of the heart, and escape through the pulmonary vessels into the alveoli. A few mature in the bronchi but the majority pass over the trachea to reach the small intestine. The males are passed in the faeces. The fertilized females penetrate into the mucosa, where they lay dozens of eggs each day. The eggs hatch in the mucosa and the rhabditiform larvae escape into the lumen and thence to the stool. So

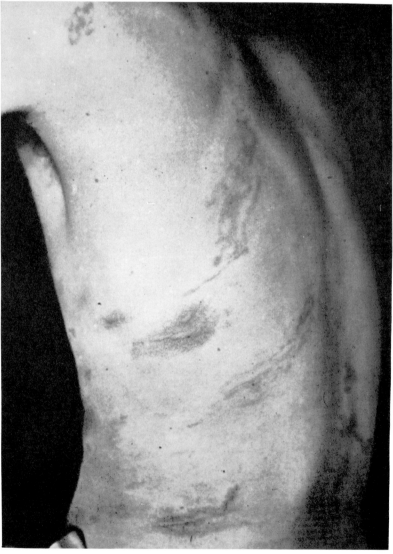

FIG. 65. Skin reactions in strongyloidiasis.

long as the environment is suitable, the free-living cycle is repeated but sooner or later filariform infective larvae are again formed. Sometimes filariform larvae are formed during the passage down the intestine and penetrate either the mucosa or the skin near the anus and repeat the tissue life-cycle; this process is called autoinfection.

In a given individual infection may persist for years.

### CLINICAL PICTURE

As a rule the intestinal infection produces no appreciable clinical signs. There may be occasional gastro-intestinal upsets and discomfort in heavy infections but there is little evidence that the worm is responsible.

The most pronounced lesions occur in the skin especially in individuals, for example ex-Far East prisoners of war, who have been infected for many years. An eruption, characterized by blotchy urticaria and arteriolar flare, and a form of 'creeping eruption', with reddened serpiginous lesions moving beneath the skin of the trunk and limbs, is common in chronic strongyloid carriers. The individual lesions are themselves transitory, tending to subside in a few hours, but the manifestations as a whole may continue for some days at a time, with long quiescent intervals between attacks. Oedema and itching of the finger tips has been recorded. Areas of violently itchy urticaria, oedema, and erythema, especially around the anal region, are also frequently attributed to strongyloid infection. It has been suggested that these arise from production of filariform larvae during passage of the rhabditiform larvae along the gut, so short-circuiting the free-living cycle. The filariform larvae penetrate the intestinal wall or perianal skin and set up dermal sensitivity reactions.

A few fatal overwhelming infections with very extensive intestinal lesions have been described in children.

### DIAGNOSIS: TREATMENT

The actively motile larvae closely resembling those of the hookworm can be seen in low power preparations of faeces.

Thiabendazole (Mintezol) is the most effective therapeutic agent. It is given in doses of 25 mg per kg body weight twice daily for 2–3 days. No starvation or purgation is necessary. Side-effects include giddiness, nausea sometimes with vomiting, and diarrhoea. The drug is expensive.

A good alternative, which is cheaper and free from side-effects in children, is mebendazole orally 100 mg twice daily for 3 consecutive days.

## LARVA MIGRANS

### CUTANEOUS (CREEPING ERUPTIONS)

The larvae of certain nematodes unnatural to man, and occasionally the larvae of *Ancylostoma duodenale* and *Necator americanus* may cause cutaneous lesions, called creeping eruptions, which result from their presence in the immediately sub-epithelial skin layers. Common causes of creeping eruptions are *Ancylostoma braziliense* and *A. caninum*, the hookworms of cats and dogs.

A minute papule may appear at the site of entry of the larva. From here the larva moves irregularly about, forming a serpiginous tunnel between the corium and the stratum granulosum of the epithelium. It may wander very slowly in this way for months and will not develop further while it remains in the unadapted host. The lesion in the proximity of the wandering larva is at first erythematous, then raised above the skin surface and finally vesicular. There is local infiltration with eosinophils and lymphocytes. The active lesion is commonly surrounded by an arteriolar flare.

It occurs most commonly in the feet, hands and buttocks. Serpiginous tunnels are burrowed by the larvae in the superficial layers of the skin. A slightly raised erythematous vesicular eruption follows, accompanied by intense pruritus. The lesions first appear as erythematous itchy papules 2–3 days after exposure and may last several weeks. They advance slowly. As the larvae advance the lesions heal behind them, becoming dried and often crusted. Secondary infection from scratching is common.

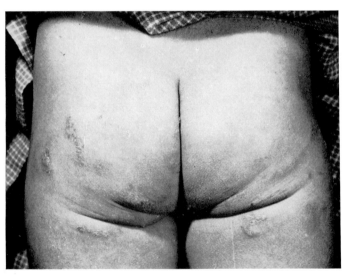

FIG. 66. Larva migrans. *A. braziliense.*
[Courtesy Dr D.R.Seaton]

More transient lesions occur occasionally in aberrant infections with filariform larvae of *Strongyloides stercoralis* (see above).

Creeping eruptions somewhat similar to those due to aberrant round worm larvae may arise from cutaneous infection with the larvae of certain flies, for instance from infection with the larva of the horse bot fly (*Gastero-philus* spp.), each lesion containing a single minute larva, which has hatched from eggs deposited on the hairs, usually of the limbs. The much larger larva of the cattle warble fly *Hypoderma bovis* may give rise to similar lesions.

Creeping eruption may be dealt with by local cauterization, by spraying the infected region with ethyl chloride or by the application of carbon dioxide snow or ethyl acetate.

Thiobendazole is the treatment of choice in larva migrans caused by helminths. It is given in a dose of 25 mg per kg body weight twice daily for 2–3 consecutive days. Alternatively, a dose of 25 mg per kg body weight may be given twice in 1 day and the dose repeated once a week for a further 3 weeks. Local itching may be relieved by antihistaminic drugs.

### VISCERAL LARVA MIGRANS

The importance of visceral larva migrans is now well established. The lesions are produced by nematode larvae which gain access to the viscera of un-adapted hosts; occasionally under unsuitable conditions they may be pro-duced by larvae of nematodes in the natural host.

In man the commonest lesions result from infection with the dog and cat ascarids *Toxocara canis* or *T. cati.*

Children especially become infected by swallowing infective eggs. The rhabditiform larvae escape into the upper small intestine and invade the mucosa, reaching the mesenteric venules and lymphatics, and eventually the viscera, usually the lungs and liver, where they are caught up. No further development takes place but the larvae remain alive for months. Single or multiple, even miliary, lesions containing secondary-stage larvae develop in this way, the number depending upon the number of eggs swallowed and hatched.

Lesions are identified at autopsy or biopsy of the appropriate tissue. They appear as minute, greyish granulomata, commonly seeded under the capsule of the liver or in the lungs, the kidneys, the heart, striated muscle, the brain, and the eye. In the eye they develop in days or weeks, as granulomata in the retina, in the vicinity of the macula. Eye lesions are nearly always unilateral.

Histological examination reveals a reaction not unlike an early tubercle, with an outer ring of lymphocytes and polymorphs, within which are layers of histiocytes and epithelioid cells which may be pallisaded or form atypical giant cells. The granuloma is eventually walled off by concentric fibrosis. In recently formed lesions the living larva lies near the centre and can be mechanically expressed. It may ultimately become necrotic or calcified.

Clinical signs depend on the number of lesions, i.e. upon the intensity of infection and upon the organ affected. There may be fever, pulmonary infiltration, hepatomegaly and sometimes encephalitis. The eye granulomata on the retina are sometimes mistaken for a retinoblastoma. General reactions include considerable eosinophilia.

Rarely, larvae from *A. braziliense* or *A. caninum,* which have escaped from the skin into the circulation may cause similar lesions; these have also been reported in autoinfections with *S. stercoralis.*

Diagnosis depends on identification of larvae in the tissues. Tentative diagnosis can be made by fluorescent antibody techniques (after absorption with *Ascaris* extracts, to exclude cross reactions) Intradermal tests using extracts of *T. canis* adults are useful for epidemiological surveys.

Treatment is not always satisfactory. Thiabendazole in the dosage given for larva migrans is probably the best drug. Diethylcarbamizine in doses of 3 mg per kg body weight thrice daily for 3 weeks may also be effective. In view of possible allergic reactions, the dosage should be small to begin with and increased gradually, as in filariasis (see p. 81).

Mebendazole is under trial and appears successful.

## GNATHOSTOMIASIS

In many parts of the East, including India, Burma, Thailand, and China, infections with this nematode have now been reported. Infection follows the ingestion of raw fish flesh containing the encysted third-stage larva of *Gnathostoma spinigerum.*

The commonest sign is a single, slowly migratory, subcutaneous swelling which may appear anywhere including the abdominal wall, the chest, the face, or the hands (including the fingers) and feet. The swelling is of variable size. It may remain intermittently in one area for days or weeks or wander from one region to another. It is usually itchy but painless, occasionally accompanied by severe boring pain. It is firm and non-pitting and suppuration is rare. Histologically there is intense inflammatory eosinophilic infiltration and the worm may sometimes be visible. Occasionally it may be seen through the skin and can then be removed. The worm has been removed from the *cervix uteri* in a case of leucorrhoea. It has recently been demonstrated as a cause of eosinophilic meningitis and myeloencephalitis.

The swelling is caused by the migration of the immature adult (about 6 mm × 0.8 mm). There is a high eosinophilia and various other systemic signs have been reported in individual cases, including paroxysmal coughing, haematuria, and spontaneous pneumothorax.

Diagnosis is made by finding the adult or by the use of specific antigens for skin reactions.

Removal of the worm usually leads to cure, since there is rarely more than one worm present.

No chemotherapy has proved fully successful although relief has been obtained with the usual doses of diethylcarbamazine.

The reservoir animals are dogs and cats. The adults live in the stomach. Eggs are passed in the faeces, hatch in water, and the larvae are ingested by *Cyclops.* Fish eat the cyclops and the third-stage larva encysts in their muscles. The infection of man thus occurs only in areas where raw fish is regularly consumed.

## EOSINOPHILIC MENINGO-ENCEPHALITIS

Eosinophilic meningitis occurs sporadically and occasionally in small epi demics in certain Pacific Islands, including Tahiti and Hawaii, and in South-east Asia, including Vietnam and Thailand.

In most cases the condition results from the invasion of the central nervous system by developing adults of nematodes, the commonest of which is *Angiostrongylus cantonensis,* the rat lung worm. Infection occurs through ingestion as food of raw freshwater crustaceans (prawns), crabs, slugs, and land snails containing the larvae of the worm. A recent case in Thailand was caused by the developing adult of *Gnathostoma spinigerum.* The pathogenic action of the worms arises from mechanical damage to the brain substance and secondary inflammatory allergic reactions in the vicinity of the parasites. The disease has been experimentally reproduced in rhesus monkeys by feeding them with *A. cantonensis* larvae.

The clinical picture of fever and signs of meningeal and brain involvement, with cerebrospinal fluid under pressure and containing many cells, predominantly eosinophils, develops 3 or more weeks after eating the infected intermediate host.

Recovery is spontaneous in most cases, with few sequelae. Occasionally some paresis of the eye muscles and even mental changes may persist.

Diagnosis is often clinical. Specific serological tests using haemagglutination techniques are under trial. The worm has been found in the brain and cord at autopsy.

There is no specific treatment but adrenal corticosteroids in the usual doses have proved useful during the period of severe illness.

## TRICHURIASIS

*Trichuris trichiura,* the whip-worm, is a common nematode parasite of man. It is world-wide in its distribution and is especially prevalent in the tropics. The adult worms are of two sexes; they measure from 30 to 50 mm in length; the anterior part of the worms is slender and filiform and the posterior two-fifths is bulky and fleshy. The worms attach themselves by their heads to the mucosa, chiefly of the caecum and upper large bowel. The female worms discharge characteristic barrel-shaped, bile-stained ova, which have a plug at each end.

Infection results from swallowing eggs which have become embryonated some 2 weeks after being passed to the exterior in the stools. The embryos emerge, attach themselves to the bowel wall, and grow into adult worms. The presence of the latter usually causes no symptoms or gross pathology. Exceptionally massive lower bowel infestations with this worm have caused bloody diarrhoea, anaemia, and prolapse of the rectum, especially in malnourished children. The diagnosis is made by finding the eggs in the stools.

Mebendazole, 100 mg orally twice daily for 3 days, is highly effective in moderate infections and is the drug of choice.

Thiabendazole, 25 mg per kg body weight, repeated at 12-hour intervals for 2–3 days is stated to clear this infection in about half of those treated with it.

Dichlorvos in slow resin release formula as a single dose of 12 mg per kg body weight is about as effective but has some disquieting side-effects.

### CAPILLARIASIS

Human capillariasis is relatively uncommon, but large numbers of cases have been recorded over the last decade in North Luzon, the Philippines. The worm concerned has been named *Capillaria philippinensis*; it is similar to but not identical with *C. hepatica*. The clinical history was usually one of several months' irregular but intractable diarrhoea, with progressive weakness, loss of weight, emaciation, dehydration and, in untreated cases, eventual death. Oedema of the ankles is common, sometimes extending to the thighs and lower trunk. The stools containing the worm eggs are watery, greenish, non-offensive, containing some faecal matter but no blood or mucus. There is vague abdominal pain, usually epigastric and sometimes griping. In severe cases evidence of intestinal malabsorption can be demonstrated; there is increased faecal fat excretion (a mean of 25 g daily) and decreased xylose excretion. Total serum protein and albumin concentrations are low in severe cases and excretion of tagged albumin has been found to be greatly increased. Some patients are anaemic, others not. Eosinophil counts are raised in some, not in others.

At autopsy in the Philippines cases there was found flattening and sometimes obliteration of villi of the small intestine, especially in the jejunum. Infections were heavy. Parasites were present in the lumen and intestinal wall, mostly in the jejunum. There were scattered local haemorrhages but little obvious reaction to the worms, which were attached either with both anterior and posterior ends free, or with the anterior filiform end inserted (as is the case with *Trichuris*).

The epidemiology of the outbreak is not yet fully worked out. The infection is acquired by eating raw fish and crustaceans found in scattered areas of small lakes and rivers.

Diagnosis is made by finding the eggs and sometimes adults in the stool.

Treatment consists of replacement of fluid and electrolytes and iron, when needed.

Thiabendazole is effective in doses of 25 mg per kg body weight twice daily for 2–3 days. Egg counts in the stools fall notably by the third day from the beginning of treatment and adults were extruded.


## ANISAKIASIS

Anisakiasis (herring worm disease), is one of the very few infections which may result from eating raw salt-water fish. The disease is caused by eating fish infected with the nematode worm *Anisakis* spp. It is common in the Far East, notably Japan, and was once common in Holland and occurred in Denmark. Infected fish have recently been discovered off small islands in Indonesia but no human cases have so far been reported from this country.

The larvae of the worm ingested in the fish penetrate the walls of the stomach and small intestine, giving rise to acute granulomatous reactions and causing local oedema. The surface ulcerates, with bleeding and eventually a submucosal abscess may form, containing the larva. The patient complains of abdominal pain and discomfort, resembling those of peptic and duodenal ulceration. There is commonly high eosinophilia.

Diagnosis is frequently made at operation for suspected stomach and intestinal ulceration. In resections of the intestine, the ascarid larva may be dissected out.

It measures 20 × 1 mm and has a tooth at the anterior end.

A fluorescent antibody test, using larval sections as antigen, has been used successfully for serological diagnosis.

There is no specific treatment.

Smoking, pickling, and salting the herrings or the other occasional hosts does not usually kill the infective larvae. On the other hand, deep freezing seems to be lethal. The disease has thus become rare in Holland today. It is still common in rural fishing areas of Japan, where it is believed many cases remain undetected.


## HEPATIC FLUKE INFECTIONS

### CLONORCHIASIS

Clonorchiasis is the name given to a state of infection of the bile passages with the trematode *Clonorchis sinensis*.

## GEOGRAPHICAL DISTRIBUTION

The infection occurs only in the Far East, in some parts of which it is very prevalent. It is endemic throughout most of China and in Vietnam, Taiwan, Korea, and Japan, wherever raw freshwater fish is eaten.

## AETIOLOGY

*C. sinensis* has been recovered from the livers of man, dogs, cats, pigs, and of a number of other animals. The adult flukes measure from 10 to 25 mm in length and from 3 to 5 mm in breadth. They contain both male and female genitalia. The golden-brown, operculated eggs are of a truncated ovoid shape and measure 27–35 μm by 11–20 μm; they are discharged via the common bile duct and are mature when discharged in the stools, each containing a miracidium. Miracidia emerge from the eggs when they are ingested by certain water-snails of several genera, including *Bythinia*. After a multiplicative cycle of development within the liver gland of the snail, cercariae emerge into the surrounding water; these penetrate into one of a number of freshwater fish and encyst in the muscles, becoming metacercariae within a few weeks. Man and the other definitive hosts become infected by consuming viable metacercariae in the flesh of the raw fish; the metacercariae excyst in the duodenum, ascend the common bile duct, and mount up the bile capillaries where they finally lodge and mature. Adults may also invade the pancreatic ducts. The number of adult worms in a case of heavy infection is very large.

The presence of the worms in the biliary canals causes trauma and local inflammatory reaction; after a time there appear crypt-like dilatations of the canals in which lie a number of worms. There is a localized hyperplasia of the biliary epithelium with marked pericholangitic fibrosis; new bile capillaries develop as branching, tree-like structures. Masses of eggs may escape into the parenchyma and set up granulomatous reactions which eventually become walled off by fibrosis, with consequent distortion of the lobular pattern. The changes in the liver ultimately depend on the number of worms and the duration of the infection. Light infections produce only minor effects. Heavy infections cause biliary stasis and lead to hepatic engorgement and enlargement, fatty parenchymal changes, and finally fibrosis. The syndrome of portal hypertension associated with splenomegaly may develop, especially in alcoholic individuals. Carcinoma of the liver or pancreas may occur.

Pathological changes leading to fibrosis and sclerosis of the ducts may be initiated in the pancreas as a result of invasion by adults.

'Toxic' effects of the infection include emaciation and cachexia especially in children. Eosinophilia varies from 10 to 40 per cent.

## CLINICAL PICTURE

The symptoms are proportional to the degree of infection. In light infections they are negligible; in heavy infections they are those of a chronic catarrhal cholangitis, with progressive enlargement of the liver, some icterus in moderately infected cases, becoming very severe in the emaciated, heavily infected individual. Emaciation is progressive. Systemic manifestations, including chronic diarrhoea, tachycardia, vertigo, tremors, cramps, lassitude, and mental depression, sometimes occur. These are thought to be a result of impaired liver function due to a long-continued heavy infestation.

Diagnosis depends on the discovery of the eggs in the faeces or in the fluid aspirated from the duodenum.

Skin tests, using antigens made from adults, have been used successfully in China. After injection of 0.1 ml of the antigen intradermally a large wheal surrounded by flare develops within 20 minutes. Differentiation from other fluke infections may be made from skin tests using serial dilutions of specific antigens.

### TREATMENT

There is no satisfactory specific treatment for clonorchiasis. A course of sodium antimonyl tartrate, given intravenously, has been stated to reduce the number of worms. Chloroquine has been used with some success in doses of 300–400 mg (base) daily, until the eggs disappear from the faeces, but for not longer than 40 days. This regime is often accompanied by severe side effects. Bithionol is unreliable. Some success has been claimed using Hetol, but this drug has been withdrawn from the market.

Prophylaxis consists of the proper cooking before consumption of all freshwater fish in the areas of endemicity of the parasite. Eating raw, salted, pickled, or partially cooked fish may lead to infection.

## FASCIOLA HEPATICA

The non-embryonated, operculated eggs of the sheep liver fluke *Fasciola hepatica* are passed in the faeces of sheep, cattle, and other ungulates. Miracidia escape in water and invade *Limnaea* snails. Cercariae are produced in a week, escape and encyst as metacercariae on vegetation including grass and water cress. Mammals are infected by ingesting the metacercariae which excyst in the duodenum and pass through the wall across the peritoneal cavity to reach the bile ducts via the liver parenchyma and periportal connective tissue. Adults mature in the biliary tract about 4 months after infection.

Pathological changes occur in the walls of the invaded bile ducts. The epithelium hypertrophies and desquamates, the duct wall hypertrophies and later fibroses. Cystic dilatations of the duct are formed and adults erode with masses of eggs into the parenchyma, setting up granulomatous reactions and, later, fibrosis. Abscesses commonly form about the eggs. The liver at first enlarges. Later it shrinks as fibrosis develops. After many years the complications of fibrosis, including portal hypertension, may develop.

Ectopic larvae may be distributed to any tissue so that adults and associated lesions may be found in the blood vessels, the brain, the orbit, or in subcutaneous abscesses.

Pharyngeal fascioliasis *(halzoun)* is described in the Middle East, resulting from the lodgement of immature adults in the mucosa following the eating of mutton or goat flesh. Serious obstruction of the air passage may result.

General reactions to the infection may be severe and include fever, coughing, abdominal pain, and tenderness over the liver, especially in the right hypochondrium or over the gall bladder. Referred pain in the right shoulder is common; there is also persistent diarrhoea, vomiting of bile-stained fluid, and frequent sweating. An irregular urticarial rash appears from time to time. There may be anaemia and leucocytosis. Eosinophilia is high.

Latent phases, which exist for months or years are common. The acute phase is caused by the presence of adults in the bile ducts, usually leading to cholangitis.

Diagnosis is made by the discovery of the eggs in the faeces; eggs do not appear until about 4 months after infection. Complement fixation tests and skin reactions, using specific adult worm antigens, become positive late.

Treatment is unsatisfacory. Chloroquine, bithionol, and emetine have been tried with equivocal results.

## OPISTHORCHIASIS (FELINEUS AND VIVERRINI)

Infections with *Opisthorcis (felineus* or *viverrini)* occur in north-eastern Europe, the U.S.S.R., India, Thailand, and Japan.

Operculated elongated ovoid embryonated eggs ($30 m \times 10 \mu m$) are passed in the faeces and hatch after ingestion by the appropriate snail (*Bythinia* spp.), from which cercariae are discharged in about 2 months. These penetrate through the skin of fish and eventually form metacercariae in the muscles. Man and other animals including the cat and the dog become infected on eating raw fish flesh. The metacercariae excyst in the duodenum and the larvae migrate up the ampulla of Vater to the distal ducts where they attach themselves and mature. Eggs escape back to the faeces about 4 months after infection.

The pattern of pathological changes resembles that of clonorchiasis, but advanced periportal hepatic fibrosis and associated syndromes are much less common. Concentrations about masses of eggs and debris in the dilated and distended bile ducts and gall bladder frequently cause signs of obstructive cholangitis and cholecystitis.

CLINICAL PICTURE

The liver fluke infections present in four clinical forms, or stages, as described by the Harinasutas for opisthorchiasis in Thailand.

1. Symptomless. Light or early infection. Eggs are present in the stools but there are no physical signs or symptoms. In some areas these represent the bulk of those infected.

2. Mild. The patient has irregular bouts of flatulence and indigestion. There is no anorexia. The liver is not enlarged and not painful or tender. There is no jaundice. This mild syndrome is seen in people with moderate or light infection which has persisted for some months or years.

3. Moderate. There is a mild cholangitis which may be persistent, or recurrent, with symptom-free intervals. The syndrome is commonest in the 15–40 age group. The patient complains of indigestion and especially flatulence, which are continuous or intermittent. There are occasional episodes of mild fever, with pain localized over the liver region and epigastrium. The liver is often palpable, firm, and slightly tender. In the more severe cases there is occasional vomiting and diarrhoea. Jaundice is common, but not severe, with a total serum bilirubin content of not more than 5–6 mg per 100 ml. The syndrome may persist for months, disappear, and reappear at intervals, which may last for several years.

4. Severe. This syndrome is the equivalent of relapsing cholangitis. The patient is ill and feels ill. There are two or three severe episodes during the year, lasting a few weeks or several months. In between, the patient returns to a condition of indifferent health. In the active episodes there are severe anorexia, indigestion, and pronounced and aggravating flatulence, with dull aching pain in the right hypochondrium and the epigastrium, often most severe in the evening. There is moderate remittent fever. The liver is moderately enlarged, tender, and firm. The spleen may be palpable, and becomes enlarged considerably if portal hypertension develops following hepatic fibrosis. Jaundice is moderate to severe (serum bilirubin ranging from 10–30 mg per 100 ml) arising from interhepatic biliary obstruction or, in later stages, the complication of carcinoma of the bile ducts. Serum albumin concentration is low; globulins are raised; the ESR is raised. The white cell count is high, often 20,000 cells per $mm^3$ or more, mostly polymorphs. The faeces are usually pale where the major factor is obstruction; with hepatocellular damage the colour is yellow. The faeces may contain blood and/or mucus. There may be diarrhoea or the passage of two or three bulky stools in the day. There are relatively few eggs in the stool.

Complications include obstructive jaundice, portal hypertension from biliary fibrosis accompanied by ascites, and oesophageal and gastric venous varices. Adenocarcinoma of the bile ducts appears in some cases, usually in the intrahepatic ducts, occasionally in the common bile duct.

Diagnosis is based on the recovery of the eggs in faeces or duodenal juice or on skin tests similar to those used for the detection of clonorchis infection.

Chloroquine has been used in the treatment of opisthorchiasis. It is clinically ineffective in cases of cirrhosis, in which the administration of choline may bring some relief.

Dosages recommended vary widely. In Thailand 300 mg chloroquine (base) is given daily for 2–6 months. The drug is believed to act on the adults in the bile ducts but the eggs show morphological changes soon after the beginning of treatment.

Side-reactions are common. They can be alleviated by oral glucose and mixed vitamins of the B group. Nausea and anorexia predominate, with consequent loss in weight. Some patients complain of dizziness and vertigo. Headache and insomnia are common. There may be allergic pruritus or skin reactions. No changes in the leucocyte or erythrocyte counts have been reported. Blurring of vision may occur in these long-term chloroquine dosage regimens; sometimes retinopathy may develop.

Bithionol has been tried with equivocal results. Dehydroemetine has been used with little success. Emetine is no longer used. Trials of Hetol (Hexachloroparaxylol) have given good results, but the drug has been withdrawn.

Secondary infection of biliary vessels is treated with tetracycline.

## INTESTINAL FLUKES

These trematodes are widely distributed in wild and domestic animals and infection of man is often only accidental. Their life-cycles have many points in common. Adults are leaf-shaped hermaphrodite motile worms varying in length from minute to 7–10 cm. They are attached by muscular suckers to the intestinal wall. Eggs which are operculate and contain an undeveloped ovum, are passed in the faeces. After 2–3 weeks, hatching takes place either in water or in a freshwater mollusc intermediate host and the miracidia escape to infect an appropriate snail, from which cercariae are eventually discharged. These encyst to form metacercariae either on vegetation or in another host, usually a reptile, fish, or a second mollusc. Man is infected by ingesting the metacercariae. The larva is released in the small intestine and matures into the adult.

Two sub-orders occur in man, namely *Amphistomata* and *Distomata*. The former are relatively unimportant clinically. *Watsonius watsoni* has been reported only once in man, but *Gastrodiscoides hominis* occurs fairly frequently in India where it is a natural infection of the pig. In man it is found in the caecum and ascending colon and gives rise in heavy infections to mucous dysentery or diarrhoea.

The more important distomata are discussed below.

*Fasciolopsis buski*

This is a common parasite of man and pigs and occasionally of dogs in China, Taiwan, Thailand, and elsewhere in the Far East.

Adults measure up to 7 cm long and are normally attached to the duodenal and jejunal mucosa. In very heavy infections they may be present in the stomach and the large intestine. Adults mature in the small intestine in about 3 months. Eggs containing miracidia are passed in the faeces. They hatch in water after about a fortnight and enter *Planorbis* snails. The cercariae produced from the snail encyst on water vegetables and develop into infective metacercariae. Man is infected by ingesting metacercariae encysted on the roots of the lotus and on the water caltrop.

The large flukes cause direct damage to the intestinal wall. Inflammatory cellular reactions and local accumulations of eosinophils appear at the point of attachment where ulceration and abscesses sometimes follow. Haemorrhage may occasionally occur as a result of erosion of mucosal vessels. Excessive secretion of mucus is common in heavy infections. Local obstruction of the gut has also been recorded.

The toxic effects of infection are severe. Oedema of presumably allergic origin occurs in the face and legs and ascites is common. Anorexia, diarrhoea, and vomiting may be persistent. An eosinophilia of moderate degree is common, associated with neutropenia. Death may result, especially in children.

Treatment consists of the oral administration of tetrachlorethylene in the usual doses (see p. 172).

*Echinostoma ilocanum*

The adult is about 1.0–1.5 cm long and is attached to the jejunal wall. Eggs are passed in the faeces. Man is infected by eating molluscs (snails and clams) containing metacercariae.

The pathological changes in the host are confined to the intestine and are similar to those induced by *Fasciolopsis*.

*Heterophyes heterophyes*

The adult measures about 0.5–0.75 cm and is attached to the wall of the small intestine. The eggs, each of which contains a fully developed miracidium, are passed in the faeces. Cercariae are formed in *Melania* snails, and enter fish. Man is infected by eating raw fish flesh containing metacercariae.

Mild inflammatory cellular reactions appear at the point of attachment of the worms and in areas in which the adult has invaded the mucosa. Superficial necrosis of the mucosa occurs with excess mucus secretion. Diarrhoea results. Occasionally the eggs reach the mesenteric lymphatics and pass to the brain and the heart; in the latter they cause tissue responses involving the myocardium and cardiac valves. *H. katsuradai*, which occurs in Japan, produces similar effects.

It is claimed in Egypt that many cases can be cured by oral administration of piperazine compounds in the usual doses. Tetrachlorethylene is an alternative.

### *Metagonimus yokogawai*

This is a natural parasite of fish-eating birds and mammals.

Man is infected accidentally. The adult is very small and attached to the wall of the duodenum. It may penetrate the mucosa and oviposit in the submucosal tissues. Mature eggs are passed in the faeces. Man becomes infected by eating raw fish flesh containing metacercariae. Other members of the family may establish themselves in many definitive hosts, including man; the second intermediate hosts are usually fish but may be frogs or shrimps. The snail involved is *Melania* spp.

The pathological processes induced by these infections are much the same as in infection with *Heterophyes* spp., except that the adults invade the deeper layers of the mucosa possibly because they are incompletely adapted to man. Eosinophilic and polymorphic infiltrations of the intestinal wall associated with erosion of the mucosa and excessive mucus secretion occur at or near the site of attachment or about eggs laid in the submucosal tissues.

Eggs may reach the intestinal venules and lymphatics and get carried to the brain, spinal cord, and the heart, where they initiate granulomatous reactions giving rise to local damage and functional disturbances. There is often relatively little tissue reaction to the invasion of the mucosal tissues by the adults, which never undergo effective encapsulation.

There is no specific treatment, but success has been reported with big doses of chloroquine, as for opisthorchiasis.

## 'LUNG' FLUKE INFECTION

## PARAGONIMIASIS

Endemic haemoptysis is a condition due to infection of the lungs and other tissues with the trematode parasite *Paragonimus westermani*. The resultant disease is characterized by an insidious onset, cough with the expectoration of blood-tinged sputum containing ova, pains in the chest and dyspnoea, bronchiectasis, and fibrosis of the lung tissue.

### GEOGRAPHICAL DISTRIBUTION

Paragonimiasis of man occurs throughout the Far East; sporadic cases of infection have been recorded in South America; it is prevalent in localized areas of West Africa including Zaïre.

*P. westermani* has been recovered from the lungs of man, of many carnivora, and of some other animals. The adult flukes measure 7.5–12 mm in lenth, 4–6 mm in breadth, and 3.5–5 mm in thickness. They contain both male and female genitalia and produce oval golden-brown-coloured, operculated eggs measuring 80–120 $\mu$m by 60–80 $\mu$m. The immature eggs classically are expectorated with the sputum, or are swallowed with it and are passed in the faeces. After their escape they mature in water over a period of some weeks; a larva (miracidium) then emerges from each egg and enters one or other of several species of snails of the genus *Melania*. Within the liver glands of the snail there is a multiplicative cycle of development, with the production finally of cercariae. The cercariae emerging from the snail enter into crayfish or crabs; in these they encyst in the muscles and other tissues and grow into metacercariae. Man and the other definitive hosts become infected by consuming viable metacercariae in these creatures; on being swallowed the metacercariae excyst in the small intestine, penetrate its wall, and actively pass through the abdominal cavity, the diaphragm, and the pleura into the lungs, where they lodge peripherally. A cyst-like capsule of inflammatory and fibrous tissue forms around each parasite. Within 6 weeks the parasites reach maturity and start producing eggs. The capsule swells and ruptures into a bronchiole; the contained eggs, together with inflammatory cells and blood, are expectorated in the sputum. It is unusual for more than twenty parasites to be present in human lungs. In addition to the site of election, the lungs, aberrant flukes may lodge in the liver, the walls of the intestine, the peritoneum and mesentery, the abdominal lymph glands, the muscle or skin of the abdominal wall, the diaphragm, and the pleura. In addition they have been recovered from organs remote from the abdomen or the chest, such as the brain and cord; their presence in the latter sites causes various manifestations of injury to the central nervous system.

CLINICAL PICTURE

At the time of infection and during the migration of the metacercariae there are no symptoms. The onset of symptoms is associated with the development of the inflammatory reaction around the pasasites and their eggs in the tissues. Usually it is insidious but there may be some initial fever. There is a cough, which is soon associated with increased expectoration of a sputum which is viscous and flecked with blood. There may be haemoptysis after a spasm of coughing, which often is associated with severe pain in the chest. There is increasing shortness of breath, with evidence of a progressive bronchitis and bronchiectasis; there may be a pleural effusion; and, as the condition continues, there is increasing radiological evidence of fibrosis in the lungs.

The symptoms caused by the presence of parasites in the abdomen vary with their location. Those present in the walls of the intestine cause symptoms of enteritis, those in the liver of hepatitis; those in lymph glands may lead to abscess formation; those parasites in the abdominal wall or skin tend to discharge their ova by rupture of their containing capsules to the exterior. In the central nervous system the parasites may give rise to Jacksonian attacks, encephalitis, meningitis, and myelitis with palsies of various types.

Though the symptoms of paragonimiasis are most severe during the first 6 or 7 years of infection, fresh symptoms may continue to appear for the 20 years that some of the parasites may survive.

### DIAGNOSIS

This is established only on recovery and identification of the characteristic eggs. In the sputum masses of eggs can often be picked out as faintly seen rust-brown points. Parasites lodged in the superficial tissues of the abdominal wall may be removed by biopsy. Eggs may sometimes be found in the stools as the result of swallowing sputum or in those cases where there are intra-abdominal lesions.

X-rays of the lungs do not afford a definitive diagnosis of the condition, but yield information of value in assessing its extent and progress.

### TREATMENT

Bithionol (Bitin) is very active in dealing with the infection and is the drug of choice. A dose of 30–50 mg per kg body weight is given every other day in divided doses, for a period of 20–30 days. Stools and sputum are freed of eggs in a few days and symptoms improve rapidly. Sputum has remained negative for eggs 6 months after the finish of treatment. Side-effects are not severe; they include diarrhoea, abdominal pain, nausea, vomiting, and an urticarial rash. A derivative, Bitin-S, has been introduced successfully in doses of 10–20 mg per kg, orally, every other day on 10–15 occasions.

Chloroquine has also been used successfully for treating the infection. Complications need symptomatic local treatment.

## CYCLOPHYLLIDEAN TAPEWORMS

### INTRODUCTION

A number of cestode worms have been recorded as parasites of man. Some of them are relatively common and, of these, a few pass one stage of their life cycles as strictly human parasites; some are parasitic in other animals and occur only incidentally in man. The commonest cestode parasites of man in the tropics and subtropics are the large cyclophyllidean tapeworms *Taenia saginata* and *T. solium* and the dwarf tapeworms *Hymenolepis nana* and *H. diminuta.*

With the notable exception of *T. solium,* of which both the adult and the larval stages may infest man, the worms mentioned occur solely in the adult stage as intestinal parasites. It is very doubtful if their presence in the bowel causes symptoms of consequence, or that any material ill-health results from it. Infections with the large tapeworms usually are single and only rarely multiple; in the case of the dwarf tapeworms commonly they are multiple. The adult worms attach themselves by their heads to the mucosa of the small intestine only for the purpose of anchorage. They have no buccal cavity or alimentary tract and, therefore, they do not suck blood or other nutriment from the point of their attachment. The strobila hangs down from its head within the lumen of the intestine. The worms derive their sustenance by surface absorption from the intestinal contents with which they are in contact. It has been claimed that in particularly susceptible persons the presence of tapeworms may cause allergic manifestations, possibly due to absorption of the metabolites of the worms; but such symptoms are rarely seen in otherwise healthy persons. The presence of an adult tapeworm infection of the bowel is usually brought to the notice of the patient by the passage of segments of the worm.

### TAENIA SAGINATA

This, the common beef tapeworm, occurs in beef-eating peoples all over the world irrespective of climate. The adult worm is a strict human parasite; it is large, white, segmented, and ribbon-like. It may measure up to 12 metres in length, and the gravid segments measure about $2 \times 1.5$ cm. It is made up of a head and neck and of segments numbering sometimes over 1000. The head, which is of pin-head size, is provided with four sucking discs (but no hooks) by means of which it adheres to the mucosa of the upper small intestine. From the neck, immature segments continuously develop; as these immature segments are pushed down the body by the formation of fresh segments they grow in size and develop within them both male and female organs. The male organs of a mature segment fertilize the female organs in an adjacent mature segment; the testes then degenerate. The uterus of the fertilized segments becomes loaded with morphologically characteristic eggs. The gravid segments are barrel-shaped muscular structures which break off from the lower end of the worm singly or in groups of two or three; these for a time contract and writhe on escaping to the exterior through the anus and empty themselves of eggs in the process. They issue from the anus unexpectedly, or they may be passed with the stools. It is on seeing the extruded segments that the patient becomes aware of the infection.

After obtaining muscular relaxation of an extruded segment, by immersion in water for half an hour, a central-stemmed uterus with fifteen to twenty lateral branches containing many eggs, and with a lateral pore, can be seen if the segment is firmly squeezed between two glass slides. By this means a diagnosis not only of the presence of the parasite but of its species can be established. It is important to differentiate a harmless *T. saginata* from the potentially highly dangerous *T. solium* infection.

The eggs survive for some time but perish unless swallowed by cattle; in the tissues of bovidae they give rise to cysticerci, each containing the head of a future worm in a small cyst. The beef is now 'measly'. Consumption of viable cysticerci results in the development of the adult worm *T. saginata* in the small intestine. There is usually only a single worm, but sometimes several may be present. The diagnosis is made by looking for extruded gravid segments; only exceptionally, when a segment has ruptured, will the eggs be seen in the stools.

## TREATMENT

Mepacrine hydrochloride is effective and is useful if it is desired to obtain the worm intact. The patient is starved for 48 hours and a duodenal tube is passed the night before treatment. A solution of the drug (1 g for an adult) in warm water is given through the tube, followed by 30 g magnesium sulphate. The tube is then withdrawn. Purgation takes place within 2 hours and the worm is usually passed whole.

Dichlorophen (Antiphen) and its associated derivatives are active taenicides. An effective adult dose is 6 g orally, repeated after 24 hours; this need not be preceded by lengthy starvation or be followed by purgation. The drug digests the immature and upper segments of the worm, only gravid segments being passed in the stools immediately after treatment. The head is not passed intact and cannot be recognized, so it is not possible to be sure that it has been eradicated until at least 3 months have elapsed after the treatment.

A dose of two tablets (each 0.5 g) of Niclosamide (Yomesan) is given after food without preparation or purging and repeated after 1 hour. The tablets are chewed before being swallowed; children 2–8 years—one tablet repeated after 1 hour. Three months' freedom from recurrence of the passage of segments indicates successful treatment.

An illness associated with high fever may be associated with the spontaneous dislodgement of a tapeworm.

## TAENIA SOLIUM

This worm in its developmental stages superficially much resembles *T. saginata*. The adult is a strict parasite of man but, in contradistinction to *T. saginata*, the larval cysticercoid stage, while it normally occurs in the pig, unfortunately can also develop in man. It is this fact which renders infection with the parasite potentially highly dangerous.

The adult worm differs from that of *T. saginata* in that the head is armed with hooks in addition to four suckers. The worm is slightly smaller and the gravid segments are more squat and contain a central, stemmed uterus with less than a dozen lateral branches. The eggs contained in the gravid segments of either species are morphologically identical.

Infection with the adult worm follows the consumption of viable cysticerci (*Cysticercus cellulosae*) in 'measly' pork. The contained heads attach themselves to the mucosa of the upper small bowel and segments grow from the neck. The gravid segments are passed intact through the anus. The segments containing the eggs are consumed by pigs and ensure the maintenance of the parasite.

If man swallows eggs liberated from disintegrating gravid segments of his own or another's intestinal worm, like the pig, he develops cysticercosis. The larvae liberated from the eggs penetrate the mucosa of the small bowel and are carried in the circulation to various tissues where they encyst and form cysticerci. Light human infections, the result of swallowing a few eggs, possibly are fairly frequent but escape notice unless a cyst is so located that it causes physical signs. Heavy infestations, with hundreds of cysticerci, cause very grave manifestations chiefly due to the presence of the cysticerci in the central nervous system.

The cysticerci in man lodge in the connective tissues, voluntary muscles, and the central nervous system. While alive they rarely cause trouble, but they begin to die and degenerate within 3–5 years. Those dying in muscle often calcify and can then be seen radiologically. Those dying in the central nervous system may not calcify and so cannot always be seen radiologically; but as they degenerate they swell and cause disintegrating cellular changes in the surrounding nerve tissue. These result in a wide range of clinical manifestations, such as Jacksonian epileptic attacks, psychiatric disturbances, and

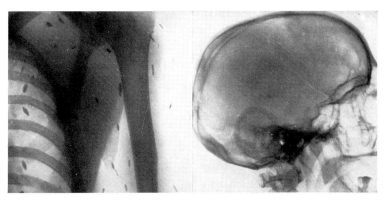

FIG. 67. *T. solium* cysticercosis. Dead cysts calcified in musculature (a), but rarely seen to be calcified in brain (b).

[From E.Noble Chamberlain, *A Textbook of Medicine,* John Wright & Sons Ltd., Bristol, 1951]

mental deterioration. Cerebral cysticercosis is a grave condition; the prognosis is a bad one, as with the death of increasing numbers of cysticerci over a period of years the effects tend to be cumulative.

One explanation sometimes advanced for the massive infection with cysticerci seen in certain individuals is that such people actually harboured an intestinal infection with an adult *T. solium*. By retroperistalsis, during some temporary intestinal disorder, one or more gravid segments were carried back up the small bowel and disintegrate. The eggs liberated their embryos, which penetrate the bowel wall, causing the extremely heavy infection.

### DIAGNOSIS

The diagnosis of an infection with an adult tapeworm is made by recovery and identification of the gravid segments passed out of the bowel.

A diagnosis of cysticercosis is made by the palpation of cysticerci, usually in the subcutaneous tissues; by biopsy of these and identification of the hooked head of the future worm in each of them; and by X-raying the general musculature and seeing calcified cysticerci in it. X-ray of the skull usually reveals nothing of specific significance.

### TREATMENT

The eradication of the adult worms from the intestine is attempted along the lines indicated in the treatment for *T. saginata* infestation. The treatment should not be delayed when this infection is detected. Every precaution must be taken to ensure that dissemination of the eggs does not occur. For this reason, mepacrine, which causes the expulsion of the whole unbroken worm, is preferred to dichlorophen or niclosamide, which digest the segments and may thus liberate the eggs. Nevertheless there have so far been no reports of cysticercosis following the use of the latter drugs.

The treatment of cerebral cysticercosis is palliative. Jacksonian epilepsy is controlled by sedatives such as the barbiturates. An individual cyst causing a localizing lesion may be removed from the brain, but this is rarely practicable.

### HYMENOLEPIS NANA AND H. DIMINUTA

The dwarf tapeworms are common and are cosmopolitan in their distribution throughout the subtropics and tropics. *H. nana* is a small worm measuring at most 40 mm in length and 1 mm in breadth. The tiny head is provided with four suckers and ring of hooks. The gravid segments liberate their contained eggs in the bowel and the eggs are passed in the faeces. It is by finding them there that a diagnosis of the infection is made. Infection results from swallowing the embryonated eggs and there is no cycle of larval development in an intermediate host. In addition to man, rats and mice harbour this parasite, but

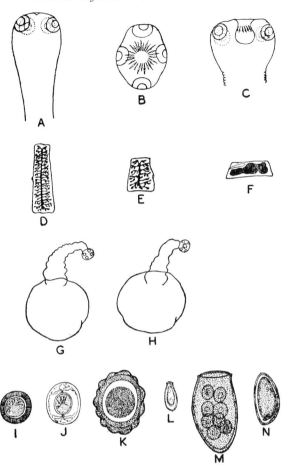

FIG. 68

A.   Head of *T. saginata* ( × 10).
B.   Head of *T. solium*, end on view ( × 25).
C.   Head of *H. nana* ( × 80).
D.   Gravid segment of *T. saginata* ( × 1⅓).
E.   Gravid segment of *T. solium* ( × 1⅓).
F.   Gravid segment of *H. nana* ( × 17).
G.   *Cysticercus bovis* with evaginated head and neck ( × 3).
H.   *C. cellulosae* ( × 3).
I.   *Taenia* egg.
J.   *H. nana* egg.
K.   *Ascaris* egg.
L.   *Clonorchis* egg.
M.   *Paragonimus* egg.
N.   *Enterobius* egg.
     (I to N; × 330).

(Drawn by David Dagnall)

murine strains of the parasite do not usually cause a human infection; the human strains are passed from man to man. Several worms are normally present; very heavy infections with *H. nana* sometimes occur, possibly as a result of internal autoinfection. Such heavy infections, which are commonly found only in very young children, may cause severe toxaemia, diarrhoea, nervous manifestations, and even convulsions.

*H. diminuta* is a common parasite of rats, mice, and other similar small rodents. It is not uncommonly found in man. It is rather larger than *H. nana*, and its maximum diameter is about 4 mm. It further differs from that worm in requiring an intermediate arthropod host for the development of its larval stage, which is a cysticercoid. The rat flea *Xenopsylla cheopis* is one among many arthropods which serve this purpose. Man is infected by swallowing the infected arthropod. Multiple infection is not uncommon; a diagnosis is made by finding the eggs in the stools.

The eggs of *H. nana* are ovoid or spherical, 30–40 $\mu$m in diameter. The embryo is small and surrounded by thick, semi-fluid material bounded externally by a very thin eggshell. The eggs of *H. diminuta* (70–80 $\mu$m in diameter) are larger but otherwise identical.

The treatment used for the other tapeworm infestations removes these worms.


## ECHINOCOCCUS GRANULOSUS (HYDATID) AND E. MULTILOCULARIS

The adult worm lives in the small intestine of the definitive host (dog, jackal, wolf, cat) which itself becomes infected by ingesting larva-containing viscera of intermediate hosts, especially sheep and cattle. Eggs are discharged in the faeces of the definitive host and are swallowed by man either as a result of direct contamination or following contact with dogs or other infected animals.

Oncospheres hatch out in the duodenum and the larvae migrate through the wall, reaching the mesenteric vessels and eventually becoming lodged in tissue capillaries, especially in the liver and, less frequently, in the lungs. A few larvae (often only one or two) survive in the tissues and go on, over months and years, to form the characteristic 'hydatid cysts'.

These are unilocular cysts with a double wall composed of an outer laminated layer and an inner nucleated 'germinal' layer. From the latter, as the cyst grows, are budded rounded cellular masses, which eventually become cystic. These are the 'brood capsules', from the inner wall of which scolices with rostellar hooklets bud and invaginate. Brood capsules may remain attached to the parent cyst wall or float free in its milky fluid contents as the so called 'hydatid sand'. Some cysts are sterile and may never produce brood capsules, others never produce scolices. If the wall of the original cyst (the 'mother' cyst) is ruptured, some of the brood capsules escape as exogenous or 'daughter' cysts and become seeded in contiguous tissues.

Cysts are unilocular in the vast majority of cases except in certain geographical regions where multilocular cysts occur (called alveolar hydatids). These are now believed to result from infection with a separate species, *Echinococcus multilocularis,* which infects small wild carnivores and rodents.

In the multilocular form of the infection the tissue cellular reactions are more vigorous but there is less fibrous reaction. Cysts contain multiple small cavities with scanty fluid containing discoloured crumpled membrane and occasional scolices. Central necrosis is not uncommon. The cuticle is deficient and fibrous capsulation incomplete.

The clinical picture of hydatid infection results largely from local pressure effects due to the cyst and from immunosensitivity reactions resulting from the host reaction to the worm.

On lodgement in the tissue the larva becomes surrounded by cellular infiltration, consisting of lymphocytes, plasma cells, and eosinophils. Later, cellular fibrous tissue envelops the cyst as a capsule. The cyst wall may eventually calcify. Pus is produced only when the dead larva has become secondarily infected.

In the tissues where the cysts are developing, local damage occurs which may or may not lead to functional disturbances. Large cysts may develop in the liver or the lungs without causing physical signs; they are often discovered by accident. On the other hand, growing cysts in the same tissues or in other areas may cause early clinical signs. Cysts developing in bone tend to become syncitial and invade the bone structure, leading to erosion, cavitation, and sometimes spontaneous fracture.

Hydatid of the liver sometimes leads to hepatomegaly which is often symptomless but must nevertheless be differentiated from amoebic liver involvement or hepatic tumour.

Compression signs are particularly common in the lungs, where they are frequently accompanied by pleural effusion. Rupture of the cyst into the bronchi may lead to relief or set off an anaphylactic reaction.

Ectopic spread of 'daughter' cysts may occur after rupture of a 'mother' cyst, leading to localizing lesions in the brain and elsewhere.

Infection with *Echinococcus* spp. leads to the development of sensitivity in the host. This does not affect the clinical picture so long as the cyst is well localized. Serious anaphylactic complications including shock may develop, however, if there is leakage of cyst fluid, following rupture or surgical interference.

Eosinophilia is appreciable and persistent, varying from 10 to 25 per cent, and rising sharply in 'anaphylactic' episodes. Complement-fixing antibodies and precipitins can be demonstrated in the blood serum, using as antigen sterile hydatid cyst fluid or alcoholic extract of brood capsules.

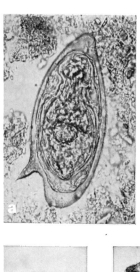
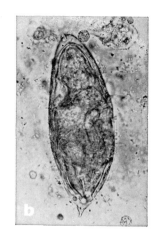
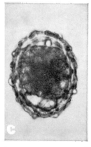
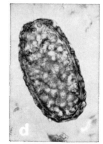
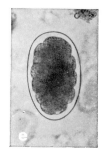
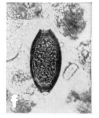
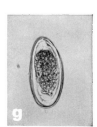
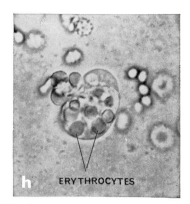

FIG. 69

### DIAGNOSIS AND TREATMENT

The antigens referred to above may also be used for a highly specific diagnostic skin test, the Casoni reaction, to perform which 0.1 ml of antigen is injected intradermally into the arm of the suspected individual. A positive reaction develops in about 20 minutes as a large wheal several centimetres in diameter, with many pseudopodia, and always surrounded by a brilliant red arteriolar flare.

The antigens may also be employed in complement–fixation reactions using the patient's serum or spinal fluid and in precipitation reactions with serum. The former test is highly specific in the presence of living hydatid larvae, the latter much less so.

X-ray examination of the suspected tissues is often helpful, especially in late cases where the cyst wall may be calcified, and in hydatid of bone, in which bone tissue is distorted and riddled with cavities; there may be spontaneous fractures.

Most cases require surgical treatment. Exploration should not be carried out unless everything is prepared for full interference. Operative procedure

---

Fig. 69. The unit of measurement used in microscopy is a micrometre ($\mu$m) and is a thousandth part of a millimetre. In the absence of a special measuring eyepiece some indication of the size of objects under the microscope can often be obtained by comparison with an erythrocyte (just over 7 $\mu$m). In the Figure the eggs (a–g) are reproduced to the same scale for comparison. The amoeba (h) is approximately one and a half times the scale of the eggs.

a. *Schistosoma mansoni*. The egg is oval, measures approximately 140 × 50 $\mu$m, has a lateral spine, contains a ciliated larva and is found in faeces.

b. *S. haematobium*. The egg is oval, measures approximately 140 × 50 $\mu$m, has a terminal spine, contains a ciliated larva and is found in urine.

c. *Ascaris lumbricoides* (fertile). The egg is round or oval, brownish in colour, measures approximately 60 × 45 $\mu$m, has an irregular (wart-like) coat, contains an unsegmented ovum and is found in faeces.

d. *A. lumbricoides* (infertile). The egg is usually more elongated than the fertile egg, has a thinner coat, contains an ovum that has atrophied, marked by numerous refractile granules which fill the egg, and is found in faeces.

e. *Ancylostoma duodenale* and *Necator americanus*. The egg is oval with broadly rounded ends, colourless, measures approximately 60 × 40 $\mu$m and contains a segmented ovum (2–8 cells) when freshly passed in faeces. The egg shown has developed to contain about 16 cells due to delay in examination.

f. *Trichuris trichura*. The egg is barrel-shaped, with a plug at each end (like a tray with handles), brown in colour, measures approximately 50 × 25 $\mu$m, contains an unsegmented ovum and is found in faeces.

g. *Enterobius vermicularis*. The egg is asymmetrical, one side being flattened, is colourless, measures approximately 50 × 25 $\mu$m, contains a tadpole-like larva (larva with small tail) and is not usually found in faeces but on perianal skin.

h. *Entamoeba histolytica*. The unencysted amoeba varies greatly in size and shape, being capable of amoeboid movement. The outer layer of ectoplasm is clear while the inner mass of endoplasm tends to be dense. In the unstained specimen (as pictured) it is necessary to see ingested erythrocytes before a positive diagnosis is made. The picture shows an amoeba containing erythrocytes (two labelled). Three others can be seen adhering to the outside.

aims at removal of the aspirated cyst (often refilled with a weak solution of formalin), with suitable precautions for preventing contamination of the tissues by the contents, an accident that may lead to severe anaphylaxis.

Attempts have been made in some inoperable cases to desensitize the patient over a long period by injection of antigens.

Anthelmintic drugs are useless.

## PSEUDOPHYLLIDEAN TAPEWORMS

### DIPHYLLOBOTHRIUM LATUM

*Diphyllobothrium latum* is a geographically widely spread fish tapeworm found mostly in cold lakes, including those at high levels in the tropics, as in Uganda, Central Africa, Zaïre, and Madagascar. It is found also in Switzerland, eastern Mediterranean countries, and as far east as Japan. The parasite has been introduced by immigrants into Canada and by fish breeders into South America.

The eggs are discharged in the faeces of humans infected with the adult worms. They mature in water for about 2 weeks and hatch an oncosphere which is taken up by a copepod, usually *Cyclops* spp., in the haemocoele of which the procercoid stage evolves. The copepod is ingested by a freshwater fish in the muscles of which the plerocercoid or sparganum larva develops. Man becomes infected by ingesting uncooked fish flesh containing sparganum (plerocercoids). The adult worm, which may reach 9 metres in length, is made up of 3000–4000 hermaphrodite proglotids containing masses of eggs. It matures in about 3 months. It inhabits the small intestine, to the mucosa of which it is attached by a small hookless scolex with two spatulate sucking lips (the 'bothria'). Multiple infections are common. Other hosts include the dog, the cat, and the pig.

In multiple infections there may be mechanical intestinal irritation and occasionally obstruction. Systemic 'toxic' effects may be considerable and include abdominal pain and discomfort and diarrhoea. Emaciation may result; convulsions are common in children. Allergic manifestations are frequent, including a high degree of eosinophilia and localized oedema. The blood white cell count is frequently raised.

In some cases megaloblastic anaemia resembling pernicious anaemia may be present, possibly as a result of competition between the worm and the host for vitamin $B_{12}$. The administration of extracts of adult worms, which contain large amounts of vitamin $B_{12}$, or the exhibition of Castle's extrinsic factor, will relieve the anaemia. The administration of folic acid may also prove successful.

Diagnosis is made by identification of the eggs in the faeces or of the adult worm after treatment with anthelmintics.

The adults may be effectively removed by dosage with niclosamide or dichlorophen (see p. 570).

### DIPHYLLOBOTHRIUM (SPARGANUM) MANSONI

Endemic areas are mainly South-east Asia.

Ingestion by man of copepods infected with procercoid larvae of other pseudophyllidean tapeworms, consumption of raw fish, frog, fowl, or snake flesh containing already developed sparganum larvae (derived from several worms grouped together as *Sparganum mansoni*) or direct contact with flesh containing spargana (for instance the use of raw frog meat as a poultice) may be followed by the appearance of spargana (sparganosis) in almost any tissue except bone. There is some lymphocytic and eosinophilic infiltration about the actively moving larva. After its death the cellular response increases and the worm becomes replaced by caseous or purulent material. The larvae usually lie in the connective tissue planes, especially in the subcutaneous and orbital tissues. The affected region is swollen and intensely painful. Elephantiasis may result from lymphatic obstruction subsequent to involvement of the local glands.

Treatment is local. Injection into orbital lesions of 2–4 ml of 40 per cent ethyl alcohol, plus a local anaesthetic such as epinephrine-free procaine, is said to be effective. Subcutaneous single lesions may be excised. In infections with one form of larva which proliferates by branching, extensive lesions may develop, and local treatment is impracticable. Some success has been claimed for standard intravenous courses of novarsenobenzol.

# 36

# YAWS, BEJEL (ENDEMIC SYPHILIS) AND PINTA

## YAWS

### DEFINITION

Framboesia, pian. A contagious disease caused by *Treponema pertenue* characterized by lesions in the skin and bones which are granulomatous in the early stages and later destructive.

### GEOGRAPHICAL DISTRIBUTION

The disease is unevenly distributed within the tropics, in northern South America, the West Indies, north and equatorial Africa, India, Pakistan, Bangladesh, Burma, Thailand, Malaysia, Indonesia, the Philippines, Panama, Mexico, northern Australia, and Sri Lanka. It is at present largely limited by mass control measures, designed originally by the World Health Organization and run by local agents, which have been highly successful but which are, nevertheless, largely holding programmes. The infection rapidly returns to high endemicity in the community if surveillance fails. It is for this reason that the disease is considered in some detail below, despite its relative infrequency.

### AETIOLOGY

*The causative organism*

The organism *T. pertenue* is a motile spirochaete about 20 μm long and having eight to twenty corkscrew spirals. It is morphologically indistinguishable from the causative organisms of syphilis (*T. pallidum*) and pinta (*T. carateum*). It has not been successfully cultivated *in vitro* but can be transmitted to rabbits and monkeys. There is controversy over its exact relationship to *T. pallidum*. Many authorities regard it as a modified form, rather than as a separate species.

*Transmission*

The organism is spread chiefly by direct contact with an infective human case. It cannot survive for long outside the body, but there is some evidence to suggest that infective material may remain in the soft moist earth floors of native huts for long enough to spread the infection. There is no animal reservoir. It is believed that the organism cannot penetrate the unbroken skin and that the usual portal of entry is a cut or abrasion.

### General

*Yaws is not a venereal disease.* It is most common in sparsely clothed and insanitary agricultural communities. Such conditions encourage transmission by contact. It is relatively uncommon in towns and cities. The reverse is true for syphilis.

Yaws is usually acquired in young childhood. Children under 1 year old are rarely affected; congenital transmission has not been demonstrated.

The majority of cases occur before puberty. The disease may be acquired by non-immune adults who have not had it in childhood. Yaws in adults is, however, usually a manifestation of earlier infection.

Coloured races are much more frequently infected than white. This is probably due mainly to difference in standards of hygiene.

The disease primarily effects the skin, its appendages, and bone. It does not cause arterial lesions such as seen in syphilis.

### Immunity

An attack of yaws may confer some resistance to a further infection. This tends to persist even after the active disease has ceased, but it is not always complete; for instance, a mother may become reinfected from the child while suckling. Treatment may also interfere with the progress or development of immunity and be followed by reinfection.

Individuals who have acquired yaws and developed an immunity to it frequently show considerable resistance to syphilis, and vice versa.

### Classification

In what follows the terms 'primary', 'secondary', and 'tertiary' are used to describe the lesions of yaws. The adjective 'primary' in relation to the initial lesion in yaws is self-explanatory. Opinion is divided, however, concerning the use of 'secondary' and 'tertiary'. So long as the classification is made in terms of the nature and behaviour of the lesion and not strictly in terms of time of appearance in relation to the initial lesion, these descriptions are acceptable.

There are striking differences between secondary and tertiary lesions which justify their separation. The important distinction to the clinician is that secondary skin lesions are, like the primary, highly infective, whereas most tertiary lesions are not. Moreover, the granulomatous secondary eruption is self-limited and tends to heal without scarring or involving surrounding structures, whereas the tertiary granuloma is progressive and involves contiguous tissues leading to destruction, scarring, and deformity. Secondary and tertiary lesions of bones differ in similar respects, the former being non-destructive and likely to resolve spontaneously, the latter destructive and permanent.

Tertiary lesions occur late in the disease and are never present contemporaneously with secondary lesions; the latter do not appear after the development of tertiary lesions.

PATHOLOGY

The basic lesion in yaws is a granuloma. in the primary phase the lesion arises at the site of infection. Subsequent manifestations presumably result from distribution of the organism in the blood-stream. The treponema can be found in the primary lesion and in most typical secondary lesions, except those of bone. It cannot as a rule be isolated from tertiary lesions.

Lesions arise in either the skin and subcutaneous tissues or in bone. In primary and secondary skin yaws the deeper structures are not usually involved as they are in the later stages. Visceral lesions have been described by some authors but occur very rarely if at all. The central nervous system is not affected.

The histological pictures presented by the primary and secondary florid lesions are identical. The appearance of the lesion at a particular site depends on the thickness of the epithelium and the looseness or otherwise of the underlying tissue.

In its earliest stages the epidermis is slightly thickened and the underlying tissue is loosely infiltrated with lymphocytes and plasma cells. As the lesion progresses it forms a papule in which the epithelium is thickened and hypertrophied branching epithelial papillae project deep into the corium. The granulomatous tissue develops immediately beneath the epithelium.

The infiltration progresses and eventually the overlying epithelium thins. Most lesions remain covered with epithelium but some may ulcerate, especially those situated in moist areas, and the exuded serous fluid eventually coagulates over the surface.

Treponemata are numerous in the upper regions of the lesion; they are not usually present in the crust formed after ulceration.

The edges of the lesion are formed by raised, slightly hyperkeratotic epithelium in which the cells are frequently oedematous and degenerate.

Unless there is secondary sepsis, healing is followed by restoration of the epithelium of any ulcerated area and eventually by recovery of pigmentation. Primary lesions may leave a thin tissue-paper scar or heal without scarring. The small lesions of secondary yaws frequently heal without scarring.

The granulomata of the later stages of yaws are similar to those of the early stages but the process spreads to involve deep tissues and the histological picture becomes complicated by the development of proliferating fibrous tissue, epithelioid cells, and sometimes giant cells. Healing occurs with scarring.

The principal active bone lesions in secondary yaws are rarefaction, particularly in the cortex of long bones, and periostitis with deposit of new bone. Rarefaction may be diffuse or focal and involve the periosteal deposits. Secondary bone changes tend to involve several bones at the same time.

Ulceration of the skin overlying secondary bone lesions is unusual. Organization of periosteal deposits and thickening of the cortex associated with bony expansion (especially in the bones of the legs) may remain after resolution of the lesions.

Active bone lesions may reappear during relapses of the disease and be followed by the same restoring processes, so that the clinical picture in a given case may be the result of repeated progress and recession of the lesions.

Tertiary lesions are destructive and may lead to deformity, osteomyelitis, and sinus formation. They are usually confined to a few bones only, unlike secondary lesions which tend to be multiple.

CLINICAL PICTURE

*Incubation period and primary lesion*
There may be no history of a primary lesion. When present, it appears 3–6 weeks after exposure.

It is most common on the legs or buttocks in areas where trauma is likely to occur.

The early stage of the primary lesion is not often seen. It appears first as a small erythematous macule which is slightly infiltrated. Within a few days a papule is formed or sometimes a group of papules surrounded by erythema. The lesion enlarges rapidly to several centimetres in diameter. The skin covering it usually remains intact but may ulcerate. In ulcerated lesions serous fluid oozes to the surface and dries as a thin yellowish film forming a yellow or grey crust over the lesion. After some weeks or months the non-ulcerated yaw heals completely or leaves a thin, light-coloured tissue-paper scar.

The lesion is usually painless; it may be itchy and scratching may lead to secondary infection.

The primary yaw is often still active when the secondary lesions first appear and may persist through the secondary period.

*Secondary skin lesions*
In the untreated case secondary lesions usually appear in a few weeks or months after the appearance of the primary lesion. They may be associated with general constitutional disturbances.

In the majority of cases the secondary eruption closely resembles the primary, except that individual lesions are somewhat smaller. The lesions may be single or multiple, grouped round the region of the primary yaw, or scattered in irregular groups over the body. There may be one or many. They often appear in successive crops. A second crop may appear before the first has healed, so that lesions in various stages of evolution may be present at the same time.

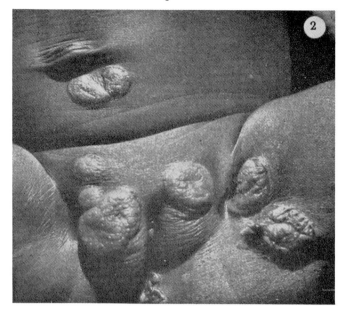

FIG. 70. Typical secondary eruption.

[Courtesy *Transactions Royal Society of Tropical Medicine and Hygiene* and Dr C.J.Hackett]

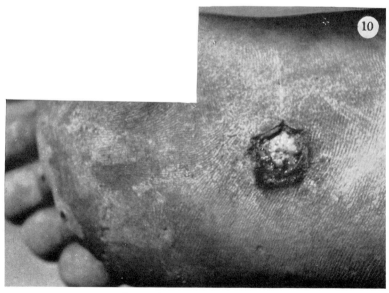

FIG. 71. Secondary plantar lesions.

[Courtesy *Transactions Royal Society of Tropical Medicine and Hygiene* and Dr C.J.Hackett]

Lesions are most commonly found on the face, especially around the mouth, in the axillae, the vulval cleft, the anus, or on the buttocks. They are rare on the scalp. They are frequent at mucocutaneous junctions but uncommon on mucous membranes proper, although they may be seen on the palate.

Ulceration may occur and crusts form which may be secondarily infected, especially near moist surfaces such as the mouth or vulva. Most lesions remain lightly covered with epithelium throughout their development.

Individual lesions may last only a few weeks or many months; they tend to heal spontaneously in due course and leave somewhat depigmented areas with little or no scarring. Sometimes the eruption subsides completely for a time and then reappears. Quiescent intervals may last weeks or years.

Secondary lesions are not usually painful unless they develop in certain special areas where the tissues are unusually firm, such as the soles of the feet and palms of the hands. They may, however, be very itchy and secondary infection from scratching is common especially about the mouth and genitalia.

In the anal or vulval regions the lesions are often florid, moist, and somewhat flattened with overhanging edges, resembling syphilitic condylomata. In the feet where the connective tissue is firm and the epithelium tough, the granulomatous tissue commonly presents on the medial or lateral aspects of the sole where the epithelium is thinner. These lesions are intensely painful and interfere with walking. The attempts made by patients so affected to walk on the inner or outer aspects of their soles, depending on which is the more involved, has given the name 'crab yaws' to this particular manifestation of the disease.

Ulceration may also occur directly through the thick plantar skin and is extremely painful and incapacitating. In such cases the picture is highly characteristic. The granulomatous tissue looks as though it has literally burst through the thickened hyperkeratotic epithelium which is cracked and turned back at the edges of the ulcer. In the course of weeks or months the granulomatous tissue may resolve and a considerable cavity may be left in the plantar epithelium, giving a punched-out appearance. Scattered irregular hard nodules of hyperkeratotic epithelium often form and eventually fall out, leaving holes. This condition is known as 'clavus'. The plantar skin is often irregularly thickened, hyperkeratotic, dry, hard, irregularly peeling ('moth eaten'), cracked, and fissured; secondary bacterial infection is common. There is often notable irregular depigmentation.

Lesions in the palms follow the same general course as those in the soles. Framboesial onychia may develop on the toes or fingers if the nail bed becomes involved.

Florid lesions of the type described above are the commonest secondary lesions. They may be absent or accompanied by other skin lesions which are caused by similar tissue changes, but differ greatly in appearance. Occasionally groups of small depigmented macules or papules with desquamating boundaries may form and recede. In some areas, often on the face about the mouth, the lesions may be circinate and closely resemble fungal infections. On the anterior aspect of the knees or thighs and sometimes on the abdomen the skin may lose its natural gloss and become leathery, desquamated, and peppered with small non-ulcerating papules. The local reaction of the epithelium may be especially vigorous on the hands and hyperkeratosis is extreme, so that small prominences or horns of dry hard epithelium may form and occasionally ulcerate. These lesions are commonly painless but may be extremely itchy.

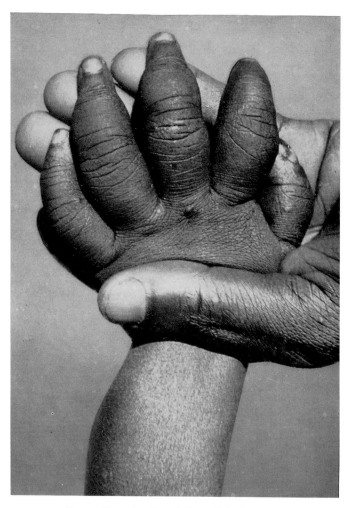

FIG. 72. Secondary bone lesions: clinical aspects.

Girl aged 3. Multiple dactylitis and swelling of radius.

[After Dr C.J.Hackett, *Bone Lesions of Yaws*, Blackwell Scientific Publications, Oxford, 1951]

The granulomatous process may involve muscle tendons, especially those in the wrist, with the development of prominent painless ganglia which may arise and subside spontaneously.

*Secondary bone lesions*
Many cases of yaws undergo spontaneous recovery in the secondary eruptive stage. A considerable proportion, however, develop bone lesions which may be the first indication of the disease.

Changes are usually multiple and involve the whole or most of the shaft of the bone. They develop rapidly and resolve spontaneously, usually in a few weeks or months. Relapses are common. Bones most involved are the long bones of the legs and forearms, especially the ulna. Involvement of the bones of the hands is also common, producing an acute polydactylitis.

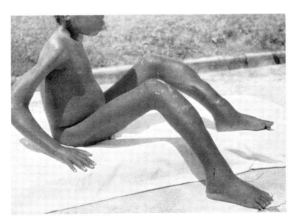

FIG. 73. Deformed tibiae in a case of yaws.

The affected areas are tender, painful, and often oedematous. The local aching and pain are severe and the function of the part may be seriously affected.

Radiographic examination reveals two main forms of lesions; focal cortical rarefactions and periosteal changes including the deposit of new bone. These lesions commonly occur together. The rarefaction disappears on healing, or is replaced by dense bone formation; the periosteal deposits may become organized with consequent thickening and irregularity of the bones involved.

Secondary bony changes are rare in the skull except for the involvement of the nasal processes of the maxillary bones, leading to the curious hard thickening of the face on either side of the bridge of the nose known as 'goundou'. In this condition the nasal processes of the maxillae are covered with thickened fibrous periosteum and new bone.

The joints are not commonly involved, although there may occasionally be some excess free fluid. Epiphysial changes are not produced by yaws *per se*.

### Late or tertiary lesions

These are seen in patients in whom the disease has been allowed to progress untreated or inadequately treated. On the whole, the tertiary lesions appear some years after the secondary manifestations. They may appear in very young children but are not usually observed before the fifth year. Most cases with tertiary lesions have a history of having had yaws at an earlier age. Occasionally there is no such history; in such cases it is presumed that the earlier stages of the infection have been latent or so mild as to be overlooked.

Tertiary lesions, like secondary, are essentially lesions of the skin, subcutaneous tissues, and bones.

A common late lesion is gummatous granuloma which causes ulceration of the skin and frequently involves the deeper tissues, including bone. The lesion is diffuse and may be first noticed as a growing subcutaneous nodule, especially in the legs and other regions where the bones lie close beneath the skin. Ulceration is common. The ulcer is indolent and slowly progressive; it closely resembles that of late syphilis. It may be secondarily infected and eventually heals with heavy scarring and deformity. Such scarring is one of the gravest manifestations of the disease.

Various other changes occur in skin and subcutaneous tissue which are regarded as tertiary manifestations of yaws. These include juxta-articular nodules, which are painless, firm, subcutaneous tumours commonly found in the neighbourhood of the larger joints, particularly the knees.

Tertiary palmar and plantar lesions are described in which scarring and contractures may develop. The soles show irregular extensive thickening of the epithelium with patchy desquamation and deep fissuring.

### Tertiary bone lesions

Certain bone lesions occur in yaws endemic areas which are usually ascribed to the infection, although proof of their origin is often lacking. These may lead to considerable destruction and deformity. Unlike the secondary lesions, they tend to develop in a few rather than many bones.

The characteristic radiographic pattern is one of well-defined local cortical rarefaction; the rarefied areas are roughly oval and often contain debris or spicules of dead bone. There may also be localized periostitis with new bone formation, as distinct from the more generalized periosteal changes of the secondary lesions.

Local pain is rarely as severe as in secondary lesions and may be absent.

Nodules on the skull occur in some cases in the older age groups. These result from irregular thickening and rarefaction of the skull bones, particularly the outer table. Ulceration of the overlying skin may occur with sinus formation. Similar nodules may sometimes be seen on the sternum and the clavicles. The latter, and the ribs, may be thickened.

Spontaneous fractures of long bones may occasionally occur at the site of tertiary lesions.

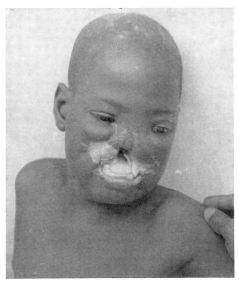

FIG. 74. Gangosa.

The most advanced and destructive lesions develop in the face and involve especially the nasal processes of the maxillary bones. In some cases the hard palate is destroyed, following ulceration of the associated mucous membrane. This condition in its various stages is known as 'gangosa'. It occurs irregularly within yaws endemic areas. The lips and skin over the maxillae ulcerate, the bone and cartilage beneath are absorbed and ultimately may disappear. Healing occurs with the most hideous scarring.

### COURSE AND PROGNOSIS

A few weeks to months after the appearance of the primary lesion, secondary lesions of various kinds, predominantly the granulomatous eruptions, develop and may persist, subside, and reappear in succession of overlapping or separate crops for 2–3 years. Secondary bone lesions commonly appear contemporaneously with secondary eruptions. After some time many cases become free of the secondary skin lesions; in others they may reappear at irregular intervals for years.

It is probable that most individuals overcome their infection at this stage and recover completely. In others the disease may be resolved during a latent secondary stage. In some the disease becomes latent and either slowly disappears or reappears after a long interval either as further secondary eruptions or in tertiary form. In others, there is a continuous progression to the destructive lesion of the tertiary stage which may appear within 2 years of the onset.

There is no way of telling whether tertiary lesions are likely to develop in a given early case, although it has been said that they appear more commonly in subjects in whom the earlier manifestations were poorly developed.

There is often no history of a primary eruption. The first sign of the disease may be a crop of secondary lesions.

Secondary lesions, especially about the lips or in the soles, may appear in older children and adults who have had more generalized eruptions in early childhood. Some of these cases may represent new infections. In others the disease may have been latent and relapsed. These later recurrences are important in maintaining the infection in a community.

The prognosis of yaws depends on the duration of the disease and the point at which active treatment was administered. In the primary and secondary stages treatment is very successful and permanent cure may be achieved. Spontaneous recovery may occur at any stage.

The effect of treatment on tertiary lesions is slow, but the progress of the lesion may be checked.

## DIAGNOSIS

### Clinical

The clinical diagnosis of an individual case of primary or secondary yaws is usually easy. The co-existence of other cases in an endemic area and the clinical history are important indications. In mass surveys in endemic areas the important feature of clinical diagnosis is to distinguish the infective case which is capable of maintaining the infection in the community. Broadly speaking, infective cases include all those with primary or secondary skin lesions. There may be latent cases which may present no active lesions at the time of examination.

It may sometimes be difficult to distinguish certain lesions of yaws from those of syphilis, pinta, or bejel and from mycobacterial ulcers.

Skin lesions due to causes other than treponemata should present little difficulty. Pus infections, scabies, fungus infection, various dermatological conditions such as lupus, seborrhoea, acne, and psoriasis may cause some confusion. The nodular lesions of leprosy may closely resemble yaws in some cases and may exist contemporaneously. Leishmanial skin lesions, particularly espundia, may be mistaken for tertiary yaws but should be distinguished by finding *Leishmania* in the tissues.

The differentiation from syphilis may be difficult; the conditions may occasionally exist contemporaneously. *Yaws is not congenital.* Lesions in the newborn or in very young infants should be regarded as syphilis, not yaws. The primary lesion of yaws is extragenital, only slightly indurated and, if near a moist surface, may be covered with a crust; in syphilis it is commonly genital, firmly indurated, and not crusted. The history of a primary lesion is much commoner in yaws than syphilis. The position of the primary and the age of onset should be important leads to the diagnosis of yaws from syphilis. The age group at the onset of syphilis is much older than in yaws. Although the macular and papular lesions of yaws may closely resemble those of syphilis, the florid primary and secondary lesions have no syphilitic counterpart. The mucous membranes proper are only occasionally involved in yaws, commonly in syphilis. Changes in the spinal fluid are common in syphilis, rare in yaws (see below). Yaws is much more common in rural populations.

The diagnosis of yaws from pinta may be difficult (see p. 595). The lesions of the hands and feet, for instance, may be indistinguishable.

The diagnosis from bejel may present difficulties (see p. 593).

Difficulty may be experienced in separating the late ulcerating granulomata of yaws, in which treponemata are rarely found, from tropical ulcer and mycobacterial ulcers. In the tropical ulcers, which are commonly single and sharply defined, the exudate contains fusiform bacilli, spirochaetes, and pyogenic bacteria in abundance. The exudate from the yaws is relatively free from organisms and rarely contains fusiform bacilli. In mycobacterial ulcers, acid-fast organisms, singly or in clumps, are usually present in the granulomatous surface and the tissue at the edges (see p. 395).

*Laboratory diagnosis*

*The treponema.* Exudate from primary or secondary skin lesions usually contains the treponema, which can be identified most easily by dark-ground examination of a wet coverslip preparation. The crust should be removed from the suspected lesion and the surface, if obviously secondarily infected, cleaned with saline. It is then lightly scraped, and fluid is gently expressed and examined. Dried preparations fixed by passing through a flame can be stained with Giemsa's stain.

*Serological reactions.* The Wasserman and Kahn reactions become positive in yaws about 3 weeks after the appearance of the primary lesion and may reach their maximum intensity in about another month, or sometimes after a much longer period. Thereafter they remain strongly positive throughout the disease until the late healing tertiary stages, when they become negative. The reactions are weakened and sometimes rendered negative by successful treatment.

Simple and rapid flocculation tests, such as that described by Ide, are now often used in the field investigation of yaws. Most of them give results very closely in accord with the Kahn reaction.

In the vast majority of cases the Wassermann or Kahn reaction is negative in the cerebrospinal fluid even when that in the blood is strongly positive.

## TREATMENT

Penicillin is the drug of choice in the treatment of yaws either in individual cases or in mass campaigns.

It is given intramuscularly in the form of procaine penicillin G in oil plus 2 per cent aluminium monostearate (PAM).

1. For treatment of individual cases the following dosage regimes are advised:

Adults:      1.2 million units, intramuscularly; given twice, with an interval of
             3–5 days between doses. Total dose: 2.4 million units.

Children:   0.6 million units intramuscularly; given twice, with an interval of
(5–15       3–5 days between doses. Total dose: 1.2 million units.
years)

Children:   0.3 million units intramuscularly. Total dose: 0.3 million units.
(under 5
years)

2. For mass treatment campaigns, adults and children aged 5–15 years are commonly given a single intramuscular dose of 1.2 and 0.6 million units respectively. Children under the age of 5 receive 0.3 million units.

Former popular chemotherapeutic compounds, including arsenicals and bismuth preparations, are not now used.

## EFFECT OF TREATMENT

Treatment with penicillin has a remarkable effect on primary and secondary skin and bone lesions in individual cases. Clinical healing is sometimes complete in a week or a fortnight.

Single dose treatment may produce equally startling results but to be permanently effective, full dosage is necessary.

In mass treatment, single dosage therapy is adequate provided some follow-up is carried out.

Relapses may occur after a full course of treatment with any therapeutic agent but the chance of relapse in a given case after proper treatment is small. Relapses occur most frequently in the first year after treatment. Full therapy is required in relapsing cases.

## CONTROL

The most satisfactory way to control the spread of yaws in a given district is the identification and treatment of infective cases. Mass treatment with penicillin must be well organized, economic, regular, and continuous in order to cover relapses and infective lesions appearing in missed latent cases. The usual field technique includes census of the population, followed by a diagnostic survey, followed in turn by mass treatment, the establishment of treatment centres, and regular visits by technicians trained to recognize fresh infective cases and treat them. In a highly endemic area the continuous control of infective cases by chemotherapy is the only effective measure.

## BEJEL (ENDEMIC SYPHILIS)

### DEFINITION

This disease is believed to be a form of endemic non-venereal syphilis, caused by *T. pallidum* and almost always contracted in infancy or early childhood. It could theoretically be transmitted venereally but this event must be extremely rare as high immunity has usually been developed by puberty. Congenital cases have very occasionally been reported.

### GEOGRAPHICAL DISTRIBUTION

The infection develops in Bedouin Arabs in the Middle East and in parts of eastern Europe (so-called 'Bosnian' endemic syphilis), North Africa, and West and Central Africa.

### AETIOLOGY

The causative organism is *T. pallidum*. Early lesions are seen in young children, usually first in the oropharyngeal areas, later in the skin and as ulcerations in any part of the body. All these lesions, especially those in the mouth and pharynx are highly infective and are spread in the local closed communities, via common drinking vessels, kissing, suckling, etc. Active lesions last 2 or 3 years and are later succeeded by tertiary lesions especially on the face and limbs. These finally cause severe scarring, bone damage and deformity with extensive areas of skin depigmentation. The late stages are not infective.

### PATHOLOGY

The basic lesion is a slowly developing granulomatous reaction indistinguishable histologically from that seen in syphilis and yaws. Depigmentation in treated lesions is often excessive and is a characteristic of the disease. Lymph glands draining the infected area are often involved in similar but less vigorous granulomatous changes.

The immunological serum reactions resemble those of syphilis.

### CLINICAL PICTURE

The lesions seen in young children are the modified equivalent of the secondary lesions of syphilis. Earliest lesions are usually seen in the mouth or oropharyngeal area. They develop as painful raised plaques on the mucous membranes, especially on the mucocutaneous functions around the mouth. They are also common on the floor of the mouth, the palate, fauces, pharynx, and larynx. Ulceration, usually with relatively little bleeding, is common and scarring may occur later. The lesions in the larynx lead to a characteristic hoarseness, which may become permanent after scarring. These lesions swarm with *Treponema* and are highly infective.

Local lymph glands are enlarged and may be tender, especially where there is secondary infection. At various intervals over months, and sometimes repeatedly over 2–3 years, crops of skin rashes occur. These are mostly maculopapular and may closely resemble those of secondary yaws, especially in moist areas in the oral and anogenital regions. Not infrequently, they appear as circinate papules and eruptions, again resembling yaws. They are highly infective.

The early lesions tend to clear in 2–3 years with or without scarring. The superficial rashes often leave irregular and sometimes extensive areas of depigmentation, which are of considerable concern to the patient.

The disease now becomes latent, although in occasional cases the process is continuous. Some cases appear to recover completely in this stage. In others, after some years, gummatous lesions appear. They often begin cutaneously but spread to deeper tissues and frequently involve underlying bone on the lower limbs and especially in the head. They progress eventually to bone destruction and hideous scarring. In the head the final result resembles advanced 'gangosa' in yaws with the maxilla, palate, and nasal bones and cartilage destroyed.

These late lesions are commonly preceded by deep nagging pain in the bones, particularly the long bones and those of the face, in which changes similar to those in yaws occur, including rarefaction and periostitis followed by laying down of periosteal bone.

Severe plantar and palmar lesions are common, leading to massive keratosis, sometimes lateral ulceration and overall depigmentation. These lesions closely resemble those of late yaws and pinta. Juxta-articular nodules also occur.

### DIAGNOSIS

The geographical area is important. The early appearance of lesions, especially oropharyngeal, in infants and young children and absence of evidence of venereal transmission are characteristic. Smears of lesions in the early stages and in skin lesions will demonstrate large numbers of *Treponemata*. The Wasserman reaction becomes positive after the first few months and remains so.

### TREATMENT

Penicillin, as prescribed for yaws, is successful in the early stages in infants and young children.

Mass campaigns using penicillin as in yaws have had some success in reducing the incidence of the infection but are hampered by the nomadic habits of many of the tribes in which the disease occurs.

## PINTA

### DEFINITION

A condition caused by *Treponema carateum*, resulting in skin lesions resembling those of endemic syphilis (bejel) and certain forms of yaws.

### DISTRIBUTION

Pinta is found in dirty poor rural areas in Central and South America, including Southern Mexico, British Honduras, Venezuela, Colombia (where it is called 'carate'), Peru, Brazil, Ecuador, and in some Caribbean Islands, especially Cuba, Puerto Rico, and Haiti. A similar disease has been reported in Indonesia, Iraq, and North Africa.

### AETIOLOGY

The causative agent is *T. carateum* which is morphologically indistinguishable from *T. pertenue*. It has not been cultivated, but has recently been transmitted to chimpanzees. It is believed that *T. carateum* may be a separate species of *Treponema* from *T. pallidum*, although many of the clinical effects and serological properties closely resemble those of endemic, non-venereal syphilis.

Lesions are rare in children under the age of 1 year. In parts of Mexico, where the disease is most highly endemic, many overt cases occur in people under 20 years of age, but evidence of infection is found in the majority of the population at more advanced ages. The infection is acquired most commonly in childhood or adolescence, probably transmitted by contact in a similar way to yaws. Like yaws, pinta is found most frequently in dark-skinned populations and rarely in Europeans.

It produces a much weaker cross-immunity with syphilis than does yaws; coincident infection with syphilis occurs. Venereally transmitted syphilis does not protect against pinta.

### PATHOLOGY

The basic lesion is a slowly developing subcutaneous granulomatous reaction, together with hypertrophy and eventual atrophy of the overlying skin and various colour changes produced by redistribution of dermal pigment. In early lesions pigment is lost from the germinal layers of the epithelium and may become concentrated and widely diffused in the upper layers of the corium. In the later stages there may be complete depigmentation of epithelium and corium.

Lymph glands draining the areas of skin involved may be enlarged and show a mild granulomatous reaction and characteristic accumulation of melanin throughout the tissues.

Visceral lesions, including changes in the heart and large vessels, and changes in the spinal fluid, have been described but have not been clearly differentiated from those of syphilis.

The blood Wassermann and similar reactions are negative in the early stages of pinta, becoming positive in most cases after some months. The reactions are positive in the majority of long-standing cases. They are sometimes positive in the spinal fluid, but it is not certain whether such changes arise from the pinta itself or concomitant syphilis.

CLINICAL PICTURE

The lesions occur on the skin and only rarely on mucous membranes. In the early stages there are no constitutional symptoms. Primary lesions ('empeine') are believed to appear at the point of infection. In experimental infections they develop in 1–8 weeks, commencing as intensely itching, slightly raised, erythematous papules which spread slowly, often developing small satellite papules. In the course of some months a raised infiltrated plaque is formed, sharply demarcated and covered with laminar scales. In dark-skinned individuals the lesion is slatey grey or even blue. The plaque slowly spreads, becoming ovoid or irregular in outline as the satellite lesions are absorbed into it.

For a long time the primary lesion may be the only one present. Eventually, after 4–12 months, other lesions appear, indicating some general spread of the infection. These later lesions, or 'pintids', develop in much the same way as the primary, starting as small papules and developing into plaques with actively growing edges which tend to become confluent. Large irregular areas of skin may become involved.

The plaques show a variety of colour changes. In the early stages the erythematous reaction is striking and on fair skins the lesions are pink because of erythema and the disappearance of pigment from the epithelium. Accumulation of pigment in the corium may give a bluish or blackish tinge to the lesions which stand out against the surrounding skin.

Pintids may be few and confined to the extremities, or multiple involving most of the trunk and limbs. They appear successively during the secondary stage, so that lesions in all stages of development may be present at any one time in the same patient.

The initial lesion usually persists during the development of pintids. In some cases lesions may undergo spontaneous recession. In others the dermal development may be continuous and uninterrupted. Sometimes the disease subsides completely, becoming latent and remaining so for years, eventually reappearing as cutaneous lesions commonly in the extremities.

Pintids are painless but may be very itchy and become secondarily infected. Moderate local glandular enlargement is common.

In the late stages the initial lesion and pintids eventually become depigmented and the skin over them atrophic. They remain slightly erythematous and continue to grow. Other depigmented, atrophic, lightly erythematous areas may appear which fuse to cover larger and larger areas of the body, especially in the extremities.

Lesions which appear following latency tend to be less generalized and are mainly confined to the distal portion of the extremities, especially the dorsal surface of the hands and forearms, the wrist, and the heels. The lesions are commonly arranged symmetrically. Those in the wrists are often disposed in roughly triangular areas with the apex pointing up the arm.

The late lesions comprise a superficial achromic dermatitis scattered over a dark background. The skin over the depigmented areas may be normal, in which case the area is often ringed with dark pigment. More commonly it is atrophic, smooth, or slightly desquamated.

In the palmar and plantar regions there is often diffuse or scattered loss of pigment, sometimes with irregular spots of hyperpigmentation. The skin surface may be unchanged or atrophic and desquamating. In some cases there is notable palmar and plantar hyperkeratosis, occasionally with contractures, conical depressions in the horny layer, and fissuring, presenting a picture very closely resembling that of yaws.

In the late stages juxta-articular nodules may form and changes in the cerebrospinal fluid similar to those in syphilis and also aortitis have been reported.

### DIAGNOSIS

The geographical distribution of the disease is important. The slowly growing lesions and changes in pigmentation, especially the white atrophied lesions of the tertiary stage, are characteristic. Many other conditions, including yaws and certain fungus infections, for example, *Tinea versicolor*, may produce irregular scattered depigmentation of the skin but these changes are seldom symmetrical. Piebald albinism is congenital.

Laboratory diagnosis can be made by finding the *Treponema carateum* in the biopsies or smears from lesions. The organisms are numerous in the epidermis in primary lesions and pintids. They may also be present in late lesion in the rete mucosum.

### TREATMENT

Penicillin, administered as in yaws, is successful in the early stages. In the later depigmented stages the skin reaction may be modified but nothing can be done regarding the colour changes. Treatment has little effect on the blood Wassermann reaction in late cases but may render it negative in early cases.

# APPENDIX

## SOME VACCINATIONS IN THE TROPICS

### CHILDREN

The following is an example of a schedule adapted for a children's clinic in the tropics. (Yellow fever or cholera vaccinations are used during epidemics.)

| Time | Vaccine | Route | Comments |
| --- | --- | --- | --- |
| Pregnant mother: first antenatal visit | Tetanus toxoid | Intramuscular | Where neonatal infection is likely |
| Newborn | BCG | Intradermal | Where prevalence is high |
| 3 months | Smallpox* | Multiple pressure or scarification | See notes. In endemic area. Should be first vaccination the child receives except BCG |
| | DPT (Diph. Pert. Tet.) | Intramuscular | First dose. Wait for 2–3 weeks after smallpox vaccination. Second dose after 6 weeks; third dose after 6 months |
| | Poliomyelitis | Oral | First dose. Second dose after 6 weeks; third dose after 6 months. Can be given at same time as DPT. See notes |
| 9–12 months | Measles | Intradermal | Seek advice. Single dose of attenuated live vaccine' or single dose killed vaccine followed by single dose live vaccine 6 weeks later |
| Fifth year | Smallpox | Multiple pressure or scarification | Primary. See notes. In non-endemic areas, if required. |
| | Poliomyelitis | Oral | Booster dose |
| | Tetanus toxoid | Intramuscular | Booster dose |

* The success of the global smallpox eradication campaign may necessitate a review of the situation in relation to smallpox vaccination in many countries.

## ADULTS

(See notes below regarding pregnant women.)

| Vaccine | Route | Comments |
|---|---|---|
| Smallpox | Multiple pressure or scarification | See notes. Primary and revaccination every 3–5 years. Certificate valid for 3 years |
| Yellow fever* | Subcutaneous | See notes. After 10 days certificate valid for 10 years |
| Cholera* | Subcutaneous. 2 doses, 0.5 and 1.0 ml vaccine a week apart. Booster after 6 months with single dose of 1.0 ml | After 6 days, *valid for 6 months only*. Repeat at 6-monthly intervals if exposure continued. Vaccination is advisable on entering cholera areas and is demanded in individuals recently exposed in endemic areas |
| Typhoid (T) (Monovalent) | Intradermal. Single dose or two doses 2 weeks apart | Local and general reaction mild |
| Tetanus toxoid | Intramuscular | Two or three injections 4–6 weeks apart (if not previously immunized), booster every 3–5 years if exposed |

* For expatriates and, during epidemics, also for indigenous populations (children and adults).

## NOTES ON VACCINATION

1. Pregnant women should not be vaccinated for smallpox, yellow fever, or measles, owing to risk of foetal damage.

2. In infants under 3–6 months of age immune bodies against attenuated viruses (especially yellow fever and measles) are sometimes developed poorly or the virus may be affected by immune bodies acquired from the mother.

It is therefore better to delay the use of these vaccines until 9–12 months of age.

Smallpox vaccine is effective at an earlier age.

3. An interval of 3–4 weeks should be allowed between the administration of live vaccines and between the use of DPT and a live vaccine, other than poliomyelitis vaccine.

4. *Smallpox and yellow fever vaccines*

(a) Smallpox and yellow fever vaccines should not be given together. If smallpox is given first (which is advisable) wait 3 weeks before giving yellow fever vaccine. If yellow fever is given first, wait a minimum of 4 days (usually 2–3 weeks) before giving smallpox vaccine.

Do not give smallpox vaccine to persons, especially children, with eczema or other severe skin rashes. Remember that the virus can be spread to other members of the family with eczema.

(b) Until recently most countries demanded a valid smallpox vaccination certificate (within 3 years of vaccination or revaccination) on entry. See footnote on page 598.

If vaccination is for some reason not advisable the doctor should provide a certificate indicating why.

Yellow fever vaccination is advisable for visitors in endemic areas. It is demanded in any person entering a 'receptive area' (for instance, Pakistan, Bangladesh, or India and the Far East) after recently leaving a known endemic region. Many endemic areas require a valid vaccination certificate before entry. The certificate is valid for 10 years.

# INDEX